Advances in Intensive Care

Advances in Intensive Care

Editor: Rafael Nash

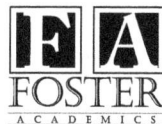

FA FOSTER
A C A D E M I C S

www.fosteracademics.com

www.fosteracademics.com

FOSTER
ACADEMICS

Cataloging-in-Publication Data

Advances in intensive care / edited by Rafael Nash.
    p. cm.
Includes bibliographical references and index.
ISBN 978-1-63242-637-6
1. Critical care medicine. 2. Emergency medicine. 3. Intensive care units. I. Nash, Rafael.
RC86.7 .A38 2019
616.025--dc23

Foster Academics,
118-35 Queens Blvd., Suite 400,
Forest Hills, NY 11375, USA

ISBN 978-1-63242-637-6 (Hardback)

Contents

Preface..IX

Chapter 1   **Posttraumatic stress symptoms in families of cancer patients admitted to**
the intensive care unit..1
Miyuki H. Komachi and Kiyoko Kamibeppu

Chapter 2   **Hospital resuscitation teams: a review of the risks to the healthcare worker**.........................8
Stephen M. Vindigni, Juan N. Lessing and David J. Carlbom

Chapter 3   **Accuracy of Critical Care Pain Observation Tool and Behavioral Pain Scale to**
assess pain in critically ill conscious and unconscious patients.................................16
Paolo Severgnini, Paolo Pelosi, Elena Contino, Elisa Serafinelli,
Raffaele Novario and Maurizio Chiaranda

Chapter 4   **Combined inhibition of C5 and CD14 efficiently attenuated the inflammatory**
response in a porcine model of meningococcal sepsis...24
Bernt C. Hellerud, Hilde L. Orrem, Knut Dybwik, Søren E. Pischke,
Andreas Baratt-Due, Albert Castellheim, Hilde Fure, Grethe Bergseth,
Dorte Christiansen, Miles A. Nunn, Terje Espevik, Corinna Lau,
Petter Brandtzæg, Erik W. Nielsen and Tom E. Mollnes

Chapter 5   **Unexpected intensive care transfer of admitted patients with severe sepsis**.........................33
Gabriel Wardi, Arvin R. Wali, Julian Villar, Vaishal Tolia,
Christian Tomaszewski, Christian Sloane, Peter Fedullo, Jeremy R. Beitler,
Matthew Nolan, Daniel Lasoff and Rebecca E. Sell

Chapter 6   **One-year resource utilisation, costs and quality of life in patients with acute**
respiratory distress syndrome (ARDS)..42
Joachim Marti, Peter Hall, Patrick Hamilton, Sarah Lamb, Chris McCabe,
Ranjit Lall, Julie Darbyshire, Duncan Young and Claire Hulme

Chapter 7   **Use of wearable devices for post-discharge monitoring of ICU patients**...........................53
Ryan R. Kroll, Erica D. McKenzie, J. Gordon Boyd, Prameet Sheth,
Daniel Howes, Michael Wood and David M. Maslove

Chapter 8   **The nocturnal acoustical intensity of the intensive care environment**.............................61
Lori J. Delaney, Marian J. Currie, Hsin-Chia Carol Huang, Violeta Lopez,
Edward Litton and Frank Van Haren

Chapter 9   **Presence of chest tubes does not affect the hemodynamic efficacy of standard**
cardiopulmonary resuscitation...69
Gu Hyun Kang, Hyun Youk, Kyoung Chul Cha, Yoonsuk Lee, Hyung Il Kim,
Yong Sung Cha, Oh Hyun Kim, Hyun Kim, Kang Hyun Lee and Sung Oh Hwang

Chapter 10   **Decreasing skeletal muscle as a risk factor for mortality in elderly patients with sepsis**...75
Keita Shibahashi, Kazuhiro Sugiyama, Masahiro Kashiura and Yuichi Hamabe

Chapter 11   **Clinically integrated multi-organ point-of-care ultrasound for undifferentiated respiratory difficulty, chest pain, or shock**..82
Young-Rock Ha and Hong-Chuen Toh

Chapter 12   **Clinical outcomes of patients undergoing primary percutaneous coronary intervention for acute myocardial infarction requiring the intensive care unit**...................101
Ken Parhar, Victoria Millar, Vasileios Zochios, Emilia Bruton,
Catherine Jaworksi, Nick West and Alain Vuylsteke

Chapter 13   **Sepsis-induced cardiac dysfunction and β-adrenergic blockade therapy for sepsis**...........................110
Takeshi Suzuki, Yuta Suzuki, Jun Okuda, Takuya Kurazumi, Tomohiro Suhara,
Tomomi Ueda, Hiromasa Nagata and Hiroshi Morisaki

Chapter 14   **Light irradiation for treatment of acute carbon monoxide poisoning**..120
Taku Tanaka, Takeshi Kashimura, Marii Ise, Brandon D. Lohman and
Yasuhiko Taira

Chapter 15   **Factors associated with increased pancreatic enzymes in septic patients**..128
Anis Chaari, Karim Abdel Hakim, Nevine Rashed, Kamel Bousselmi,
Vipin Kauts, Mahmoud Etman and William Francis Casey

Chapter 16   **Perspective on optimizing clinical trials in critical care: how to puzzle out recurrent failures**.............................134
Bruno François, Marc Clavel, Philippe Vignon and Pierre-François Laterre

Chapter 17   **Long-term recovery following critical illness in an Australian cohort**..145
Kimberley J. Haines, Sue Berney, Stephen Warrillow and Linda Denehy

Chapter 18   **Extrasystoles for fluid responsiveness prediction in critically ill patients**............................155
Simon Tilma Vistisen, Martin Buhl Krog, Thomas Elkmann,
Mikael Fink Vallentin, Thomas W. L. Scheeren and Christoffer Sølling

Chapter 19   **Seizure prophylaxis in the neuroscience intensive care unit**...163
Sushma Yerram, Nakul Katyal, Keerthivaas Premkumar,
Premkumar Nattanmai and Christopher R. Newey

Chapter 20   **Interleukin-6 is a key factor for immunoglobulin-like transcript-4-mediated immune injury in sepsis**...............................173
De Wen Zhang and Jian He

Chapter 21   **The impact of smoking on patient outcomes in severe sepsis and septic shock**...............179
Fahad Alroumi , Ahmed Abdul Azim, Rachel Kergo,
Yuxiu Lei and James Dargin

Chapter 22   **Management of patients with high-risk pulmonary embolism**...190
Takeshi Yamamoto

Chapter 23   **Hepcidin predicts response to IV iron therapy in patients admitted to the intensive care unit**...199
Edward Litton, Stuart Baker, Wendy Erber, Shannon Farmer, Janet Ferrier,
Craig French, Joel Gummer, David Hawkins, Alisa Higgins, Axel Hofmann,
Bart De Keulenaer, Julie McMorrow, John K. Olynyk, Toby Richards,
Simon Towler, Robert Trengove and Steve Webb

Chapter 24   **The prognostic performance of qSOFA for community-acquired pneumonia**.....................................205
Fumiaki Tokioka, Hiroshi Okamoto, Akio Yamazaki, Akihiro Itou and
Tadashi Ishida

Chapter 25   **Immunosenescence in neurocritical care**..213
Shigeaki Inoue, Masafumi Saito and Joji Kotani

Chapter 26   **How to manage various arrhythmias and sudden cardiac death in the cardiovascular intensive care**...223
Yoshinori Kobayashi

Permissions

List of Contributors

Index

Preface

This book has been an outcome of determined endeavour from a group of educationists in the field. The primary objective was to involve a broad spectrum of professionals from diverse cultural background involved in the field for developing new researches. The book not only targets students but also scholars pursuing higher research for further enhancement of the theoretical and practical applications of the subject.

Intensive care, also known as critical care, refers to the care and treatment meant for saving the life of critically ill patients. The patients admitted in an intensive care unit are usually the ones who are almost on the verge of death. A coronary care unit (CCU) is a common type of intensive care unit especially designed to take care of critically ill heart patients. Some of the severe heart conditions in which constant monitoring and intensive care are required include heart attacks, cardiac dysrhythmia, atrial fibrillation, unstable angina and heart block. There is a constant availability of telemetry and electrocardiographs in the coronary care units for the proper and regular assessment of the condition of the heart. This book is a valuable compilation of topics, ranging from the basic to the most complex advancements in the field of intensive care. It brings forth some of the most innovative concepts and elucidates the unexplored aspects of intensive care. The extensive content of this book provides the readers with a thorough understanding of the subject.

It was an honour to edit such a profound book and also a challenging task to compile and examine all the relevant data for accuracy and originality. I wish to acknowledge the efforts of the contributors for submitting such brilliant and diverse chapters in the field and for endlessly working for the completion of the book. Last, but not the least; I thank my family for being a constant source of support in all my research endeavours.

Editor

Posttraumatic stress symptoms in families of cancer patients admitted to the intensive care unit

Miyuki H. Komachi[1*] and Kiyoko Kamibeppu[2]

Abstract

Background: Families of cancer patients in the ICU often experience severe stress. Understanding their experience is important for providing family-centered care during this difficult period. Little is known about the experience of families of cancer patients admitted to the ICU. This study evaluated the prevalence of posttraumatic stress symptoms (PTSS) among families of cancer patients admitted to the ICU.

Methods: We carried out a longitudinal study at a teaching and advanced treatment hospital. Participants were 23 family members of 23 ICU patients. Family members provided demographic data, electronic medical records of patients, and completed the Impact of Event Scale-Revised (IES-R), the Center for Epidemiologic Studies Depression Scale (CES-D), and the State-Trait Anxiety Inventory Form X (STAI-state, trait).

Results: Mean total IES-R total score, IES-R re-experience score, IES-R avoidance score, and STAI-state score within 24 h of ICU admission and 3 months later differed significantly. The IES-R score of families of patients with recurrent cancer was significantly higher than the score of families of patients with an original cancer diagnosis ($t = 2.63$, $p = 0.029$). For two-way analysis of variance, time point was significantly associated with IES-R score ($F = 1.751$, $p = 0.011$, $df = [1]$).

Conclusions: Families of recurrent cancer patients admitted to the ICU experience serious PTSS within 24 h of admission. It is important that appropriate psychiatric support be provided to family members of these patients.

Keywords: Intensive care, Family, Posttraumatic stress disorder, Cancer, Recurrence

Background

When patients with cancer are admitted to the ICU after invasive surgical procedures, they receive high-quality, specialized medical treatment [1].

According to a survey of healthcare facilities and a bedside overview in Japan, the number of operations performed on patients with cancer increased from 2010 to 2014, and the number of ICU beds at the cancer institute hospital of Japanese Foundation for Cancer Research occupied by these patients increased from 2011 to 2014 [2, 3]. Results of an investigation in Japan revealed that 40 % of patients in the ICU died of cancer [4].

Patients admitted to the ICU may not be able to communicate for several reasons such as sedation, ventilator use, delirium, or coma. Families of patients in the ICU experience severe stress [5]. Recent studies show that family members experience severe mental stress during the initial period after a patient's admission to the ICU in Brazil, Europe, and the USA [6–8].

Some studies reported that families of patients in the ICU with cancer in Japan have psychiatric stress [9]. Families of patients with recurrent cancer experienced more severe psychological shock than families of patients with original cancer at a general ward in Japan and Spain [10, 11]. The results of these studies may indicate that families of patients admitted to the ICU with recurrent cancer may experience a severe psychological burden. However, few studies have quantitatively analyzed the psychiatric stress of family members of cancer patients admitted to the ICU with recurrent disease.

It is also important to study posttraumatic stress of family members on a continuous basis, from early ICU

* Correspondence: mhasegawa-tky@umin.ac.jp
[1]Division of Health Sciences, Graduate School of Health and Welfare Sciences, International University of Health and Welfare, 1-3-3 Minamiaoyama Aoyama 1-Chome Tower 4th and 5th floor, Minato-ku, Tokyo 107-0062, Japan
Full list of author information is available at the end of the article

admission until the patient leaves the ICU to determine if stress experienced at an early point is a predictive factor for posttraumatic stress after 3 months [12]. The aims of this study were (1) to investigate the prevalence of families with PTSS and associated symptoms within 24 h of ICU admission and after 3 months and (2) to examine the prevalence of families with PTSS among patients with an original diagnosis of cancer compared with patients with a diagnosis of recurrent cancer at the same time points.

Methods

Setting and participants

This longitudinal study was performed and consecutively recruited at a teaching and advanced treatment hospital. We conducted the survey and collected pertinent medical records in the medical/surgical ICU (23 beds).

Inclusion criteria for patients were ICU planned admission after original or recurrent cancer surgery. The only exclusion criterion for patients was living alone. Inclusion criteria for family members included (1) the family member visited the patient in the medical/surgical ICU within 24 h of admission; (2) the family member was the patient's spouse, child, parent, sibling, or relative; (3) the family member granted permission to be surveyed by a physician and a ICU staff; (4) the family member was older than 20 years; (5) the family member was able to provide informed consent; and (6) the family member was able to communicate in Japanese. Exclusion criteria for family members included (1) being under treatment for a mental or physical disease and (2) being a caregiver for other family members.

We fully explained our research and asked for a list of participants who satisfied the inclusion criteria for patients and family members. We requested that participants return the study questionnaires sent by mail within 24 h (time point 1: T1) and 3 months later (time point 2: T2) to avoid placing pressure on them to complete the information in front of us and to protect the participants' anonymity. Within 2 weeks of T2, a postcard with a written reminder about filling out the follow-up questionnaire for T2 was sent to participants. Thereafter, the questionnaire and pre-stamped/pre-addressed envelopes to encourage people to return the questionnaires for T2 were sent to participants. We asked participants to fill out questionnaires within 24 h of a family member's admission to the ICU and 3 months later. Postmarks of all questionnaires analyzed were the day of or the day after the participant was recruited at T1 and T2.

Data collection

To investigate the psychiatric conditions of family members quantitatively, we used data of subjects gathered from electronic medical records and self-reported questionnaires.

The questionnaires asked the following: demographics of the family (age, sex, number of live-in members, education level, marital status, family relationship to patient, and household income); the number of family members who had ever died in an ICU; personal history of mental disorder, other family members' history of mental disorder, experience with loss of a family member, other experience with loss, occurrence of a recent stressful event, and history of traumatic stress. For this latter variable, we used an event checklist that was published in the Clinical-Administered posttraumatic stress disorder (PTSD) scale for DSM-IV [13].

The following were collected from electronic medical records: patient demographics (age and sex); clinical characteristics (APACHE II score) [14], length of ICU stay, reason for admission to ICU, number with complications, number who died during ICU stay, and history of ICU admissions.

In addition, participants were asked to complete the existing measures of the Japanese-Language Version of the Impact of Event Scale-Revised (IES-R-J, hereafter referred to as IES-R) [15, 16], the Center for Epidemiologic Studies Depression Scale (CES-D) [17, 18], and the Spielberger's State-Trait Anxiety Inventory Form X (STAI-state, trait) [19, 20].

The IES-R was used to measure PTSS in the families of cancer patients admitted to the ICU [15, 16]. The IES-R has been tested in various studies, including the survey of the Great Hanshin-Awaji Earthquake, and is accepted as a reliable and valid scale for measurement of symptoms related to PTSD among Japanese subjects [15]. The IES-R items comprised three dimensions (eight intrusion items, eight avoidance items, and six hyperarousal items) described in the DSM-IV-TR to categorize PTSS [21]. It consisted of 22 statements that the responder rated on a 5-point scale (0 to 4) in terms of response to a specific stressful life event in the past week. Every PTSS score and the total score on the IES-R were measured. Cronbach's coefficient alpha of IES-R in our study was 0.96. Cronbach's coefficient alpha values of the three IES-R subscales of intrusion, avoidance, and hyperarousal, were 0.94, 0.76, and 0.87, respectively.

Regarding cutoffs for IES-R and CES-D scores, IES-R total scores above 25 represent high risk of PTSD [15], and CES-D scores above 16 represent high risk of clinical depression [18].

Ethical considerations

This study was approved by the ethics committees of the Graduate School of Medicine of the University of Tokyo.

Data analysis

Descriptive statistics were used for descriptive data. We used the Wilcoxon signed-rank test and the t test to compare variables related to psychopathology between the two time points and term of cancer diagnosis (original diagnosis/recurrence). Furthermore, we used two-way analysis of variance (ANOVA) to examine the main effect and interaction in terms of cancer diagnosis (original diagnosis/recurrence) and time point (T1/T2) on the IES-R score. Power analysis was conducted. Statistical significance was set at $p < 0.05$ [22]. All statistical analyses were done using SPSS 17.0 (SPSS, Chicago, IL).

Results

Of the 26 families who agreed to participate and received questionnaires, 23 participants returned the questionnaires at T1. A total of 23 families were analyzed at T1, and 18 families were analyzed at T2 (Fig. 1).

Table 1 shows the demographics and clinical characteristics of patients and their accompanying family members and patients' primary causative diseases for ICU admission.

The measures of anxiety, depression, and symptom characteristics of PTSS by time point and cancer status are shown in Tables 2 and 3.

Mean total IES-R score and STAI-state score differed significantly from T1 to T2 (IES-R score $z = -2.43$, $p = 0.04$, $r = -0.57$, post hoc = 0.73; STAI-state $t = 2.41$, $p = 0.04$, $r = 0.51$, post hoc = 0.53). The percentage of family members whose IES-R scores were above the PTSD high-risk threshold of 25 was 21.7 % (5 of 23) at T1 and 11.1 % (2 of 18) at T2. The percentage of family members whose CES-D scores were above the clinical depression high-risk threshold of 16 was 21.2 % (7 of 23) at T1 and 16.7 % (3 of 18) at T2.

At T1, 14 of 23 (60.9 %) ICU admissions were for original cancer diagnoses and 9 of 23 (39.1 %) were for recurrent cancer diagnoses. At T2, 11 of 18 (61.1 %) ICU admissions were for original cancer diagnoses and 7 of 18 (38.9 %) were for recurrent cancer diagnoses.

Within 24 h of ICU admission, the mean IES-R score of families of patients with original and recurrent cancer

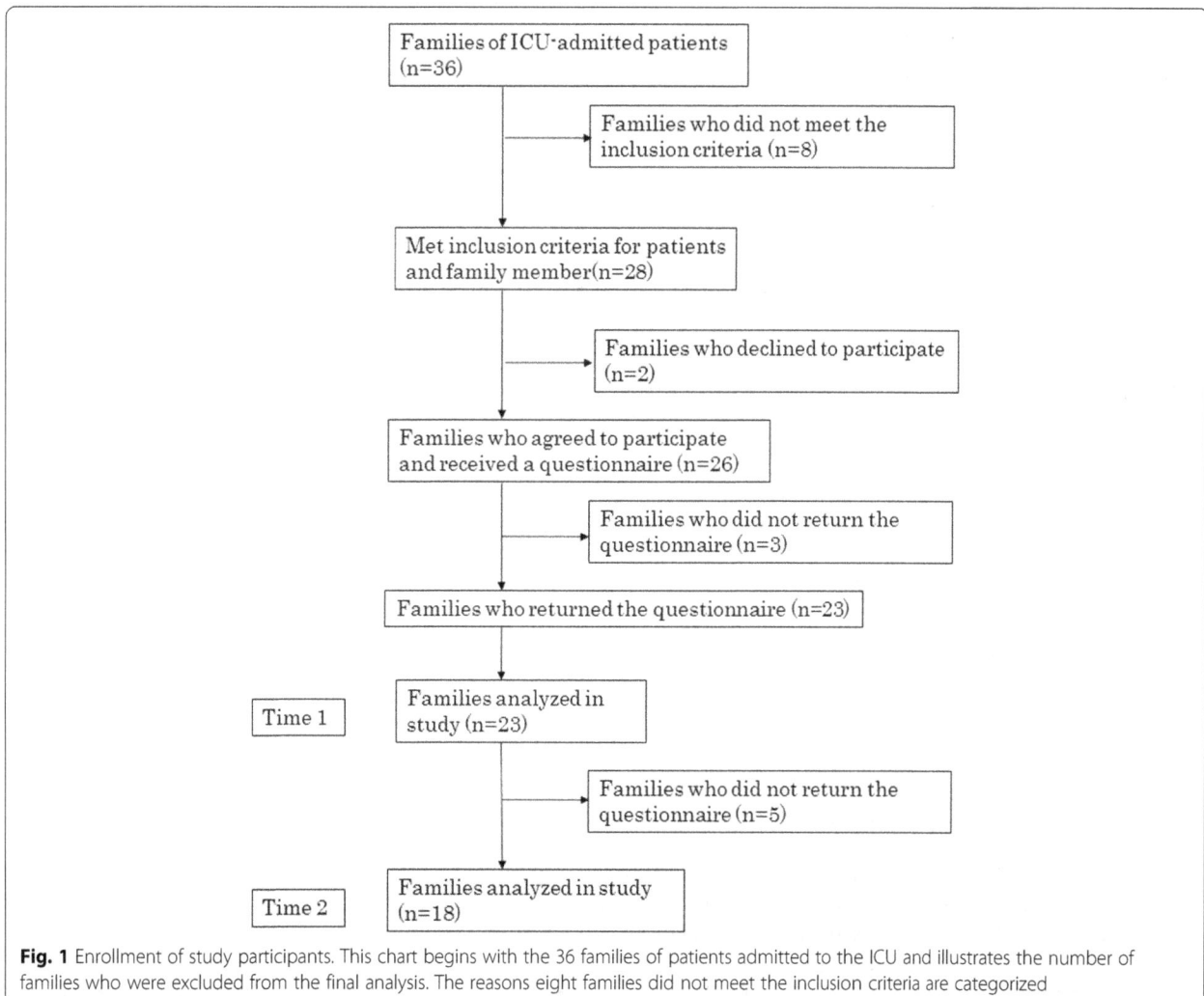

Fig. 1 Enrollment of study participants. This chart begins with the 36 families of patients admitted to the ICU and illustrates the number of families who were excluded from the final analysis. The reasons eight families did not meet the inclusion criteria are categorized

Table 1 Characteristics of family members (*n* = 23) and patients admitted to the ICU (*n* = 23)

Family member characteristics	n	%	Mean	SD	Median	Range
Age			53.3	12.4	54.0	28-79
Number who lived with patient in ICU			3.0	1.1	3.0	1-7
Sex						
Female	18	78.3				
Education level						
High school degree or higher	20	87.0				
Marital status						
Married	21	91.3				
Relationship to patient						
Spouse	13	56.5				
Child	3	13.0				
Parent	2	8.7				
Sibling	5	21.7				
Other	0					
Household income						
<3 million yen	2	8.7				
3 million - 10 million yen	18	78.2				
>10 million yen	3	13.0				
Unclear	0					
Subject has a history of mental illness - yes	1	4.3				
Family has a family member with a history of mental illness - yes	1	4.3				
Family has experienced loss of a family member (spouse, child, parent, or sibling) - yes	19	82.6				
Family has experienced loss of a relative - yes	16	69.6				
Family has experienced a stressful event within the past month - yes	13	56.5				
Family has encountered a traumatic event in the past - yes	12	52.2				
Patient characteristics	n	%	Mean	SD	Median	Range
Age			60.6	14.8	63.0	20-78
APACHE II score			8.3	4.1	8.0	2-16
Length of ICU stay (hours)			79.4	46.1	48.0	48-169
Sex						
Female	7	30.4				
Number with complications	14	60.9				
Number who died during ICU stay	0	0				
Patient was admitted to ICU in the past - yes	2	8.7				
Primary causative diseases for ICU admission by type of admission						
Hepato-biliary-pancreatic cancer	6					
Esophageal cancer or other alimentary canal cancer	6					
Lung cancer	0					
Other underlying causes of cancer	4					
Cancer recurrence	7					
Total	23					

admissions was 14.3 and 29.3, respectively. IES-R scores for families of patients with recurrent cancer diagnoses were significantly higher than scores for families of patients with original cancer diagnoses (*z* = -2.63, *p* = 0.029, *r* =-1.42, post hoc = 0.99). In terms of STAI-trait,

a significant difference was observed between original and recurrent cancer diagnoses (*t* = 2.08, *p* = 0.037, *d* = 0.49, post hoc = 0.48).

At 3 months, the mean IES-R score of families of patients with original and recurrent cancer admissions

Table 2 Psychometric assessment of family members of ICU patients by time point

	Time point 1 ($n = 23$)			Time point 2 ($n = 18$)			p	t or z	r or d	post hoc
	Mean	SD	Median	Mean	SD	Median				
IES-R (total)	15.0	13.3	13.50	11.0	11.19	10.50	0.04[b]	−2.43	−0.57	0.73
Re-experience	6.79	7.17	4.0	4.42	5.06	3.4	0.06[b]	−1.98	−0.47	0.59
Arousal	4.83	5.70	32	2.13	3.18	1.8	0.38[b]	−0.44	−0.10	0.12
Avoidance	5.29	6.81	3.8	4.46	4.19	3.4	0.09[b]	−0.95	−0.22	0.22
CES-D	14.62	8.12	12.00	13.15	8.55	12.00	0.22[b]	−0.61	−0.14	0.14
STAI (state)	48.88	13.59	45.0	43.72	11.65	43.0	0.04[a]	2.41	0.51	0.53
STAI (trait)	45.11	5.3	38.0	–	–	–	–	–	–	–

IES-R Impact Event Scale-Revised, *CES-D* the Center for Epidemiological Studies Depression Scale, *STAI* the Spielberger's State-Trait Anxiety Inventory
[a]Paired *t* test
[b]Wilcoxon signed-rank test

was 10.0 and 16.2, respectively. There were no significant differences between these groups at 3 months (z = -0.12, p = 0.38, r = -0.53, post hoc = 0.56).

Two-way analysis of variance was used to assess the presence of differences in IES-R scores by time point (within 24 h/3 months later) and cancer status (original cancer/recurrent cancer). Time point was significantly associated with IES-R score (F = 1.751, p = 0.011, df = [1], f = 0.4, post hoc = 0.35). There was no significant main effect of cancer status or interaction effect of time point and cancer status (F = 1.751, p = 0.206, df = [1], f = 0.28, post hoc = 0.19).

Discussion

Mean IES-R total scores in this study were as high as those seen in a previous study of families of patients with unplanned ICU admissions [23]. These family members felt severe psychiatric stress regarding expectations of death of the patient [24].

In addition, we revealed that the severity of PTSS of family members varied by the causative disease of the patient admitted to the ICU. Patients with unplanned ICU admissions had a higher disease severity than patients with recurrent cancer ICU admissions (APACHE II score of unplanned ICU admission was 20.4; APACHE

Table 3 Psychometric assessment of family members of ICU patients by cancer status

		Original n=14 (60.9%)			Recurrence n=9 (39.1%)			p	t or z	r or d	post hoc
		Mean	SD	Median	Mean	SD	Median				
Time point 1 (n=23)	IES-R (total)	14.3	10.8	5.5	29.3	10.3	19.0	0.029[b]	-2.63	-1.42	0.99
	Re-experience	4.3	5.7	3.2	22.5	11.4	20.4	0.031[b]	-1.8	-0.43	0.39
	Arousal	2.8	3.4	2.6	10.3	5.4	8.4	0.028[b]	-1.5	-0.35	0.28
	Avoidance	4.5	4.18	3.45	20.8	10.6	19.2	0.038[b]	-2.06	-0.49	0.48
	CES-D	10.36	8.12	10.0	16.89	9.78	16.0	0.075[b]	-1.78	-0.42	0.37
	STAI (state)	44.44	15.34	44.0	49.78	14.67	45.0	0.005[a]	1.88	0.44	0.40
	STAI (trait)	37.43	8.41	36.5	46.56	11.78	44.0	0.037[a]	2.08	0.49	0.48
		Original n=11 (61.1%)			Recurrence n=7 (38.9%)			p	t or z	r or d	post hoc
		Mean	SD	Median	Mean	SD	Median				
Time point 2 (n=18)	IES-R (total)	10.0	7.56	8.0	16.2	15.34	12.0	0.38[b]	-0.12	-0.53	0.56
	Re-experience	4.8	5.0	4.2	10.6	9.8	6.8	0.28[b]	-0.44	-0.10	0.07
	Arousal	2.0	2.8	1.9	7.3	6.7	4.7	0.34[b]	-0.36	-0.09	0.06
	Avoidance	4.6	4.3	4.3	11.4	8.4	7.8	0.30[b]	-0.36	-0.09	0.06
	CES-D	11.0	8.61	9.0	13.6	4.89	12.0	0.12[b]	-1.57	-0.37	0.30
	STAI (state)	39.0	11.95	39.0	49.14	12.55	49.0	0.08[a]	1.78	0.42	0.37

IES-R Impact Event Scale-Revised, *CES-D* the Center for Epidemiological Studies Depression Scale, *STAI* the Spielberger's State-Trait Anxiety Inventory
[a]Paired *t* test
[b]Wilcoxon signed-rank test

II score of this study was 9.7) [23]. However, the PTSS of family members of patients with recurrent cancer ICU admissions was as severe as that of family members of patients with unplanned ICU admissions [23]. Thus, the psychiatric stress level of family members of patients with recurrent cancer ICU admissions was similar to that of family members of patients with unplanned ICU admissions despite the finding that the condition of patients with unplanned ICU admissions was more critical.

In early ICU admissions, this study also showed that family members of patients with recurrent cancer had more severe PTSS and anxiety than family members of patients with an original cancer diagnosis. A previous study reported that the low QOL of family members of recurrent cancer patients admitted to the general ward was related to the fact that the family members had believed the patient's original cancer had been cured during the first admission [10]. Another study showed that families of patients with recurrent cancer felt fear when recalling the side effects the patient experienced during treatment of the original cancer [11]. These results indicated that family members of patients with cancer recurrence have a stronger psychiatric shock than family members of patients with original cancer. The results of this study were similar to these previous studies.

Recent studies have addressed the development of typical PTSD reactions and anxiety in relatives of ICU-treated adult patients. The current results showed that psychiatric shock and anxiety were reduced between early ICU admission and 3 months later. These results support the findings of Paparrigopoulos et al. (2006), who demonstrated that families of patients admitted to the ICU for various causes over a 6-month period have a high level of distress at ICU admission, but this distress level decreases 6 months later [25]. The Previous studies in Brazil and China showed that families of patients with recurrent cancer demonstrated development of typical PTSD reactions that were similar to those seen in families of patients with ICU admissions for various causes [6, 24]. In terms of depression, the results of this study differed from findings of Paparrigopoulos et al. [25].

Based on the cutoffs for IES-R and CES-D, even at T2, the percentages of families who were at high risk of PTSD and clinical depression were 11.1 % (2 of 18) and 16.7 % (3 of 18), respectively. These findings indicate that some families experience psychiatric burden for long periods, and psychiatric assessment and intervention are needed for families of patients admitted to the ICU due to exacerbation of cancer.

Families of patients with recurrent cancer were predisposed to anxiety, relative to families of patients with original cancer. A previous study reported that families of recurrent cancer patients have lower QOL than families of original cancer patients [10]. However, only

few reports to date have compared the character traits of families of recurrent cancer patients and families of original cancer patients. The current study contributes to the scientific literature by offering insight into the relationship between cancer recurrence and development of psychiatric symptoms in family members of recurrent cancer patients.

Limitations

This study has several limitations. First, this study was conducted at the medical/surgical ICU in a teaching and advanced treatment hospital. This could introduce selection bias regarding the state of the family. Second, this study was conducted by healthcare professionals providing high-quality medical care to severely ill patients and their families. This may have been a source of possible bias. Third, the questionnaire of this study was a Japanese self-administered questionnaire, which means that findings might be underestimated or overestimated. Fourth, the possibility of recall bias cannot be ruled out, especially as families were under a great deal of stress when completing the questionnaire. Fifth, the sample size of this study was small, and a larger sample size should be considered for future study designs. Sixth, this study was not able to evaluate PTSD because it did not involve any diagnostic interview. Finally, changes regarding PTSD diagnosis recently proposed in DSM-V were not taken into account [26]. The fact that the DSM-V expands the DSM-IV-TR's three symptom clusters to four symptom clusters, it needs to be considered when interpreting the results of this study.

Conclusions

Our results showed a difference in PTSS in family members of a cancer patient being admitted to the ICU with regard to cancer status from within 24 h to 3 months. However, some family members still have PTSS and depression 3 months later. It is necessary to protect families from mental distress after patients are discharged from the ICU. It is important that appropriate psychiatric support be provided to family members of these patients.

Abbreviations
ANOVA, two-way analysis of variance; CAPS, the Clinical-Administered post-traumatic stress disorder scale; CES-D, the Center for Epidemiologic Studies Depression scale; IES-R, Impact of Event Scale-Revised; PTSD, Posttraumatic stress disorder; PTSS, Posttraumatic stress symptoms

Acknowledgements
We appreciate the contribution of the families who participated in the research.

Funding
The authors have disclosed no financial relationships related to this article.

Authors' contributions
MK conceived the study, collected the data, performed the data analysis, and drafted manuscript. KK helped design the study, helped with data interpretation, and critically revised the manuscript. Both authors read and approved the final manuscript.

Competing interests
The authors declare that they have no competing interests.

Author details
[1]Division of Health Sciences, Graduate School of Health and Welfare Sciences, International University of Health and Welfare, 1-3-3 Minamiaoyama Aoyama 1-Chome Tower 4th and 5th floor, Minato-ku, Tokyo 107-0062, Japan. [2]Department of Family Nursing, Division of Health Sciences and Nursing, Graduate School of Medicine, The University of Tokyo, 7-3-1 Hongo, Bunkyo-ku, Tokyo 113-0033, Japan.

References
1. Kawasaki S, Abe I. Outcome and prognosis of patients admitted to the intensive care unit. J Jpn Soc Intensive Care Med. 2007;14:299–307.
2. Center for Cancer Control and Information Service. Registration and statistics of Cancer. [Cited 2016 June 07]. Available from: http://ganjoho.jp/reg_stat/statistics/index.html.
3. The cancer institute hospital of JFCR. Clinics and departments, anesthesiology/pain service. [Cited 2016 June 07]. Available from: http://www.jfcr.or.jp/hospital/department/clinic/central/icu/feature.html.
4. Kinoshita S, Miyashita M. Evaluation of end-of-life cancer care in the ICU: perceptions of the bereaved family in Japan. Am J Hospice Palliat Med. 2013;30:225–30.
5. White DB, Engelberg RA, Wenrich MD, et al. Prognostication during physician-family discussions about limiting life support in intensive care units. Crit Care Med. 2007;35:442–48.
6. Fumls RRL, Ranzani OT, Martins PS, et al. Emotional disorders in pairs of patients and their family members during and after ICU stay. PLOS ONE. 2015;10(1):e0115332.
7. Sundararajan K, Martin M, Rajagopala S, et al. Posttraumatic stress disorder in close Relatives of Intensive Care Unit Patients' Evaluation (PRICE) study. Aust Crit Care. 2014;27:183–7.
8. McAdam JL, Fontaine DK, White DB, et al. Psychological symptoms of family members of high-risk intensive care unit patients. Am J Crit Care. 2012;21: 386–94.
9. Suzuki K, Hirai K. Experience of families making a decision about therapeutic principles of cancer patients admitted to the ICU unexpectedly. Japanese Nursing Association. Nursing Academy: Adult Health Nursing I. 2009;39:184–6.
10. Morishita M, Kamibeppu K. Quality of life and satisfaction with care among family caregivers of patients with recurrent or metastasized digestive cancer requiring palliative care. Support Care Cancer. 2014;22:2687–96.
11. Vivar CG, Whyte DA, McQueen A. 'Again': the impact of recurrence on survivors of cancer and family members. J Clin Nur. 2010;19:2048–56.
12. Harvey AG, Bryant RA. Dissociative symptoms in acute stress disorder. J Trauma Stress. 1999;12:673–80.
13. Asukai N, Hirohata S, Kato H, et al. Psychometric properties of the Japanese-Language Version of the Clinician-Administered PTSD Scale for DSM-IV [in Japanese with English Abstract]. Jpn J trauma Stress. 2003;1:47–53.
14. Knaus WA, Draper EA, Wagner DP, et al. APACHE II: A severity of disease classification system. Crit Care Med. 1985;13:818–29.
15. Asukai N, Kato H, Kawamura N, et al. Reliability and validity of the Japanese-language version of the Impact of Event Scale-Revised (IES-R-J): four studies of different traumatic events. J Nerv Ment Dis. 2002;190:175–82.
16. Weiss DS. The Impact of Event Scale-Revised. In: Assessing psychological trauma and PTSD. 2nd ed. New York: The Guilford Press; 2004. p. 168–89.
17. Radloff LS. The CES-D scale, a self-report depression scale for research in the general population. Appl Psychol Meas. 1977;1:385–401.
18. Shima S, Kano T, Kitamura T. New depression self-assessment scale. Clin Psychiatry. 1985;27:17–24.
19. Spielberger CD, Gorsuch RL, Lushene RE. Manual for the State–Trait Anxiety Inventory (Self-Evaluation Questionnaire). Palo Alto: 7 Consultant Psychologists Press; 1970.
20. Nakazato K, Mizuguchi K. Development of new anxiety scale: STAI. Jpn J Psychosom Med. 1982;22:107–12.
21. American Psychiatric Association. Diagnostic and Statistical Manual of Mental Disorders. 4th ed. Washington DC: American Psychiatric Association; 2003.
22. Armitage P, Berry G, Matthew JNS. Statistical Methods in Medical Research. 4th ed. Oxford: Blackwell; 2002.
23. Komachi M, Kamibeppu K. Acute stress symptoms in families of patients admitted to the intensive care unit during the first 24 hours following admission in Japan. Open J Nursing. 2015;5:325–35.
24. Chui WYY, Chan SW. Stress and coping of Hong Kong Chinese family members during a critical illness. J Clin Nurs. 2007;16:372–81.
25. Paparrigopoulos T, Melissaki A, Efthymiou A, et al. Short-term psychological impact on family members of intensive care unit patients. J Psychosom Res. 2006;61:719–22.
26. American Psychiatric Association. Diagnostic and Statistical Manual of Mental Disorders. 5th ed. Arlington: American Psychiatric Association; 2013.

2

Hospital resuscitation teams: a review of the risks to the healthcare worker

Stephen M. Vindigni[1*], Juan N. Lessing[2] and David J. Carlbom[3]

Abstract

Background: "Code blue" events and related resuscitation efforts involve multidisciplinary bedside teams that implement specialized interventions aimed at patient revival. Activities include performing effective chest compressions, assessing and restoring a perfusing cardiac rhythm, stabilizing the airway, and treating the underlying cause of the arrest. While the existing critical care literature has appropriately focused on the patient, there has been a dearth of information discussing the various stresses to the healthcare team. This review summarizes the available literature regarding occupational risks to medical emergency teams, characterizes these risks, offers preventive strategies to healthcare workers, and highlights further research needs.

Methods: We performed a literature search of PubMed for English articles of all types (randomized controlled trials, case-control and cohort studies, case reports and series, editorials and commentaries) through September 22, 2016, discussing potential occupational hazards during resuscitation scenarios

Results: The literature search identified six potential occupational risk categories to members of the resuscitation team—infectious, electrical, musculoskeletal, chemical, irradiative, and psychological. Retrieved articles were reviewed in detail by the authors.

Conclusion: Overall, we found there is limited evidence detailing the risks to healthcare workers performing resuscitation. We identify these risks and offer potential solutions. There are clearly numerous opportunities for further study in this field.

Keywords: Code blue, Code team, Cardiopulmonary resuscitation, CPR, Advanced cardiac life support, Hospital rapid response teams, Medical emergency teams, Occupational medicine

Background

"Code blue" events are cardiopulmonary resuscitation efforts that occur in hospital settings. A dedicated multidisciplinary resuscitation team rapidly convenes at the bedside, initiates cardiopulmonary resuscitation (CPR), and performs an assessment of the situation. Cardiac defibrillation, establishment of intravenous (IV) access, placement of an advanced airway, blood draws, and medication administration, among other tasks, are integrated into these code situations. Multiple hospital staff are frequently present including physicians at all training levels, medical students, nurses, critical care staff, laboratory technicians, social workers, and clergy; increasingly, patient family members are also at the bedside.

The primary goal of resuscitation efforts is revival of the patient, and there is extensive literature discussing the management of cardiopulmonary arrest. There is, however, a dearth of literature commenting on the risks to the code team performing the resuscitation. One author experienced severe neck pain diagnosed as an epidural cervical hematoma following multiple rounds of CPR during a code. This event prompted a literature search to see if other providers experienced similar ill health effects, but we were able only to identify one editorial in the nursing literature that broadly discussed code-related occupational hazards [1]. Thus began our review of the available literature, which revealed many risk categories, which include

* Correspondence: stephen.vindigni@gmail.com
[1]Division of Gastroenterology, Department of Medicine, University of Washington, 1959 NE Pacific Street, Box 356424, Seattle, WA 98195-6424, USA
Full list of author information is available at the end of the article

infectious, electrical, musculoskeletal, chemical, irradiative, and psychological components (Table 1).

Through better understanding of the potential harms to resuscitation teams, we have the opportunity to mitigate or prevent them. The aim of this review is to summarize the available literature regarding occupational risks to medical emergency teams, characterize these risks, offer preventive strategies, and highlight the need for further research.

Materials and methods

We performed a review of peer-reviewed publications with a broad systematic literature search using PubMed to identify articles that discuss potential occupational hazards during resuscitation scenarios. Only articles published in English were reviewed. PubMed was searched for all historical articles through September 22, 2016. A medical librarian assisted with developing the literature search strategy. All identified articles were reviewed by two authors (SV, JL) with relevant information abstracted. Additional articles were identified from the reference sections. Based on review of the articles found, six risk areas were identified. Using this information, the search strategy was further refined to use the following keywords: "occupational exposure" or "code blue" or "resuscitation" or "trauma team" or "cardiopulmonary resuscitation" or "CPR" and "electric" or "chemical" or "musculo" or "musculoskeletal" or "psych" or "mental" or "infectious" or "infection" or "radiation." We reviewed all study types including randomized controlled trials, cohort and case-control studies, reviews, case reports and case series, and editorials. In total, 6266 studies were identified in the literature with 73 meeting the criteria to be included and reviewed across six categories (Fig. 1).

Results and discussion

Infectious risks

Multiple studies have discussed the benefits of universal precautions in healthcare settings, including during code situations. While focus has traditionally been placed on viral hepatitis (e.g., hepatitis B and C) and human immunodeficiency virus (HIV), providers are at risk for exposure to multiple infectious agents via cutaneous, mucosal, and percutaneous routes. In the late 1980s and 1990s, significant focus was on the risk of HIV exposure with multiple studies making strong arguments for universal precautions during code situations [2].

Table 1 Risks to in-hospital resuscitation teams and potential preventive strategies to mitigate risk

Risk category	Specific risks and potential exposures	Potential preventive actions and solutions
Infectious	□ Percutaneous/needlestick injuries □ Respiratory/airborne exposures □ Contact exposures □ Emerging/re-emerging infections	□ Convenient sharps disposal □ Use of needles with safety features □ Blood-borne pathogens training for all employees □ Reporting of needlestick injuries with post-exposure medical evaluations and prophylaxis □ Breathing filter during mask ventilation □ Clearly defined roles for staff regarding: who is responsible for blood draw, central line placement, etc.
Electrical	□ Shock during defibrillation □ ICD misfiring □ Fire generation near oxygen-rich atmospheres	□ Standard maintenance of defibrillators □ Training of resuscitation team members on the use of defibrillators □ Placing a donut magnet over ICDs; consider including on code cart □ Clear announcement of impending defibrillation □ Preferential use of gel adhesive pads instead of hand-held paddles. If paddles are used, avoidance of excess amounts of conduction gel □ Consider removal of supplemental oxygen from bed prior to defibrillation
Musculoskeletal	□ Neck/back injuries during/following chest compressions □ Falls while running to code situations	□ Training to providers on proper posture and chest compression technique □ Adjust height of bed during chest compressions and/or use of step stools □ Adequate number of chest compressors to allow recovery and reduce resuscitator fatigue
Chemical	□ Risks of chemical warfare	□ Programs for decontamination of victims of chemical warfare
Irradiative	□ Exposure during cross-table cervical spine radiographs with manual cervical spine stabilization, generally in trauma patients □ Brachytherapy patients	□ Maximize distance between provider and radiation beam □ Use of lead-lined gloves, lead aprons, thyroid shields, and glasses
Psychological	□ Traumatic stress with short- and long-term mental and physical impact	□ Stress management programs □ De-briefing following resuscitation efforts, ideally within less than 72 h and in a non-threatening manner □ Counseling and related programs for depression, PTSD and, overall mental health well-being □ Implementation of "death rounds"

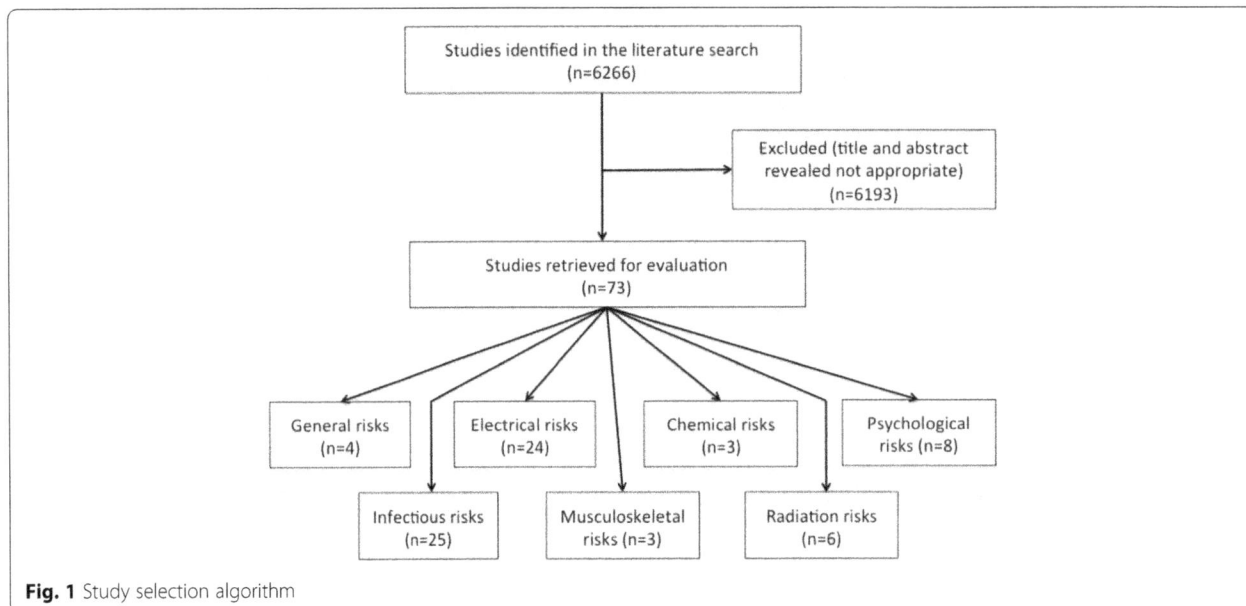

Fig. 1 Study selection algorithm

While the incidence of needlestick injuries among healthcare workers during routine medical care has been well documented in the literature, code situations undoubtedly present a higher risk. During resuscitative attempts, multiple providers are using needles for venipuncture, arterial blood gas sampling, and emergent placement of central venous catheters, often during active patient motion related to repositioning or CPR efforts. Despite this, very little has been published on the topic of needlestick injuries during resuscitation. One case report describes a resident physician who sustained a needlestick injury while attempting to place a central line; he appropriately reported the injury and received post-exposure prophylaxis [3]. But outside of this case report, no additional data was found. While not a needle exposure, there is one case report of a critical care nurse who sustained a puncture wound during chest compressions through contact with a patient's sternotomy wires following prior cardiac surgery; there were no reported infectious complications [4].

Given the perceived increased risk of parenteral exposure, measures beyond universal precautions are essential, including the use of safer syringes using newer engineered controls. These devices have a mechanism that retracts or covers the exposed needle to prevent accidental exposure following patient intervention [5, 6].

There is also the increasing use of intraosseous (IO) catheters leading the American Heart Association (AHA) to endorse IO cannulation as an appropriate means of access during resuscitation in the patient without available IV access [7]. While there are no documented adverse events to resuscitation teams, we anticipate these devices are safer and likely pose less risk to healthcare providers when compared to emergent femoral or other central line access placement.

Another area for potential infectious risk is respiratory exposure. While earlier resuscitation efforts included mouth-to-mouth resuscitation—with very rare documentation of infectious agent transmission—newer guidelines focus on chest compressions and no longer include direct mouth-to-mouth contact without the use of a protective barrier [8–10]. Historical concerns included a multitude of oral-to-oral infectious agents, including tuberculosis, HIV, herpes simplex, and *Helicobacter pylori*; these risks are no longer present [11]. In hospital-based settings, ventilation is performed through a bag-valve mask. Mask ventilation may contribute to the spread of infection exposing chest compressors to infectious air particles, but this is uncommon; a breathing filter may eliminate this risk [12]. The act of intubation and suctioning prior to intubation likely increases the risk of airborne or respiratory exposure, as seen during the severe acute respiratory syndrome (SARS) outbreak of 2003, but following intubation, manual ventilation and suctioning did not significantly increase risk [13]. Despite this, there is still at least a low-level risk present as providers are in contact with patient secretions.

Contact transmission is also rare. Theoretically, there may be increased exposure in patients with methicillin-resistant *Staphylococcus aureus* or vancomycin-resistant *enterococci*, but if universal precautions are implemented with gloves (and ideally gowns), this risk is reduced. First responders in the field may be at greater risk given the lack of a controlled setting with one case report describing a firefighter exposed to a child's oral secretions leading to *Streptococcus pyogenes* cellulitis at the site of an abrasion [8, 14]. There are no documented inpatient complications during resuscitation efforts.

Finally, there is always concern for emerging or re-emerging infections. Recent examples have been avian influenza, SARS, and Ebola virus disease [15–17]. These events are rare and unpredictable. There is one case report describing exposure to the H1N1 influenza virus when an endotracheal tube leaked during open-chest cardiac massage resulting in aerosolization of the virus [15]. Ulrich and Grady also describe the ethical concerns around cardiopulmonary resuscitation in Ebola patients and stress the importance of personal protective equipment and training of healthcare workers [16]. They also raise the difficult question of futility of CPR in Ebola-affected patients, particularly in the setting of higher risks to rescuers; they acknowledge Ebola can present with a spectrum of symptoms and some patients may benefit from CPR more than others.

In general, infections tend to be at the forefront of most providers' minds when they think about the risks related to resuscitation efforts. Despite this, true documented transmission is rare with percutaneous injury the most concerning and should be even less of a risk with accessible sharp containers and the aforementioned use of safer, advanced syringe devices. Additionally, there should be clearly assigned roles for who will be performing procedures involving sharps so as not to create confusion and ensuring only trained healthcare workers are performing needle-based interventions.

Electrical risks

Although significantly less common than a needlestick injury, there is a risk of electrical injury to code teams, particularly during defibrillatory shocks administered for treatment of ventricular fibrillation and pulseless ventricular tachycardia rhythms. These risks are particularly important as access to defibrillators by bystanders and non-healthcare providers in community settings (e.g., department stores, airports, etc.) has become increasingly common. A systematic review identified 29 adverse events during defibrillator use [18]. Excluding intentional or misuse of defibrillators (e.g., attempted suicide), three incidents were associated with faulty equipment (e.g., crack in paddles, inappropriate discharge) and four occurred during training or maintenance of equipment (e.g., accidental discharge). Fifteen accidental shocks during resuscitation could not be attributed to faulty equipment. Most were due to healthcare workers coming into contact with the patient or the stretcher, with few cases attributed to arc discharge between paddles and the patient's chest. The most common adverse effects were burns and tingling sensations [19]. The use of adhesive gel pads has limited the need for hand-held paddles, which has further reduced the risk of inadvertent shock [20].

Many studies have stressed the importance of limiting interruptions of chest compressions to reduce falls in coronary and cerebral perfusion pressure. To accomplish this, charging the defibrillator while compressions are ongoing is now recommended [21, 22]. Eliminating this delay ensures greater compression fraction (i.e., the percentage of time during which chest compressions are being delivered) but may also increase the risk of contact with the patient during defibrillation. Edelson et al. performed a multi-center, retrospective study of defibrillator charging by analyzing CPR-sensing defibrillator transcripts for pre-shock pauses and total hands-off time [21]. With charging during CPR, hands-off time was decreased and only one shock was administered with chest compressions ongoing; the compressor was unaffected. The data supports the AHA recommendation that defibrillator charging during chest compressions is safe [23].

More recently, there has been the suggestion of maintaining chest compressions during defibrillation with the hypothesis that the shock risk is low if gloves are worn by providers [24, 25]. Studies analyzing the electrical resistance of nitrile gloves used during codes compared to unused, control gloves found that gloves became degraded during wear and especially during active chest compressions (e.g., microscopic tearing, conductive moisture). There was a decrease in resistive protection; therefore, gloves were considered inadequate electrical insulation for ongoing contact with the patient during defibrillation [26]. Additional studies have shown similar results with vinyl and nitrile gloves [27, 28]. Lemkin asserts that the leakage current does not determine the risk of defibrillation, particularly since the amount of energy transferred is dependent on total energy delivered, voltage, and resistance of the patient [29]. Using cadavers to map rescuers' voltage exposure during defibrillation, he concluded hands-on defibrillation poses a risk to chest compressors without a clear negative impact of lifting hands for < 5 s on patients. The study results are debated as an overestimation of risk, but currently active hands-on defibrillation cannot be endorsed, and brief compression pauses are still recommended during shock delivery [30, 31]. The development of a "resuscitation blanket"—a layer between the patient's chest and rescuers' hands to prevent shock exposure—has been proposed but has not been incorporated into practice [32].

An additional potential electrical exposure is the firing of implantable cardioverter defibrillators (ICDs) during resuscitation. Clements presents a case report of a 75-year old man with pulseless electrical activity undergoing CPR [33]. The ICD was found to deliver four shocks during CPR that had no effect on the resuscitators; however, one shock was delivered during cardiac massage resulting in a shock to the massager and an inability to return to work for at least 30 min. The cardiac massage was hypothesized to mimic a shockable rhythm. An additional case report by Siniorakis describes a chest compressor who received an ICD-related shock that threw him against a wall resulting in neck and back pain [34]. The "electrical noise" generated by chest compressions was believed to have been interpreted by the ICD as ventricular fibrillation. Other case reports describe ICD-related paresthesias [35]. The current guidance is placement of a donut magnet over the ICD to eliminate the risk of ICD firing.

Despite the above risks, the incidence of significant shocks is low, and while defibrillation is considered a risk to healthcare workers, the fear of significant shock injury (as often inaccurately depicted by Hollywood) is unwarranted.

An additional rare electrical risk to note is fire related to defibrillation performed near flammable material, such as oxygen [18, 36]. Historical reports suggested removal of oxygen masks during defibrillation; however, more recent recommendations assert the low risk of fire is outweighed by the risks of delayed defibrillation and possible endotracheal dislodgement [37–39].

Musculoskeletal risks

The act of performing chest compressions is a strenuous task for even the fittest of healthcare workers. There are multiple potential injuries that can be sustained from shoulder to neck to back injuries. Musculoskeletal strain may not be apparent at first, tempered by the rush of adrenaline during a code situation but may become more evident in the days following a resuscitation effort.

There is a dearth of published literature discussing the musculoskeletal impact of CPR on the resuscitator. Cheung et al. performed a prospective, observational, interview-based study of medical emergency teams to assess physical injuries during hospital emergencies [40]. Injuries included back or shoulder pain following chest compressions, slipping en route to a resuscitation code, and exposure to urine, feces, blood, or vomitus. Of 17 injuries recorded, only one required treatment and time off from work. The injury rate was 13 per 1000 emergency team participants. Based on these results, the risk of injury was overall low and injuries that did occur were usually minor and without short- or long-term effect on daily activities [40].

Jackson and Sturrock describe a case of "resuscitation shoulder" or the partial tear of a rotator cuff experienced by a resident physician after performing repetitive and prolonged chest compressions on several patients over three consecutive nights while on call [41]. Similar injuries have been described following repetitive athletic pursuits.

Anecdotally, these authors are aware of a resident who developed an anterior cruciate ligament tear following a fall while running to a code. As mentioned above, one author developed acute neck pain following multiple rounds of vigorous CPR during an overnight code. He ultimately developed neurological symptoms with tingling in his fingers and was found to have a cervical epidural hematoma that was managed conservatively with improvement in symptoms. There is also a news media story of a paramedic developing a myocardial infarction (MI) while performing CPR on a patient experiencing an MI [42].

The effect of rescuer fatigue during prolonged codes has also been discussed with decreased compression depth achieved [43]. It can be hypothesized that as resuscitators develop fatigue, they may develop altered posture and increase the risk of musculoskeletal strain or sprain.

Additional factors to consider include space availability as limited by room size and number of providers in the room, bed type (emergency stretcher vs. standard hospital bed), height of the bed and availability of step stools for shorter providers, length of the code, improper rescuer positioning, and patient characteristics (e.g., obesity). These factors may predispose and/or increase the risk of injury during a resuscitation. In addition to prevention of musculoskeletal strain, a recent simulation study found the use of a step stool (23 cm in height) was associated with improved compression depth [44].

Chemical risks

We did not identify any literature focused on chemical risks during in-hospital resuscitation. There are a few publications commenting on the risk of chemical exposure to rescuers in mass causality or chemical warfare scenarios, but not in hospital settings. Depending on the chemical agent, patients may be at higher risk of cardiopulmonary arrest. Since healthcare providers have the potential to be exposed to victims of chemical warfare, protocols should be established to prepare for decontamination of these patients and ensure the protection of healthcare workers [45]. Interestingly, a study on the performance of paramedics wearing chemical protective suits found impairment of fine motor skills (e.g., IV cannulation, subcutaneous epinephrine injection) but overall successful resuscitation (e.g., defibrillation, tracheal intubation), despite delays imparted by wearing the suit [46]. This scenario may be translated to inpatient codes in the rare event of a chemical outbreak.

Radiation risks

Radiation risk is equally uncommon during resuscitation efforts. A rare exception is for patients who arrest during a radiographic examination, although the imaging study would be terminated in this setting. Most publications commenting on radiation risk relate to trauma patients who present in the emergency department and are being stabilized, which is a different scenario than a true cardiopulmonary arrest. In these trauma situations, there is possible radiation exposure to healthcare workers if manual cervical spine stabilization is required and cervical spine radiographs are taken, but more often, the patient is stabilized and images are obtained quickly with healthcare staff in a protected area and often wearing leaded protective equipment. Lead aprons, leaded gloves, thyroid shields, and glasses should be available for use during radiographic studies of trauma patients in these rare situations [47].

An additional potential radiation exposure is when resuscitation efforts are required in patients with implanted radioactive sources, such as in brachytherapy, for treatment of various cancers. For these patients undergoing surgery, Basran et al. suggest the use of lead-based gloves and use of dosimetry to measure exposure [48]. In known patients with active radioactive sources who code, these protective approaches may also apply.

Psychological risks
Resuscitation efforts, even if successful, may have a dramatic psychological impact on resuscitation team members. While the greatest literature on the mental health impact of rescuers is related to disasters and mass tragedy, such as following the 9/11 response, there is less evidence on the psychological impact of in-hospital resuscitations. As resuscitations are often unexpected, it may be difficult for healthcare workers to adapt and there is a risk of personal crisis and traumatic stress [49]. Stress can also have physical effects, including headache, chronic pain, and hypertension with the potential for absenteeism, impaired decision-making, and effects both at work and home [49, 50].

With the premise that nurses may experience long-term stress effects following a resuscitation, Cudmore performed a survey of nurses exploring the perceived need for debriefing following the resuscitation of a patient [51]. Nurses supported a formal debriefing session, particularly if the resuscitation was difficult or upsetting, such as involving a child, more than one patient, or related to major trauma or burns. Gamble discussed a framework for debriefing including introduction of resuscitation team members, discussion of case facts, an emotional description of the events and nurse response, identification of learning opportunities, and summing up a plan of action [52]. Based on our review, there are no studies focused on physician response to stress following resuscitation.

While not immediately related to resuscitation efforts, some institutions have implemented "death rounds" to discuss the emotions surrounding a patient death. While generally focused in a palliative care setting more commonly than a code blue scenario, the presence of a supportive environment to discuss difficult situations is likely to be beneficial [53–55].

Limitations
The greatest limitation (and significant finding) of this review is a lack of published literature on this topic. Of existing literature, the quality and rigor is variable as numerous cited studies are case reports rather than higher levels of evidence, such as randomized controlled trials or meta-analyses. While our literature review was thorough, it is possible additional risk categories exist. Given that medical errors and description of workplace injuries are often underrepresented in the literature, we anticipate that there are significantly more episodes of resuscitation harms that have not been documented nor published, especially the psychological impact to providers imparted by these stressful situations.

Conclusions
As the population ages, inpatient medical teams will continue to be engaged in resuscitation scenarios, possibly with increased frequency. This orchestrated resuscitation possesses inherent risks for the providers that include infectious, electrical, musculoskeletal, chemical, irradiative, and mental health threats. For each of these, strategies can be taken to reduce, if not prevent, risk. In addition to identifying these risks and potential preventive approaches, this review also highlights the overall lack of evidence of this topic area. While the patient is appropriately the focus during resuscitation efforts, we must not neglect the providers who need to remain in good health for the next code blue echoed over the loud speaker.

Abbreviations
AHA: American Heart Association; CPR: Cardiopulmonary resuscitation; HIV: Human immunodeficiency virus; ICDs: Implantable cardioverter defibrillators; IO: Intraosseous; IV: Intravenous; MI: Myocardial infarction; SARS: Severe acute respiratory syndrome

Acknowledgements
The authors would like to acknowledge Kristen DeSanto, MSLS, clinical librarian at the University of Colorado, who assisted with identifying articles for inclusion in this review.

Funding
The authors declare no support from any organization for the submitted work and no financial relationships with any organizations that might have an interest in the submitted work.

Disclaimer
The findings and conclusions in this report are those of the author(s) and do not necessarily reflect the views of the University of Washington or University of Colorado.

Authors' contributions

All authors were involved in the conception and design of the review, the assessment of articles, and the manuscript drafting and revising, and all provided final approval of the version submitted.

Competing interests

The authors declare that they have no competing interests.

Author details

[1]Division of Gastroenterology, Department of Medicine, University of Washington, 1959 NE Pacific Street, Box 356424, Seattle, WA 98195-6424, USA. [2]Division of General Internal Medicine, Department of Medicine, University of Colorado, 13001 E 17th Place, Aurora, CO 80045, USA. [3]Division of Pulmonary, Critical Care and Sleep Medicine, Department of Medicine, University of Washington, 1959 NE Pacific Street, Seattle, WA 98195-6424, USA.

References

1. McCabe E. Code team hazards. Nurs Manag. 1997;28(3):48K–L.
2. Lewandowski C, Ognjan A, Rivers E, et al. Health care worker exposure to HIV-1 and HTLV I-II in critically ill. Ann Emerg Med. 1992;21(11):1353–9.
3. Henderson DK. Management of needlestick injuries: a house officer who has a needlestick. JAMA. 2012;307(1):75–84.
4. Steinhoff JP, Pattavina C, Renzi R. Puncture wound during CPR from sternotomy wires: case report and discussion of perresuscitation infection risks. Heart Lung. 2001;30(2):159–60.
5. Higginson R, Parry A. Needlestick injuries and safety syringes: a review of the literature. Br J Nurs. 2013;22(8):S4. S6-8, S10
6. Trim JC. A review of needle-protective devices to prevent sharps injuries. Br J Nurs. 2004;13(3):144. 146-53
7. American Heart Association. Web-based integrated guidelines for cardiopulmonary resuscitation and emergency cardiovascular care—part 7: adult advanced cardiovascular life support. 2010 June 15, 2017]; Available from: ECCguidelines.heart.org
8. Mejicano GC, Maki DG. Infections acquired during cardiopulmonary resuscitation: estimating the risk and defining strategies for prevention. Ann Intern Med. 1998;129(10):813–28.
9. Rinker AG Jr. Disease transmission by mouth-to-mouth resuscitation. Emerg Med Serv. 2001;30(1):89–90.
10. Sun D, Bennett RB, Archibald DW. Risk of acquiring AIDS from salivary exchange through cardiopulmonary resuscitation courses and mouth-to-mouth resuscitation. Semin Dermatol. 1995;14(3):205–11.
11. Wenzel V, Idris AH, Dorges V, et al. The respiratory system during resuscitation: a review of the history, risk of infection during assisted ventilation, respiratory mechanics, and ventilation strategies for patients with an unprotected airway. Resuscitation. 2001;49(2):123–34.
12. Chan MT, Chow BK, Chu L, Hui DS. Mask ventilation and dispersion of exhaled air. Am J Respir Crit Care Med. 2013;187(7):e12–4.
13. Raboud JSA, McGeer A, Bontovics E, Chapman M, Gravel D, Henry B, Lapinsky S, Loeb M, McDonald LC, Ofner M, Paton S, Reynolds D, Scales D, Shen S, Simor A, Stewart T, Vearncombe M, Zoutman D, Green K. Risk factors for SARS transmission from patients requiring intubation: a multicentre investigation in Toronto. Canada PLoS One. 2010;5(5):e10717.
14. Valenzuela TD, Hooton TM, Kaplan EL, Schlievert P. Transmission of 'toxic strep' syndrome from an infected child to a firefighter during CPR. Ann Emerg Med. 1991;20(1):90–2.
15. Cunha BA, Syed U, Thekkel V, Davis M. Unusual nosocomial exposure to H1N1 influenza virus via open-chest cardiac. Infect Control Hosp Epidemiol. 2010;31(7):775–6. doi: 10.1086/653817.
16. Ulrich CM, Grady C. Cardiopulmonary resuscitation for Ebola patients: ethical considerations. Nurs Outlook. 2015;63(1):16–8. doi: 10.1016/j. outlook.2014.11.011.
17. Fowler RA, Guest CB, Lapinsky SE, et al. Transmission of severe acute respiratory syndrome during intubation and mechanical ventilation. Am J Respir Crit Care Med. 2004;169(11):1198–202. doi: 10.1164/rccm. 200305-715OC.
18. Hoke RS, Heinroth K, Trappe HJ, Werdan K. Is external defibrillation an electric threat for bystanders? Resuscitation. 2009;80(4):395–401. doi: 10. 1016/j.resuscitation.2009.01.002.
19. Gibbs W, Eisenberg M, Damon SK. Dangers of defibrillation: injuries to emergency personnel during patient resuscitation. Am J Emerg Med. 1990; 8(2):101–4.
20. Petley GW, Cotton AM, Deakin CD. Hands-on defibrillation: theoretical and practical aspects of patient and rescuer. Resuscitation. 2012;83(5):551–6. doi: 10.1016/j.resuscitation.2011.11.005.
21. Edelson DP, Robertson-Dick BJ, Yuen TC, et al. Safety and efficacy of defibrillator charging during ongoing chest compressions. Resuscitation. 2010;81(11):1521–6. doi: 10.1016/j.resuscitation.2010.07.014.
22. Steen S, Liao Q, Pierre L, Paskevicius A, Sjoberg T. The critical importance of minimal delay between chest compressions and subsequent defibrillation: a haemodynamic explanation. Resuscitation. 2003;58(3):249–58.
23. Emergency Cardiovascular Care Committee, Task Forces of the American Heart Association. 2005 American Heart Association guidelines for cardiopulmonary resuscitation and emergency cardiovascular care. Circulation. 2005;112(24 Suppl):IV1–203.
24. Kerber RE. "I'm clear, you're clear, everybody's clear": a tradition no longer necessary for defibrillation? Circulation. 2008;117(19):2435–6.
25. Lloyd MS, Heeke B, Walter PF, Langberg JJ. Hands-on defibrillation: an analysis of electrical current flow through rescuers in direct contact with patients during biphasic external defibrillation. Circulation. 2008;117(19):2510–4.
26. Deakin CD, Lee-Shrewsbury V, Hogg K, Petley GW. Do clinical examination gloves provide adequate electrical insulation for safe hands-on defibrillation? I: resistive properties of nitrile gloves. Resuscitation. 2013;84(7):895–9.
27. Petley GW, Deakin CD. Do clinical examination gloves provide adequate electrical insulation for safe hands-on defibrillation? II: material integrity following exposure to defibrillation waveforms. Resuscitation. 2013;84(7):900–3.
28. Sullivan JL, Chapman FW. Will medical examination gloves protect rescuers from defibrillation voltages. Resuscitation. 2012;83(12):1467–72.
29. Lemkin DL, Witting MD, Allison MG, et al. Electrical exposure risk associated with hands-on defibrillation. Resuscitation. 2014;85(10):1330–6.
30. Kulstad E, Garrett M, Naiman M, Garrett F. Overestimated electrical exposure risk associated with hands-on defibrillation? Resuscitation. 2015;92:e15.
31. Lemkin DL, Bond MC, Witting MD, Lemkin MA. Reply to letter: "overestimated electrical exposure risk associated with hands-on defibrillation?". Resuscitation. 2015;92:e17–8.
32. Yu T, Ristagno G, Li Y, et al. The resuscitation blanket: a useful tool for "hands-on" defibrillation. Resuscitation. 2010;81(2):230–5.
33. Clements PA. Hazards of performing chest compressions in collapsed patients with internal cardioverter defibrillators. Emerg Med J. 2003;20(4):379–80.
34. Siniorakis E, Hardavella G, Arvanitakis S, et al. Accidental shock to rescuer from an implantable cardioverter defibrillator. Resuscitation. 2009;80(3):293–4.
35. Stockwell B, Bellis G, Morton G, et al. Electrical injury during "hands on" defibrillation—a potential risk of internal cardioverter defibrillators. Resuscitation. 2009;80(7):832–4.
36. Miller PH. Potential fire hazard in defibrillation. JAMA. 1972;221(2):192.
37. Theodorou AA, Gutierrez JA, Berg RA. Fire attributable to a defibrillation attempt in a neonate. Pediatrics. 2003;112(3 Pt 1):677–9.
38. McAnulty GR, Robertshaw H. Risk of fire outweighed by need for oxygen and defibrillation. J Accid Emerg Med. 1999;16(1):77.
39. Cantello E, Davy TE, Koenig KL. The question of removing a ventilation bag before defibrillation. J Accid Emerg Med. 1998;15(4):286.
40. Cheung W, Gullick J, Thanakrishnan G, et al. Injuries occurring in hospital staff attending medical emergency team (MET). Resuscitation. 2009;80(12):1351–6.
41. Jackson CE, Sturrock R. Resuscitation shoulder—a complication of cardiac arrest. England: Rheumatology (Oxford); 2007. p. 1040–1.
42. Bentz L. Detroit paramedic has heart attack while giving CPR to man having heart attack. Atlanta: CNN; 2013.
43. McDonald CH, Heggie J, Jones CM, Thorne CJ, Hulme J. Rescuer fatigue under the 2010 ERC guidelines, and its effect on cardiopulmonary resuscitation (CPR) performance. Emerg Med J. 2013;30(8):623–7.
44. Cheng A, Lin Y, Nadkarni V, et al. The effect of step stool use and provider height on CPR quality during pediatric cardiac arrest: a simulation-based multicentre study. CJEM. 2017;2017:1–9.
45. Brennan RJ, Waeckerle JF, Sharp TW, Lillibridge SR. Chemical warfare agents: emergency medical and emergency public health issues. Ann Emerg Med. 1999;34(2):191–204.

46. MacDonald RD, LeBlanc V, McArthur B, Dubrowski A. Performance of resuscitation skills by paramedic personnel in chemical protective suits. Prehosp Emerg Care. 2006;10(2):254–9.

47. Weiss EL, Singer CM, Benedict SH, Baraff LJ. Physician exposure to ionizing radiation during trauma resuscitation: a prospective clinical study. Ann Emerg Med. 1990;19(2):134–8.

48. Basran PS, Baxter P, Beckham WA. Reducing radiation risks to staff for patients with permanently implanted radioactive sources requiring unrelated surgery. J Appl Clin Med Phys. 2015;16(5):5372.

49. Flannery RB Jr, Everly GS Jr. Crisis intervention: a review. Int J Emerg Ment Health. 2000;2(2):119–25.

50. Caine RM, Ter-Bagdasarian L. Early identification and management of critical incident stress. Crit Care Nurse. 2003;23(1):59–65.

51. Cudmore J. Do nurses perceive that there is a need for defusing and debriefing following the resuscitation of a patient in the accident and emergency department. Nurs Crit Care. 1996;1(4):188–93.

52. Gamble M. A debriefing approach to dealing with the stress of CPR attempts. Prof Nurse. 2001;17(3):157–60.

53. Smith L, Hough CL. Using death rounds to improve end-of-life education for internal medicine residents. J Palliat Med. 2011;14(1):55–8.

54. Khot S, Billings M, Owens D, Longstreth WT Jr. Coping with death and dying on a neurology inpatient service: death rounds as an educational initiative for residents. Arch Neurol. 2011;68(11):1395–7.

55. Hough CL, Hudson LD, Salud A, Lahey T, Curtis JR. Death rounds: end-of-life discussions among medical residents in the intensive care unit. J Crit Care. 2005;20(1):20–5.

3

Accuracy of Critical Care Pain Observation Tool and Behavioral Pain Scale to assess pain in critically ill conscious and unconscious patients

Paolo Severgnini[1*], Paolo Pelosi[2], Elena Contino[1], Elisa Serafinelli[1], Raffaele Novario[1] and Maurizio Chiaranda[1]

Abstract

Background: Critically ill patients admitted to intensive care unit (ICU) may suffer from different painful stimuli, but the assessment of pain is difficult because most of them are almost sedated and unable to self-report. Thus, it is important to optimize evaluation of pain in these patients. The main aim of this study was to compare two commonly used scales for pain evaluation: Critical Care Pain Observation Tool (CPOT) and Behavioral Pain Scale (BPS), in both conscious and unconscious patients. Secondary aims were (1) to identifying the most relevant parameters to determine pain scales changes during nursing procedures, (2) to compare both pain scales with visual analog scale (VAS), and (3) to identify the best combination of scales for evaluation of pain in patients unable to communicate.

Methods: In this observational study, 101 patients were evaluated for a total of 303 consecutive observations during 3 days after ICU admission. Measurements with both scales were obtained 1 min before, during, and 20 min after nursing procedures in both conscious (n.41) and unconscious (n.60) patients; furthermore, VAS was recorded when possible in conscious patients only. We calculated criterion and discriminant validity to both scales (Wilcoxon, Spearman rank correlation coefficients). The accuracy of individual scales was evaluated. The sensitivity and the specificity of CPOT and BPS scores were assessed. Kappa coefficients with the quadratic weight were used to reflect agreement between the two scales, and we calculated the effect size to identify the strength of a phenomenon.

Results: CPOT and BPS showed a good criterion and discriminant validity ($p < 0.0001$). BPS was found to be more specific (91.7 %) than CPOT (70.8 %), but less sensitive (BPS 62.7 %, CPOT 76.5 %). COPT and BPS scores were significantly correlated with VAS ($p < 0.0001$). The combination of BPS and CPOT resulted in better sensitivity 80.4 %. Facial expression was the main parameter to determine pain scales changes effect size = 1.4.

Conclusions: In critically ill mechanically ventilated patients, both CPOT and BPS can be used for assessment of pain intensity with different sensitivity and specificity. The combination of both BPS and CPOT might result in improved accuracy to detect pain compared to scales alone.

Keywords: Pain, Critical Care Pain Observation Tool, Behavioral Pain Scale, Critical ill patients, Intensive care unit, Pain management

* Correspondence: paolo.severgnini@uninsubria.it
[1]Department of Biotechnologies and Sciences of Life, Intensive Care Unit–
ASST Sette Laghi–Ospedale di Circolo Fondazione Macchi, University of
Insubria, Viale Luigi Borri 57, 21100 Varese, Italy
Full list of author information is available at the end of the article

Background

Pain management in critically ill patients is a complex process, but relevant to the clinical management. Pain is highly underestimated although it seems to be the patients' worst memory in intensive care unit (ICU) [1, 2] even after 5 years from ICU discharge [3]. The perception of pain in ICU patients is mainly associated with respiratory therapy, positioning of nasogastric tube, venous and arterial catheters, and lack of mobilization [2]. However, patients are usually unable to self-report their pain due to sedative drugs and intubation, likely leading to its underestimation [4, 5]. Pain with agitation and delirium has been reported to negatively affect outcome of mechanically ventilated patients [6]. Thus, it is required to have valid and reliable methods to assess pain in unconscious patients to optimize treatment [7]. There is no one standard approach to evaluate pain in ICU, and the proposed tools actually used have several advantages and disadvantages. In conscious patients, self-report, i.e., visual analog scale (VAS) is the gold standard for pain assessment [8]. In unconscious patient, new methods have been developed to assess pain by using behavioral scales [9–11]. In unconscious patients, two scales have been proposed to assess pain in ICU patients: Behavioral Pain Scale (BPS) [12] and Critical Care Pain Observation Tool (CPOT) [13]. However, the potential superiority of each of them for assessment of pain in mechanically ventilated patients is not well established [14, 15]. The main difference between CPOT and BPS is the evaluation of body movements and muscle tension. We hypothesized that CPOT is more sensitive and accurate to assess pain compared to BPS in critically ill patients being specifically focused on muscular tension.

The aims of the present study were the following: (1) to compare CPOT and BPS separately, in conscious and unconscious critically ill mechanically ventilated patients; (2) to identify the most relevant parameters to determine pain scales changes during nursing procedures; (3) to compare both pain scales with VAS; and (4) to identify the best combination of scales for evaluation of pain in patients unable to communicate.

Methods

This was a prospective, mono-centric study registered at ClinicalTrials.gov (ID NCT01669486). The study was conducted in the ICU at "Ospedale di Circolo Fondazione Macchi Varese". The study was revising by the local Ethical Committee (protocol n.0003412), and informed consent was obtained from the relatives or patients according to local regulations.

The staff is made up of 12 doctors and 28 nurses for 12 beds in a general intensive care unit. The patients-nurse ratio is 2:1 by day and 3:1 by night. The medical staff is also completed by five physicians in training. The most active phase of nursing care was made every morning and every afternoon. The nurses performed maneuvres for taking care of hygiene, therapy administration, and continuous monitoring of vital parameters. They are graduated in nursing after 3 years at university school and 2 years of master in intensive care. The medical staff is provided by physician graduated in medicine and surgery and specialized in anesthesia and intensive care after 5 years in training. The medical staff during the study was responsible for the assessment of pain through the acquisition of the behavioral scale scores. Assessments have been carried out by medical staff trained to identify the presence of pain with two scales. These observations were not blinded. In the morning, nurses provide patients' passive turning, cleaning, and repositioning; they perform airway suctioning, medications, and catheter management. In the afternoon, nurses provide only patient cleaning and repositioning. To get standardized measurements before, during, and after the maximum level of pain stimuli, we analyzed the behavioral scale scores during the nursing care performed in the morning [16].

The patients were evaluated with the Glasgow Coma Scale (GCS) and Sedation Agitation Scale (SAS). The conscious patients were identified with a GCS >10 and SAS = 4 (avoiding too agitated and too sedated patients to determine VAS).

Pain evaluation was performed in conscious and unconscious patients before, during, and 20 min after nursing care [17, 18]. Inclusion criteria were (1) need of invasive mechanical ventilation and (2) admission in ICU longer than 24 h. Exclusion criteria were (1) age <18 years old, (2) infusion of neuromuscular blocking agents, (3) any diseases causing tetraplegic and paraplegic condition as well as lateral neurological signs, and (4) pregnancy. After the enrollment day, every morning, the patients were evaluated for inclusion and exclusion criteria and, if feasible, we repeated the observations until tracheal extubation time, for a maximum of three observations for patient. We collected patients' characteristics within 24 h after ICU admission, including age, gender, medical or surgical, SAS [19], and severity of illness by Acute Physiology and Chronic Health Evaluation (APACHE) and Simplified Acute Physiology Score (SAPS II). Pain assessment was performed by the CPOT and BPS scales in conscious and unconscious patients, while VAS in conscious patients only. In this study, the conscious patients were identified with a GCS greater than 10 and the patients that were able to answer with the VAS scale. The CPOT scale includes four behavioral indicators: facial expression, body movements, muscle tension, and compliance with the ventilator (Table 1). Each item is scored from 0 to 2 for a possible total score range from 0 to 8 points [15]. The BPS includes three behavioral indicators: facial expression, upper limb movements, and compliance with the ventilator (Table 1).

Table 1 Behavioral Pain Scale, Critical Care Pain Observation Tool, Behavioral Pain Scale and Critical Care Pain Observation Tool combination

BPS score		CPOT score				BPS and CPOT combination score
Facial Expression		Facial Expression				
Relaxed	1	Relaxed, neutral	0			1
Partially Tightened	2	Tense	1			3
Fully tightened Grimacing	3 or 4	Grimacing	2			5 or 6
Upper Limb Movement		Body Movement		Muscle Tension		
No movement	1	Absence of movements	0	Relaxed	0	1
Partially bent	2	Protection	0 or 1	Tense, rigid	0 or 1	3 or 4
Fully bent with finger flexion Permanently retracted	3 or 4	Restlessness	0, 1, or 2	Very tense, or rigid	0, 1, or 2	5, 6, 7, or 8
Ventilator Compliance		Ventilator Compliance				
Tolerating movement	1	Tolerating ventilator	0			1
Coughing but tolerating for the most of time	2	Coughing but tolerating	1			3
Fighting ventilator Unable to control ventilation	3 or 4	Fighting ventilator	2			5 or 6

The table shows the Behavioral Pain Scale (BPS) (first column), the Critical Care Pain Observation Tool (CPOT) scores (second column), and the BPS and CPOT combination score (third column). The individual BPS and CPOT scores for each raw were summed. The BPS and CPOT combination score was obtained from the individual BPS and CPOT combination score from each raw. This combined BPS and CPOT score ranges from 3 to 20

Each item is scored from 1 to 4 for a possible score range from 3 and 12 points [12]. The VAS is a linear scale and identifies the pain by the self-report of patient, and it is considered the gold standard for evaluation of pain in conscious patients. In agreement with the literature [8], VAS ≥3 was used as a cutoff value to determine patients with pain. The combination of both BPS and CPOT scales was obtained by summing arithmetically the two scales normalized (Table 1). The two scales were normalized to convert the numeric scores from each scale. We compared CPOT subscale Body Movement and Muscle Tension with BPS subscale Upper Limb Movement and we summed the point of subscales. We considered a BPS score 3-4 and CPOT score 0-1-2 like absence pain; a BPS score 5-6-7 and CPOT score 3-4 like moderate pain; and a BPS score 8-9-10-11-12 and CPOT score 5-6-7-8 like severe pain.

Statistical analysis

The statistical calculations were performed with in MedCalc for Windows, version 12.1.4.0. First, we calculate the sample size. The sample size calculation determined the number of the patients to enroll, and it was calculated a "priori" and based on 0.05 type I error and 0.20 type II error with a difference expected of 10 % order of magnitude in the area under the curve (AUC) area. We evaluated the validity to both scales, as criterion validity and discriminant validity. Discriminant validity refers to the ability of an instrument to measure the presence or the absence of the variable. In this study, the discriminant was correlated with the mean scores of both scales

before and during the nursing care, 20 min after and during the procedure, and before and 20 min after the procedure, in conscious and unconscious patients. This correlation was calculated with Wilcoxon coefficient, which is a non-parametric test to determinate whether two samples come from the same statistical population, in the presence of ordinal values and continuous distribution. Box plot is a way to describe groups of numerical data through their quartiles. Criterion validity refers to the ability of an instrument to accurately measure the phenomenon of interest, in this case, the measurement of pain. It was evaluated by correlating the observed CPOT and BPS scores to the "gold standard" of pain measurement, i.e., VAS, when possible in conscious patients, and using the Spearman rank correlation coefficient (rs). Additionally, the sensitivity and the specificity of CPOT and BPS scores with ROC curve were assessed, only in conscious patients. The best discriminating between real and false positive is obtained by a curve passing in the upper left corner of at x/Y graphic ($x = 1 -$ specificity, $y =$ sensibility). In this case, the true positive corresponds to 100 % and the false positive correspond to 0 %. The AUC measures the ability of the scales to discriminate between patients who did or did not feel pain. The accuracy of individual scales was evaluated using calculation of sensitivity multiplied by the prevalence of positive to the sum of the observations (VAS ≥3, presence of pain) added to the specificity multiplied by the prevalence of negatives (VAS <3, absence of pain). Kappa coefficients with the quadratic weight were used to reflect agreement between the two scales [20], in conscious and unconscious patients. The Cohen's Kappa is statistical co-efficient that represents the degree of accuracy and reliability in a statistical classification; it is a concordance index calculated according to the ratio between the agreements in excess of the maximum obtainable [21]. The effect size is a quantitative measure of the strength of a phenomenon, for example, the correlation between two variables. We used this test to identify the most important subscale both BPS and CPOT, in conscious and unconscious patients. Cohen classified effect size as small (0.2–0.5), medium (0.5–0.8), large (0.8–1.3), and very large (>1.3) [22].

The level of significance accepted was a P value <0.05.

Results

In the study period (Fig. 1), 253 patients were admitted to the ICU and 162 patients met entry criteria. Among them, 61 patients were excluded (29 patients refused consent and 32 patients required sedation during the nursing care); thus, a total of 101 patients, 41 conscious and 60 unconscious patients, were included into the final analysis. In this study, the sample size was 75 patients/observations. In the enrollment phase, we needed to consider 101 patients to obtain 75 observations in conscious patients

with VAS scale. The clinical characteristics of the patients are reported in Table 2. None patients presented delirium assessed through CAM-ICU scale. The analgesia and sedation of patients were obtained with the administration of midazolam (mean i.v. dose in unconscious patients was 0.04 ± 0.03 mg/kg/h, while in conscious patients 0.03 ± 0.028 mg/kg/h) and morphine (mean i.v. dose in unconscious patients 0.069 ± 0.12 mg/kg/h, while in conscious 0.061 ± 0.12 mg/kg/h) or propofol 2 % (mean i.v. dose in unconscious patients 0.14 ± 0.10 mg/kg/h, while in conscious patients 0.12 ± 0.10 mg/kg/h) and remifentanil (mean i.v. dose in unconscious patients 0.03 ± 0.01 mg/kg/h, while in conscious patients 0.02 ± 0.01 mg/kg/h) and they were kept constant during the procedure, minimizing any possible influence on the evaluation of pain. We interrupted the sedation to evaluate the level of consciousness of patients, when possible and useful, only after the nursing procedures and after the evaluation of the patients, not to interfere with the application of the scales.

The medical patients were affected to respiratory failure, from pulmonary edema and pneumonia. The surgical ones instead included patients undergoing abdominal, vascular, and thoracic surgery and multiple trauma. In addition to usual devices like central lines, arterial line, gastric tube,

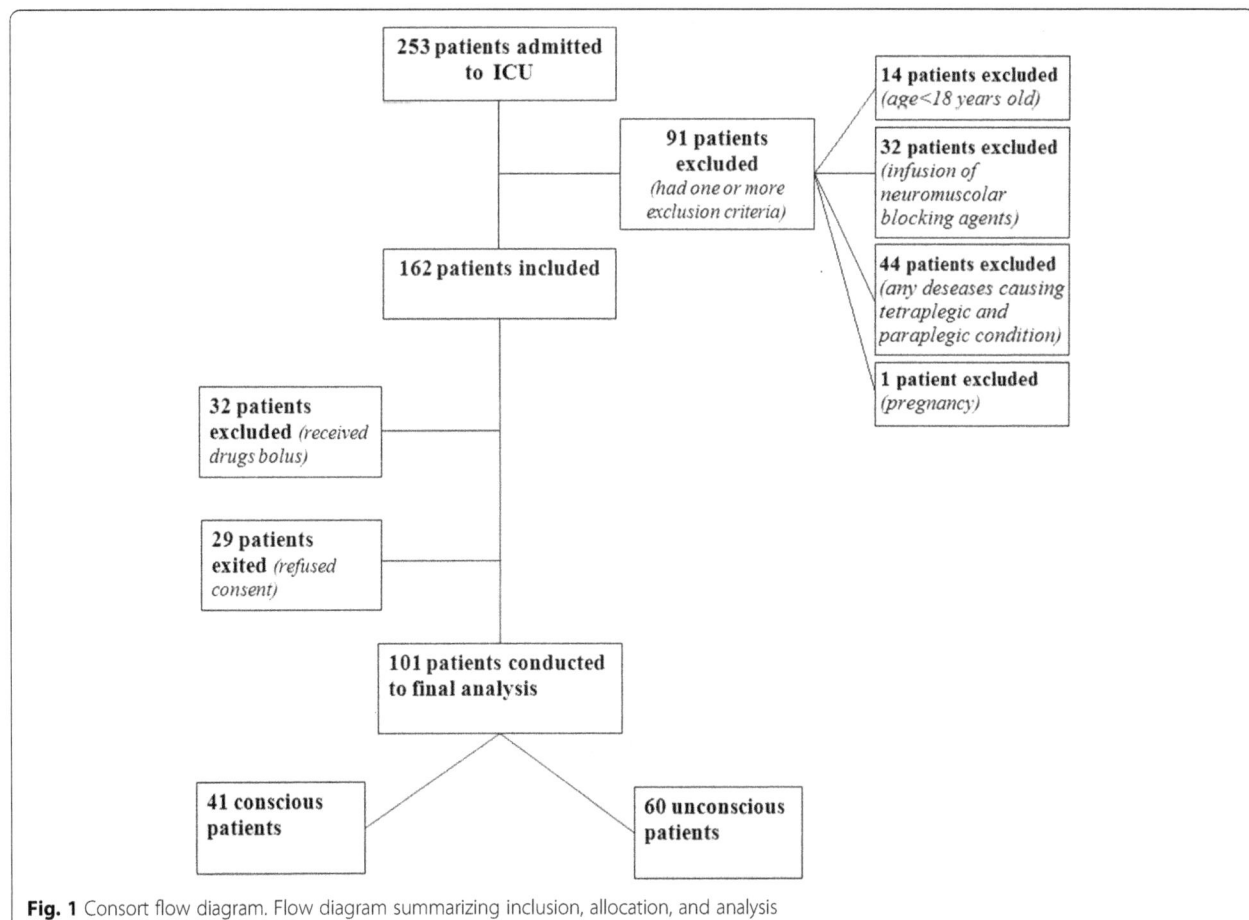

Fig. 1 Consort flow diagram. Flow diagram summarizing inclusion, allocation, and analysis

Table 2 Clinical characteristics of the patients at the time of enrollment

Age (years)		65 ± 16.7
Gender (M/F)		64/37
APACHE II (mean ± SD)		15.7 ± 7.1
SAPS II (mean ± SD)		43.5 ± 13.4
SAS (mean ± SD)		3.0 ± 1.1
CAM ICU		(−) n: 101; (+) n: 0
Patient category	Medical (n)	33
	Surgical (n)	68
Outcome	ICU discharge (n)	88
	Died (n)	13

Data are expressed as mean ± standard deviation
APACHE II acute physiology and chronic health evaluation, *SAPS II* simplified acute physiology score, *SAS* sedation agitation scale, *CAM ICU* confusion assessment method for the intensive care unit; *ICU* intensive care unit, *(+)* presence, *(-)* absence, *(n)* number

tracheal tube, and urinary catheter, these patients presented additionally surgical incisions, drainages, and open abdomen treatment.

We calculated discriminant validity for BPS and CPOT in overall, conscious and unconscious patients. BPS showed a statistically significant difference during nursing care (overall $Z = -12.3$, $p < 0.0001$; conscious $Z = -6.93$, $p < 0.0001$; unconscious $Z = -10.68$, $p < 0.0001$) and during and after nursing care (overall $Z = -12.6$, $p < 0.0001$; conscious $Z = -6.78$, $p < 0.0001$; unconscious $Z = -11.15$, $p <$

0.0001). We observed similar results with CPOT (during: overall $Z = -12.09$, $p < 0.0001$; conscious $Z = -6.48$, $p < 0.0001$; unconscious $Z = -10.62$, $p < 0.0001$; during and after, overall $Z = -12.81$, $p < 0.0001$; conscious $Z = -6.64$ $p < 0.0001$; unconscious $Z = -11.36$, $p < 0.0001$).

Figure 2 shows changes in CPOT and BPS during nursing in overall, conscious and unconscious patients; both CPOT and BPS values increased during nursing while decreased at the end of procedure to come back to original status.

We compared the two scales in three different moments, with the Cohen's Kappa, before $k = 0.69$, during = 0.64, after = 0.66; a k-value larger than 0.6 showed a good correlation.

Among different individual parameters for CPOT and BPS, in overall, conscious and unconscious patients, facial expression was the most important one for pain detection with effect size 1.4 while the other parameters presented an effect size more less (BPS scale Upper Limb Movement = 0.84, Ventilator Compliance = 0.99; CPOT scale Muscle Tone = 0.71, Body Movement = 0.60 and Ventilator Compliance = 1.09).

The criterion validity of BPS and CPOT scale showed a strong correlation with VAS, including all measurements (BPS rs = 0.56; $p < 0.0001$ CPOT rs = 0.48; $p < 0.0001$).

Sensitivity and specificity to both scales and their combination are shown in Table 3 into three different moments. During the nursing care, in particular, we found a low

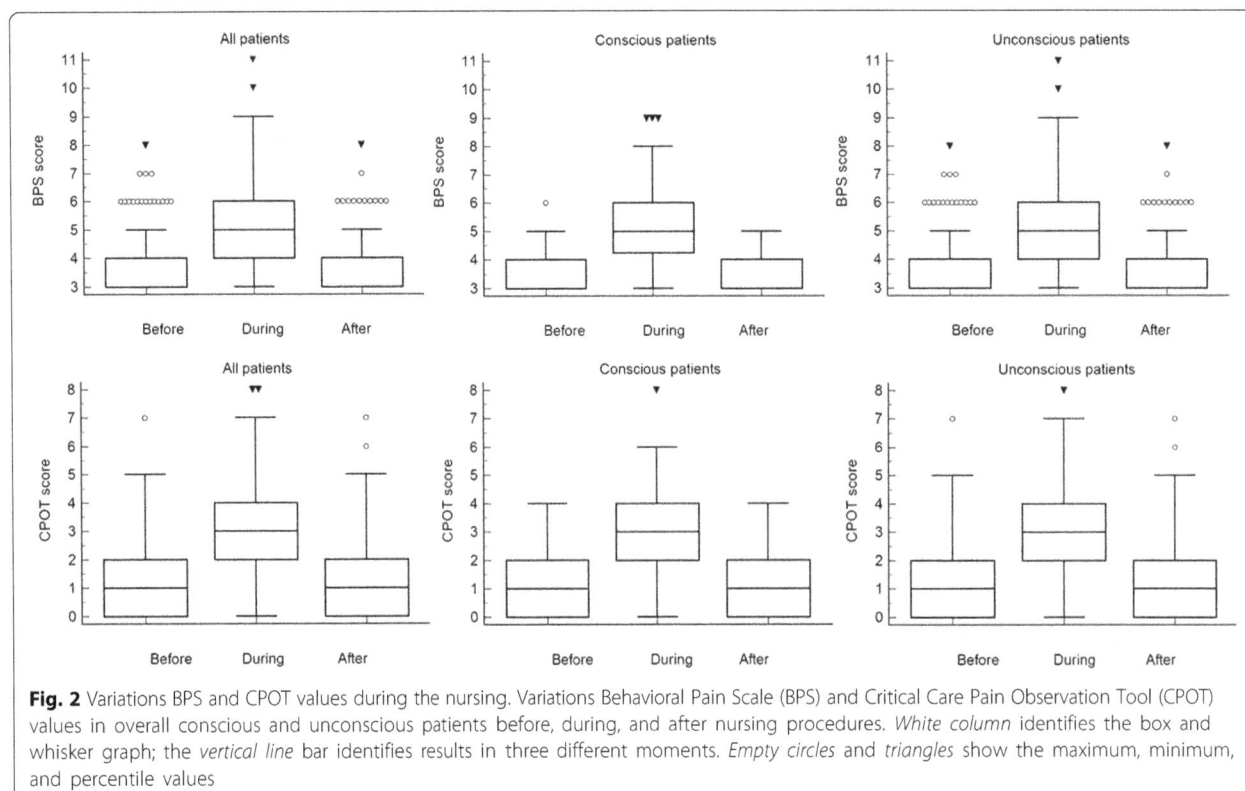

Fig. 2 Variations BPS and CPOT values during the nursing. Variations Behavioral Pain Scale (BPS) and Critical Care Pain Observation Tool (CPOT) values in overall conscious and unconscious patients before, during, and after nursing procedures. *White column* identifies the box and whisker graph; the *vertical line* bar identifies results in three different moments. *Empty circles* and *triangles* show the maximum, minimum, and percentile values

Table 3 The table shows results of CPOT and BPS sensitivity and specificity

		Before	During	After	Overall	Cutoff value
BPS	Sensitivity	79.2	62.8	62.5	84.8	
	Specificity	61.2	91.7	60.8	52.3	5
	AUC	0.71	0.83	0.6	0.76	
CPOT	Sensitivity	25	76.5	33.3	48.5	
	Specificity	91.3	70.8	60.8	88.2	2
	AUC	0.57	0.8	0.5	0.7	
BPS and CPOT combination score	Sensitivity	70.8	80.4	79.2	50.5	
	Specificity	58.8	75	37.2	89	7
	AUC	0.65	0.84	0.55	0.74	

Sensitivity and specificity of BPS, CPOT as well as the association of both scales (BPS and CPOT combination score) compared to patient self-report before, during and after nursing maneuvers. Overall are all patients regardless of the stage of nursing, by entering into a single database all the measurements

BPS Behavioral Pain Scale, *CPOT* Critical Care Pain Observation Tool

sensitivity for BPS (BPS sensitivity 62.8 % and specificity 91.7 %, accuracy 72.04 %), and low specificity for CPOT (CPOT sensitivity 76.5 % and specificity 70.8 %, accuracy 74.68 %). The ROC curve obtained with the association of both BPS and CPOT scales, summing arithmetically the two scales normalized (Fig. 3), showed during the nursing specificity 75 % and sensitivity 80.4 %, with an accuracy 78.67 % with a AUC = 0.84.

Discussion

In the present study, we evaluated two different pain scales in unconscious and conscious critically ill mechanically ventilated patients during nursing care. We found that (1) CPOT and BPS separately increased during nursing care in both unconscious and conscious patients and were significantly correlated; (2) facial expression showed greater changes for pain assessment; (3) in conscious patients, during nursing care, BPS showed higher specificity, and lower sensitivity compared to CPOT; and (4) the combination of both BPS and CPOT resulted in improved accuracy to detect pain compared to individual pain scales. Thus, against our expectations, our data suggest that CPOT was actually equivalent to BPS in sensitivity and

accuracy for pain evaluation because none scale have better sensitivity and specificity to each other (BPS sensitivity 62.8 % and specificity 91.7 %, CPOT sensitivity 76.5 %, and specificity 70.8 %).

Our data suggest that using both BPS and CPOT during nursing care or other painful intervention might improve the evaluation of pain. To our knowledge, this is the first study suggesting that the combination of BPS and CPOT may be considered as a valuable tool for pain assessment in mechanically ventilated critically ill patients [15, 23, 24].

In the present study, we evaluated patients requiring mechanical ventilation and admitted to a general ICU. Thus, our results may be more easily applicable to a mixed population of critically ill patients. Few previous studies simultaneously recorded BPS and CPOT as well as VAS [15, 25, 26]. We compared both BPS and CPOT with VAS in conscious patients during nursing care, but our findings can be applied also to unconscious patients, being the pain assessment and the level of analgesia similar in both groups. These scales are normally used to evaluate pain in unconscious patients. Based on our own data, we demonstrated that BPS and CPOT might provide information about pain in unconscious patients,

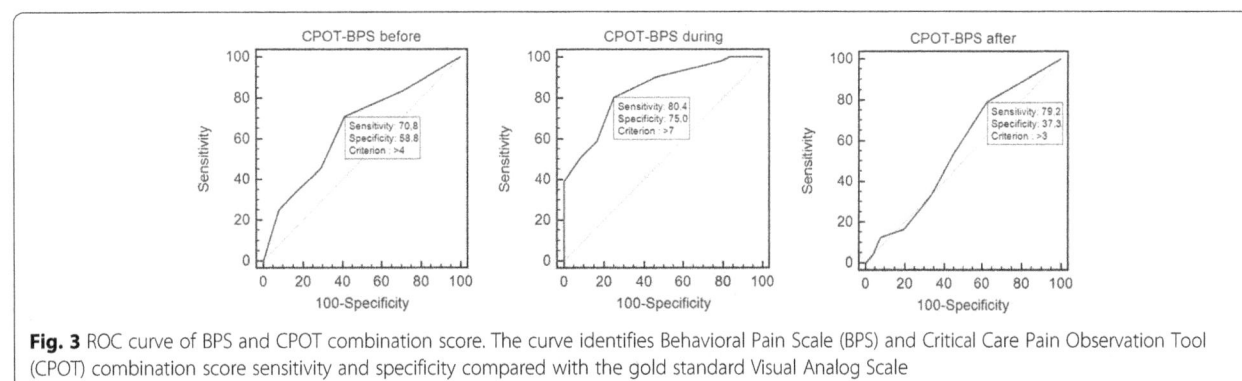

Fig. 3 ROC curve of BPS and CPOT combination score. The curve identifies Behavioral Pain Scale (BPS) and Critical Care Pain Observation Tool (CPOT) combination score sensitivity and specificity compared with the gold standard Visual Analog Scale

as shown by the correlation between VAS and BPS and CPOT. First, we showed a correlation between VAS and BPS and CPOT in conscious patients. Secondly, we obtained similar finding in unconscious patients.

Our results are in line with those reported in previous studies showing that both BPS and CPOT increase during nursing care and return back to baseline in a short period of time [27]. The diagnostic performance of both CPOT and BPS worsened after nursing care, suggesting that these scores might be affected by clinical maneuvres. Procedures like passive mobilization, i.e., turning and repositioning, and suctioning have been shown to increase pain. Conversely, active mobilization, i.e., rehabilitation, might be associated with less pain. In the present study, nursing procedures included turning and repositioning, but not routine suctioning and rehabilitation. Rehabilitation was not considered in the present study, since it might not induce pain due to active movements, better controlled by conscious patients only. Both BPS and CPOT have been evaluated in both unconscious and conscious patients. Pain assessment was similar in unconscious and conscious patients, suggesting that nursing care is painful independent of the level of sedation and analgesia [25]. Different individual items are included in BPS and CPOT. Muscular tone movement of arms and legs are included in CPOT but not BPS. Facial expression and ventilator compliance are recorded in both scales, although using different individual scores. We found that facial expression was the most important parameter related to pain assessment, in agreement with previous literature [15, 24]. It is important to note that facial expression is also easier to be scored at bedside. Furthermore, BPS and CPOT showed a good criterion and discriminant validity as previously reported [24–27], but BPS showed higher specificity but lower sensitivity compared to CPOT and so we cannot have considered CPOT superior to BPS, contrary to our hypothesis.

Thus, we hypothesized that of both BPS and CPOT, scales might result in improved accuracy to detect pain compared to each scale alone. The accuracy was evaluated by summing the scores of both scales for each individual observation. We found that during nursing care, the combination of BPS and CPOT resulted in better sensitivity. On the other hand, its specificity was higher than CPOT but lower than BPS. However, it was not possible to assess the best type of combination between the two scales, due to the higher prevalence of true positive cases and the limited sample size. In our study we did not find patients with delirium, and this may have been due to the optimization of the level of sedation.

Our study has limitations to be addressed. First, we evaluated only nursing care and no other possible painful maneuvers like suctioning. Second, the pain scales used are subjective to the operator and not objective. However, only one trained assessor evaluated pain for each patient. Third, we did not found any case of delirium in our analyzed patients, and this may be due to the level of sedative drugs applied, and/or to the feasibility of the CAM-ICU application in our population of critically ills patients.

Fourth, a relatively small group of patients was analyzed. Further studies are required to confirm our results in a larger population of patients.

Conclusions
Both CPOT and BPS scales are applicable to detect pain in conscious and unconscious critically ill mechanically ventilated patients, but with different sensitivity and specificity. The association of both scales might improve the efficiency for pain assessment. The level of consciousness does not affect the perception of pain during nursing care.

Abbreviations
APACHE: Acute Physiology and Chronic Health Evaluation; AUC: Area under the curve; BPS: Behavioral Pain Scale; CPOT: Critical Care Pain Observation Tool; ICU: Intensive care unit; rs: Spearman score; SAPS II: Simplified Acute Physiology Score; SAS: Sedation Agitation Scale; SD: Standard deviation; VAS: Visual analog scale; Z: Wilcoxon score

Acknowledgements
The author would like to specially thank all medical and nursing staff in the department of critical care unit for their collaboration and assistance with data collection. An important thank to patients who participated to the study.

Funding
We had no external funding sources; each author has funded the research with their own funds.

Authors' contributions
SP and PP conceived the study, participated in its design as well as coordination, and drafted the manuscript. EC participated as a local investigator, participated in the design of the study, and helped to draft the manuscript. ES participated as a local investigator and helped to draft the manuscript. NR participated in the design of the study and performed the statistical analysis. All authors read and approved the final manuscript.

Author's information
-Severgnini Paolo, MD is the coordinator of steering committee. Azienda Ospedaliera Fondazione Macchi ASST Sette Laghi, Intensive Care Unit–Department of Biotechnologies and Sciences of Life, University of Insubria, Varese, Italy
-Pelosi Paolo, MD, FERS is a member of steering committee. IRCCS AOU San Martino-IST, Department of Surgical Sciences and Integrated Diagnostics, University of Genoa, Genoa, Italy
-Elena Contino, MD is a member of steering committee. Azienda Ospedaliera Fondazione Macchi ASST Sette Laghi, Intensive Care Unit–Department of Biotechnologies and Sciences of Life, University of Insubria, Varese, Italy
-Elisa Serafinelli, MD is a member of steering committee. Azienda Ospedaliera Fondazione Macchi ASST Sette Laghi, Intensive Care Unit–Department of Biotechnologies and Sciences of Life, University of Insubria, Varese, Italy
-Novario Raffaele, PH is a member of steering committee, participated in the design of the study and performed the statistical analysis. Azienda Ospedaliera Fondazione Macchi ASST Sette Laghi, Medical Physics Unit–

Department of Biotechnologies and Sciences of Life, University of Insubria, Varese, Italy
-Chiaranda Maurizio, MD, PhD is a member of steering committee. Azienda Ospedaliera Fondazione Macchi ASST Sette Laghi, Anesthesia and Intensive Care Unit "A"– Department of Biotechnologies and Sciences of Life, University of Insubria, Varese, Italy

Competing interests
The authors declare that they have no competing interests.

Author details
[1]Department of Biotechnologies and Sciences of Life, Intensive Care Unit– ASST Sette Laghi–Ospedale di Circolo Fondazione Macchi, University of Insubria, Viale Luigi Borri 57, 21100 Varese, Italy. [2]Largo R. Benzi 10, 16132 Genova, Italy.

References
1. Granja C, Lopes A, Moreira S, et al. Patients' recollections of experiences in the intensive care unit may affect their quality of life. Crit Care. 2005;9(2): R96–109.
2. Gelinas C. Management of pain in cardiac surgery ICU patients: have we improved over time? Intensive Crit Care Nurs. 2007;23(5):298–303.
3. Zetterlund P, Plos K, Bergbom I, et al. Memories from intensive care unit persist for several years—a longitudinal prospective multi-centre study. Intensive Crit Care Nurs. 2012;28(3):159–67.
4. Russell S. An exploratory study of patients' perceptions, memories and experiences of an intensive care unit. J Adv Nurs. 1999;29(4):783–91.
5. Cullen L, Greiner J, Titler MG. Pain management in the culture of critical care. Crit Care Nurs Clin North Am. 2001;13(2):151–66.
6. Dale CR, Kannas DA, Fan VS, et al. Improved analgesia, sedation, and delirium protocol associated with decreased duration of delirium and mechanical ventilation. Ann Am Thorac Soc. 2014;11(3):367–74.
7. Lindenbaum L, Milia DJ. Pain management in the ICU. Surg Clin North Am. 2012;92(6):1621–36.
8. Chanques G, Viel E, Constantin JM, et al. The measurement of pain in intensive care unit: comparison of 5 self-report intensity scales. Pain. 2010; 151(3):711–21.
9. Puntillo KA, Morris AB, Thompson CL, et al. Pain behaviors observed during six common procedures: results from Thunder Project II. Crit Care Med. 2004;32(2):421–7.
10. Mateo OM, Krenzischek DA. A pilot study to assess the relationship between behavioral manifestations and self-report of pain in postanesthesia care unit patients. J Post Anesth Nurs. 1992;7(1):15–21.
11. Li D, Puntillo K, Miaskowski C. A review of objective pain measures for use with critical care adult patients unable to self-report. J Pain. 2008;9(1):2–10.
12. Payen JF, Bru O, Bosson JL, et al. Assessing pain in critically ill sedated patients by using a behavioral pain scale. Crit Care Med. 2001;29(12):2258–63.
13. Gelinas C, Fortier M, Viens C, et al. Pain assessment and management in critically ill intubated patients: a retrospective study. Am J Crit Care. 2004;13(2):126–35.
14. Liu Y, Li L, Herr K. Evaluation of two observational pain assessment tools in Chinese critically ill patients. Pain Med. 2015;16(8):1622–8.
15. Ahlers SJ, van Gulik L, van der Veen AM, et al. Comparison of different pain scoring systems in critically ill patients in a general ICU. Crit Care. 2008;12(1):R15.
16. Gelinas C, Fillion L, Puntillo KA, et al. Validation of the critical-care pain observation tool in adult patients. Am J Crit Care. 2006;15(4):420–7.
17. Aissaoui Y, Zeggwagh AA, Zekraoui A, et al. Validation of a behavioral pain scale in critically ill, sedated, and mechanically ventilated patients. Anesth Analg. 2005;101(5):1470–6.
18. Jeitziner MM, Schwendimann R, Hamers JP, et al. Assessment of pain in sedated and mechanically ventilated patients: an observational study. Acta Anaesthesiol Scand. 2012;56(5):645–54.
19. Riker RR, Picard JT, Fraser GL. Prospective evaluation of the Sedation-Agitation Scale for adult critically ill patients. Crit Care Med. 1999;27(7):1325–9.
20. Landis JR, Koch GG. The measurement of observer agreement for categorical data. Biometrics. 1977;33(1):159–74.
21. Sim J, Wright CC. The kappa statistic in reliability studies: use, interpretation, and sample size requirements. Phys Ther. 2005;85(3):257–68.
22. Sullivan GM, Feinn R. Using effect size-or why the P value is not enough. J Grad Med Educ. 2012;4(3):279–82.
23. Barr J, Fraser GL, Puntillo K, et al. Clinical practice guidelines for the management of pain, agitation, and delirium in adult patients in the intensive care unit. Crit Care Med. 2013;41(1):263–306.
24. Gelinas C, Puntillo KA, Joffe AM, et al. A validated approach to evaluating psychometric properties of pain assessment tools for use in nonverbal critically ill adults. Semin Respir Crit Care Med. 2013;34(2):153–68.
25. Pudas-Tahka SM, Axelin A, Aantaa R, et al. Pain assessment tools for unconscious or sedated intensive care patients: a systematic review. J Adv Nurs. 2009;65(5):946–56.
26. Puntillo K, Pasero C, Li D, et al. Evaluation of pain in ICU patients. Chest. 2009;135(4):1069–74.
27. Rijkenberg S, Stilma W, Endeman H, et al. Pain measurement in mechanically ventilated critically ill patients: Behavioral Pain Scale versus Critical-Care Pain Observation Tool. J Crit Care. 2015;30(1):167–72.

Combined inhibition of C5 and CD14 efficiently attenuated the inflammatory response in a porcine model of meningococcal sepsis

Bernt C. Hellerud[1,2*], Hilde L. Orrem[1], Knut Dybwik[3], Søren E. Pischke[1], Andreas Baratt-Due[1], Albert Castellheim[4], Hilde Fure[5], Grethe Bergseth[5], Dorte Christiansen[5], Miles A. Nunn[6], Terje Espevik[7], Corinna Lau[5], Petter Brandtzæg[2,8], Erik W. Nielsen[3,9] and Tom E. Mollnes[1,5,7,9]

Abstract

Background: Fulminant meningococcal sepsis, characterized by overwhelming innate immune activation, mostly affects young people and causes high mortality. This study aimed to investigate the effect of targeting two key molecules of innate immunity, complement component C5, and co-receptor CD14 in the Toll-like receptor system, on the inflammatory response in meningococcal sepsis.

Methods: Meningococcal sepsis was simulated by continuous intravenous infusion of an escalating dose of heat-inactivated *Neisseria meningitidis* administered over 3 h. The piglets were randomized, blinded to the investigators, to a positive control group ($n = 12$) receiving saline and to an interventional group ($n = 12$) receiving a recombinant anti-CD14 monoclonal antibody together with the C5 inhibitor coversin.

Results: A substantial increase in plasma complement activation in the untreated group was completely abolished in the treatment group ($p = 0.006$). The following inflammatory mediators were substantially reduced in plasma in the treatment group: Interferon-γ by 75% ($p = 0.0001$), tumor necrosis factor by 50% ($p = 0.01$), Interleukin (IL)-8 by 50% ($p = 0.03$), IL-10 by 40% ($p = 0.04$), IL-12p40 by 50% ($p = 0.03$), and granulocyte CD11b (CR3) expression by 20% ($p = 0.01$).

Conclusion: Inhibition of C5 and CD14 may be beneficial in attenuating the detrimental effects of complement activation and modulating the cytokine storm in patients with fulminant meningococcal sepsis.

Keywords: Endotoxin, Chemokines, Complement, Cytokines, Immune response, *Neisseria meningitidis*, Septic shock, Toll-like receptor

Background

Fulminant meningococcal sepsis is a rapid and devastating infection caused by *Neisseria meningitidis*, characterized by whole-body inflammation and severe disturbances in homeostasis leading to high mortality despite optimal antimicrobial and intensive care treatment [1–3]. Within 12–24 h after onset of the first symptoms, the number of meningococci in the circulation may reach levels as high as 10^8/mL in the plasma [3]. A massive and complex inflammatory response is triggered, which in turn is harmful to the body and leads to multi-organ failure [1–3]. Treatment-resistant septic shock caused by profound vasodilation and declining cardiac function is the principal cause of death [1–3]. Activation of TLR4-MD2 by lipopolysaccharide (LPS) is considered the most important inflammatory mechanism in meningococcal sepsis [4, 5]. However, different clinical trials aiming to reduce the inflammatory response caused by LPS have failed to

* Correspondence: bernt.christian@hellerud.com
[1]Department of Immunology, Oslo University Hospital Rikshospitalet, and K.G. Jebsen IRC, University of Oslo, N-0027 Oslo, Norway
[2]Department of Pediatrics, Oslo University Hospital Ullevål and University of Oslo, Oslo, Norway
Full list of author information is available at the end of the article

improve the outcome in patients with severe sepsis. This includes studies attempting to neutralize LPS or attenuate the response to LPS by blocking different steps of the inflammatory mechanisms, including binding of LPS to TLR4-MD2 or blocking the effect of individual inflammatory mediators like IL-1β and tumor necrosis factor (TNF) [6–9].

Molecular structures of meningococci other than LPS activate different parts of the innate immune system, including the complement system and additional TLRs beside TLR4-MD2 [10]. CD14 serves as a cofactor for several of the TLRs, including TLR4 and TLR2 [11, 12]. Complement is a plasma cascade system with diverse inflammatory effects, driven mainly by activation products which react with leukocyte surface receptors [13, 14]. It can be activated through three initial routes, namely the classical, lectin, and alternative pathway. Activation of all three initial pathways merges and leads to activation of the common complement factors C3 and C5. Further, activation of C5 leads to formation of C5a and the terminal C5b-9 complex (TCC) [15]. C5a is a potent anaphylatoxin with diverse inflammatory effects including stimulation of cytokine production, upregulation of adhesion molecules, paralysis of neutrophils, and increased vascular permeability [16]. TCC incorporates into bacterial lipid membranes as the membrane attack complex and may cause lysis of pathogens, in particular *Neisseria* species. TCC may also be formed in the fluid phase as a soluble form (sC5b-9) and then serves as a valuable marker of complement activation.

We have hypothesized that a combined inhibition of complement and CD14 will efficiently attenuate the inflammatory response in various clinical situations including sepsis [17]. Previously, we demonstrated that upstream inhibition of the inflammatory response by combined blocking of CD14 and complement strongly attenuates a wide range of inflammatory responses induced by meningococci in an ex vivo whole blood model [10]. A reinforced inhibitory effect on a broad spectrum of inflammatory mediators by the combined inhibition has recently also been proven in porcine *E. coli* induced sepsis [18] and mouse and pig polymicrobial sepsis where survival was also increased [19, 20].

The aim of the present study was to investigate the effect of blocking both C5 and CD14 on the inflammatory response induced in vivo in a porcine model of meningococcal sepsis. The model has been developed by our group as the first large animal model simulating meningococcal sepsis and has been proven to be a valuable tool to study inflammatory mechanisms of the disease and potential interventions [5, 21, 22].

Methods

Interventional drugs

For inhibition of porcine CD14, a recombinant variant of a well-established anti-porcine CD14 mouse monoclonal IgG2b antibody (Mil2) was used. This novel anti-porcine CD14 antibody (rMIL2) was recently constructed by our group as a mouse-human chimeric, IgG2/IgG4 hybrid antibody keeping the antigen binding site the same as for Mil2 [23]. Thus, rMIL2 exerts comparable ex vivo and in vivo CD14 binding and inhibition efficacies as the original murine clone, demonstrated by competitive binding tests and cytokine release assays. The original Mil2 clone was used in our initial intervention studies of porcine sepsis [18, 24–26]. The inflammatory response was successfully inhibited, but this clone was hampered by undesired effect or functions mediated by the IgG2b Fc part of Mil2 and consequently induced an anaphylactoid-like reaction. In contrast, the IgG2/4 rMIL2 was completely inert with respect to such functions [22] and successfully used in a subsequent study [20] and in the present one. Endotoxin-free recombinant OmCI (coversin), a 16.8-kDa protein, was provided by Akari Therapeutics Plc (London, UK) [27].

Bacteria

The international reference strain *N. meningitidis* 44/76 (H44/76) was obtained from the National Institute of Public Health, Oslo, Norway. It is characterized as B:15:P1.7,16:L3,7,9 and was originally isolated from a female patient with lethal meningococcal septic shock [28]. Meningococci were grown overnight on Columbia agar and resuspended in sterile PBS. For safety reasons, bacteria were heat inactivated at 57 °C for 30 min, and then frozen at −70 °C until used.

Animals and experimental groups

Piglets (*Sus scrofa domesticus*, outbred stock) of either sex, weighing 6 kg (range 5.5–6.5 kg) were used. All piglets were clinically healthy and thus none were excluded from the study. The piglets were randomized into two groups, each consisting of 12 animals: an intervention and a positive control group. In addition, two sham control piglets that received saline instead of bacteria were included as reference. The groups were blinded for the investigators. The number of piglets in each group was decided according to previous analysis and experience showing that at least 10 animals in each group were needed to demonstrate differences [5, 18].

Anesthesia and surgery

The piglets were pre-medicated with 2–3 mg intranasal midazolam at the animal housing facility before transport to laboratory. At the laboratory, venous access was established in one of the ears and thereafter 10–15 mg/kg ketamine was given intravenously (i.v.) before oral intubation using a 4.9-mm inner diameter tube with cuff. After intubation, an i.v. infusion of propofol (10 mg/kg/h) and fentanyl (50 µg/kg/h) was started and mechanical ventilation was established. A 5 F pulmonary artery catheter (Baxter Edwards Laboratories, Irvine, CA) was inserted via the left external jugular vein and guided into a distal pulmonary artery by pressure wave-form analysis. A cannula was inserted in the left carotid artery for continuous recording of arterial pressure and intermittent blood sampling. A urinary catheter was inserted into the urinary bladder via a cystotomy. After the completion of surgery and insertion of catheters, the animals were placed on their right side, remaining in this position for the rest of the experiment.

Experimental design

After induction of anesthesia and surgery, the intervention group received first a bolus of coversin (1 mg/kg) and thereafter a bolus of rMIL2 (5 mg/kg), administered about 10 min before induction of sepsis. Excess coversin from the bolus not bound to C5 is rapidly removed from circulation [27]. Therefore, to bind C5 synthesized by piglets during the experiment, coversin was infused at 0.2 mg/h throughout the experimental course. Sepsis was induced by i.v. infusion of increasing numbers of *N. meningitidis*. Septic shock was obtained according to the Third International Consensus Definitions for Sepsis and Septic shock, as vasopressors were needed to keep the blood pressure above 65 mmHg [29]. Due to the influence of vasopressors, cardiovascular parameters could not be included as scientific readouts. There was no difference between the positive control group and the intervention group regarding the amount of vasopressors needed to keep the blood pressure above 65 mmHg.

To limit the need for inhibitors, the size of the pigs used in the present study was reduced from about 30-kg to about 6-kg piglets compared to previously published studies employing the porcine model of meningococcal sepsis [5, 21]. However, we found that in these piglets a state of fulminant sepsis was reached within a shorter time than in the larger animals. Thus, the observational period was shortened from 4 h in the previous studies to 3 h in the present study.

Each piglet received a total of 8.4×10^9 bacteria/kg. The positive control group received the same volume of saline as the intervention group. The sham animals also received the same volume of saline. Blood samples were drawn before i.v. infusion of intervention agents (Tbasis), before start of bacterial infusion (T0), and 60, 120, and 180 min after induction of sepsis (T60, T120, and T180). All animals received the same background infusion of Ringer's acetate, i.e., 10 mL/kg/h during surgery and until 60 min after induction of sepsis, and

thereafter 20 mL/kg/h to 120 min and 30 mL/kg/h to 180 min after induction of sepsis. In addition, 10% glucose was given i.v. at 5 mL/kg/h throughout the experimental course to avoid hypoglycemia. Inotrop and vasopressor therapy were given when needed as a therapy for severe and lethal hypotension.

Functional complement activity

A commercially available enzyme immune assay (Complement system Screen WIESLAB®; Euro Diagnostica, Malmö, Sweden) was used to test functional activity of the classical complement pathway. The kit detects human complement activity, but has been shown to cross-react efficiently with pig [30]. Samples were analyzed in serum, prepared after 1-h clotting, centrifuged, and immediately aliquoted and stored at −70 °C.

Complement activation

Soluble TCC (sC5b-9) was measured using multiplex xMAP technology (Bio-Plex® Multiplex System, Bio-Rad Laboratories, Inc. Hercules, CA) as previously described [18, 31]. Samples were analyzed in EDTA-plasma prepared immediately after blood sampling. Whole blood was placed on crushed ice, centrifuged within 30 min at 1500 g at 4 °C for 20 min, immediately aliquoted, and stored at −70 °C.

Cytokines

The cytokines TNF, IL-1β, IL-4, IL-6, IL-8, IL-10, and IL-12p40 and Interferons (INF)-α and INF-γ were analyzed in EDTA-plasma obtained as described for soluble TCC above, using multiplex technology (ProcartaPlex, eBioscience, Bender MedSystems GMbH, Vienna, Austria).

Leukocyte activation

Leukocyte activation was measured by flow cytometry. In pig whole blood, neutrophils are clearly discriminated from mononuclear cells, but lymphocytes and monocytes cannot be separated by forward/side scatter dot plots. For measurement of wCD11R3 on neutrophils (the pig ortholog to human CD11b), blood was collected at Tbasis and T180, anticoagulated with EDTA, and stained with mouse anti-porcine wCD11R3 FITC clone 2 F4/11 or the isotype-matched mouse IgG1-FITC negative control Ab (AbD Serotec, Oxford, UK). The samples were incubated for 15 min in the dark, and red cells were lysed with 0.16 M NH₄Cl/10 mM NaHCO₃-/0.12 mM EDTA (Tritiplex III) for 8–10 min in the dark at ambient temperature. Samples were centrifuged at 300 g for 5 min at 4 °C, and the cells were washed with PBS, 0.1% BSA (Biotest, Dreieich, Germany). The samples were then resuspended in PBS, 0.1% BSA before flow cytometry (FACSCalibur; Becton Dickinson, Franklin

Lakes, NJ). Values are given in mean fluorescence intensity (MFI).

Data presentation and statistical analysis

Statistical analyses were performed with GraphPad Prism version 6 (GraphPad Software, San Diego, CA). The positive control group was compared with the treatment group using two-way ANOVA. Area under the curve (AUC) was used as a single measure of the total difference between groups in the amount of each cytokine secreted.

The difference in wCD11R3 upregulation on granulocytes in the intervention group and the positive control group was measured at only one time-point (T180) in addition to baseline and was analyzed by Student's t test. For all statistical analyses, $p < 0.05$ was considered statistically significant. Two sham animals were included as references.

Results

Complement activation

TCC was used as a measure of complement activation at the different time points during the experiment. In the positive control group, TCC increased from mean 273 (±87; 95% CI) complement arbitrary units (CAU)/L at T0 to mean 1233 (±871) CAU/L at T180 ($p = 0.01$) (Fig. 1, upper panel), confirming systemic activation of complement. No increase of TCC was seen in the treatment group. Complete inhibition of complement activity in the treatment group after administration of coversin was further confirmed at T60 by the classical pathway WIESLAB® assay, which detects the total complement activity of the classical and terminal pathway (Fig. 1, lower panel).

Cyotokines

IFN-γ: In the positive control group, IFN-γ increased from <lower detection limit (LDL) at T0 to mean 16 (±7.5) pg/mL at T120 and 14 (±6.4) pg/mL at T180 (Fig. 2). In the treatment group, IFN-γ increased from <LDL at T0 to mean 2 (±2.3) pg/mL at T120 and 8 (±5.3) pg/mL at T180. The difference between the groups was statistically significant ($p = 0.0001$), and the area under the curve (AUC) was 75% lower in the treatment group than in the positive control group. No increase was seen in sham animals.

TNF: In the positive control group, TNF increased from <LDL at T0 to mean 44 (±15.1) ng/mL at T120 (Fig. 2). Thereafter, the level declined to mean 13 (±4) ng/mL at T180. In the treatment group, TNF increased from <LDL to a plateau of mean 17 (±6.4 and ±10) ng/mL at T120 and T180. The difference between the groups was

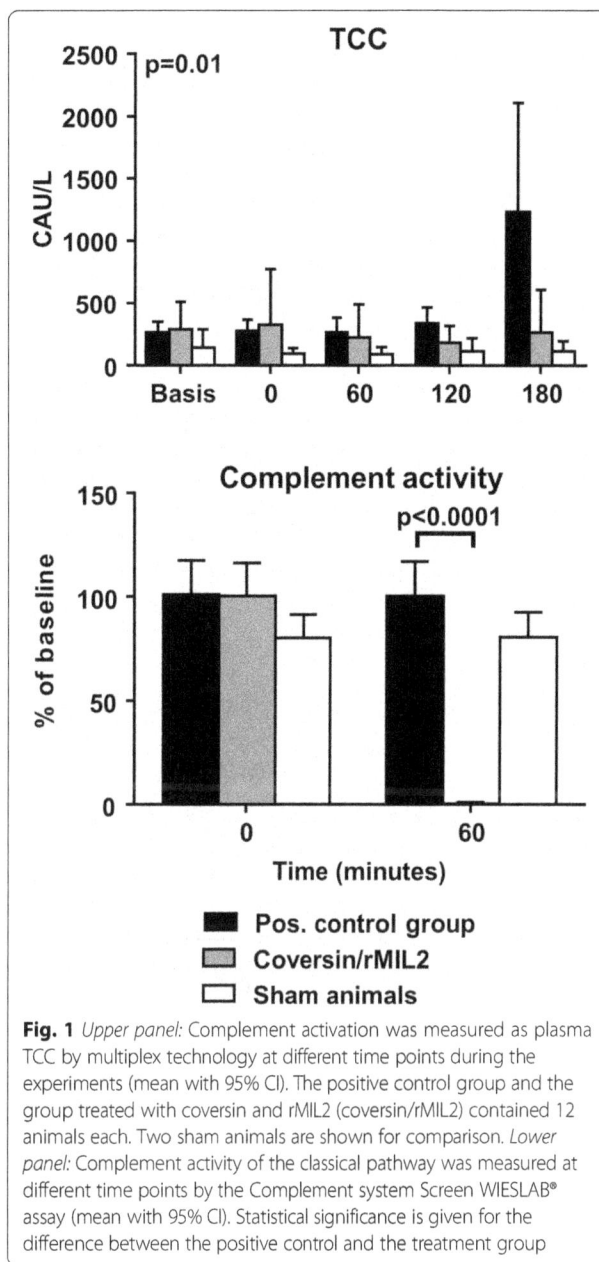

Fig. 1 *Upper panel:* Complement activation was measured as plasma TCC by multiplex technology at different time points during the experiments (mean with 95% CI). The positive control group and the group treated with coversin and rMIL2 (coversin/rMIL2) contained 12 animals each. Two sham animals are shown for comparison. *Lower panel:* Complement activity of the classical pathway was measured at different time points by the Complement system Screen WIESLAB® assay (mean with 95% CI). Statistical significance is given for the difference between the positive control and the treatment group

statistically significant ($p = 0.01$), and the AUC was 50% lower in the treatment group than in the positive control group. No increase was seen in sham animals.

IL-1β: In the positive control group, IL-1β increased from <LDL at T0 to mean 0.1 (±0.05) ng/mL at T120 and 0.9 (±0.5) ng/mL at T180 (Fig. 2). In the treatment group, IL-1β increased from <LDL at T0 to mean 0.08 (±0.01) ng/mL at T120 and 0.6 (±0.3) ng/mL at T240. The AUC was 30% lower in the treatment group than in the positive control group but the difference between the groups was not significant ($p = 0.2$). No increase was seen in sham animals.

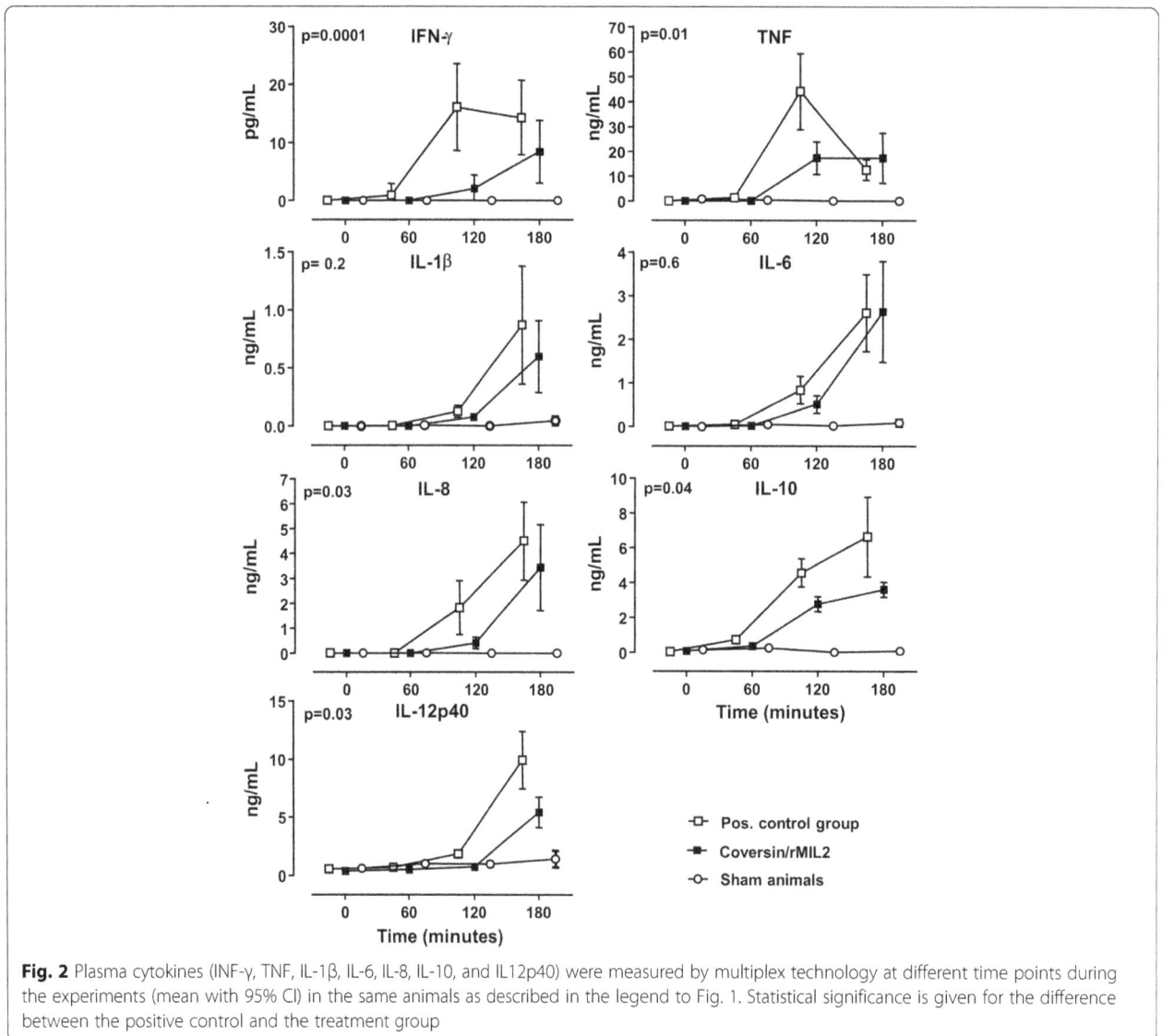

Fig. 2 Plasma cytokines (INF-γ, TNF, IL-1β, IL-6, IL-8, IL-10, and IL12p40) were measured by multiplex technology at different time points during the experiments (mean with 95% CI) in the same animals as described in the legend to Fig. 1. Statistical significance is given for the difference between the positive control and the treatment group

IL-6: In the positive control group, IL-6 increased from <LDL at T0 to mean 0.8 (±0.3) ng/mL at T120 and 2.6 (±0.9) ng/mL at T180 (Fig. 2). In the treatment group, IL-6 increased from <LDL at T0 to mean 0.5 (±0.2) ng/mL at T120 and 2.6 (±1.1) ng/mL at T180. The AUC was 15% lower in the treatment group than in the positive control group, but the difference between the groups was not significant ($p = 0.6$). No increase was seen in sham animals.

IL-8: In the positive control group, IL-8 increased from <LDL at T0 to mean 1.8 (±1) ng/mL at T120 and 4.5 (±1.6) ng/mL at T180 (Fig. 2). In the treatment group, IL-8 increased from <LDL at T0 to 0.4 (±0.2) ng/mL at T120 and 3.4 (±1.7) ng/mL at T180. The difference between the groups was statistically significant ($p = 0.03$), and the AUC was 50% lower in the treatment group

than the positive control group. No increase was seen in sham animals. One animal of the treatment group showed excessively increased IL-8 level at T180 right before it died (83 ng/mL). This value was 33 SD higher than the mean value of the rest of the treatment group. Thus, it was regarded as an outlier and excluded from statistical analysis.

IL-10: In the positive control group, IL-10 increased from mean 0.05 (±0.01) ng/mL at T0 to 4.6 (±0.8) ng/mL at T120 and 6.6 (±2.3) ng/mL at T180 (Fig. 2). In the treatment group, IL-10 increased from mean 0.1 (±0.01) to 2.8 (±0.4) ng/mL at T120 and 3.6 (±0.4) ng/mL at T180. The difference between the groups was statistically significant ($p = 0.04$), and the AUC was 40% lower in the treatment group than the positive control group. No increase was seen in sham animals.

IL-12p40: In the positive control group, IL-12p40 increased from mean 0.5 (±0.01) ng/mL at T0 to 1.8 (±0.3) ng/mL at T120 and 10.0 (±2.5) ng/mL at T180 (Fig. 2). In the treatment group, IL-12p40 increased from mean 0.4 (±0.01) ng/mL at T0 to 0.7 (±0.1) ng/mL at T120 and 5.4 (±1.2) ng/mL at T180. The difference between the group was statistically significant ($p = 0.03$), and the AUC was 50% lower in the treatment group than the positive control group. No increase was seen in sham animals.

IFN-α and IL-4 were not increased in any of the groups (data not shown).

Granulocyte activation

wCD11R3: In the positive control group, wCD11R3 increased from mean MFI 51 (±9) at T0 to MFI 700 (±150) at T180, whereas in the treatment group wCD11R3 increased from mean MFI 46 (±14) at T0 to MFI 568 (±68) at T180 (Fig. 3). The difference between the two groups was significant ($p = 0.01$).

Discussion

Fulminant meningococcal sepsis is associated with a massive, rapid, and harmful inflammatory activation that is rarely seen in other conditions. CD14-mediated activation of the Toll-like receptor system and activation of complement are the two best characterized parts of the innate immune system participating in this inflammatory response. Previously, we have performed extensive studies

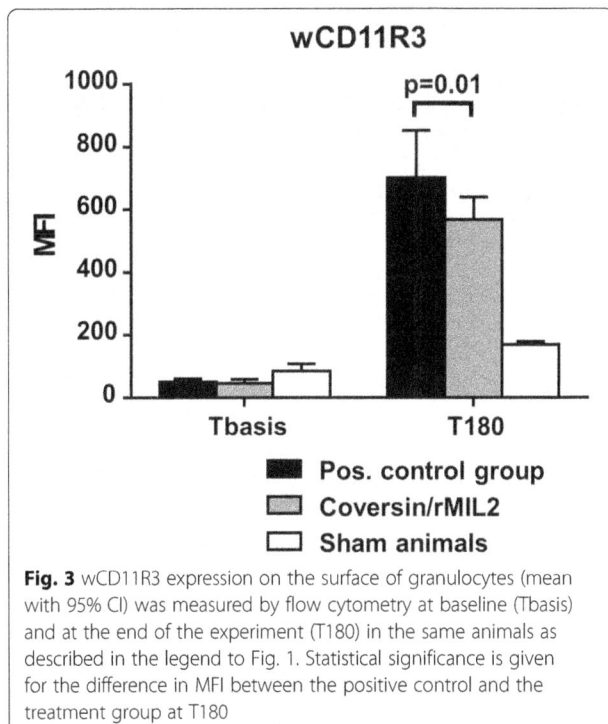

Fig. 3 wCD11R3 expression on the surface of granulocytes (mean with 95% CI) was measured by flow cytometry at baseline (Tbasis) and at the end of the experiment (T180) in the same animals as described in the legend to Fig. 1. Statistical significance is given for the difference in MFI between the positive control and the treatment group at T180

on the effect of blocking CD14 and complement individually and together in both in vitro and in vivo inflammatory models [10, 18, 32]. The results from these studies have clearly demonstrated attenuation of the inflammatory response when these two parts of the innate immune system are blocked together, compared to separate blocking. Thus, based on the previous studies, and not least in order to limit the total number of animals used, this study was designed to investigate only the effect of combined CD14 and complement inhibition in meningococcal sepsis. This combined blocking of C5 and CD14 significantly and efficiently attenuated the inflammatory response induced by *N. meningitidis* in vivo.

Sustained high-grade activation of complement continuing until death despite optimal antibiotic and conventional supportive treatment is a characteristic for non-surviving patients with fulminant meningococcal sepsis [33]. Persistent high levels of complement-derived inflammatory molecules may contribute to the development of the systemic inflammatory response syndrome (SIRS). The potent anaphylatoxin C5a is considered the most important of these mediators, and thus blocking complement at the level of C5 is an interesting approach in fulminant meningococcal sepsis. Abolished delivery of C5a will attenuate the inflammatory response, while simultaneous administration of antibiotic treatment ensures killing of meningococci despite the lack of C5b-9 lysis. Also, activation of complement C3 is maintained when C5 is blocked, leaving C3-mediated opsonophagocytosis active for clearance of bacteria.

In the present study, we reproduced the systemic complement activation seen in patients with fulminant meningococcal sepsis. For the first time, it is demonstrated that this complement activation can be efficiently abolished by a C5 inhibitor in vivo, suggesting that such treatment can have a potential role as adjuvant treatment in patients with fulminant meningococcal sepsis.

Combined treatment with C5 and CD14 inhibition was applied to tackle two important inflammatory mechanisms at the earliest possible stage during immune recognition of meningococci. The goal of inhibiting the innate immune response in cases of fulminant meningococcal sepsis should be to interfere with the initial pro-inflammatory signals. This is to avoid further escalation of the cytokine response and prevent development of "point of no return." Then it is impossible to reverse the highly disturbed pathophysiology of this condition. Presently, the most effective method to downregulate plasma cytokine level in patients with fulminant meningococcal sepsis is appropriate antibiotic treatment. The bacterial load as determined by number of *N. meningitidis* DNA molecules per milliliter plasma is reduced by 50% within 3 to 4 h after initiation of antibiotic treatment [34]. In parallel, key inflammatory cytokines and chemokines are reduced by 50% in plasma within 1 to 3 h [35, 36]. Even though the present study simulated a situation without antibiotics and escalating number of meningococci, the combined blocking of C5 and CD14 alone obtained a substantial attenuation of the release of several key cytokines, i.e., INF-γ, TNF, IL-8, IL-10, and IL-12p40. Our present experiments suggest that combined C5 and CD14 inhibition might reduce the cytokine production in patients and add to the effect of antibiotics per se.

The inhibitory effects on TNF and IL-10 by the combined treatment are of particular interest. TNF was efficiently but transiently inhibited in the initial phase, in a way that abolished the high peek in TNF concentration otherwise seen in the positive control group as well as in previous studies [18, 21]. TNF is a strong inductor of the acute phase response in SIRS and is the most extensively studied cytokine in sepsis [37]. High levels of TNF in the initial phase of sepsis have been associated with early hemodynamic deterioration [37, 38]. Thus, attenuated increase of TNF in the initial phase of sepsis development may be particularly beneficial. There is evidence that with progression of sepsis anti-inflammatory mechanisms become increasingly important [37, 39, 40]. IL-10 is the most potent anti-inflammatory cytokine, being substantially increased in meningococcal sepsis [41–43]. Sustained high levels of IL-10, and in particular sustained high IL-10/TNF ratio have been demonstrated to be associated with high mortality in meningococcal sepsis as well as in other infectious diseases [39, 44, 45]. IL-10 is responsible for extensive changes in the function of monocytes in meningococcal sepsis [43, 46]. Based on these observations, we assume that it may be beneficial to decrease the level of IL-10 in meningococcal sepsis, like we obtained with the combined treatment in this study. Furthermore, we suggest that the balance between TNF and IL-10 may be altered in a favorable way in the initial as well as later stages of sepsis development by the combined treatment. This may be in contrast to isolated inhibition of pro-inflammatory cytokines like TNF and IL-1β, which has been tried without success [40]. Given the substantial amounts of cytokines released "downstream" of the innate immune recognition phase, it is perhaps not surprising that inhibition of only one of these does not have an effect on the clinical course of the fulminant form of the disease. Thus, "upstream" inhibition of bottle-neck molecules of the main pattern recognition systems, like complement and CD14/TLRs, is a rational approach for broad-acting attenuation of the inflammatory response induced by meningococci.

Further, we suggest that the efficient inhibition of the chemokine IL-8 that we obtained initially in this study can be beneficial with respect to the prognosis. High levels of IL-8 have been described to predict fatal sepsis [47–50]. IL-8 attracts leukocytes to the site of inflammation, and high levels of IL-8 are likely to contribute to the profound leukopenia characteristic of severe meningococcal sepsis.

The significantly reduced expression of granulocyte wCD11R3 (the porcine ortholog to human CD11b) in the treatment group implies that combined treatment influenced white blood cell function not only by decreasing cytokine release but also by decreasing expression of surface molecules. In complex with CD18, wCD11R3 constitutes complement receptor 3 (CR3), which is active in phagocytosis of bacteria. Phagocytosis per se is obviously beneficial in meningococcal disease in order to clear bacteria from the circulation. However, it does not need to be as efficient in the presence of antibiotics, and a limited decrease of phagocytosis may possibly be beneficial due to less induced oxidative burst, which otherwise may be harmful to surrounding tissue [32].

Conclusions
We suggest that the course of meningococcal sepsis observed in piglets in the present study represents a realistic model of the situation in patients with fulminant meningococcal sepsis. We demonstrate that efficient complement inhibition can be obtained in this model. Furthermore, we find that combined inhibition of the two key innate immune systems, complement with the central component C5 and the TLRs with the co-receptor CD14, can modulate the inflammatory response in fulminant meningococcal sepsis, provided the C5 and CD14 inhibition is initiated early. Modulation of this inflammatory response may be of potential benefit in patients with meningococcal sepsis.

Acknowledgements
We thank Ernst Arne Høiby and Berit Nyland at the National Institute of Public health, Oslo, Norway, for providing the inactivated meningococci.

Funding
This work was supported to T.E.M. by The Research Council of Norway, The Odd Fellow Foundation, The Simon Fougner Hartmann Family Fund, and the European Community's Seventh Framework Programme under grant agreement no. 602699 (DIREKT).

Authors' contributions
BCH, HLO, SP, ABD, AC, TE, EWN, PB, and TEM designed the research. BCH, HLO, KD, SP, ABD, and EWN performed the research. HF, GB, and DC performed the laboratory analysis. MAN supplied the coversin. CL made the mouse-human chimeric anti-porcine CD14 IgG2/4 antibody. BCH and TEM analyzed the data. BCH wrote the paper, and all authors contributed to revising the paper. All authors read and approved the final manuscript.

Competing interests
The authors declare that they have no competing interests.

Author details
[1]Department of Immunology, Oslo University Hospital Rikshospitalet, and K.G. Jebsen IRC, University of Oslo, N-0027 Oslo, Norway. [2]Department of Pediatrics, Oslo University Hospital Ullevål and University of Oslo, Oslo, Norway. [3]Department of Anesthesiology, Nordland Hospital and Nord University, Bodø, Norway. [4]Department of Anesthesiology and Intensive Care Unit, Institution of Clinical Science, Sahlgrenska Academy, University of Gothenburg, Gothenburg, Sweden. [5]Research Laboratory, Nordland Hospital, Bodø, Norway. [6]Akari Therapeutics Plc, London, UK. [7]Centre of Molecular Inflammation Research and Department of Cancer Research and Molecular Medicine, Norwegian University of Science and Technology, Trondheim, Norway. [8]Institute of Clinical Medicine, Faculty of Medicine, University of Oslo, Oslo, Norway. [9]Faculty of Health Sciences, K.G. Jebsen TREC, University of Tromsø, Tromsø, Norway.

References
1. Stephens DS, Greenwood B, Brandtzaeg P. Epidemic meningitis, meningococcaemia, and Neisseria meningitidis. Lancet. 2007;369:2196–210.
2. van Deuren M, Brandtzaeg P, van der Meer JW. Update on meningococcal disease with emphasis on pathogenesis and clinical management. Clin Microbiol Rev. 2000;13:144–66.
3. Brandtzaeg P, van Deuren M. Classification and pathogenesis of meningococcal infections. Methods Mol Biol. 2012;799:21–35.
4. Sprong T, Stikkelbroeck N, van der Ley P, Steeghs L, van Alphen L, Klein N, Netea MG, van der Meer JW, van Deuren M. Contributions of Neisseria meningitidis LPS and non-LPS to proinflammatory cytokine response. J Leukoc Biol. 2001;70:283–8.
5. Hellerud BC, Nielsen EW, Thorgersen EB, Lindstad JK, Pharo A, Tonnessen TI, Castellheim A, Mollnes TE, Brandtzaeg P. Dissecting the effects of lipopolysaccharides from nonlipopolysaccharide molecules in experimental porcine meningococcal sepsis. Crit Care Med. 2010;38:1467–74.
6. Iskander KN, Osuchowski MF, Stearns-Kurosawa DJ, Kurosawa S, Stepien D, Valentine C, Remick DG. Sepsis: multiple abnormalities, heterogeneous responses, and evolving understanding. Physiol Rev. 2013;93:1247–88.
7. J5studyGroup. Treatment of severe infectious purpura in children with human plasma from donors immunized with Escherichia coli J5: a prospective double-blind study. J Infect Dis. 1992;165:695–701.
8. Hillmen P, Muus P, Roth A, Elebute MO, Risitano AM, Schrezenmeier H, Szer J, Browne P, Maciejewski JP, Schubert J, et al. Long-term safety and efficacy of sustained eculizumab treatment in patients with paroxysmal nocturnal haemoglobinuria. Br J Haematol. 2013;162:62–73.
9. Opal SM, Laterre PF, Francois B, LaRosa SP, Angus DC, Mira JP, Wittebole X, Dugernier T, Perrotin D, Tidswell M, et al. Effect of eritoran, an antagonist of MD2-TLR4, on mortality in patients with severe sepsis: the ACCESS randomized trial. JAMA. 2013;309:1154–62.
10. Hellerud BC, Stenvik J, Espevik T, Lambris JD, Mollnes TE, Brandtzaeg P. Stages of meningococcal sepsis simulated in vitro, with emphasis on complement and Toll-like receptor activation. Infect Immun. 2008;76:4183–9.
11. Lee CC, Avalos AM, Ploegh HL. Accessory molecules for Toll-like receptors and their function. Nat Rev Immunol. 2012;12:168–79.
12. Zanoni I, Granucci F. Role of CD14 in host protection against infections and in metabolism regulation. Front Cell Infect Microbiol. 2013;3:32.
13. Ehrnthaller C, Ignatius A, Gebhard F, Huber-Lang M. New insights of an old defense system: structure, function, and clinical relevance of the complement system. Mol Med. 2011;17:317–29.
14. Kolev M, Le Friec G, Kemper C. Complement—tapping into new sites and effector systems. Nat Rev Immunol. 2014;14:811–20.
15. Muller-Eberhard HJ. Molecular organization and function of the complement system. Annu Rev Biochem. 1988;57:321–47.
16. Ward PA. Role of C5 activation products in sepsis. ScientificWorldJournal. 2010;10:2395–402.
17. Mollnes TE, Christiansen D, Brekke OL, Espevik T. Hypothesis: combined inhibition of complement and CD14 as treatment regimen to attenuate the inflammatory response. Adv Exp Med Biol. 2008;632:253–63.
18. Barratt-Due A, Thorgersen EB, Egge K, Pischke S, Sokolov A, Hellerud BC, Lindstad JK, Pharo A, Bongoni AK, Rieben R, et al. Combined inhibition of complement C5 and CD14 markedly attenuates inflammation, thrombogenicity, and hemodynamic changes in porcine sepsis. J Immunol. 2013;191:819–27.
19. Huber-Lang M, Barratt-Due A, Pischke SE, Sandanger O, Nilsson PH, Nunn MA, Denk S, Gaus W, Espevik T, Mollnes TE. Double blockade of CD14 and complement C5 abolishes the cytokine storm and improves morbidity and survival in polymicrobial sepsis in mice. J Immunol. 2014;192:5324–31.
20. Skjeflo EW, Sagatun C, Dybwik K, Aam S, Urving SH, Nunn MA, Fure H, Lau C, Brekke OL, Huber-Lang M, et al. Combined inhibition of complement and CD14 improved outcome in porcine polymicrobial sepsis. Crit Care. 2015;19:415.
21. Nielsen EW, Hellerud BC, Thorgersen EB, Castellheim A, Pharo A, Lindstad J, Tonnessen TI, Brandtzaeg P, Mollnes TE. A new dynamic porcine model of meningococcal shock. Shock. 2009;32:302–9.
22. Barratt-Due A, Johansen HT, Sokolov A, Thorgersen EB, Hellerud BC, Reubsaet JL, Seip KF, Tonnessen TI, Lindstad JK, Pharo A, et al. The role of bradykinin and the effect of the bradykinin receptor antagonist icatibant in porcine sepsis. Shock. 2011;36:517–23.
23. Lau C, Gunnarsen KS, Hoydahl LS, Andersen JT, Berntzen G, Pharo A, Lindstad JK, Ludviksen JK, Brekke OL, Barratt-Due A, et al. Chimeric anti-CD14 IGG2/4 Hybrid antibodies for therapeutic intervention in pig and human models of inflammation. J Immunol. 2013;191:4769–77.
24. Thorgersen EB, Hellerud BC, Nielsen EW, Barratt-Due A, Fure H, Lindstad JK, Pharo A, Fosse E, Tonnessen TI, Johansen HT, et al. CD14 inhibition efficiently attenuates early inflammatory and hemostatic responses in Escherichia coli sepsis in pigs. FASEB J. 2010;24:712–22.
25. Thorgersen EB, Pischke SE, Barratt-Due A, Fure H, Lindstad JK, Pharo A, Hellerud BC, Mollnes TE. Systemic CD14 inhibition attenuates organ inflammation in porcine Escherichia coli sepsis. Infect Immun. 2013;81:3173–81.
26. Egge KH, Thorgersen EB, Pischke SE, Lindstad JK, Pharo A, Bongoni AK, Rieben R, Nunn MA, Barratt-Due A, Mollnes TE. Organ inflammation in porcine Escherichia coli sepsis is markedly attenuated by combined inhibition of C5 and CD14. Immunobiology. 2015;220:999–1005.
27. Hepburn NJ, Williams AS, Nunn MA, Chamberlain-Banoub JC, Hamer J, Morgan BP, Harris CL. In vivo characterization and therapeutic efficacy of a C5-specific inhibitor from the soft tick Ornithodoros moubata. J Biol Chem. 2007;282:8292–9.
28. Holten E. Serotypes of Neisseria meningitidis isolated from patients in Norway during the first six months of 1978. J Clin Microbiol. 1979;9:186–8.
29. Singer M, Deutschman CS, Seymour CW, Shankar-Hari M, Annane D, Bauer M, Bellomo R, Bernard GR, Chiche JD, Coopersmith CM, et al. The third international consensus definitions for sepsis and septic shock (sepsis-3). JAMA. 2016;315:801–10.
30. Salvesen B, Mollnes TE. Pathway-specific complement activity in pigs evaluated with a human functional complement assay. Mol Immunol. 2009;46:1620–5.
31. Bongoni AK, Lanz J, Rieben R, Banz Y. Development of a bead-based multiplex assay for the simultaneous detection of porcine inflammation markers using xMAP technology. Cytometry A. 2013;83:636–47.
32. Lappegard KT, Christiansen D, Pharo A, Thorgersen EB, Hellerud BC, Lindstad J, Nielsen EW, Bergseth G, Fadnes D, Abrahamsen TG, et al. Human genetic deficiencies reveal the roles of complement in the inflammatory network: lessons from nature. Proc Natl Acad Sci U S A. 2009;106:15861–6.
33. Brandtzaeg P, Mollnes TE, Kierulf P. Complement activation and endotoxin levels in systemic meningococcal disease. J Infect Dis. 1989;160:58–65.
34. Ovstebo R, Brandtzaeg P, Brusletto B, Haug KB, Lande K, Hoiby EA, Kierulf P. Use of robotized DNA isolation and real-time PCR to quantify and identify close correlation between levels of Neisseria meningitidis DNA and lipopolysaccharides in plasma and cerebrospinal fluid from patients with systemic meningococcal disease. J Clin Microbiol. 2004;42:2980–7.
35. Waage A, Brandtzaeg P, Halstensen A, Kierulf P, Espevik T. The complex pattern of cytokines in serum from patients with meningococcal septic shock. Association between interleukin 6, interleukin 1, and fatal outcome. J Exp Med. 1989;169:333–8.
36. Moller AS, Bjerre A, Brusletto B, Joo GB, Brandtzaeg P, Kierulf P. Chemokine patterns in meningococcal disease. J Infect Dis. 2005;191:768–75.

37. Chaudhry H, Zhou J, Zhong Y, Ali MM, McGuire F, Nagarkatti PS, Nagarkatti M. Role of cytokines as a double-edged sword in sepsis. In Vivo. 2013;27:669–84.

38. Waage A, Halstensen A, Espevik T. Association between tumour necrosis factor in serum and fatal outcome in patients with meningococcal disease. Lancet. 1987;1:355–7.

39. Gogos CA, Drosou E, Bassaris HP, Skoutelis A. Pro- versus anti-inflammatory cytokine profile in patients with severe sepsis: a marker for prognosis and future therapeutic options. J Infect Dis. 2000;181:176–80.

40. Schulte W, Bernhagen J, Bucala R. Cytokines in sepsis: potent immunoregulators and potential therapeutic targets—an updated view. Mediators Inflamm. 2013;2013:165974.

41. Riordan FA, Marzouk O, Thomson AP, Sills JA, Hart CA. Proinflammatory and anti-inflammatory cytokines in meningococcal disease. Arch Dis Child. 1996;75:453–4.

42. Bjerre A, Brusletto B, Hoiby EA, Kierulf P, Brandtzaeg P. Plasma interferon-gamma and interleukin-10 concentrations in systemic meningococcal disease compared with severe systemic Gram-positive septic shock. Crit Care Med. 2004;32:433–8.

43. Gopinathan U, Brusletto BS, Olstad OK, Kierulf P, Berg JP, Brandtzaeg P, Ovstebo R. IL-10 immunodepletion from meningococcal sepsis plasma induces extensive changes in gene expression and cytokine release in stimulated human monocytes. Innate Immun. 2015;21:429–49.

44. van Dissel JT, van Langevelde P, Westendorp RG, Kwappenberg K, Frolich M. Anti-inflammatory cytokine profile and mortality in febrile patients. Lancet. 1998;351:950–3.

45. Wu HP, Chen CK, Chung K, Tseng JC, Hua CC, Liu YC, Chuang DY, Yang CH. Serial cytokine levels in patients with severe sepsis. Inflamm Res. 2009;58:385–93.

46. Gopinathan U, Ovstebo R, Olstad OK, Brusletto B, Dalsbotten Aass HC, Kierulf P, Brandtzaeg P, Berg JP. Global effect of interleukin-10 on the transcriptional profile induced by *Neisseria meningitidis* in human monocytes. Infect Immun. 2012;80:4046–54.

47. Mera S, Tatulescu D, Cismaru C, Bondor C, Slavcovici A, Zanc V, Carstina D, Oltean M. Multiplex cytokine profiling in patients with sepsis. APMIS. 2011;119:155–63.

48. Bozza FA, Salluh JI, Japiassu AM, Soares M, Assis EF, Gomes RN, Bozza MT, Castro-Faria-Neto HC, Bozza PT. Cytokine profiles as markers of disease severity in sepsis: a multiplex analysis. Crit Care. 2007;11:R49.

49. Macdonald SP, Stone SF, Neil CL, van Eeden PE, Fatovich DM, Arendts G, Brown SG. Sustained elevation of resistin, NGAL and IL-8 are associated with severe sepsis/septic shock in the emergency department. PLoS One. 2014;9:e110678.

50. Halstensen A, Ceska M, Brandtzaeg P, Redl H, Naess A, Waage A. Interleukin-8 in serum and cerebrospinal fluid from patients with meningococcal disease. J Infect Dis. 1993;167:471–5.

Unexpected intensive care transfer of admitted patients with severe sepsis

Gabriel Wardi[1*], Arvin R. Wali[2], Julian Villar[3], Vaishal Tolia[4,5], Christian Tomaszewski[5], Christian Sloane[5], Peter Fedullo[6], Jeremy R. Beitler[6], Matthew Nolan[5], Daniel Lasoff[5] and Rebecca E. Sell[6]

Abstract

Background: Patients with severe sepsis generally respond well to initial therapy administered in the emergency department (ED), but a subset later decompensate and require unexpected transfer to the intensive care unit (ICU). This study aimed to identify clinical factors that can predict patients at increased risk for delayed transfer to the ICU and the association of delayed ICU transfer with mortality.

Methods: This is a nested case-control study in a prospectively collected registry of patients with severe sepsis and septic shock at two EDs. Cases had severe sepsis and unexpected ICU transfer within 48 h of admission from the ED; controls had severe sepsis but remained in a non-ICU level of care. Univariate and multivariate regression analyses were used to identify predictors of unexpected transfer to the ICU, which was the primary outcome. Differences in mortality between these two groups as well as a cohort of patients directly admitted to the ICU were also calculated.

Results: Of the 914 patients in our registry, 358 patients with severe sepsis were admitted from the ED to non-ICU level of care; 84 (23.5%) had unexpected ICU transfer within 48 h. Demographics and baseline co-morbidity burden were similar for patients requiring versus not requiring delayed ICU transfer. In unadjusted analysis, lactate ≥4 mmol/L and infection site were significantly associated with unexpected ICU upgrade. In forward selection multivariate logistic regression analysis, lactate ≥4 mmol/L (OR 2.0, 95% CI 1.03, 3.73; $p = 0.041$) and night (5 PM to 7 AM) admission (OR 1.9, 95% CI 1.07, 3.33; $p = 0.029$) were independent predictors of unexpected ICU transfer. Mortality of patients who were not upgraded to the ICU was 8.0%. Patients with unexpected ICU upgrade had similar mortality (25.0%) to those patients with severe sepsis/septic shock (24.6%) who were initially admitted to the ICU, despite less severe indices of illness at presentation.

Conclusions: Serum lactate ≥4 mmol/L and nighttime admissions are associated with unexpected ICU transfer in patients with severe sepsis. Mortality among patients with delayed ICU upgrade was similar to that for patients initially admitted directly to the ICU.

Keywords: Sepsis, Severe sepsis, Septic shock, Lactate, Unexpected ICU transfer, Mortality

Background

Severe sepsis and septic shock are responsible for over 750,000 inpatient stays and over 215,000 deaths annually in the USA [1]. Early goal-directed therapy (EGDT) was shown to reduce mortality in patients with severe sepsis and septic shock compared to the then-standard therapy [2]. While further studies have challenged the necessity of strict adherence to the algorithms of EGDT as standard of care evolves, prompt identification, early administration of antibiotics, source control, and aggressive fluid resuscitation have improved outcomes for patients with sepsis [3–6]. Many emergency departments (ED) have adopted bundled care strategies to identify, treat, and improve management of sepsis, which have been shown to decrease mortality in these patients [7].

Some patients with severe sepsis respond well initially to aggressive care, but later decompensate. Early identification of this subset of patients could help ensure

* Correspondence: gwardi@ucsd.edu
[1]Department of Emergency Medicine and Division of Pulmonary, Critical Care and Sleep Medicine, UC San Diego Health System, 200 West Arbor Drive, San Diego, CA 92103, USA
Full list of author information is available at the end of the article

assignment to the appropriate level of care on admission and avoid subsequent delayed escalations of care associated with worse outcomes [8]. However, identification of these patients remains a challenge. Prior research has evaluated general patient characteristics for all-comers admitted from the ED at risk of delayed escalation to the ICU, and this includes tachypnea, sepsis, elevated lactate, non-sustained hypotension, and fever [9–12]. However, risk factors for unexpected decompensation and ICU transfer in patients admitted with severe sepsis have not been specifically examined.

The aim of the current study, therefore, is to identify risk factors that predict unexpected upgrade to the ICU within 48 h of hospital admission in patients with severe sepsis presenting to the ED and to quantify the association between delayed ICU upgrade and in-hospital mortality.

Methods
Study design, setting, definitions, and population
We performed a retrospective cohort study of patients presenting with severe sepsis or septic shock to two urban hospitals within the same university system, between July 2012 and September 2014. Our institutional review board approved this study with waiver of informed consent, IRB# 151413. One hospital is a quaternary care center while the other functions as a safety-net hospital with a total combined annual ED census of approximately 60,000 patients per year. Provider staffing of both emergency departments is based on expected patient census and did not change over the study period. Our hospital system adopted a bundled care initiative, referred to as "Code Sepsis," designed to rapidly identify and treat patients with suspected severe sepsis or septic shock. The major components of our bundle care protocol are summarized in Table 1. Our institution had a 79% compliance with core measures of the protocol from 2012 to 2014, with an increase to 90% compliance by 2014.

All patients identified by our bundled care initiative between July 2012 and September 2014 were eligible for inclusion. Patient data initially were reviewed and recorded by a senior critical care attending physician (P.F.) to confirm diagnosis of severe sepsis or septic shock. Patients were considered to have severe sepsis if they met all three of the following criteria: (1) at least two-fourths systemic inflammatory syndrome criteria (SIRS) (heart rate >90, white blood cell count $>12 \times 10^3/\mu L$ or $<4 \times 10^3/\mu L$ or >10% immature bands, temperature >38 °C or <36 °C, or respiratory rate >20), (2) either a confirmed or suspected infection, (3) and had evidence of end-organ damage defined as any one of the following: (a) bilateral pulmonary infiltrates with new (increased) oxygen requirement to keep saturation >90% or $PaO_2/FiO_2 < 250$ mm Hg in absence of pneumonia, <200 mm Hg in presence of pneumonia, (b) systolic blood pressure (SBP) <90 or mean arterial pressure <65 or SBP

Table 1 Summary of key aspects in our bundled care initiative

Identification:

  A. Any 2 of the following (at least 2 required)

    (1) Temp >38.3 °C (100.9 °F) or <36.0 °C (96.8 °F)

    (2) Heart rate >90/min

    (3) Respiratory rate >20 breaths per min

AND

  B. Evidence of hypoperfusion (at least 1 required)

    (1) MAP <65 mmHg

    (2) SBP 40 mmHg below baseline

    (3) Acutely altered mental status

    (4) Oxygen saturation <92%

    (5) Exam suggestive of hypoperfusion

AND

  C. Suspected infection source

  Management:

    Phase 1:

      Ensure adequate intravenous access

      Weight-based IV fluid bolus

      Repeat serum lactate 3 h after first specimen obtained

      Administer broad-spectrum IV antibiotics in parallel

      If persistent hypotension OR failure to clear lactate by 10%, start phase 2

    Phase 2:

      Obtain central venous access

      Obtain ScvO2

      Transduce CVC to measure a CVP

      Insert arterial catheter

      Additional volume resuscitation

      Begin vasopressor

      Contact nursing/house supervisor and ICU team

      Serial lactate and ScvO2 (every 6 h)

      Consider transfusion to hematocrit of 30 if ScvO2 < 65% after volume resuscitation and pressor initiation

      Consider corticosteroids if vasopressor-dependent hypotension

decrease >40 mm Hg from baseline, (c) urine output <0.5 mL/kg/h for >2 h or creatinine increase >2.0 mg/dL or doubling of baseline creatinine, (d) bilirubin >4.0 mg/dL, (e) platelets $<80,000 \times 10^3/\mu L$ or >50% reduction from baseline, (f) international normalized ratio >1.5 or activated partial thromboplastin time >60 s, (g) pH < 7.30 or lactate > 4 mmol/L, or (h) acute alteration in mental status.

Septic shock was defined as a MAP < 65 mm Hg following a 20 mL/kg fluid bolus for at least 2 h or the need for vasoactive medications to ensure a MAP > 65 mm Hg.

The inclusion criteria were age ≥ 18, initiation of our bundled care plan during their ED stay, and admission to the wards from the ED. The exclusion criteria were admission directly to the ICU from the ED, direct admission/transfer to the wards without any care in the ED, initiation of our bundled care initiative for sepsis after admission to an inpatient unit, and patients with active hospice, comfort-only, or end-of-life care at the time of admission to the hospital. Our institution uses Society of Critical Care Medicine guidelines for admission to the ICU [13]. Thus, for patients with sepsis, ICU admission indications included the presence of hemodynamic instability and/or shock, the requirement for vasoactive medications or invasive blood pressure measurement, the need for mechanical ventilation, profound mental status changes, and/or a high level of nursing requirements only available in the ICU. Attending physician clinical judgment may override general guidelines dictating admission to the ICU.

Patients were classified as either "needing early escalation" or "not needing early escalation" based on their course over the first 48 h of admission. A 48-h window was selected based on prior studies have found that significant progression and potential decompensation of septic patients in the ED typically occurs by this point [11, 12]. Patients were classified as "needing early escalation" if admitted to a non-ICU level of care from the ED but subsequently upgraded to ICU level within the first 48 h or if they died in the wards within 48 h of admission. Patients were classified as "not needing early escalation" if no ICU upgrade was required during this time. Patients who required ICU care more than 48 h after admission to the wards were classified as "not needing early escalation."

We evaluated the following candidate predictor variables for their association with needing early escalation: age, sex, initial and worrisome vital signs while in the ED (maximal heart rate, maximal temperature, maximal respiratory rate, minimal systolic blood pressure), maximal shock index (heart rate divided by systolic blood pressure), initial laboratory results in the ED (white blood cell count, serum bicarbonate, serum lactate, both as a continuous and dichotomized variable with a cutoff of 4 mmol/L, sodium, creatinine), Charlson co-morbidity index, length of stay in the ED (defined as from entry to the transition of care to the accepting service), day or night admission time (5 PM to 7 AM was considered a night admission), weekday (Monday to Friday) or weekend admission, residence in a nursing facility, active malignancy, immunosuppression (recent or chronic steroid use, HIV positive with CD4 < 200, organ transplantation, or active use of immunosuppressive medications), time to antibiotics after arrival to the ED, and volume of fluid administered per kilogram within 6 h of meeting criteria for severe sepsis or septic shock. Vital status at hospital discharge was also recorded. All data were reviewed and

retrospectively extracted by three reviewers (G.W., A.W., and V.T.), who were involved in the study design and not blind to the study hypotheses. Data were abstracted into a standardized collection sheet devised by the authors (G.W., R.S.). Ten percent of charts were independently evaluated to assess inter-rater agreement and yielded a kappa greater than 0.85 for all variables.

Statistical analysis

Data analysis was performed using SPSS Statistics version 22 (SPSS, Armonk, NY). Univariate analysis was performed using two-sample t tests, chi-squared tests and Fisher exact test as appropriate. A two-sided alpha of <0.05 was considered statistically significant. A forward selection multivariate logistic regression model was performed to identify independent predictors of ICU upgrade within 48 h. An entry probability of F set at 0.05 for entry and 0.10 for removal were used. For this model, the number of candidate predictor variables was limited to no more than 1 variable per 10 patients experiencing the primary endpoint. The following 8 variables were considered in the forward selection model-building process: serum lactate ≥4 mmol/L, presence of pneumonia, time to antibiotic administration, nighttime admission, Charlson co-morbidity index, shock index, quantity of fluid administered, and age. These variables were selected based upon prior studies that have shown that these are risk factors for unexpected ICU transfer, significant biological plausibility, or significant findings in the univariate analysis [10–12, 14]. A separate multivariable logistic model was used to determine if unexpected ICU transfer was an independent risk factor for death and included the following four variables: serum lactate ≥4 mmol/L, time to antibiotic administration, volume of fluids resuscitation, and shock index.

The sensitivity and specificity of select variables (initial serum lactate and night admission) found to be statistically significant in multivariate analysis were calculated. We also created a receiver operator characteristic curve to determine the optimal statistical cutoff point for initial serum lactate for maximal predictive value.

Results

Patient population characteristics

Of the 998 patients who met the criteria for severe sepsis or septic shock, 914 were identified in the ED (Fig. 1). Of these, 358 had severe sepsis and were admitted to the wards. The remaining 556 patients were admitted directly to the ICU. When compared to patients directly admitted to the ICU from the ED, patients admitted to non-ICU level of care had lower mean initial lactate (2.8 vs. 4.1 mmol/L; $p < 0.005$) and shock index (1.02 vs. 1.11; $p = .002$) and received

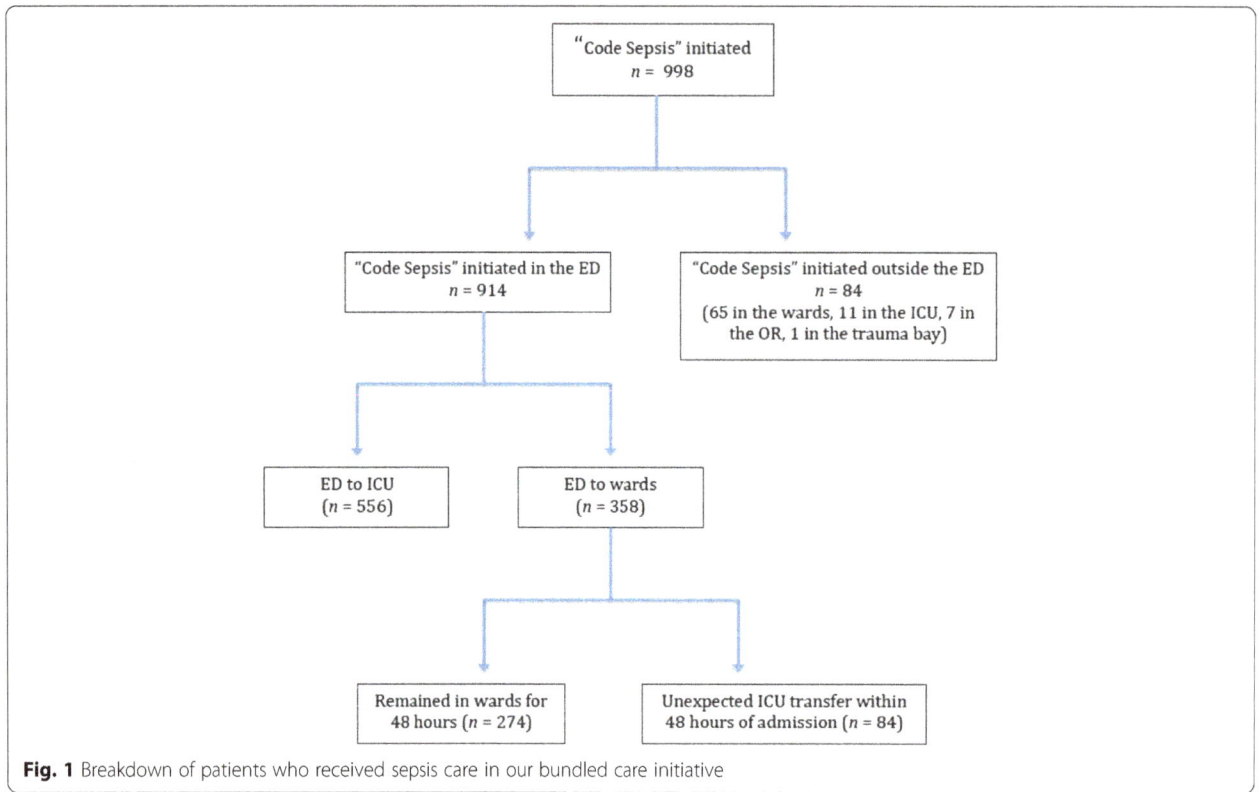

Fig. 1 Breakdown of patients who received sepsis care in our bundled care initiative

less fluid in the first 6 h (33 vs. 40 mL/kg; $p < 0.005$) as seen in Table 2.

Predictors of early escalation to the ICU

Of the 358 patients admitted first to non-ICU level of care, 84 (23.5%) had an unexpected upgrade to the ICU within 48 h of admission. Univariate analysis (Table 3) revealed that higher initial lactate level was significantly associated with unexpected ICU transfer within 48 h (3.7 vs. 2.6 mmol/L; $p = 0.011$). The cutoff value of triage serum lactate levels that maximized correct prediction of unexpected ICU transfer was 4.44 mmol/L, which had a sensitivity of 0.282 and a specificity of 0.873. Serum lactate ≥4 mmol/L was found in 28.2% of patients with unexpected transfer versus in 16.7% of patients who remained in the wards ($p = 0.039$). The odds of experiencing early ICU transfer doubled for patients with an initial lactate level ≥4 mmol/L (OR 2.0, 95% CI 1.05, 3.66; $p = 0.024$). Patients with a genitourinary source were less likely to have delayed admission to the ICU; patients with pneumonia were more likely to decompensate on the floor ($p = 0.03$). Importantly, markers of bundle compliance and adherence to current resuscitation guidelines did not differ significantly as there was no difference in the time to antibiotic administration (96.6 vs. 113.1 min; $p = 0.136$) or volume of fluid administered in the first 6 h (35.7 vs. 32.4 mL/kg; $p = 0.167$) between the bundle compliant and bundle non-compliant groups.

The sensitivity and specificity of lactate ≥4 mmol/L for early escalation to the ICU were 0.282 and 0.833, and night admission had a sensitivity and specificity of 0.595 and 0.509, respectively.

In forward selection multivariate logistic regression analysis, lactate ≥4 mmol/L (OR 2.0, 95% CI 1.03, 4.37; $p = 0.003$) and night admission (OR 1.9, 95% CI 1.07, 3.33; $p = 0.029$) were independently associated with early escalation to ICU level of care within 48 h of admission (Table 4).

Early ICU transfer and mortality

Overall, 43 of the 358 patients who were admitted to the wards (12.0%) did not survive to discharge. Death before discharge was significantly more likely among patients admitted to the wards who required early ICU upgrade compared to those without early upgrade (25 vs. 8%; $p < .005$). In unadjusted logistic regression analysis, early escalation to the ICU was associated with significantly higher mortality compared to non-escalation (OR 3.8, 95% CI 1.92, 7.20; $p < 0.005$). When adjusting for lactate ≥4 mmol/L, age, time to antibiotics, and SI, the association of delayed escalation with mortality remained highly significant (OR 4.2, 95% CI 1.87, 9.241; $p < 0.005$).

The in-hospital mortality of patients who were admitted from the ED directly to the ICU was 24.6%; this was nearly identical to the patients who had unexpected transfer to the ICU ($p = 0.943$). Despite this similar

Table 2 Baseline characteristics of patients with either severe sepsis or septic shock treated in the ED with our bundled care initiative

	ED directly to ICU	ED towards (including delayed ICU transfers within 48 h)	p value
Number	556	358	
Age, years	58.8 (±18)	58.4 (±18)	0.785
Sex, %male (n)	57.6% (320)	55.3% (198)	0.337
Triage SBP (mm Hg)	105 (±28)	112 (±28)	0.001
Shock index (SBP/HR)	1.11 (±0.33)	1.02 (±0.30)	0.002
Triage HR (BPM)	111 (±29)	110 (±23)	0.662
Fluids per kg within 6 h of presentation	40.1 (±20.7)	33.2 (±18.9)	<0.005
Initial lactate (mmol/L)	4.1 ± 3.4	2.8 ± 2.3	<0.005
% with septic shock at presentation (n)	55.6% (310)	0% (0)	<0.005
Site of infection%, (n)			<0.005
Abdominal	14.9% (83)	17.6% (63)	
Cardiac	1.3% (7)	1.1% (4)	
Central nervous system	1.1% (6)	1.4% (5)	
Genitourinary	21.9% (122)	31.3% (112)	
Musculoskeletal	7.0% (39)	13.4% (48)	
Pulmonary	24.8% (138)	22.3% (80)	
Unknown/others[a]	28.9% (161)	12.9% (46)	
Mortality,% (n)	24.6% (137)	12.0% (43)	<0.005

[a]Others include patients with multiple organ system infections, catheter-related infections, head and neck infection, and neutropenic fever without definitive source

mortality rate, patients who had delayed ICU admission received less fluid volume administered in the first 6 h (35.7 mL/kg versus 40.1 mL/kg; $p = 0.020$) and lower shock index (0.99 versus 1.09; $p = 0.013$) and none were in shock at time of admission (0 versus 55.6%; $p = <0.005$). Serum lactate values were not statistically different however (3.7 versus 4.1 mmol/L; $p = 0.357$) nor was the percentage of patients with lactate ≥4 mmol/L (28.2% versus 34.3%; $p = 0.351$). In multivariate logistic regression analysis controlling for these variables, delayed ICU admission, compared to direct ICU admission, was not independently associated with increased mortality (OR 1.40, 95% CI 0.73, 2.67; $p = 0.309$).

Discussion

Bundled care initiatives have been effective in the early identification and management of patients with severe sepsis and septic shock, yet some patients still unexpectedly decompensate and require ICU transfer after initial admission to the ward [7]. We found that an initial serum lactate ≥4 mmol/L was associated with a more than doubling of adjusted odds for early ICU transfer. Patients admitted between 5 PM and 7 AM were also more likely to have unexpected ICU upgrade in the multivariate logistic regression analysis. Patients with a delayed ICU transfer had a significant increase in mortality

with an adjusted odds ratio of 4.2 compared to those that did not need early escalation; however, mortality was nearly identical when compared to patients directly admitted to the ICU.

Although numerous studies have evaluated factors associated with unexpected ICU admission, ours is unique in that it evaluates patients with suspected severe sepsis or septic shock who receive early, evidence-based aggressive care. Two prior studies have attempted to identify characteristics of infected patients from the ED that could predict unexpected transfer to the ICU. One evaluated patients with suspected infection (defined as blood cultures drawn in the ED or within 3 h of admission) and found that respiratory compromise, congestive heart failure, peripheral vascular disease, systolic blood pressure <100 mmHg, tachycardia, or elevated creatinine levels all predicted unanticipated ICU transfer within 48 h [15]. Caterino et al. studied patients who were given a discharge diagnosis of "sepsis" and performed a multivariate regression analysis of 78 patients and found that a lower bicarbonate and lack of fever were associated with unexpected ICU transfer [16].

Two previously published studies evaluated the development of septic shock in septic patients admitted from the ED. Glickman et al. investigated the progression of

Table 3 Results of univariate analysis of factors of unexpected ICU transfer in patients with severe sepsis initially admitted to the wards

	Early escalation to ICU (n = 84)	No escalation to ICU with 48 h (n = 274)	p
Patient characteristics			
Age, years	58.5 (±18.3)	58.2 (±16.0)	0.872
Sex, % male (n)	54% (45)	56% (153)	0.781
Charlson co-morbidity index	3.44 (±2.11)	3.01 (±2.51)	0.125
% immunocompromised (n)	67% (183)	58% (49)	0.152
% from nursing home (n)	13% (36)	14% (12)	0.855
% with active malignancy	30% (82)	32% (27)	0.787
Infection site,% (n)			0.03
Abdominal	17% (14)	18% (49)	
Cardiac	1% (1)	1% (3)	
Central nervous system	0% (0)	2% (5)	
Musculoskeletal	10% (8)	14% (39)	
Genitourinary	21% (18)	34% (94)	
Pulmonary	28% (24)	21% (56)	
Other/unknown/multiple	23% (19)	10% (27)	
Vital signs			
Triage temperature (°C)	37.3 (±1.0)	38.1 (±5.5)	0.190
Triage heart rate (BPM)	109 (±23)	110 (±24)	0.580
Triage systolic blood pressure (mm Hg)	113 (±27)	111 (±24)	0.612
Triage shock index (HR/SBP)	0.98 (±0.32)	1.03 (±0.28)	0.235
Minimum SBP during ED stay (mm Hg)	93 (±21)	94 (±21)	0.809
Maximal HR during ED stay (BPM)	120 (±24)	115 (±23)	0.072
Maximal RR during stay (RPM)	25 (±6)	25 (±11)	0.975
Laboratory results			
Sodium (mEq/L)	134 (±5)	133 (±11)	0.600
Creatinine (mg/dL)	1.70 (±1.5)	2.04 (±1.6)	0.692
Bicarbonate (mEq/L)	22 (±4.7)	23 (±4.3)	0.218
Lactate (mmol/L)	3.7 (±3.2)	2.6 (±1.8)	0.011
% with lactate > = 4 mmol/L	28.1%	16.7%	0.039
White count (×10^9/L)	13.2 (±8.4)	11.3 (7.8)	0.051
Interventions			
Time to antibiotics (min)	96.6 (±89.9)	113.1 (±86.7)	0.136
Fluids administered in 1st 6 h (mL/kg)	35.7 (±18.5)	32.4 (±19.0)	0.167
Temporal impact			
Time in ED (min)	543 (±310)	646 (±411)	0.339
% admission during weekday (n)	70% (192)	76% (64)	0.334
% admission at night (n)	60% (50)	49% (134)	0.060
Mortality % (n)	25% (21)	8% (22)	<0.005

disease in hemodynamically stable septic patients without organ dysfunction to septic shock [11]. They found that the majority of patients who progressed to septic shock did so within 48 h and had an increased 30-day mortality versus in the group who did not progress to septic shock. The authors identified older age, female sex, presence of fever, anemia, comorbid lung disease, and vascular access device infection as risk factors. Capp et al. performed a retrospective chart review study to evaluate factors associated of the development of septic

Table 4 Results of forward selection multivariate logistic regression analysis to determine patient characteristics of unexpected ICU transfer

Variable	OR (95% CI)	p
Lactate ≥4 (mmol/L)	2.0 (1.03, 3.73)	0.041
Nighttime admission (5 PM—7 AM)	1.9 (1.07, 3.33)	0.029

OR are presented as odds of early escalation of care to the ICU

shock in septic patients admitted from the ED within the first 48 h [12]. The authors found approximately 8% of patients with sepsis progressed to septic shock at 48 h. Identified factors included a lactate >4 mmol/L, female gender, non-persistent hypotension, a bandemia of at least 10%, and a history of coronary artery disease. While our results have some similarities to these studies, ours is unique in that patients with sepsis (but not severe sepsis) were excluded and all patients received upfront, aggressive care. To our knowledge, no prior studies thus far have evaluated predictors of delayed ICU admission in a relatively ill patient population who received bundle care. That lactate >4 mmol/L was associated with the development of septic shock in the study by Capp further strengthens its use in determining which patients are at increased risk of unexpected ICU transfer. Furthermore, in the sensitivity analysis we performed to identify the serum lactate value that best predicts unexpected transfer to the ICU, we found that a lactate of 4.44 mmol/L had the best discriminatory value. We do not advocate adoption of this specific threshold in clinical decision-making, recognizing that sensitivity may be prioritized over specificity when screening for potentially fatal critical illness. Yet, this finding further strengthens using lactate values as a measure of severity of illness in septic shock. Indeed, prior research has shown that patients with serum lactate ≥4 mmol/L without hypotension had similar mortality to those with "overt" shock (defined as persistent hypotension after a 20 mL/kg fluid bolus) [17].

We also found that admission at night was an independent risk factor for unexpected ICU transfer. Staffing levels are lower at night in our ED, wards, and ICU that may partially explain this. Furthermore, certain hospital services, such as ultrasound and other diagnostic modalities, are not readily available at night, which may also contribute. This could be similar to the "weekend" effect—the increase in mortality seen in patients over the weekend compared to weekdays—that is well described in patients with acute medical conditions [18]. This "weekend" effect was also seen in a recent national database study that showed septic patients were more likely to have early in-hospital mortality—but not overall mortality—if admitted during the weekend [19]. Although the "weekend" effect was not shown in our analysis, we believe the similarities between this and night

admission (e.g., lower staffing levels, less specialists and diagnostic modalities immediately available) suggests that patients fare poorer when less resources are available.

It has been previously shown that patients who have an unanticipated delayed upgrade to the ICU have higher mortality rates compared to those admitted to the ICU directly from the ED. Parkhe et al. found that a delayed ICU admission (defined as more than 24 h after initial admission) had a significantly higher mortality rate (35%) at 30 days than patients directly admitted to the ICU (9.1%) [20]. Similar studies have shown comparable results that are independent of the severity of illness at the time of admission [21]. However, in our cohort, delayed ICU admission was not independently associated with increased mortality. Differences in illness severity, threshold for ICU admission, inclusion of patients with septic shock, and hospital-specific sepsis protocols with early, aggressive may account for this discrepancy in findings.

Limitations

We acknowledge several limitations in our study. It is retrospective and dependent upon chart review for data collected from a single hospital system, and thus, findings should be considered associations rather than causal relationships. As the patients in this study were identified by the medical staff in our ED, we suspect there were patients who met the inclusion criteria and would have benefited from aggressive care but did not have the bundled care initiative started. Furthermore, patients who received management in our bundled care initiative, but who did not meet criteria for severe sepsis or septic shock, were also excluded. We also did not include certain variables, such as bilirubin, degree of bandemia, lactate trends over time, and coagulation profile in our study, which prior research has shown to correlate with adverse events and increased mortality in patients with significant abnormalities in these variables [22, 23]. Finally, our data predate the most recent definition of sepsis and septic shock in our investigation ("Sepsis 3") [24]. We acknowledge that the change in definitions could change the outcomes in our study. However, a high number of hospital systems use the "Sepsis 2" definitions of severe sepsis and septic shock, thus making our results applicable to general practice standards. Furthermore, numerous professional societies have not yet officially adopted the definitions in Sepsis 3.

Conclusions

Serum lactate ≥4 and night admission were independently associated with increased probability of unexpected upgrade to the ICU in patients with severe sepsis. Unexpected ICU transfer was associated with a significant increase in mortality when compared to those in this population who remained in the wards for at least 48 h. Mortality was the same as for patients who were directly admitted to the ICU despite controlling for indices of illness in the group who were initially admitted to the wards. Prospective studies are needed to validate these results and this hypothesis.

Abbreviations
ED: Emergency department; EGDT: Early goal-directed therapy; ICU: Intensive care unit; MAP: Mean arterial pressure; OR: Odds ratio

Acknowledgements
The authors have no additional acknowledgements.

Funding
This work has not received any funding from any grant or other financial support. It was completed at the University of California, San Diego. It was presented at the American Thoracic Society Annual Meeting in San Francisco 5/2016.

Authors' contributions
GW, AW, VT, RS, CS, and CT conceived the study and design. GW, AW, VT, and PF performed the data collection. GW, AW, and VT oversaw the conduct of the trial. GW, AW, and VT managed the data, including quality control. JV and JB provided the statistical advice. GW and AW drafted the manuscript, and all authors contributed substantially to its revision. GW takes responsibility for the paper as a whole. All authors read and approved the final manuscript.

Authors' information
GW is a fellow in the Division of Pulmonary, Critical Care and Sleep Medicine and Department of Emergency Medicine at the University of California, San Diego. AW is a medical student at the University of California, San Diego. JV is a fellow in the Division of Pulmonary, Critical Care Medicine at Stanford University. VT is an associated professor in the Departments of Emergency Medicine and Internal Medicine at the University of California, San Diego. CT is a professor in the Department of Emergency Medicine at the University of California, San Diego. CS is a professor in the Department of Emergency Medicine at the University of California, San Diego. PF is a professor in the Division of Pulmonary, Critical Care, and Sleep Medicine at the University of California, San Diego. JB is an assistant professor in the Division of Pulmonary, Critical Care, and Sleep Medicine at the University of California, San Diego. MN is a resident in the Department of Emergency Medicine at the University of California, San Diego. DL is a fellow in the Division of Medical Toxicology at the University of California, San Diego. RS is an assistant professor in the Division of Pulmonary, Critical Care, and Sleep Medicine at the University of California, San Diego.

Competing interests
The authors declare that they have no competing interests.

Author details
[1]Department of Emergency Medicine and Division of Pulmonary, Critical Care and Sleep Medicine, UC San Diego Health System, 200 West Arbor Drive, San Diego, CA 92103, USA. [2]University of California San Diego School of Medicine, 9500 Gilman Drive, La Jolla, CA 92093-0602, USA. [3]Division of Pulmonary and Critical Care Medicine, Stanford University School of Medicine, M121-L, Stanford, CA 94305-5119, USA. [4]Department of Internal Medicine, University of California, San Diego, 200 West Arbor Drive, San Diego, CA 92103, USA. [5]Department of Emergency Medicine, University of California, San Diego, 200 West Arbor Drive, San Diego, CA 92103, USA. [6]Division of Pulmonary, Critical Care, and Sleep Medicine, University of California, San Diego, 200 W Arbor Drive, San Diego, CA 92103, USA.

References
1. Gaieski DF, Edwards JM, Kallan MJ, et al. Benchmarking the incidence and mortality of severe sepsis in the United States. Crit Care Med. 2013;41(5):1167–74.
2. Rivers E, Nguyen B, Havstad S, et al. Early goal-directed therapy in the treatment of severe sepsis and septic shock. N Engl J Med. 2001;345(19):1368–77.
3. Arise Investigators, ANZICS Clinical Trials Group. Goal-directed resuscitation for patients with early septic shock. N Engl J Med. 2014;2014(371):1496–506.
4. Mouncey PR, Osborn TM, Power GS, Harrison DA, Sadique MZ, Grieve RD, Jahan R, Harvey SE, Bell D, Bion JF, Coats TJ. Trial of early, goal-directed resuscitation for septic shock. N Engl J Med. 2015;372(14):1301–11.
5. ProCESS Investigators. A randomized trial of protocol-based care for early septic shock. N Engl J Med. 2014;2014(370):1683–93.
6. Gaieski DF, Mikkelsen ME, Band RA, et al. Impact of time to antibiotics on survival in patients with severe sepsis or septic shock in whom early goal-directed therapy was initiated in the ED. Crit Care Med. 2010;38(4):1045–53.
7. Nguyen HB, Corbett SW, Steele R, et al. Implementation of a bundle of quality indicators for the early management of severe sepsis and septic shock is associated with decreased mortality. Crit Care Med. 2007;35(4):1105–12.
8. Chalfin DB, Trzeciak S, Likourezos A, et al. Impact of delayed transfer of critically ill patients from the ED to the intensive care unit. Crit Care Med. 2007;35(6):1477–83.
9. Delgado M, Liu V, Pines JM, Kipnis P, Gardner MN, Escobar GJ. Risk factors for unplanned transfer to intensive care within 24 hours of admission from the ED in an integrated healthcare system. J Hosp Med. 2013;8(1):13–9.
10. Farley H, Zubrow MT, Gies J, et al. ED tachypnea predicts transfer to a higher level of care in the first 24 hours after ED admission. Acad Emerg Med. 2010;17(7):718–22.
11. Glickman SW, Cairns CB, Otero RM, et al. Disease progression in hemodynamically stable patients presenting to the emergency department with sepsis. Acad Emerg Med. 2010;17(4):383–90.
12. Capp R, Horton CL, Takhar SS, et al. Predictors of patients who present to the emergency department with sepsis and progress to septic shock between 4 and 48 hours of emergency department arrival. Crit Care Med. 2015;43(5):983–8.
13. Egol A. Guidelines for intensive care unit admission, discharge, and triage. Crit Care Med. 1999;27:633–8.
14. Keller AS, Kirkland LL, Rajasekaran SY, et al. Unplanned transfers to the intensive care unit: the role of the shock index. J Hosp Med. 2010;5(8):460–5.
15. Kennedy M, Joyce N, Howell MD, et al. Identifying infected ED patients admitted to the hospital ward at risk of clinical deterioration and intensive care unit transfer. Acad Emerg Med. 2010;17(10):1080–5.
16. Caterino JM, Jalbuena T, Bogucki B. Predictors of acute decompensation after admission in ED patients with sepsis. Am J Emerg Med. 2010;28(5):631–6.
17. Puskarich MA, Trzeciak S, Shapiro NI, et al. Outcomes of patients undergoing early sepsis resuscitation for cryptic shock compared with overt shock. Resuscitation. 2011;82(10):1289–93.
18. Bell CM, Redelmeier DA. Mortality among patients admitted to hospitals on weekends as compared with weekdays. N Engl J Med. 2001;345(9):663–8.
19. Powell ES, Khare RK, Courtney DM, et al. The weekend effect for patients with sepsis presenting to the emergency department. J Emerg Med. 2013;45(5):641–8.
20. Parkhe M, Myles PS, Leach DS, et al. Outcome of ED patients with delayed admission to an intensive care unit. Emerg Med. 2002;14(1):50–7.
21. Escarce JJ, Kelley MA. Admission source to the medical intensive care unit predicts hospital death independent of APACHE II score. JAMA. 1990; 264(18):2389–94.

22. Shapiro NI, Wolfe RE, Moore RB, et al. Mortality in ED Sepsis (MEDS) score: a prospectively derived and validated clinical prediction rule. Crit Care Med. 2003;31(3):670–5.

23. Fischer CM, Yano K, Aird WC, et al. Abnormal coagulation tests obtained in the ED are associated with mortality in patients with suspected infection. J Emerg Med. 2012;42(2):127–32.

24. Singer M, Deutschman CS, Seymour CW, et al. The third international consensus definitions for sepsis and septic shock (sepsis-3). JAMA. 2016;315(8):801–10.

One-year resource utilisation, costs and quality of life in patients with acute respiratory distress syndrome (ARDS)

Joachim Marti[1*], Peter Hall[2], Patrick Hamilton[3], Sarah Lamb[4], Chris McCabe[5], Ranjit Lall[6], Julie Darbyshire[7], Duncan Young[7] and Claire Hulme[8]

Abstract

Background: The long-term economic and quality-of-life outcomes of patients admitted to intensive care unit (ICU) with acute respiratory distress syndrome are not well understood. In this study, we investigate 1-year costs, survival and quality of life following ICU admission in patients who required mechanical ventilation for acute respiratory distress syndrome.

Methods: Economic analysis of data collected alongside a UK-based multi-centre randomised, controlled trial, aimed at comparing high-frequency oscillatory ventilation with conventional mechanical ventilation. The study included 795 critically ill patients admitted to ICU. Hospital costs were assessed using daily data. Post-hospital healthcare costs, patient out-of-pocket expenses, lost earnings of survivors and their carers and health-related quality of life were assessed using follow-up surveys.

Results: The mean cost of initial ICU stay was £26,857 (95 % CI £25,222–£28,491), and the average daily cost in ICU was £1738 (CI £1667–£1810). Following hospital discharge, the average 1-year cost among survivors was £7523 (CI £5692–£9354). The mean societal cost at 1 year was £44,077 (£41,168–£46,985), and the total societal cost divided by the number of 1-year survivors was £90,206. Survivors reported significantly lower health-related quality of life than the age- and sex-matched reference population, and this difference was more marked in younger patients.

Conclusions: Given the high costs and low health-related quality of life identified, there is significant scope for further research aimed at improving care in this in-need patient group.

Background

Intensive care units (ICU) account for an important share of hospital budgets for a relatively small volume of patients given the complex procedures involved, the use of costly technology and medications, and the involvement of highly qualified staff. Patients admitted to ICU with acute respiratory distress syndrome (ARDS), an inflammatory lung condition, are particularly resource-intensive [1–3], have high mortality and morbidity [4–8], and survivors report lower quality of life than other critically ill patients [9]. Patients with ARDS often require mechanical ventilation (MV), a particularly costly life-sustaining therapy [2]. As MV itself can cause lung injury, inflammation and even death [10], alternative ventilation strategies that better protect the lungs have been called for. Recent large trials have examined the effectiveness of high-frequency oscillatory ventilation (HFOV) as compared to conventional ventilation in

* Correspondence: j.marti@imperial.ac.uk
[1]Centre for Health Policy, Imperial College London, Praed Street, London W2 1NY, UK
Full list of author information is available at the end of the article

patients with ARDS but have not demonstrated any improvement in short-term mortality with the use of HFOV [11, 12]. A comprehensive evaluation of these alternative therapies requires the assessment of long-term mortality outcomes and the consideration of resource use and patient quality of life [13–17]. The volume of high quality data arising from recent research in this area presents new opportunities for knowledge generation beyond the core objectives of those studies.

Following discharge, recovery is challenging for survivors of ARDS as physical and neuropsychological disabilities may persist for years [6, 17–23]. In the long run, health-related quality of life (HRQL) of the survivors of ARDS and other critically ill patients has been found to be significantly lower than for the general population [1, 9, 24–32]. To date, economic studies of patients with ARDS mostly focused on ICU and hospital costs [3, 33, 34] and few studies have examined the long-term costs among ICU survivors [31, 35, 36]. Survivors of ARDS may require on-going treatments and rehabilitation following hospital discharge [1, 19, 26] as well as extensive support from carers [6], which may lead to an important economic cost to the health sector and the society as a whole [35, 37]. The measurement and reporting of costs and quality-adjusted life years (QALYs) in ICU populations is vital to allow health service and policy advances.

In this paper, we used in-hospital trial data and follow-up questionnaires of a prospective cohort of patients with ARDS to examine 1-year healthcare utilisation and quality-of-life outcomes, enabling the calculation of costs and QALYs. The economic and quality-of-life data were collected alongside the OSCAR trial [12], a multi-centre randomised, controlled trial of HFOV as compared with conventional mechanical ventilation, conducted in England, Wales and Scotland. We assessed the economic costs and benefits within the initial year following randomisation and estimated detailed costs for various parts of the care pathway (initial ICU stay, hospital stay following first ICU discharge and post-hospital resource use) and patient groups.

Methods
Patient population
The data used in this study come from the OSCAR study, a multi-centre, randomised, controlled trial of HFOV as compared to conventional MV in patients with moderate-to-severe ARDS. Patients (>16 years) who were undergoing MV were recruited in different-sized ICUs from 29 hospitals across England, Wales and Scotland and were randomised to either HFOV or conventional MV. Patients were eligible if they were expected to require at least two more days of MV and met the definition of moderate or severe ARDS. Patients were excluded if they had been on ventilation for 7 days

or more. Inclusion criteria for OSCAR and patient recruitment have been described in detail in Young et al. [12]. The study was approved by national ethics review committees and research governance departments at each centre. Patients or their representatives provided written informed consent.

Data collection
Characteristics such as age, gender, ventilation prior to enrolment, physiology and other information required to assess illness severity were collected at the time of randomisation. The Acute Physiology, Age, and Chronic Health Evaluation (APACHE II) score was used to measure the severity of illness within the first 24 h after the patient was admitted to an ICU. The APACHE II score is based on several physiological measurements and pre-admission health status and ranges from 0 to 71, with higher scores corresponding to more severe illness. The baseline ratio of the partial pressure of arterial oxygen (PaO2) to the fraction of inspired oxygen (FiO2) was also recorded as a measure of the severity of ARDS. Case report forms (CRFs) were completed by the medical and nursing staff for each day a patient was in ICU. The CRFs recorded the use of antibiotics, sedatives and muscle relaxant drugs as well as information on support for organ systems. Serious adverse events and whether the patient required a chest drain or presented radiological evidence of barotrauma were also recorded. ICU discharge date and location, ICU readmissions and hospital discharge date were available.

Following hospital discharge, questionnaires were sent to surviving patients and their carers at 6 and 12 months. Patients were asked about their use of medical services during the previous 6 months, including primary- and community-based health and social services and residential inpatient stays. The questionnaires also contained questions related to the use of aids and equipment, gross loss of earnings and other major expenses. Patients' questionnaires also recorded quality of life using the EuroQol-5D (EQ-5D) [38]. Carers' questionnaires recorded the cost of travel to and from medical services, major expenses and loss of earnings.

Data analysis
Quality of life
Patients' HRQL was measured at 6 and 12 months using EQ-5D. Health utility weights for each patient were derived from EQ-5D responses using the standard UK specific tariffs [39]. For each time period, mean utility scores were compared to those of an age- and sex-matched reference population [39].

To obtain mean QALYs at 1 year, quality of life and survival data were combined into a single metric. Patients' histories were partitioned into several periods from randomisation to 1 year, and a utility value was assigned to each of these periods [40]. For the ventilation period, we multiplied the average number of days ventilated by the utility weight of an unconscious patient reported in the EQ-5D scoring manual (–0.4) [38]. We then calculated the mean utility scores of survivors at 6 and 12 months using all available questionnaires and, assuming a linear change in HRQL between assessments, we calculated mean utility scores at two additional midpoints (3 and 9 months). The mean time in each period was obtained by calculating the area under the relevant Kaplan-Meier survival curve. The sum of the mean survival time in each state multiplied by the utility weights provided an estimate of the quality-adjusted survival at 1 year, expressed in QALYs.

Costing methodology

We used a bottom-up micro-costing approach where we assigned unit costs to volumes of resource use for each patient [41]. We analysed costs from the perspective of the health and social care sector (NHS) and from a broader societal perspective. Costing was undertaken for the various pathways of care following ICU admission: initial ICU stay, hospital stay following first ICU discharge, post-hospital NHS resource use and societal costs. ICU and hospital costs were assessed using the bottom-up approach [36, 42, 43].

Resource use associated with initial stay in ICU was assessed daily based on the number of organs supported, respiratory support, whether the patient was on renal replacement therapy, whether he/she required X-rays (to check for barotrauma) or a chest drain (pneumothorax) and use of medicines. The quantities of resource use were multiplied by their corresponding unit costs, and the sum per patient for the entire stay was calculated. The unit costs of ICU resources including cost per organ supported, radiology and the cost of pneumothorax were taken from the National Schedule of Reference Costs [44]. The costs of medicines used were taken from the British National Formulary (BNF) [45]. The daily cost of ventilation was based on a fixed and per patient cost. We assumed that ventilation machines would be used for 5 years; annual maintenance and the costs of single use circuits were also included.

Once patients were discharged from ICU, the cost of step-down and the cost of ICU readmissions were calculated using the number of days until death or discharge multiplied by the cost of the level of care required, based on various nationally available references [44, 46, 47]. If a patient was discharged to another hospital following ICU, the cost of transport was taken as that of an emergency transfer. Serious adverse events and corresponding unit costs were assessed on an individual basis. Patient-reported data on resource use were collected at 6 and

12 months. NHS resource use included further inpatient care, outpatient care, primary- and community-based care and aids and equipment provided by the NHS. The costs of attendance at medical services were calculated using national reference costs multiplied by the number of times a patient attended [44, 47]. Inpatient stays were based on the number of days admitted multiplied by the corresponding unit cost [47]. The cost of aids and equipment was taken from the NHS supply chain cost for each individual item. Costs incurred by patients and their carers included cost of travel, loss of earnings and patient out-of-pocket expenses for aids, equipment and extra expenses (home adaptations). The cost of travel to and from appointments for both carers and patients was based on the distance in miles provided in the questionnaires multiplied by the cost per petrol mile as provided by HM Revenue & Customs (HMRC) [48]. Patients and carers were asked to give the gross amount lost in earnings in the 6 months covered by each questionnaire. Cost of aids and equipment purchased by patients was directly reported in the patient questionnaire. All costs were adjusted to 2012 prices using the Hospital and Community Healthcare Services (HCHS) index published by the Personal Social Services Research Unit (PSSRU) [47]. Unit costs used in the analysis and more details on the costing strategy are provided in the supplemental appendix.

Outcomes

The primary outcomes were 1-year survival, quality of life and resource use. Resource use was measured in terms of duration of treatment in both the ICU and the hospital and in terms of health care and societal costs at 1 year, divided into the various care pathways, i.e. ICU stay, hospital stay and post-discharge period. These outcomes were presented for various subgroups of patients based on baseline demographic, physiological, and clinical characteristic, including ventilation strategy (HFOV or conventional ventilation). Total cost per 1-year survivor was obtained by dividing the sum of ICU, hospital, and post-hospital costs for all patients by the number of patients remaining alive 1 year post-randomisation. The 1-year incremental cost effectiveness ratio (ICER) of HFOV as compared to conventional MV was also calculated. The ICER was obtained by dividing the difference between the average 1-year costs in the HFOV group, and the average 1-year cost in the conventional ventilation group by the difference between average health outcomes (QALYs) gained in the HFOV group and those gained in the conventional ventilation group [49].

Statistical analyses

Patient characteristics are presented using means and standard deviations (SD) for continuous variables and proportions and percentages for categorical variables. We compared baseline characteristics of 1-year survivors and non-survivors using Student's t tests for continuous variables and chi-squared tests for categorical variables. No corrections were made for multiple testing. Cost data are presented using means, 95 % confidence intervals, median and interquartile range. HRQL at 6 and 12 months and quality-adjusted survival were summarised using means and 95 % confidence intervals. HRQL of survivors was compared to population reference values using Student's t tests. We first estimated mean post-hospital costs based on complete cases. To obtain total costs at 1-year for each patient, missing data on post-hospital costs among 1-year survivors was addressed by multiple imputation using chained equations. We used a truncated model in which costs were constrained to be equal or above zero and generated ten datasets. Estimates from each imputed dataset were combined following Rubin's rule [50]. All p values were two-sided, and a significance level of less than 0.05 was used. R 3.0.2 and Stata 12 (Statacorp, College Station, TX, USA) were used for the analyses.

Results

Patients

A total of 795 patients underwent randomisation. A flow chart of the study population is presented in Fig. 1. Among the 795 patients included in the analysis, 343 patients died in ICU and 47 died in hospital after ICU discharge (in-hospital mortality rate of 49.1 %). Of the 405

remaining patients, 17 died between hospital discharge and the 12 months follow-up. Thus, the 1-year mortality rate was 51.2 %. A total of 234 patients completed the cost and quality-of-life questionnaires at 6 months, and 205 patients completed the questionnaires at 12 months (response rate of 58.9 and 52.8 %, respectively). Overall, 170 1-year survivors and 95 carers completed both the 6-month and the 12-month questionnaires. Baseline patient characteristics are displayed in Table 1. The mean age was 55 years and most patients were male (62.3 %) and had pneumonia identified as the primary cause of ARDS (58.6 %). The mean ICU length of stay (+/– SD) was 17.0+/–16.5 days, and the mean hospital length of stay was 33.6+/–43.1 days. Compared to 1-year survivors, non-survivors were older, had a higher APACHE II score, lower PaO_2:FiO_2 ratio and were less likely to have been admitted in surgery. 1-year survivors who have completed both 6 and 12 months questionnaires were younger and had lower APACHE II scores than 1-year survivors with incomplete information (unreported analysis).

Survival and quality of life

Figure 2 shows the Kaplan-Meier survival estimates at 1 year by age, APACHE II score and ventilation strategy (HFOV and conventional ventilation), based on complete follow-up data on mortality. Higher 1-year mortality was observed among older (≥ 65) patients (OR 3.98, 95 % CI 2.86–5.55) and patients with higher (>26) APACHE II score (OR 2.55, 95 % CI 1.80–3.63), after adjustment for

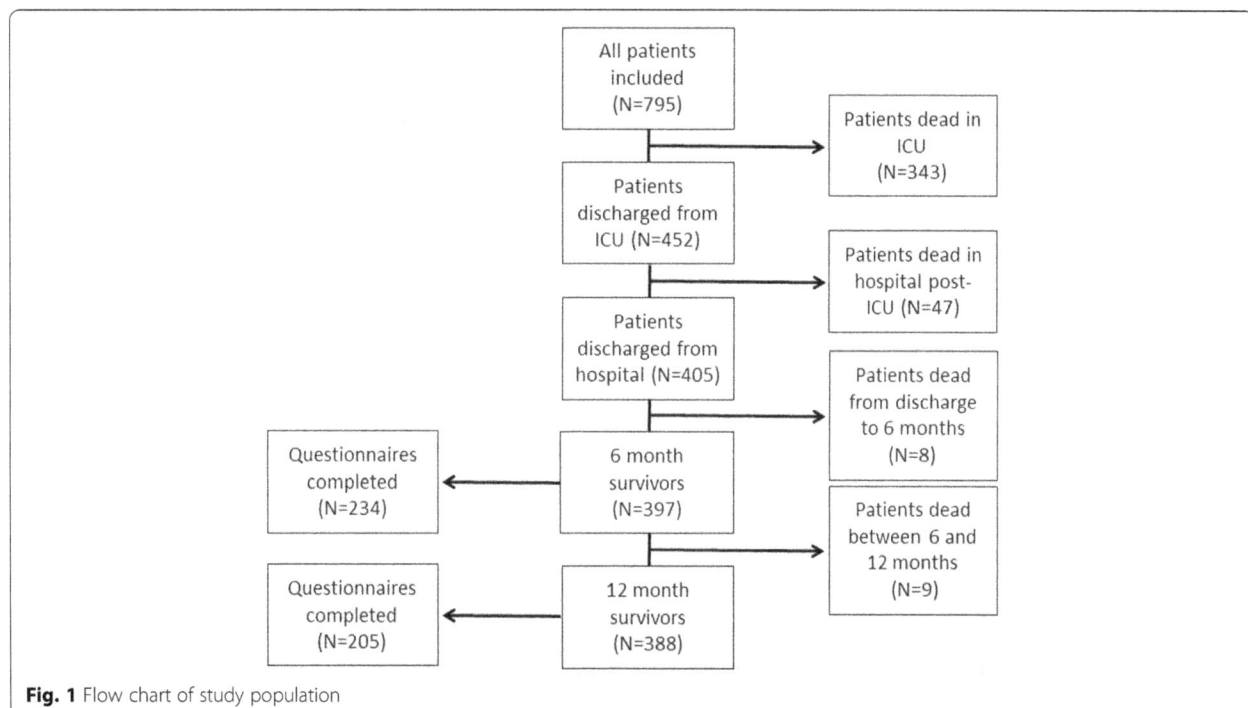

Fig. 1 Flow chart of study population

sex and PaO$_2$:FiO$_2$ ratio by logistic regression. The shape of the Kaplan-Meier curve suggests that the largest differences in mortality rates between these groups are observed within the first 30 days from randomisation and that, after 60 days, mortality rates were relatively low and stable in all groups. There was no significant difference in 1-year survival in the HFOV group as compared to the conventional ventilation group (OR 1.06, 95 % CI 0.79–1.43).

Health-related quality of life of survivors in the different age groups and for an age- and sex-matched population of reference is displayed in Table 2, separately for the 6 and 12 months follow-up. Survivors of ARDS reported significantly lower HRQL than the age- and sex-matched reference population and this difference was more marked in younger (<65 years) patients. Table 3 displays HRQL data at 6 and 12 months in various patient groups. Combining the survival and HRQL information, we obtained a mean quality-adjusted survival at 1 year of 0.27 (0.25–0.29), indicating that for every 100 patients admitted in ICU, 27 QALYs were generated over a 1-year period. Mean QALY over the period was significantly lower for older (≥65) patients and patients with higher (>26) APACHE II score, and higher in the HFOV group, as compared to the conventional ventilation group.

Costs

As shown in Table 4, the mean per-patient cost of initial ICU stay among patients with ARDS was £26,857 (95 % CI £25,222–£28,491) and the average cost per day in ICU was £1738 (95 % CI £1667–£1810). Following initial ICU discharge, the mean cost of hospital stay among ICU survivors was £19,195 (95 % CI £15,936–£22,455) at an average daily cost of £732 (95 % CI £643–£821). Overall, a patient admitted to ICU with ARDS had an expected hospital cost of £37,626 (95 % CI £34,866–£40,385), and the average daily cost of the hospital stay was £1446 (95 % CI £1406–£1486). Following hospital discharge, the average 1-year cost amongst survivors was £7523 (95 % CI £5692–£9354). This comprised costs to the NHS (£3935), including primary and community-based care, hospital and residential stays and equipment and aids paid by the NHS, and costs to the patient and their carers (£3556), including travel costs to and from appointments, earning losses and extra expenses. These estimates were based on complete case analysis. The average 1-year post-hospital cost using multiple imputed data was £6624 (95 % CI £4464–£8784). The mean societal (total) cost at 1 year was £44,077 (95 % CI £41,168–£46,985), and the total societal cost divided by the number of 1-year survivor was £90,206 (this represents the mean 1 year cost of a survivor).

In-hospital resource use in patient subgroups is displayed in Table 5. Although HFOV patients had higher 1-year costs as compared to conventional ventilation patients, the difference was not statistically significant. 1-year survivors with APACHE II score over 22 exhibited higher ICU and hospital costs and had longer hospital stays than less severely ill patients. Overall, the cost of initial ICU stay accounted for 70 % of total hospital costs. As expected, healthcare costs were skewed and exhibited high between-patient variation. We identified 10 patients with extreme (>£200,000) societal costs. These patients were relatively young on average (mean 50 years) and had long hospital stays (mean 193 days).

Discussion

In this multicentre study conducted in 29 hospitals across England, we found that adults admitted to ICU with moderate-to-severe ARDS had high 1-year mortality (51.8 %) and incurred high hospital costs (mean = £37,626; CI £34,866–£40,385). Our results are comparable to those obtained in a multi-country study where the reported daily ICU costs ranged from €1168 to €2025 [51]. However, previous ICU costing studies gave rise to a wide range of daily ICU cost estimates [51, 52], [53] due to an

Table 1 Baseline patient characteristics

Characteristic	All patients (N = 795)	1-year survivors (N = 388)	1-year non-survivors (N = 407)	P value
Age—years [SD]	55.4 [16.8]	50.2 [15.6]	60.4 [16.4]	<0.001
Female—no. (%)	300 (37.7)	148 (38.1)	152 (37.4)	0.8168
APACHE II score [SD]^a	21.8 [6.1]	20.3 [5.7]	23.2 [6.0]	<0.001
PaO2:FiO2 ratio—KPa [SD]	15.1 [5.0]	16.0 [5.2]	14.2 [4.6]	<0.001
Prime condition: Pneumonia/pneumonitis—no. (%)	466 (58.6)	220 (56.7)	246 (60.4)	0.2849
Surgery admission—no. (%)	108 (13.6)	64 (16.5)	44 (10.8)	0.0194
ICU length of stay—days [SD]	17.0 [16.5]	19.7 [15.5]	14.4 [16.9]	<0.001
Hospital length of stay—days [SD]^b	33.6 [43.1]	47.2 [48.6]	20.9 [32.3]	<0.001

APACHE Acute Physiology and Chronic Health Evaluation, *FiO2* fraction of inspired oxygen and *PaO2* partial pressure of arterial oxygen
^{a}APACHE II score calculated for 765 patients only
^{b}Five patients with missing information on hospital discharge

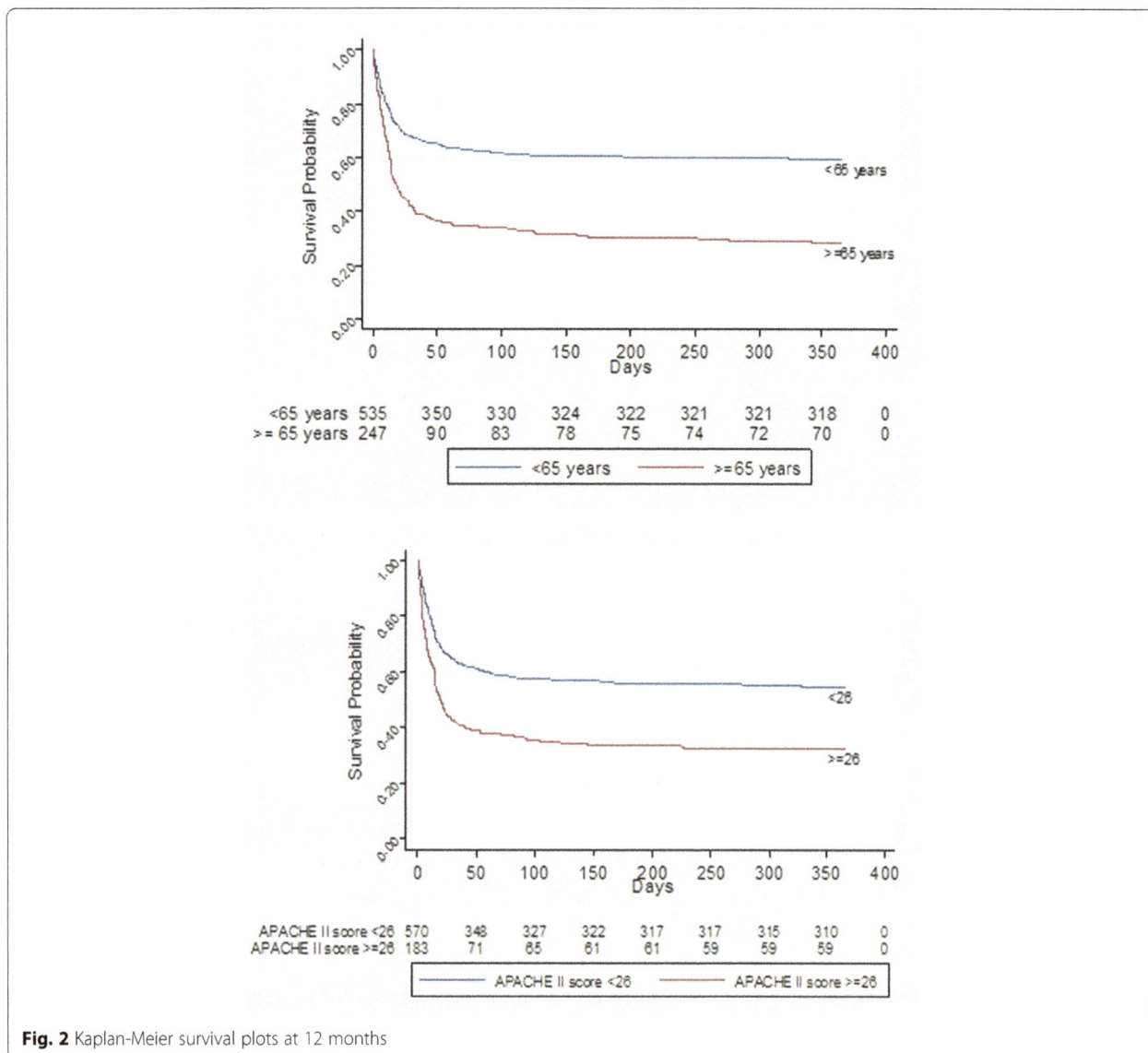

Fig. 2 Kaplan-Meier survival plots at 12 months

important variation in methodological approaches and underlying assumptions. Analyses among survivors revealed lower than normal quality of life and non-negligible resource use and costs following hospital discharge. These were equally split between health and social care costs (mean = £3935; CI £2917–£4953) and costs to the patient and their carers (mean = £3556; CI £2332–£4780). The cost per 1-year survivor was £90,206 (CI £84,536–£96,134), which is higher than figures previously published in ARDS patients [1] possibly due to

Table 2 HRQL of ARDS patients at 6 and 12 months, compared with age- and sex-matched reference values

	ARDS patients	Age- and sex-matched reference values	P value
	Mean (SD)	Mean (SD)	
EQ5D index at 6 months			
Patients under 65	0.55 (0.37)	0.85 (0.06)	<0.001
Patients 65 and above	0.62 (0.37)	0.77 (0.02)	0.003
EQ5D at 12 months			
Patients under 65	0.58 (0.35)	0.85 (0.06)	<0.001
Patients 65 and above	0.58 (0.38)	0.77 (0.02)	<0.001

Table 3 Quality of life

	6 months	12 months	Quality-adjusted survival at 12 months
	Mean EQ5D index (95 % CI)	Mean EQ5D index (95 % CI)	Mean QALY (95 % CI)
All patients	0.5622 (0.5163–0.6081)	0.5831 (0.5348–0.6314)	0.2676 (0.2457–0.2894)
Age			
<65	0.55 (0.49–0.60)	0.58 (0.53-0.64)	0.31 (0.28-0.35)
≥65	0.62 (0.52–0.71)	0.58 (0.48–0.68)	0.16 (0.12–0.21)
Gender			
Male	0.57 (0.51–0.63)	0.58 (0.52–0.64)	0.27 (0.23–0.30)
Female	0.55 (0.47–0.63)	0.59 (0.51–0.67)	0.27 (0.23–0.31)
APACHE II			
<26	0.57 (0.52–0.62)	0.57 (0.52–0.63)	0.29 (0.26–0.33)
≥26	0.48 (0.34–0.61)	0.60 (0.50–0.71)	0.16 (0.12–0.20)
PaO2:FiO2 ratio (KPa)			
<15	0.57 (0.51–0.64)	0.58 (0.51–0.65)	0.23 (0.20–0.27)
≥15	0.55 (0.48–0.63)	0.59 (0.52–0.65)	0.31 (0.27–0.35)
Ventilation method			
Conventional	0.52 (0.45–0.59)	0.55 (0.48–0.61)	0.25 (0.21–0.29)
HFOV	0.61 (0.54–0.67)	0.62 (0.55–0.69)	0.29 (0.25–0.33)

Table 4 Costs in different care pathways

Cost category	N	Mean (95 % CI)	Median	25th Centile	75th Centile
Hospital costs					
Initial ICU stay (all patients)	795				
Total cost		£26,857 (£25,222–£28,491)	£21,067	£11,654	£34,263
Daily cost		£1738 (£1667–£1810)	£1607	£1494	£1760
Post-ICU (ICU survivors)	446				
Total cost		£19,195 (£15,936–£22,455)	£7380	£2673	£20,665
Daily cost		£732 (£643–£821)	£297	£297	£1476
Hospital stay (all patients)	795				
Total cost		£37,626 (£34,866–£40,385)	£25,013	£13,991	£46,802
Daily cost		£1446 (£1406–£1486)	£1516	£1051	£1711
Post-hospital costs (1-year survivors)					
Costs to the NHS[a]	169	£3935 (£2917–£4953)	£1676	£554	£5000
Costs to the patient and their carers[b]	91	£3556 (£2332–£4780)	£395	0	£5411
Patient OOP expenses	169	£93 (£9.6–£176.4)	£0	£0	£0
Patient lost earnings	169	£2836 (£1856–£3816)	£0	£0	£2500
Carer OOP expenses	95	£565 (£305–£824)	£18	£0	£270
Carer lost earnings	93	£503 (£153–£854)	£0	£0	£0
Costs at 1 year (all patients)[c]	795	£44,077 (£41,168–£46,985)	£31,533	£20,415	£53,786
Costs at 1 year (1-year survivors)[c]	388	£54,759 (£50,357–£59,162)	£42,244	£29,170	£63,319
Cost per 1-year survivor[d]	388	£90,206 (£84,536–£96,134)			

[a]Based on 170 patients with questionnaires completed at both 6 and 12 months
[b]Based on 95 carers with questionnaires completed at both 6 and 12 months and based on 91 patients/carer questionnaires with complete information
[c]Post-hospital costs for patients with incomplete information at 6 months and/or 12 months were imputed
[d]Sum of costs among all patients, divided by the number of survivors

Table 5 Resource use in subgroups of patients with ARDS (mean [SD])

	All patients						1-year survivors					
	n	ICU cost £	ICU los days	Hosp. cost £	Hosp. los days	Total societal cost[a] £	n	ICU cost £	ICU los days	Hosp. cost £	Hosp. los days	Total societal cost[a] £
Age (years)												
<65	540	28,173 [1040]	17.8 [0.72]	40,080 [1802]	35.6 [1.8]	46,882 [1817]	318	30,808 [1262]	19.9 [0.87]	47,470 [2465]	45.3 [2.50]	55,041 [2494]
≥65	255	24,070 [1381]	15.6 [1.00]	32,429 [2153]	28.6 [2.2]	38,135 [2172]	70	28,376 [2380]	19.2 [1.85]	46,175 [4023]	52.4 [4.64]	53,481 [4137]
Gender												
Male	495	25,715 [969]	16.3 [0.67]	37,017 [1780]	31.9 [1.57]	43,728 [1804]	240	28,786 [1220]	18.7 [0.85]	46,603 [2719]	45.5 [2.45]	54,425 [2771]
Female	300	28,740 [1530]	18.4 [1.09]	38,630 [2315]	35.8 [2.76]	44,652 [2323]	148	32,938 [2156]	21.5 [1.54]	48,263 [3498]	48.4 [4.26]	55,302 [3517]
APACHE II score												
<26	577	27,160 [917]	17.3 [0.63]	38,740 [1634]	35,3 [1.73]	45,171 [1647]	310	30,058 [1224]	19.7 [0.87]	47,035 [2401]	46.8 [2.5]	54,520 [2423]
≥26	188	26,167 [1909]	16.7 [1.36]	34,226 [2979]	27.9 [2.65]	40,680 [3030]	59	34,338 [3282]	21.8 [2.3]	52,160 [5985]	50.54 [5.85]	59,962 [6194]
PaO2:FiO2 ratio (KPa)												
<15	433	26,271 [1209]	16.6 [0.85]	35,518 [1897]	29.5 [1.78]	41,958 [1926]	183	32,718 [1828]	20.9 [1.3]	50,357 [3255]	45.3 [2.9]	58,010 [3292]
≥15	362	27,557 [1134]	17.8 [0.79]	40,146 [2104]	38.0 [2.28]	46,611 [2110]	205	28,273 [1340]	18.7 [0.94]	44,450 [2827]	47.8 [3.3]	51,857 [2872]
Prime condition												
Pneumonia	466	26,245 [1022]	16.7 [0.71]	36,356 [1874]	29.9 [1.6]	42,537 [1882]	220	29,987 [1380]	19.4 [0.95]	46,480 [3098]	41.7 [2.6]	53,629 [2921]
Other	329	27,723 [1410]	17.8 [1.0]	39,424 [2138]	38.3 [2.5]	46,257 [2174]	168	30,871 [1853]	20.1 [1.3]	48,227 [2849]	53.1 [3.8]	56,239 [2921]
Surgery admission												
No	687	26,883 [892]	17.1 [0.62]	37,104 [1506]	32.0 [1.5]	43,495 [1519]	324	30,700 [1194]	19.9 [0.83]	47,135 [2406]	45.2 [2.4]	54,579 [2440]
Yes	108	26,690 [2404]	17.4 [1.7]	40,942 [4015]	42.1 [4.7]	47,779 [4065]	64	28,695 [3106]	18.9 [2.26]	47,752 [4584]	53.9 [5.61]	55,672 [4636]
Ventilation method												
Conventional	397	25,606 [1110]	16.3 [0.76]	36,148 [1756]	32.5 [1.9]	42,489 [1764]	194	28,588 [1519]	18.3 [1.02]	44,343 [2499]	44.5 [2.96]	51,842 [2522]
HFOV	398	28,105 [1249]	18.0 [0.89]	39,100 [2207]	34.2 [2.1]	45,660 [2234]	194	32,151 [1639]	21.2 [1.20]	50,130 [3480]	48.7 [3.30]	57,677 [3536]
ICU los (1-year survivors)												
≤15	–	–	–	–	–	–	198	–	–	29,071 [1792]	28.7 [1.76]	36,330 [1826]
>15	–	–	–	–	–	–	190	–	–	66,166 [3468]	65.4 [3.67]	73,965 [3509]

[a]Total societal costs estimates based on imputed data for patients with missing post-hospital cost

higher in-hospital mortality in our sample. These figures will be of use to health economic modellers in the future when evaluating ICU interventions; especially given existing evidence for the UK is scarce. Our study revealed heterogeneity in costs across patient groups, especially regarding age and disease severity, but these results were mostly driven by higher short-term mortality in older and more severely ill patients. In line with previous studies [1,

26], we found that hospital costs accounted for the largest share of the economic burden of ARDS at 1 year (81.6 %) and that the length of ICU stay was the main cost driver. However, as previously shown [17, 37], costs can still be important following hospital discharge. Survivors required extensive community-based and social care services, specific aids and equipment and incurred extra expenses related to home adaptations. In addition, indirect costs such as lost earnings caused by employment reductions and the economic value of support from caregivers were non-negligible.

The 1-year mortality was 51.8 % in our sample, which is in line with results reported in previous studies [31]. The mean health-related quality of life of 1-year survivors was significantly lower than the age- and sex-matched reference values, and the difference was particularly marked among younger patients. When survival and quality of life were combined in the full sample, we found low quality-adjusted survival at 1 year. Specifically, we found that 100 patients admitted in ICU with ARDS are expected to accrue 27 QALYs in 1 year, in line with previous estimates [24]. Overall, high mortality combined with poor quality of life among survivors gives rise to low benefit per patient 1 year post-ICU admission and high cost per survivor.

The data used in this study were collected alongside the OSCAR trial of high-frequency oscillatory ventilation (HFOV), as compared to conventional ventilation. The clinical results of the OSCAR trial have shown no significant effect of HFOV on 30-day mortality and showed no short-term benefits or harm of HFOV [12]. In this longer term economic analysis, we found no difference in survival between the HFOV and conventional ventilation group, but we found that patients in the HFOV arm had better quality of life at 6 and 12 months and had higher average costs. A comprehensive cost-effectiveness analysis alongside the OSCAR trial was published elsewhere and found no evidence of cost-effectiveness of HFOV as compared to conventional ventilation [54].

Our study has several limitations that should be noted. First, data on the use of community-based health and social care among survivors were collected retrospectively using self-completed questionnaires, which may have affected the accuracy of the data due to reporting and recall bias [55]. As is inherent with most questionnaire-based research, our study suffered from incomplete return of the quality-of-life and resource use questionnaires. Although partially mitigated against by multiple imputation, our results may therefore be biased if the return rate depends on patient health status. Specifically, if missing data are more prevalent in sicker patients, our cost estimates are likely to be biased downwards and our quality of life estimates upwards. Also, both costs and quality of life estimates were based on a linearity assumption as we had to rely on two data collection points for their calculation. Finally, we restrained our analysis to costs and outcomes incurred over 1 year. Several studies have assessed the long-term benefits of intensive care and found that ICU was a reasonably good use of resources, especially in low-risk patients, i.e. patients with lower disease severity and higher short-term survival [31, 56, 57].

The results presented here are based on longitudinal trial data collected in a large sample of ARDS patients treated in 29 different-sized ICUs, which improves external validity. In addition, the 1-year follow-up period enabled us to capture on-going risk of death beyond the typical "short-term" follow-up periods of similar studies. Additionally, we are among the first to provide estimates of societal costs following ARDS. The estimates presented in this paper, broken down in several patient groups and care settings, will be of use to health economic modellers requiring cost and utility estimates to populate decision-analytical models [58].

Conclusions

Given the high costs and low health-related quality of life identified, there is significant scope for further research aimed at improving care in this in-need patient group.

Abbreviations
APACHE, Acute Physiology, Age, and Chronic Health Evaluation; ARDS, acute respiratory distress syndrome; BNF, British National Formulary; CRF, case report form; EQ-5D, EuroQol-5D; FiO2, fraction of inspired oxygen; HCHS, Hospital and Community Healthcare Services; HFOV, high-frequency oscillatory ventilation; HMRC, HM revenue & Customs; HRQL, health-related quality of life; ICER, incremental cost effectiveness ratio; ICU, intensive care unit; MV, mechanical ventilation; NHS, National Health Service; NIHR, National Institute for Health Research; PaO2, partial pressure of arterial oxygen; PSSRU, Personal Social Services Research Unit; QALY, quality-adjusted life year; SD, standard deviation

Acknowledgements
We thank the study participants and the research team involved in the OSCAR trial.

Funding
This research was funded by the National Institute for Health Research Health Technology Assessment Programme (Award Number 06/04/01); OSCAR Current Controlled Trials number, ISRCTN10416500. This paper presents independent research funded by the National Institute for Health Research (NIHR). The views expressed are those of the author(s) and not necessarily those of the National Health Service (NHS), the NIHR or the Department of Health.

Authors' contributions
JM performed the economic and statistical analyses and drafted the manuscript. PH, PHa and RL participated in the economic and statistical analyses. CH conceived the study and participated in its design and coordination and helped to draft the manuscript. DY, SL, CM and JD participated in the design of the study. All authors read and approved the final manuscript.

Competing interests

Dr Young was a Health Technology Assessment programme commissioning board member during the study and is currently a consultant advisor for the National Institute for Health Research Efficacy and Mechanism Evaluation programme. Professor Hulme is a Health Technology Assessment commissioning board member. Professor Lamb chairs the Health Technology Assessment Clinical Evaluation and Trials Board.

Author details

[1]Centre for Health Policy, Imperial College London, Praed Street, London W2 1NY, UK. [2]Edinburgh Cancer Research Centre, University of Edinburgh, Crewe Road South, Edinburgh EH4 2XR, UK. [3]Central Manchester University Hospitals NHS Foundation Trust, Manchester, UK. [4]Oxford Clinical Trials Unit, University of Oxford, Oxford, UK. [5]Department of Emergency Medicine, University of Alberta, Alberta, Canada. [6]Warwick Clinical Trials Unit, University of Warwick, Coventry, UK. [7]Nuffield Department of Clinical Neurosciences, University of Oxford, Oxford, UK. [8]Academic Unit of Health Economics, University of Leeds, Leeds, UK.

References

1. Angus DC, et al. Healthcare costs and long-term outcomes after acute respiratory distress syndrome: a phase III trial of inhaled nitric oxide. Crit Care Med. 2006;34(12):2883–90.
2. Dasta JF, et al. Daily cost of an intensive care unit day: the contribution of mechanical ventilation*. Crit Care Med. 2005;33(6):1266–71.
3. Rossi C, et al. Variable costs of ICU patients: a multicenter prospective study. Intensive Care Med. 2006;32(4):545–52.
4. Brun-Buisson C, et al. Epidemiology and outcome of acute lung injury in European intensive care units. Intensive Care Med. 2004;30(1):51–61.
5. Carson SS. Outcomes of prolonged mechanical ventilation. Curr Opin Crit Care. 2006;12(5):405–11.
6. Cox CE, et al. Surviving critical illness: acute respiratory distress syndrome as experienced by patients and their caregivers. Crit Care Med. 2009;37(10):2702–8.
7. Derdak S, et al. High-frequency oscillatory ventilation for acute respiratory distress syndrome in adults: a randomized, controlled trial. Am J Respir Crit Care Med. 2002;166(6):801–8.
8. Rubenfeld GD, Herridge MS. Epidemiology and outcomes of acute lung injury. CHEST Journal. 2007;131(2):554–62.
9. Davidson TA, et al. Reduced quality of life in survivors of acute respiratory distress syndrome compared with critically ill control patients. JAMA. 1999; 281(4):354–60.
10. Tremblay LN, Slutsky AS. Applied physiology in intensive care medicine 1. Berlin Heidelberg: Springer; 2012. p. 343–52.
11. Ferguson ND, et al. High-frequency oscillation in early acute respiratory distress syndrome. N Engl J Med. 2013;368(9):795–805.
12. Young D, et al. High-frequency oscillation for acute respiratory distress syndrome. N Engl J Med. 2013;368(9):806–13.
13. Detsky ME, Stewart TE. Long-term outcomes of patients after acute respiratory distress syndrome: Hard work for nothing? Minerva Anestesiol. 2010;76(8):641–4. ordered 04.10.12.
14. Fessler HE, Hess DR. Does high-frequency ventilation offer benefits over conventional ventilation in adult patients with acute respiratory distress syndrome? Respir Care. 2007;52(5):595–605.
15. Griffiths JA, Gager M, Waldmann C. Follow-up after intensive care. Continuing Education in Anaesthesia, Critical Care & Pain. 2004;4(6):202–5.
16. Ip T, Mehta S. The role of high-frequency oscillatory ventilation in the treatment of acute respiratory failure in adults. Curr Opin Crit Care. 2012;18(1):70–9.
17. Wilcox ME, Herridge MS. Long-term outcomes in patients surviving acute respiratory distress syndrome. Semin Respir Crit Care Med. 2010;31(1):55–65. ordered 04.10.2012.
18. Cooper AB, et al. Long-term follow-up of survivors of acute lung injury: lack of effect of a ventilation strategy to prevent barotrauma. Crit Care Med. 1999;27(12):2616–21.
19. Herridge MS. Recovery and long-term outcome in acute respiratory distress syndrome. Crit Care Clin. 2011;27(3):685–704. ordered 04.10.2012.
20. Herridge MS, et al. One-year outcomes in survivors of the acute respiratory distress syndrome. N Engl J Med. 2003;348(8):683–93.
21. Hopkins RO, et al. Neuropsychological sequelae and impaired health status in survivors of severe acute respiratory distress syndrome. Am J Respir Crit Care Med. 1999;160(1):50–6.
22. Rothenhausler HB, et al. The relationship between cognitive performance and employment and health status in long-term survivors of the acute respiratory distress syndrome: results of an exploratory study. Gen Hosp Psychiatry. 2001;23(2):90–6.
23. Schelling G, et al. Health-related quality of life and posttraumatic stress disorder in survivors of the acute respiratory distress syndrome. Crit Care Med. 1998;26(4):651–9.
24. Angus DC, et al. Quality-adjusted survival in the first year after the acute respiratory distress syndrome. Am J Respir Crit Care Med. 2001;163(6):1389–94.
25. Chelluri L, et al. Long-term mortality and quality of life after prolonged mechanical ventilation*. Crit Care Med. 2004;32(1):61–9.
26. Cheung AM, et al. Two-year outcomes, health care use, and costs of survivors of acute respiratory distress syndrome. Am J Respir Crit Care Med. 2006;174(5):538–44.
27. Combes A, et al. Morbidity, mortality, and quality-of-life outcomes of patients requiring > or = 14 days of mechanical ventilation. Crit Care Med. 2003;31(5):1373–81.
28. Cuthbertson BH, et al. Quality of life in the five years after intensive care: a cohort study. Critical Care (London, England). 2010;14(1):R6.
29. Heyland DK, Groll D, Caeser M. Survivors of acute respiratory distress syndrome: relationship between pulmonary dysfunction and long-term health-related quality of life. Crit Care Med. 2005;33(7):1549–56.
30. Hodgson CL, et al. Long-term quality of life in patients with acute respiratory distress syndrome requiring extracorporeal membrane oxygenation for refractory hypoxaemia. Crit Care. 2012;16(5):R202.
31. Linko R, et al. One-year mortality, quality of life and predicted life-time cost-utility in critically ill patients with acute respiratory failure. Crit Care. 2010;14(2):1–9.
32. Schelling G, et al. Pulmonary function and health-related quality of life in a sample of long-term survivors of the acute respiratory distress syndrome. Intensive Care Med. 2000;26(9):1304–11.
33. Gilbertson AA, Smith JM, Mostafa SM. The cost of an intensive care unit: a prospective study. Intensive Care Med. 1991;17(4):204–8.
34. Valta P, et al. Acute respiratory distress syndrome: frequency, clinical course, and costs of care. Crit Care Med. 1999;27(11):2367–74.
35. Graf J, et al. Health care costs, long-term survival, and quality of life following intensive care unit admission after cardiac arrest. Crit Care. 2008;12(4):R92.
36. Peek GJ, et al. Efficacy and economic assessment of conventional ventilatory support versus extracorporeal membrane oxygenation for severe adult respiratory failure (CESAR): a multicentre randomised controlled trial. Lancet (London, England). 2009;374(9698):1351–63.
37. Kress JP, Herridge MS. Medical and economic implications of physical disability of survivorship. Semin Respir Crit Care Med. 2012;33(4):339–47. ordered 04.10.2012.
38. EuroQol G. EuroQol—a new facility for the measurement of health-related quality of life. Health policy (Amsterdam, Netherlands). 1990;16(3):199.
39. Kind P, Hardman G, Macran S. UK population norms for EQ-5D, vol. 172. York: University of York UK; 1999. Centre for Health Economics.
40. Billingham L, Abrams K. Simultaneous analysis of quality of life and survival data. Stat Methods Med Res. 2002;11(1):25–48.
41. Lipscomb J, et al. Health care costing: data, methods, current applications. Medical care. 2009;47(7_Supplement_1):S1–6.
42. Jegers M, et al. Definitions and methods of cost assessment: an intensivist's guide. Intensive Care Med. 2002;28(6):680–5.
43. McLaughlin AM, et al. Determining the economic cost of ICU treatment: a prospective "micro-costing" study. Intensive Care Med. 2009;35(12):2135–40.
44. NHS Reference Costs 2011 to 2012. Available from: https://www.gov.uk/government/publications/nhs-reference-costs-financial-year-2011-to-2012. Accessed Nov 2014.
45. Committee, J.F. British National Formulary. 64th ed. London: BMJ Group and Pharmaceutical Press; 2012.
46. Excellence, N.I.f.H.a.C. Rehabilitation after critical illness. Clinical Guidelines CG83. London: National Institute for Health and Clinical Excellence; 2009.
47. Curtis L. Unit costs of health and social care. 2012. Personal Social Services Research Unit.

48. HMRC. Approved mileage rates 2011/2012. Available from: http://www.
    hmrc.gov.uk/rates/travel.htm. Accessed Nov 2014.
49. Torrance GW, Drummond MF. Methods for the economic evaluation of
    health care programmes. Oxford: Oxford university press; 2005.
50. Rubin DB. Multiple imputation after 18+ years. J Am Stat Assoc. 1996;
    91(434):473–89.
51. Tan SS, et al. Direct cost analysis of intensive care unit stay in four European
    countries: applying a standardized costing methodology. Value Health.
    2012;15(1):81–6.
52. Moerer O, et al. A German national prevalence study on the cost of
    intensive care: an evaluation from 51 intensive care units. Critical Care
    (London, England). 2007;11(3):R69.
53. Cooper LM, Linde-Zwirble WT. Medicare intensive care unit use: analysis of
    incidence, cost, and payment*. Crit Care Med. 2004;32(11):2247–53.
54. Lall R, et al. A randomised controlled trial and cost-effectiveness analysis of
    high-frequency oscillatory ventilation against conventional artificial
    ventilation for adults with acute respiratory distress syndrome. 2015. The
    OSCAR (OSCillation in ARDS) study.
55. Bhandari A, Wagner T. Self-reported utilization of health care services:
    improving measurement and accuracy. Med Care Res Rev. 2006;63(2):217–35.
56. Cox CE, et al. An economic evaluation of prolonged mechanical ventilation.
    Crit Care Med. 2007;35(8):1918–27.
57. Ridley S, Morris S. Cost effectiveness of adult intensive care in the UK.
    Anaesthesia. 2007;62(6):547–54.
58. Alsarraf AA, Fowler R. Health, economic evaluation, and critical care. J Crit
    Care. 2005;20(2):194–7.

Use of wearable devices for post-discharge monitoring of ICU patients

Ryan R. Kroll[1†], Erica D. McKenzie[2†], J. Gordon Boyd[1,3], Prameet Sheth[4], Daniel Howes[1,5], Michael Wood[6], David M. Maslove[1,3,7*] and for the WEARable Information Technology for hospital INpatients (WEARIT-IN) study group

Abstract

Background: Wearable devices generate signals detecting activity, sleep, and heart rate, all of which could enable detailed and near-continuous characterization of recovery following critical illness.

Methods: To determine the feasibility of using a wrist-worn personal fitness tracker among patients recovering from critical illness, we conducted a prospective observational study of a convenience sample of 50 stable ICU patients. We assessed device wearability, the extent of data capture, sensitivity and specificity for detecting heart rate excursions, and correlations with questionnaire-derived sleep quality measures.

Results: Wearable devices were worn over a 24-h period, with excellent capture of data. While specificity for the detection of tachycardia was high (98.8%), sensitivity was low to moderate (69.5%). There was a moderate correlation between wearable-derived sleep duration and questionnaire-derived sleep quality ($r = 0.33$, $P = 0.03$). Devices were well-tolerated and demonstrated no degradation in quality of data acquisition over time.

Conclusions: We found that wearable devices could be worn by patients recovering from critical illness and could generate useful data for the majority of patients with little adverse effect. Further development and study are needed to better define and enhance the role of wearables in the monitoring of post-ICU recovery.

Keywords: Wearable devices, Medical informatics, Mobile health technologies, Validation study, Critical care, Sleep quality, Heart rate monitoring

Background

Consumer interest in personal health tracking has recently increased, leading to an industry in wearable devices now valued at more than $9 billion worldwide [1]. With more wearables in use than ever before, there has been growing enthusiasm for their potential to improve health care delivery [2]. Current clinical uses for wearable devices are mostly limited to outpatient settings, with a focus on the management of chronic diseases [3–5]. Newer generation

devices generate data that could also be useful in characterizing convalescence from acute illness. These include photoplethysmography (PPG) sensors to detect heart rate [6, 7], as well as accelerometers to track activity and movement [3, 8, 9].

Frequent heart rate tracking has the potential to identify episodes of clinical deterioration early. Accelerometer data could potentially be used to encourage mobilization, objectively measure functional status, and track progress towards rehabilitation goals. Wrist-worn accelerometers have also been used to evaluate sleep quality in healthy subjects [10, 11]. In the inpatient and intensive care unit (ICU) settings, where poor sleep has been linked with adverse outcomes [12, 13], data describing sleep quality

* Correspondence: david.maslove@queensu.ca

†Equal contributors

[1]Department of Critical Care Medicine, Queen's University and Kingston Health Sciences Centre, Kingston, Ontario, Canada

[3]Department of Medicine, Queen's University and Kingston Health Sciences Centre, Kingston, Ontario, Canada

Full list of author information is available at the end of the article

may be useful in identifying targets for sleep-promoting interventions [14].

There is little clinical evidence to inform the practice of using wearables in health care, most of which is focused on chronic conditions. Newer consumer-grade wearables have been evaluated in only a handful of studies examining their accuracy among healthy volunteers [3–5]. These studies have called for evaluations of this technology among a wider range of patient populations.

In this study, we examine the feasibility of using a common consumer-grade wearable device to monitor patients recovering from critical illness. We enrolled patients who no longer required intensive care measures but remained in the ICU prior to ward transfer, in order to best approximate post-ICU settings like the general wards, while still collecting gold standard data to validate device functionality. We report on a number of practical considerations that could affect the deployment of wearables including overall wearability, completeness of data capture, device longevity, and risk of transmitting nosocomial infections. We also evaluated the accuracy of wearables for measuring sleep quality and identifying changes in heart rate that might be clinically relevant. We hypothesized that patients recovering from critical illness would be able to wear wrist-worn devices and that useful data could be collected from these with a moderate degree of accuracy.

Methods

Patients and setting

This prospective observational study was conducted in a 33-bed general medical-surgical/trauma ICU in southeastern Ontario, between August 2015 and February 2016. Adult patients (age > 17) were included if they were receiving continuous cardiac and oxygen saturation monitoring, but were otherwise receiving ward-level treatment. Exclusion criteria included mechanical ventilation, vasopressor support, and continuous sedation or analgesia. We specifically chose to study patients who were still in the ICU, as this was the most practical way to obtain gold standard measurements of heart rate and sleep quality, which would otherwise require the use of Holter monitors and complex follow-up procedures. To reduce the potential risk of transmitting nosocomial infections, patients under contact precautions for methicillin-resistant *Staphylococcus aureus* (MRSA) and *Clostridium difficile* infections were also excluded. We also excluded patients at risk of vascular compromise of the arm on which the wearable device was to be placed, such as patients with upper extremity deep venous thrombosis, peripherally inserted central catheters, radial arterial lines, dialysis fistulas, and severe upper extremity trauma. As this was a feasibility study, a convenience sample of 50 participants was recruited.

Ethics, consent, and permissions

All participating patients, or substitute decision makers on their behalf, provided written informed consent for participation in this study. The Health Sciences Research Ethics Board at Queen's University reviewed and approved the study protocol (DMED-1818-15), and the trial was registered with clinicaltrials.gov (NCT02527408).

Device

Participating patients wore the Fitbit Charge HR device (Fitbit, San Francisco, CA, USA) for a single 24-h period (Fig. 1). The Fitbit Charge HR is a commercially available wrist-worn wearable that records heart rate, steps, and sleep quality. The study employed three size large wearable devices (15.7 to 19.3 cm wrist circumference) and three size extra-large wearable devices (19.6 to 22.6 cm wrist circumference). In an effort to reduce the risk of potential iatrogenic infection, we used disinfectant wipes to thoroughly clean wearables between uses. All devices were applied to participants by a study investigator or coordinator.

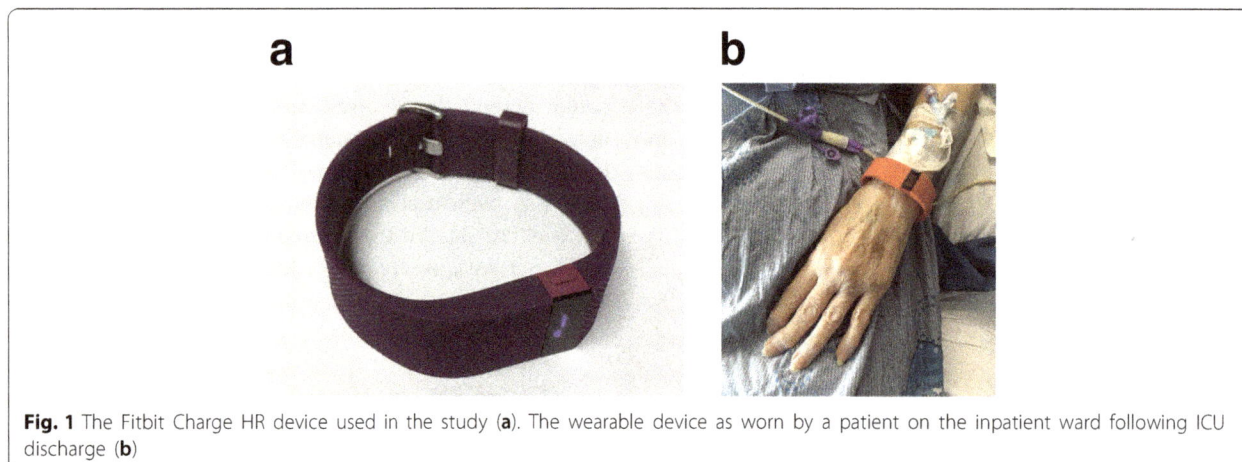

a　　　　　　　　　　**b**

Fig. 1 The Fitbit Charge HR device used in the study (**a**). The wearable device as worn by a patient on the inpatient ward following ICU discharge (**b**)

Data monitoring and capture

We used continuous pulse oximetry pulse rate recordings (SPO2-R) as a comparison measure of heart rate (HR) in order to evaluate the ability of wearables to detect both tachycardia (HR > 100 bpm) and bradycardia (HR < 50 bpm). We used SPO2-R values as a comparator as both SPO2-R and wearable device values reflect the pulse rate (rather than electrical heart rate), and because this is a widely accepted method of heart rate measurement. The wearables recorded heart rate values every 5 min, while the SPO2-R recorded heart rate values every minute. Cardiac rhythm was assessed at the time of device application, and again at the time of removal, at which time data regarding sleep quality was also collected using the Richards-Campbell Sleep Questionnaire (RCSQ) [15]. This survey uses a visual analog scale to assess sleep depth, latency, awakenings, percentage of time awake, and overall quality of sleep. The RCSQ was completed either by the patients themselves or by their designated night shift nurse, a practice previously shown to have slight to moderate agreement with self-assessment [16]. Due to the interaction between sleep and delirium in the ICU [17], patients were screened for delirium by a trained researcher using the confusion assessment method (CAM)-ICU at the time of device application, and again at the time of device removal.

Wearable-reported sleep data included time of sleep onset and awakening, sleep duration, minutes asleep, minutes awake, restless count, and a calculated measure of sleep quality. Overall sleep quality was taken as the average across sleep episodes, weighted by the duration of each sleep episode. The percentage of total sleep occurring during nighttime hours, which we defined as 22:00 to 06:00, and the percentage of nighttime hours spent asleep were calculated. For participants who had no Fitbit-detected sleep over the recording period, a score of 0 was given for all sleep parameters. Methods for obtaining wearable and SPO2-R data are reported elsewhere [18], and in the Supplementary Content (see Additional file 1).

Microbiological assessment

We conducted microbiologic sampling of the wearables used from a convenience subset of patients ($n = 16$) in order to evaluate both the risk of transmitting nosocomial pathogens from repeated application of wearables to different patients, as well as the efficacy of our disinfection practices (see Additional file 1).

Statistical analysis

In the absence of preliminary data to inform a sample size calculation, we targeted an enrollment of 50 patients, a cohort size equal to that used in a similar study of wrist-worn wearables for heart rate tracking in healthy volunteers [5]. In addition to basic descriptive statistics, we calculated the sensitivity and specificity of the wearables for detecting tachycardia and bradycardia. Based on the PPG mechanism of heart rate sensing employed in consumer-grade wearables, we hypothesized that the accuracy of wearable device heart rate tracking may be different in patients not in sinus rhythm and further analyzed these patients as a subgroup. We calculated Pearson correlation coefficients between the various wearable-derived measures of sleep quality and the RCSQ measures of sleep quality. Based on the mechanism of sleep sensing, which relies on the absence of movement, we hypothesized that the accuracy of wearables for sleep tracking may differ in patients with delirium, and further analyzed these patients as a subgroup. Statistical analyses for this study were performed using R (v 3.2.2).

Results

Patients and device wearability

We enrolled a total of 50 patients between August 2015 and January 2016 (Table 1). The median wrist circumference in our cohort was 18.6 cm (SD 1.9 cm), with 6 of the 50 patients enrolled having moderate or severe edema of the wrist at the time of device application. The size large device was used for 23 patients (46%), while the size extra-large was used for 27 patients (54%). While there were no patients for whom the wearable device could not be fitted, the fit was noted to be very tight

Table 1 Characteristics of patients included in the study ($n = 50$)

Mean heart rate (bpm)	88.3	
Mean age (years)	64	
	Patients ($n = 50$)	%
Male	26	52
Female	24	48
Admission diagnosis		
Respiratory	12	24
Sepsis	7	14
Surgical	7	14
Neurologic	11	22
Trauma	3	6
Cardiovascular	6	12
Medical	4	8
Sinus rhythm		
At start of monitoring	43	86
At end of monitoring	42	84
Personal fitness tracker size used		
Large	23	46
Extra large	27	54

in one patient, and very loose in two patients. Devices were adjusted only once at the time of application and were not re-assessed by study personnel for the duration of the 24-h recording period. No intravenous lines were re-sited in order to facilitate application, although hospital identification wristbands had to be relocated in some cases. No wearables required removal during the monitoring period as a result of patient discomfort. The wearable device was removed prior to the completion of the monitoring period in two patients; one patient was discharged earlier than expected from the ICU, while another developed a diffuse drug-associated rash. Excluding patients whose devices were removed early, the devices were unable to detect a heart rate reading 4% of the time.

Tachycardia and bradycardia detection

We identified 13 SPO2-R-confirmed readings of bradycardia among four patients, all of whom were in sinus rhythm. Further statistical analysis was not done due to this small sample. The wearable had a sensitivity of 69.5% and specificity of 98.8% for the detection of tachycardia (Table 2 and Fig. 2). Among patients not in sinus rhythm ($n = 8$), the specificity for detecting tachycardia was similar (99.5%), although sensitivity was worse (51.6%). For faster heart rates (> 150 bpm), wearable device concordance with SPO2-R was poor. However, in many such cases, the wearable device reading showed better agreement with the true heart rate measured by continuous ECG, than did the SPO2-R readings, which tended to be falsely high.

Sleep data

A summary of the sleep quality data collected by the wearables is shown in Table 3. Among the 47 participants who had complete wearable sleep data recorded, the median wearable-reported sleep duration was 6.6 h (interquartile range [IQR] 2.7–13.5 h) and the median number of sleep periods was 2 (IQR 1–4). Five participants (11%) had no wearable device documented sleep for the entirety of the 24-h monitoring period. Among the 43 participants for whom the RCSQ was completed, the median total score was

Table 2 Test performance characteristics for personal fitness tracker detection of tachycardia, as compared to SPO2-R

	Sinus rhythm	Atrial fibrillation
Sensitivity	0.695	0.516
Specificity	0.988	0.995
Positive predictive value	0.948	0.983
Negative predictive value	0.914	0.804
Accuracy	0.92	0.836

5.7/10.0 (IQR 2.7–8.0/10.0). There was a moderate correlation between wearable-derived sleep duration and total RCSQ score ($r = 0.33$, $P = 0.03$, 95% confidence interval [CI] 0.04, 0.58) (Fig. 3). The correlation between the percentage of nighttime asleep, as reported by the wearable device, and total RCSQ score was 0.36 ($P = 0.02$, 95% CI 0.07, 0.60). The correlation between the Fitbit-reported number of sleep periods and RCSQ-reported awakenings was 0.38 ($P = 0.01$, 95% CI 0.09, 0.61). There were no significant differences in wearable-reported sleep parameters between the CAM-ICU positive ($n = 8$) and CAM-ICU negative participants; however, 25% of CAM-ICU positive participants recorded no sleep over the entire 24-h monitoring period, compared to 8% of CAM-ICU negative participants.

Device reusability

Wearables were not found to be a significant source of pathogenic bacteria. Microbiologic sampling revealed bacteria consistent with commensal skin flora (*Staphylococcus epidermidis*) and/or environmental organisms (*Bacillus* species). *S. epidermidis* was only observed in samples taken prior to hydrogen peroxide disinfection, while *Bacillus* species were found in both pre- and post-disinfection specimens. Individual wearable devices were used between 5 and 13 times. There were no differences in wearable-SPO2-R heart rate correlations between the first and second half of the study ($P = 0.18$).

Discussion

The long-term adverse consequences of critical illness are increasingly being recognized as a research priority in critical care [19]. A growing body of research is now examining the determinants and potential modifiers of post-ICU recovery, including at least one study that made use of a wearable device to track patient movement and activity [20]. However, post-ICU recovery research currently lacks the richness of data available to researchers focused on the ICU stay itself since post-discharge data collection is limited to infrequent visits to follow-up clinics, or in many cases is nonexistent. New strategies are needed to collect data—ideally on a continuous basis—that better describes ICU recovery on the wards and in the patient's home environment.

To this end, we undertook an observational study to determine the feasibility of using a commercial-grade wearable device to monitor recovery after critical illness. Overall, the device was well tolerated and captured the vast majority of available data. For the detection of tachycardia, we found the wearable delivered high specificity and positive predictive value, but only low to moderate sensitivity. Much of the undercounting of fast heart rates

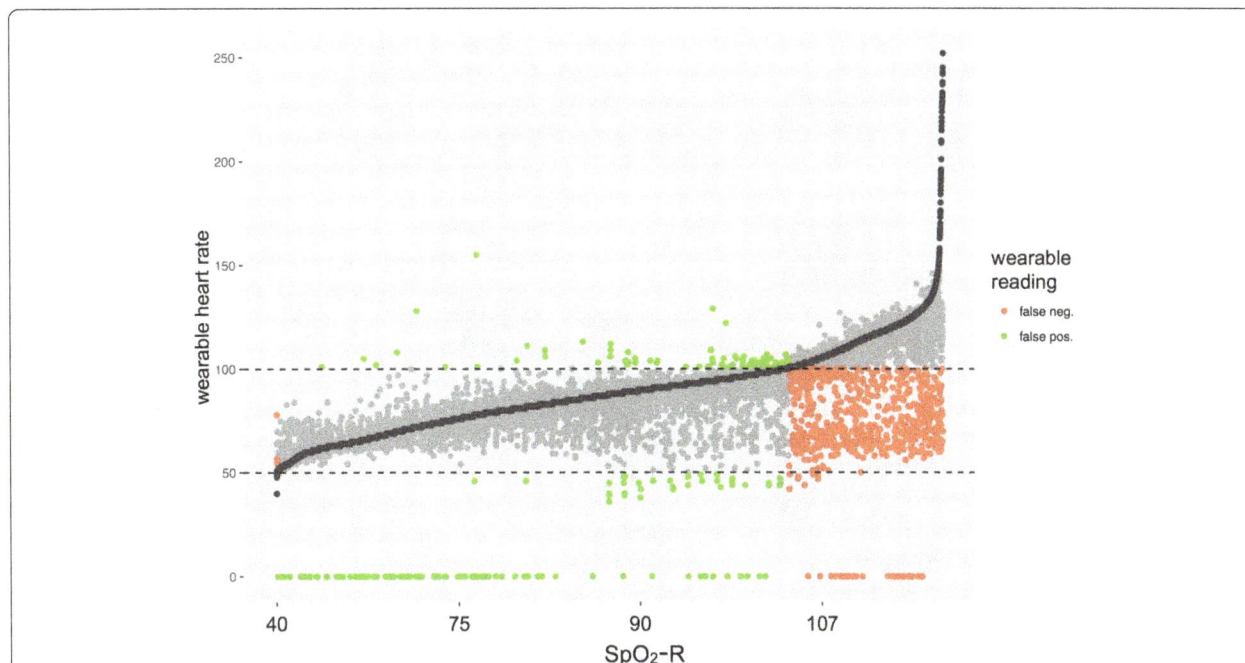

Fig. 2 Accuracy of wearable-derived heart rates for the detection of tachycardia (HR > 100) or bradycardia (HR < 50) as determined by SPO2 heart rates. The SPO2-derived values (dark gray) are shown sorted from lowest to highest heart rate. The corresponding wearable-derived heart rate is shown in either light gray (correct classification), green (false positive), or red (false negative). The majority of misclassified heart rates are false negatives for the detection of tachycardia. Some misclassification is due to wearable device readings of "0," reflecting data not captured by the device

by the wearable device was seen in patients who were not in sinus rhythm during at least some portion of the monitoring period. Compared to a validated sleep questionnaire, the wearable device had a moderate correlation with several metrics of sleep quality. Device performance

Table 3 Summary of wearable-reported and RCSQ sleep parameters

	Median	(IQR)
Wearable		
Total sleep duration, hours	6.6	(2.7–13.5)
Asleep time, hours	6.1	(2.6–12.5)
Restless count	7	(2.5–19.0)
Sleep quality A	45.8	(38.0–63.5)
# Sleep periods	2	(1.0–4.0)
22:00–6:00 sleep as % of total	50%	(15–80%)
% of 22:00–6:00 asleep	48%	(3–84%)
RCSQ		
Mean score	5.7	(2.7–8.0)
1. Sleep depth	5	(3.2–7.6)
2. Sleep latency	6.2	(2.7–8.9)
3. Awakening	5	(2.6–8.6)
4. Returning to sleep	6.4	(2.1–9.1)
5. Sleep quality	5.7	(1.6–8.6)

RCSQ Richards-Campbell Sleep Questionnaire

did not appear to degrade over time. The wearables studied did not appear to be a significant source of nosocomial pathogens, although the presence of *Bacillus* species even after device cleaning suggests that spore-forming organisms could persist on some devices. Whether or not wearables would have to be reused at all would depend on their costs—which currently are relatively low—compared to the potential cost savings achieved with better clinical outcomes. The use of wearables to monitor convalescence after ICU discharge will ultimately pertain to patients who no longer require the resources of heavily monitored settings. To that end, our results are generalizable to a large contingent of patients, including post-ICU patients cared for on the wards, as well as those who have been discharged home.

In addition to their potential use following an ICU admission, wearables may also play a role in monitoring inpatients for signs of clinical deterioration, so as to identify as soon as possible any patient needing a higher level of care. Early Warning Systems (EWS) have been developed to address a "failure to rescue" problem, in which critical illness is identified too late [21]. Wearable devices stand to enhance data collection and monitoring both prior to and following an ICU admission, and as such is of growing importance in critical care research.

Interest in the clinical use of wearable devices and mobile health technology is increasing [2, 22]. While clinical evaluations of this technology remain scarce, some

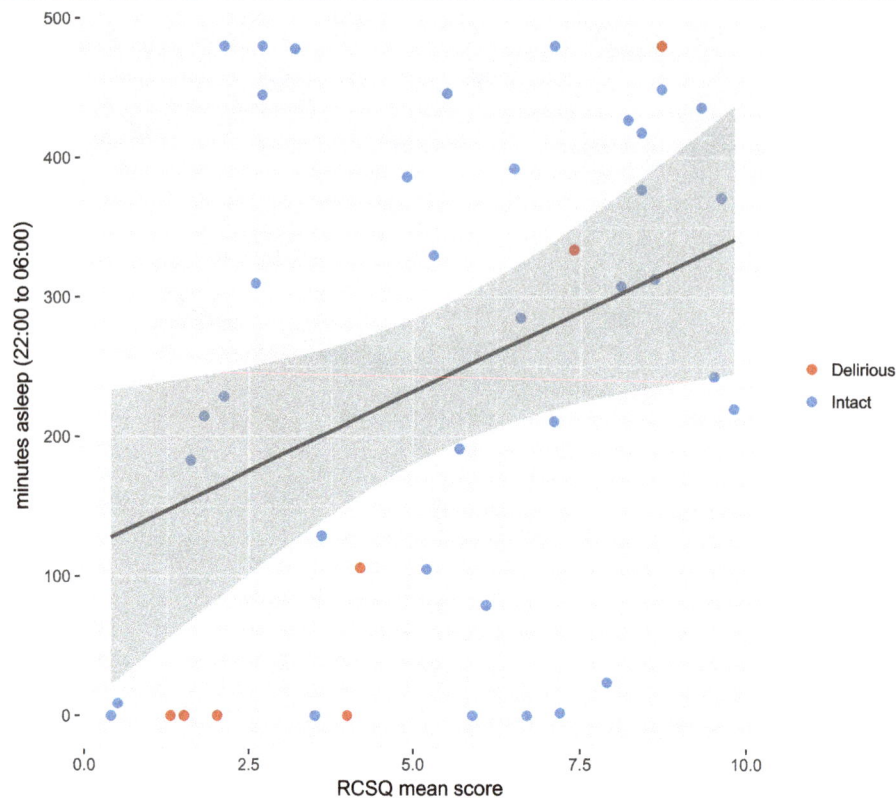

Fig. 3 Correlation between mean score on the Richards-Campbell Sleep Questionnaire (RCSQ) and wearable-derived measure of the number of minutes asleep overnight (between 22:00 and 06:00). The Pearson correlation coefficient was 0.33 (95% CI 0.04 - 0.58)

rigorous evaluations have been reported among healthy volunteers [4, 5] and among outpatients [23]. To our knowledge, this is the first study to examine the feasibility of using commercially available wearable devices among hospital inpatients to evaluate for heart rate derangements and sleep quality.

Wearables have the potential to become a useful tool in the early detection of critical illness. Heart rate is factored into the majority of EWS algorithms [24–28], and while the role of an EWS in reducing mortality remains unclear, there is evidence to suggest that these systems may be helpful [24]. Changes in heart rate may also portend changes in clinical status among ICU survivors on the wards or following hospital discharge. In this study, the high specificity but low to moderate sensitivity identified for the detection of tachycardia suggests that as currently configured, wearable-derived heart rate tracking would be highly specific, thereby mitigating alarm fatigue, but may lack sensitivity in some situations, resulting in missed detection of heart rate excursions. Ultimately, further confirmatory studies are required, which should also investigate alternate approaches to event detection, such as those based on proportional changes in heart rate. One potential limitation of wearable-enabled heart rate monitoring is a direct result of the PPG-based sensing mechanism employed, which may perform poorly in patients with a pulse deficit, such as those in atrial fibrillation.

Hospitalized patients often have a severely disrupted sleep, which may impair recovery [12]. Illness, medications, around-the-clock care activities, and environmental light and noise may contribute to perturbed sleep. Consumer-grade wearables with sleep monitoring capabilities could facilitate the routine evaluation of sleep among inpatients and the assessment of sleep-promoting interventions. Resource-intensive polysomnography (PSG) is impractical for routine sleep monitoring, and compliance with sleep questionnaires and sleep diaries is poor among inpatients [29]. Continuous data collection from wearables is passive and unobtrusive, and wearables are far less expensive than both PSG equipment and standard actigraphy devices.

Two recent studies have compared commercial-grade wearables with PSG in healthy subjects [10, 11]. Mantua et al. found a strong correlation in total sleep time between wearable-derived data and PSG, and De Zambotti et al. found good agreement between wearables and PSG in measuring sleep, despite slight but significant overestimation of total sleep by the wearable devices. Altered sleep and activity patterns among inpatients may decrease the accuracy of wearables, which rely on movement to determine wakefulness, and could overestimate sleep in inpatients, who may be awake but immobile for long periods. The wearable device used in our study only counts periods of inactivity that exceed one hour as sleep, and may not capture fragmented naps, which are common in critically ill patients [30, 31].

Our study has a number of limitations that should be considered in interpreting the results. Conclusions regarding the influence of non-sinus rhythm on the accuracy of heart rate monitoring are limited by the relatively low prevalence of this condition in the study cohort, as are the findings relating sleep with delirium, which also had a low prevalence. While we considered the absence of sleep quality measures reported to indicate an absence of sleep during the monitoring period, an alternate interpretation is that these conditions reflect a failure of data capture. It is worth noting, however, that for the cases included that recorded no sleep data, heart rate data was successfully collected, making a failure of data capture an unlikely explanation for these findings. Lastly, differences between the internal clocks of the wearables and bedside monitors may have resulted in asynchronous heart rate recordings being treated as simultaneous, although correction factors were used in the analysis, and the time differences observed were shorter than the 5 min sampling interval of the wearable device.

Conclusions

In this observational study, we compared heart rate and sleep data recorded from a commercial-grade wearable device, with data from cardiac telemetry and sleep questionnaires. Devices showed high specificity and moderate sensitivity for the detection of tachycardia, with better performance in patients in sinus rhythm. Sleep quality metrics were moderately correlated with questionnaire data.

Future research in this area should focus on improving tachycardia detection, evaluating patients on the wards and at home, integrating wearable-derived data into the study of ICU recovery, and determining the impact of integrating wearable devices into hospital-wide EWS or rapid response services. Patients with arrhythmias should be studied as a subgroup in order to better define the accuracy of wearable-based heart rate sensing in this population. Further validation of sleep quality accuracy using other comparators such as PSG or conventional actigraphy would be useful, as would assessments of the accuracy of activity tracking.

Additional file

Additional file 1: Details regarding microbiologic assessment of the wearable devices as well as specifics regarding wearble device data capture and analysis. (PDF 49 kb)

Abbreviations
CAM: Confusion Assessment Method; ECG: Electrocardiography; EWS: Early Warning System; HR: Heart rate; ICU: Intensive care unit; MRSA: Methicillin-resistant *Staphylococcus aureus*; PPG: Photoplethysmography; PSG: Polysomnography; RCSQ: Richards-Campbell Sleep Questionnaire; SPO2-R: Pulse oximetry pulse rate recordings (SPO2-R)

Acknowledgements
The authors wish to thank Miranda Hunt, Ilinca Georgescu, Tracy Boyd, and the nursing staff in the ICU at Kingston General Hospital.

Funding
This work was supported by an Innovation Fund award from the Southeastern Ontario Academic Medical Organization (SEAMO). Drs. Maslove and Boyd are supported by New Clinician Scientists awards from SEAMO.

Authors' contributions
RRK participated in primary data collection and analysis, data interpretation, and contributed to the drafting of the manuscript. EDM contributed to the analysis and interpretation of data and drafting of the manuscript. JGB contributed to the study concept and design, data analysis and interpretation, and revising of the manuscript. PS conducted the microbiologic sampling sub-study and contributed to the interpretation of results. DH contributed to the study concept and interpretation of results. MDW contributed to data collection and analysis and interpretation of results. DMM contributed to the study concept and design, data collection, data analysis, interpretation of results, and drafting of the manuscript. All authors read and approved the final manuscript.

Competing interests
The authors declare that they have no competing interests.

Author details
¹Department of Critical Care Medicine, Queen's University and Kingston Health Sciences Centre, Kingston, Ontario, Canada. ²School of Medicine, Queen's University, Kingston, Ontario, Canada. ³Department of Medicine, Queen's University and Kingston Health Sciences Centre, Kingston, Ontario, Canada. ⁴Department of Pathology and Molecular Medicine, Queen's University and Health Sciences Centre, Kingston, Ontario, Canada. ⁵Department of Emergency Medicine, Queen's University and Kingston Health Sciences Centre, Kingston, Ontario, Canada. ⁶Department of Neuroscience, Queen's University, Kingston, Ontario, Canada. ⁷Kingston Health Sciences Centre, Kingston General Hospital, Davies 2, 76 Stuart St., Kingston, Ontario K7L 2V7, Canada.

References
1. Salah H, MacIntosh E, Rajakulendran N. Wearable tech: leveraging canadian innovation to improve health: MaRS Market Insights; 2014 Mar 26. p. 1–45.

Available from https://www.marsdd.com/wp-content/uploads/2015/02/MaRSReport-WearableTech.pdf

2.   Savage N. Mobile data: made to measure. Nature. 2015;527:S12–3.

3.   El-Amrawy F, Nounou MI. Are currently available wearable devices for activity tracking and heart rate monitoring accurate, precise, and medically beneficial? Healthc Inform Res. 2015;21(4):315–6.

4.   Case MA, Burwick HA, Volpp KG, Patel MS. Accuracy of smartphone applications and wearable devices for tracking physical activity data. JAMA-J Am Med Assoc. 2015;313(6):625–6.

5.   Wang R, Blackburn G, Desai M, Phelan D, Gillinov L, Houghtaling P, et al. Accuracy of wrist-worn heart rate monitors. JAMA Cardiol. 2017;2(1):104–6.

6.   Asada HH, Shaltis P, Reisner A, Rhee S. Mobile monitoring with wearable photoplethysmographic biosensors. IEEE Eng Med Biol Mag. 2003;22(3):28–40.

7.   Tamura T, Maeda Y, Sekine M, Yoshida M. Wearable photoplethysmographic sensors—past and present. Electronics. 2014;3(2):282–302.

8.   Pantelopoulos A, Bourbakis NG. A survey on wearable sensor-based systems for health monitoring and prognosis. IEEE Trans Syst, Man, Cybern C. 2009;40(1):1–12.

9.   Di Rienzo M, Rizzo F, Parati G, Brambilla G, Ferratini M, Castiglioni P. MagIC system: a new textile-based wearable device for biological signal monitoring. Applicability in daily life and clinical setting. In: Engineering in medicine and biology society, 2005. IEEE-EMBS 2005. 27th annual international conference of the 2005 (pp. 7167–7169). Shanghai: IEEE.

10. de Zambotti M, Baker FC, Willoughby AR, Godino JG, Wing D, Patrick K, et al. Measures of sleep and cardiac functioning during sleep using a multi-sensory commercially-available wristband in adolescents. Physiol Behav. 2016;158:143–9.

11. Mantua J, Gravel N, Spencer R. Reliability of sleep measures from four personal health monitoring devices compared to research-based actigraphy and polysomnography. Sensors. 2016;16(5):646.

12. Young JS, Bourgeois JA, Hilty DM, Hardin KA. Sleep in hospitalized medical patients, part 1: factors affecting sleep. J Hosp Med. 2008;3(6):473–82.

13. Kamdar BB, Needham DM, Collop NA. Sleep deprivation in critical illness: its role in physical and psychological recovery. J Intensive Care Med. 2012;27(2):97–111.

14. Litton E, Carnegie V, Elliott R, Webb SAR. The efficacy of earplugs as a sleep hygiene strategy for reducing delirium in the ICU: a systematic review and meta-analysis. Crit Care Med. 2016;44(5):992–9.

15. Richards KC, O'Sullivan PS, Phillips RL. Measurement of sleep in critically ill patients. J Nurs Meas. 2000;8(2):131–44.

16. Kamdar BB, Shah PA, King LM, Kho ME, Zhou X, Colantuoni E, et al. Patient-nurse interrater reliability and agreement of the Richards-Campbell Sleep Questionnaire. Am J Crit Care. 2012;21(4):261–9.

17. Flannery AH, Oyler DR, Weinhouse GL. The impact of interventions to improve sleep on delirium in the ICU: a systematic review and research framework. Crit Care Med. 2016;44(12):2231–40.

18. Kroll RR, Boyd JG, Maslove DM. Accuracy of a wrist-worn wearable device for monitoring heart rates in hospital inpatients: a prospective observational study. J Med Internet Res. 2016;18(9):e253.

19. Herridge MS, Chu LM, Matte A, Tomlinson G, Chan L, Thomas C, et al. The RECOVER program: disability risk groups and 1-year outcome after 7 or more days of mechanical ventilation. Am J Crit Care Med. 2016;194(7):831–44.

20. McNelly AS, Rawal J, Shrikrishna D, Hopkinson NS, Moxham J, Harridge SD, et al. An exploratory study of long-term outcome measures in critical illness survivors: construct validity of physical activity, frailty, and health-related quality of life measures. Crit Care Med. 2016;44(6):e362–9.

21. Roney JK, Whitley BE, Maples JC, Futrell LS, Stunkard KA, Long JD. Modified early warning scoring (MEWS): evaluating the evidence for tool inclusion of sepsis screening criteria and impact on mortality and failure to rescue. J Clin Nurs. 2015;24(23–24):3343–54.

22. Semple JL, Armstrong KA. Mobile applications for postoperative monitoring after discharge. Can Med Assoc J. 2016. electronically published ahead of print; https://doi.org/10.1503/cmaj.160195.

23. Jakicic JM, Davis KK, Rogers RJ, King WC, Marcus MD, Helsel D, et al. Effect of wearable technology combined with a lifestyle intervention on long-term weight loss: the IDEA randomized clinical trial. JAMA. 2016;316(11):1161–71.

24. Smith MEB, Chiovaro JC, O'Neil M, Kansagara D, Quiñones AR, Freeman M, et al. Early warning system scores for clinical deterioration in hospitalized patients: a systematic review. Ann Am Thorac Soc. 2014;11(9):1454–65.

25. Churpek MM, Yuen TC, Park SY, Meltzer DO, Hall JB, Edelson DP. Derivation of a cardiac arrest prediction model using ward vital signs. Crit Care Med. 2012;40(7):2102–8.

26. Churpek MM, Yuen TC, Winslow C, Meltzer DO, Kattan MW, Edelson DP. Multicenter comparison of machine learning methods and conventional regression for predicting clinical deterioration on the wards. Crit Care Med. 2016;44(2):368–74.

27. Churpek MM, Yuen TC, Park SY, Gibbons R, Edelson DP. Using electronic health record data to develop and validate a prediction model for adverse outcomes in the wards. Crit Care Med. 2014;42(4):841.

28. Churpek MM, Yuen TC, Winslow C, Hall J, Edelson DP. Differences in vital signs between elderly and nonelderly patients prior to ward cardiac arrest. Crit Care Med. 2015;43(4):816–22.

29. Bano M, Chiaromanni F, Corrias M, Turco M, De Rui M, Amodio P, et al. The influence of environmental factors on sleep quality in hospitalized medical patients. Front Neurol. 2014;5(4):267.

30. Fitbit Inc. Fitbit help: how do I track my sleep? [internet]. help.fitbit.com. [accessed 2016 Oct 15]. Available from: https://help.fitbit.com/articles/en_US/Help_article/1314

31. Elliott R, McKinley S, Cistulli P, Fien M. Characterisation of sleep in intensive care using 24-hour polysomnography: an observational study. Crit Care. 2013;17(2):R46.

The nocturnal acoustical intensity of the intensive care environment

Lori J. Delaney[1,2,8]* iD, Marian J. Currie[1,2], Hsin-Chia Carol Huang[3], Violeta Lopez[4,5], Edward Litton[5,6] and Frank Van Haren[2,7]

Abstract

Background: The intensive care unit (ICU) environment exposes patients to noise levels that may result in substantial sleep disruption. There is a need to accurately describe the intensity pattern and source of noise in the ICU in order to develop effective sound abatement strategies. The objectives of this study were to determine nocturnal noise levels and their variability and the related sources of noise within an Australian tertiary ICU.

Methods: An observational cross-sectional study was conducted in a 24-bed open-plan ICU. Sound levels were recorded overnight during three nights at 5-s epochs using Extech (SDL 600) sound monitors. Noise sources were concurrently logged by two research assistants.

Results: The mean recorded ambient noise level in the ICU was 52.85 decibels (dB) (standard deviation (SD) 5.89), with a maximum noise recording at 98.3 dB (A). All recorded measurements exceeded the WHO recommendations. Noise variability per minute ranged from 9.9 to 44 dB (A), with peak noise levels >70 dB (A) occurring 10 times/hour (SD 11.4). Staff were identified as the most common source accounting for 35% of all noise. Mean noise levels in single-patient rooms compared with open-bed areas were 53.5 vs 53 dB ($p = 0.37$), respectively.

Conclusion: Mean noise levels exceeded those recommended by the WHO resulting in an acoustical intensity of 193 times greater than the recommended and demonstrated a high degree of unpredictable variability, with the primary noise sources coming from staff conversations. The lack of protective effects of single rooms and the contributing effects that staffs have on noise levels are important factors when considering sound abatement strategies.

Keyword: Critical care, Disturbance, Intensive care, Noise, Sleep disturbance, Staff

Background

Both sleep deprivation and fragmentation have been associated with a variety of adverse somatic, cognitive, and physiological effects. Patients are subjected to a cacophony of disruptive sounds in the intensive care unit (ICU) environment, and numerous studies have found an association between noise and the sleep disturbance experienced by patients [1–8]. Objective and subjective studies show that even small changes in noise levels can adversely impact sleep [1–4, 9]. For example, a 10 dB (A) (refer to list of abbreviations) increase in noise is perceived as a doubling of noise levels, while sound intensity is doubled for each 3 dB (A) increase [10]. Altered sleep architecture and circadian disturbances have been attributed to poorer patient outcomes and is potentially a precipitating cause for the onset of delirium [11–15].

There exists a number of official recommendations regarding noise levels within the hospital environment. The World Health Organization (WHO), the Environmental Protection Agency, and the International Noise Council all recommend that to reduce sleep disturbance, noise levels within hospital wards should not exceed 30 dB(A) at night [16]. However, none of these recommendations

* Correspondence: Lori.delaney@canberra.edu.au
[1]Faculty of Nursing, University of Canberra, Canberra, Australia
[2]College of Medicine, Biology and Environment, Australian National University, Canberra, Australia
Full list of author information is available at the end of the article

are specific to the ICU environment, but rather, they are generalised to the hospital environment [17].

Noises that may be disruptive to the ICU environment include conversations, monitor alarms, phone calls, doorbells, and door closures. Compared with lower acuity hospital areas, these are purported to be more frequent and intense in the ICU and result in elevated noise levels [17]. In addition to mean noise level, noise variability may also contribute to sleep disruption. Variations in noise levels may heighten the sympathetic nervous system response, increasing cortisol release, and increase sleep latency [6, 18]. Current research debates the impact of noise on the patients with polysomnography studies reporting that noise levels contributed to 15 to 20% of patient sleep disturbances [3, 4], in contrast to subjective studies which reported that noise is a significant stressor for patients [1, 5, 6, 11]. The effectiveness of interventions to reduce noise levels have been questioned with results revealing transient reductions in ambient noise levels, with limited reductions in the quantity of peak noise levels [1]. Emerging research suggests that the sound quality and the unpredictable variable changes in noise levels may be the major factor-associated adverse effects within the ICU environment which requires intervention [19, 20].

The primary aim of this study was to investigate the intensity and pattern of nocturnal noise levels such as variability and their sources within an Australian ICU compared with the recommendations stipulated by the World Health Organization (WHO). The secondary aim was to investigate whether single-patient rooms provided a significant reduction in ambient noise levels compared with open-bed areas.

Methods
Setting
This observational study was conducted in a 24-bed, open-plan designed, Australian tertiary referral ICU. The unit provides both ICU and high dependency care, including medical and surgical services, trauma and neurosurgical care and post-operative cardiothoracic care. The ICU design is characteristic of a second-generation ICU and includes two centralised open nursing stations, four isolation rooms, three two-bedded bays and four four-bedded bays, with all beds in shared bays separated by linen curtains and rooms separated by semi-partitioned walls (Fig. 1).

Data collection procedures
Noise monitoring
Six sound monitors (Extech Model SDL 600) were positioned throughout the unit: at the nursing station and in the patients' clinical environment. The placement of the sound meters was determined via cluster randomisation

and involved only the occupied patient care spaces, with sites categorised as nursing stations, single-patient rooms, two-bedded and four-bedded bays. Sound monitors were mounted adjacent to the head of patients' beds at a height of 155 cm. This position was chosen to reflect the experience of patients, minimise disruption to clinical care and reduce interference with other monitoring equipment. Noise levels were monitored for 9 h (2200–0700 h) over three weekday nights—two consecutive and one non-consecutive based on a predetermined hospital wide monitoring roster.

Sound levels were recorded in A-weighted decibels at 5-s epochs using an Extech Sound Level Monitor (Model SDL 600, frequency range 31.5 Hz–8 KHz, 30–180 dB (A)) which complied with the International Electrotechnical Commission Standards. The A-weighted filter was used as it attenuates the curve that describes loudness frequency for the human ear. All logged data were saved onto a secured digital 2-GB memory card in a spreadsheet format for subsequent analysis.

Logging of noise sources
Two research assistants completed the logging of noise sources in the ICU into predetermined categories: staff, alarms, doors, phones, wash basins, trolleys and pumps, including an 'Other' category to accommodate unexpected noise sources. To reflect the nocturnal activity in the clinical setting, the research assistants logged noise sources at four different time points: 2300 to 2400, 0200 to 0300, 0400 to 0500 and 0600 to 0700 h.

Data analysis
Data derived from the sound monitors (Extech Model SDL 600) were downloaded and exported to Microsoft Excel (2010). Descriptive statistical analysis (means and standard deviations) was undertaken using IBM SPSS software (version 20) to describe the noise levels recorded. The variability of noise levels within the ICU were calculated by determining the difference between the mean and maximum noise levels within 5-min intervals over the 9 h recording period. The noise sources logged by the research assistants for each hour were collated and reported via descriptive statistics. An analysis of variance (ANOVA) was performed to identify differences between noise levels recorded over each of the three nights and to determine if single-patient rooms were significantly quieter than shared patient spaces.

The perceived loudness of noise is a logarithmic measure and subsequently does not exhibit a linear relationship to changes in noise levels. In order to quantify the impact of the recorded noise levels, psychoacoustical analysis was undertaken in order to describe the increases in volume and the acoustical intensity that these produce (Additional file 1: Table S1) [18]. Identification

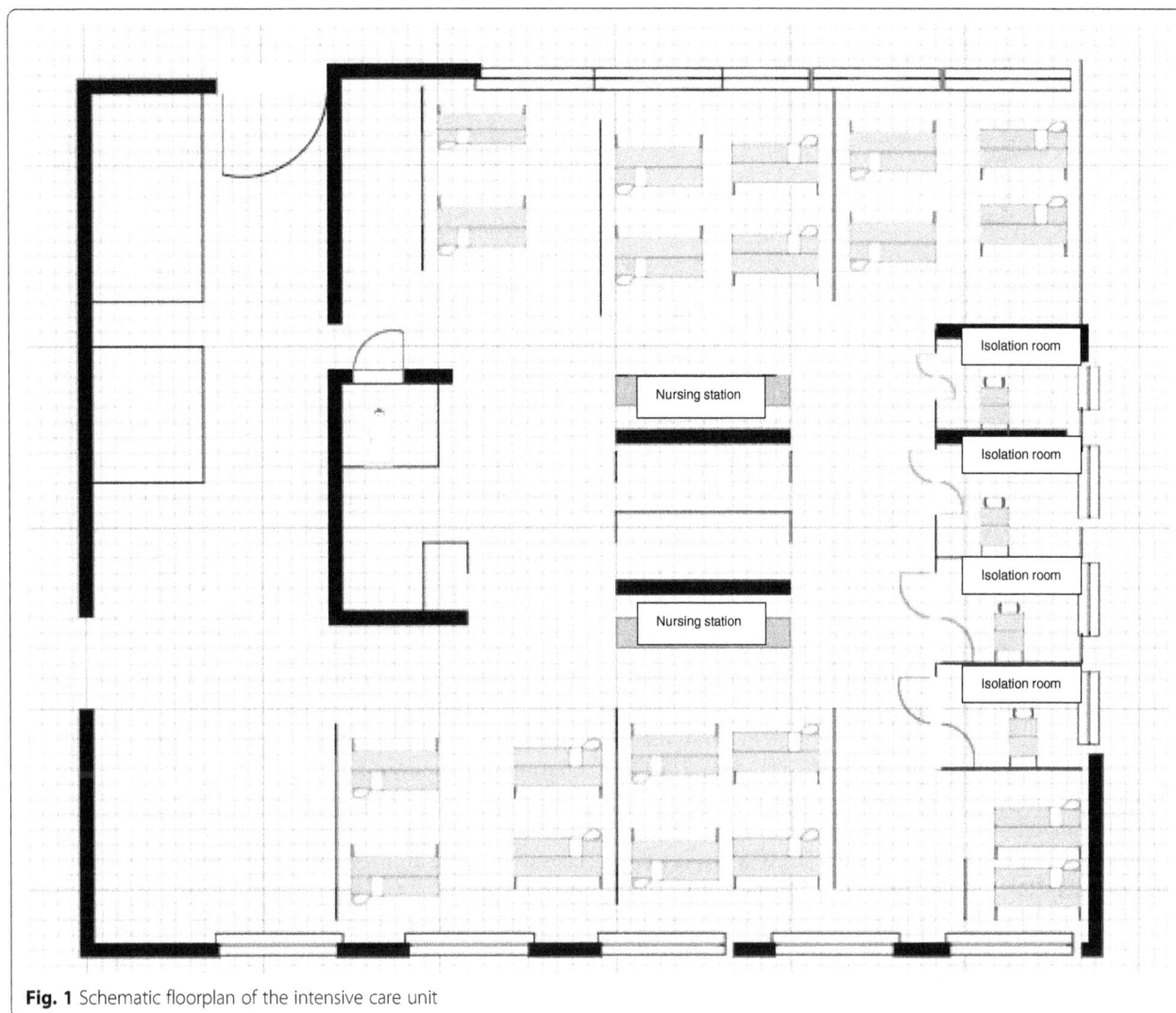

Fig. 1 Schematic floorplan of the intensive care unit

of these measures provides details of sound levels produced in the environment, whilst acoustical intensity reports a linear relationship of how many times greater the noise levels are compared to the recommended levels (30 dB A).

Ethics

The Australian Capital Territory Health Human Research Ethics Committee (ETHLR.12.253) approved the study; the need for informed consent was waived. The study was conducted in accordance with the principles outlined in the Declaration of Helsinki.

Results

A total of 18 clinical spaces, which included 16 patient care spaces and two nursing stations between June and September 2013 were monitored for nocturnal noise levels. Each bed space was occupied for the entire

monitoring period. The ambient noise levels recorded over the three nights were similar with a variance of 2.86 dB (A) (night 1 $L_{A\ mean} = 53.71 \pm 4.69$ dB (A), night 2 $L_{A\ mean} = 53.15 \pm 6.21$ dB (A) and night 3 $L_{A\ mean} = 50.85 \pm 6.18$ dB (A)) (Fig. 2). The overall ambient nocturnal noise level for the monitoring period in the ICU was 52.85 dB (A) (SD 5.89) and exceeded the WHO recommendations by 22.85 dB (A), which produces an increase in both noise volume (4.8 times greater) and acoustical intensity (192.8 times greater) than recommended.

The peak noise levels ranged from 85.5 to 98.3 dB (A). Noise levels within single-room and open-bed areas were similar to noise levels in two-bedded bays ($p = 0.37$) and four-bedded bays ($p = 0.06$) (Table 1). The primary sources of environmental noise were staff conversations and monitor alarms, which accounted for 35.4 and 34.1% of noises per hour respectively (Table 2).

The variability in ambient noise levels in the ICU is shown in Fig. 3, with frequent undulations in noise levels

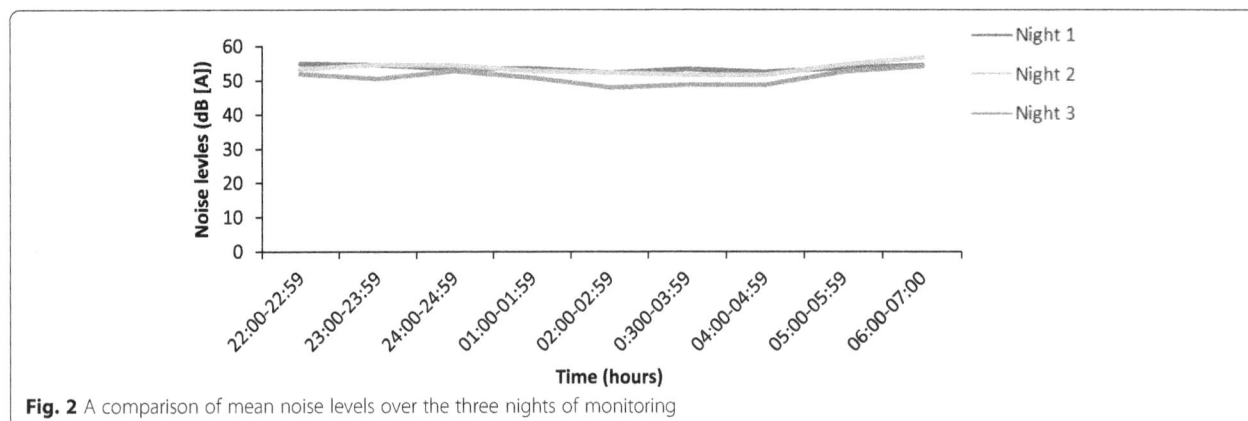

Fig. 2 A comparison of mean noise levels over the three nights of monitoring

ranging from 9.9 to 44 dB (A) above ambient noise levels. Peak noise levels >70 dB (A) were found to occur 10 times/hour (SD 11.4).

Discussion

Noise

We found that nocturnal noise exceeded the international recommendations throughout the entire monitoring period. The noise levels were of similar intensity to heavy traffic. Our results are consistent with other studies reporting noise levels in an ICU [1, 4, 6, 21–24]. The elevated ambient noise levels and the high degree of variability, in combination with the frequency of peak noises identified, are likely to contribute to sleep disruption [1–3, 21–23]. At the reported noise levels, the ICU environment is perceived to be 4.8 times louder, producing an acoustical intensity 193 times greater than the WHO recommendations. Our ICU can be classified as moderately noisy (50–60 dB (A) to very noisy (60–70 dB (A)) according to the hospital noise levels described by Pereira et al. [24] and may have adverse implications for patients in the ICU.

Sleep disturbances associated with waking, arousal and sleep-to-wake transitions are purported to occur with sound intensities ranging between 50 and 60 dB [25, 26], with spikes in noise levels identified by Gabor et al. [4] as a contributing factor to sleep disruption. Stanchina and colleagues demonstrated that noise variability between ambient noise levels and peak noises determined

the number of arousals for individuals exposed to ICU noise [19]. This indicates that noise disturbance is not only attributed to peak noises, but is also associated with frequency and unpredictability [27]. Subsequently, the capacity for patients to acclimatise to noise levels is unlikely to occur when the noise levels generated demonstrate frequent undulations and elevations in noise levels. The variability in noise levels within the ICU is likely to preclude patients' ability to acclimatise to noise within the environment and adversely impact on sleep continuity, contributing to additional physical and psychological stress. This is supported by patient reports, whereby unfamiliar and loud noises where a major causative factor in preventing their ability to sleep whilst in the ICU [28].

The resultant unpredictability of the environment has been associated with a heightened stress response secondary to autonomic stimulation and enhanced sympathetic activity, which adversely affects sleep latency. As a result, increased cortisol release inhibits melatonin secretion and thereby disrupts circadian rhythm regulation [29]. Exposure to noise sources greater than 50 dB (A) have been shown to produce cardiovascular changes such as increased heart rate variability, [30–32] along with electroencephalographic changes suggestive of

Table 1 Nocturnal noise levels within the ICU

Location	Mean (dB (A))(SD)	Min (dB (A))	Peak (dB (A))
Intensive care unit (overall)	52.9 (5.9)	40.2	98.3
Nursing station	54.8 (5.8)	42	98.3
Isolation rooms	53.5 (4.1)	47.7	96.3
Two-bedded bay	53 (6.8)	41.6	86.1
Four-bedded bay	52 (6.1)	40.2	85.5

Table 2 Sources of nocturnal noise in occurrences per hour in the ICU

Source	Mean occurrences per hour mean (SD)	Proportion of total occurrences per hour (%)
Staff	84.38 (32.77)	35.5
Alarms	81.06 (43.95)	34.1
Other	35.81 (19.96)	15.1
Doors	12.88 (12.37)	5.4
Pumps	7.19 (12.55)	3.0
Equipment	6.06 (4.64)	2.6
Trolleys	5.94 (7.19)	2.5
Wash basins	4.13 (2.55)	1.7

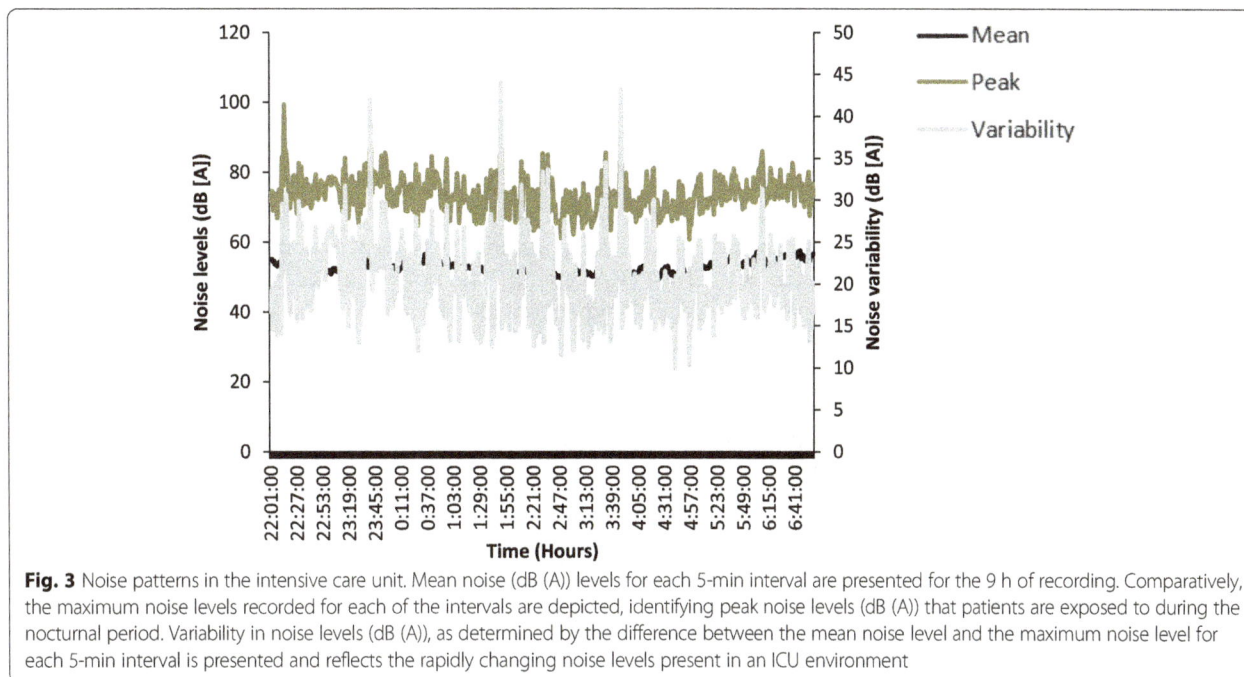

Fig. 3 Noise patterns in the intensive care unit. Mean noise (dB (A)) levels for each 5-min interval are presented for the 9 h of recording. Comparatively, the maximum noise levels recorded for each of the intervals are depicted, identifying peak noise levels (dB (A)) that patients are exposed to during the nocturnal period. Variability in noise levels (dB (A)), as determined by the difference between the mean noise level and the maximum noise level for each 5-min interval is presented and reflects the rapidly changing noise levels present in an ICU environment

arousal and lightening of sleep [33]. The association between heart rate and acoustics was reported by Hagerman et al. who identified an increase in pulse rate occurring with higher acoustical exposure, resulting in an increased incidence of readmission in a coronary care unit [34]. The variable and unpredictable changes in noise levels within the ICU are likely to impede on sleep quality and continuity, which may have further implications on cognitive function and the development of delirium.

Further, clinicians working within the environment are also susceptible to noise-induced stress, which can lead to exhaustion and irritability [35]. The emerging research on 'alarm fatigue' suggests that 72 to 99% of clinical alarms are false alarms. This contributes to staff desensitisation to alarms and has even been associated with patient deaths [36]. Further, evidence suggests that noise can impinge on concentration and clinical decision-making [36].

The use of single-patient bed spaces as a means to reduce patients' exposure to elevated and disruptive noise levels is not supported by the findings of this study, with four-bedded bays having the lowest ambient noise levels. Previous findings reported by Tegnestedt et al. further support this finding, whereby single-patient rooms were not found to have lower noise levels than shared patient spaces [37]. The reported noise levels in the single-patient rooms in this study may be reflective of the acuity of patients cared for in these rooms. Higher acuity patients require greater clinical interventions resulting in more noise being generated, whilst four-bedded bays may be more likely to be co-habited by less acute patients. In addition, behavioural modifications, such as

regulatory processes that staff engage in, in shared care spaces may contribute to a more conscientious approach to the noise generated in order to reduce its burden and impact on multiple individuals. Further, the clinical design of the single-patient rooms may also be a contributing factor, whereby alarm volumes may need to be increased in order to assure staff's ability to hear them when outside of the room or in the anteroom. In addition, the lack of noise-absorbing features may be a critical consideration that results in greater noise reverberation.

Sources of noise

The frequent ascension of noise levels in this study was observed to be associated with frequent monitor alarms, to which staff did not always respond. The impact of this on environmental noise was compounded by the ability for staff to communicate intelligibly to safeguard clinical decision-making and interventions, whereby speech needs to be 15 dB greater than the ambient noise to ensure clarity of communication. This in turn contributes to a further escalation in noise levels, known as the Lombard effect [38]. Noises produced at these levels are unlikely to provide patients with a nocturnal environment to support sleep and is problematic for clinical staff to ensure that communication is intelligible to mitigate the risk of error. This may account for the high rate of noise attributed to staff behaviour and suggests that moderating behaviour and alarm settings may have a beneficial effect on reducing nocturnal noise levels. The reported noise levels and the identified sources of noise in this study may adversely affect both patient and clinicians, and thus, there is a need for strategies to be devised and implemented to reduce the disruptions and stressors imposed by constant noise exposure.

Possible interventions

The possibility of curbing noise levels in the ICU environment by employing behaviour modification approaches to ameliorate the noise generated by staff and alarms has been previously identified. Such initiatives have included modifying alarms (tailoring parameters to patients and adjusting the volume at night) [1, 39] staff education regarding the physiological aspects of sleep and its role in recovery [39, 40] and behaviour-regulating interventions such as the use of 'yacker trackers' to identify noise increases [41]. While many of these studies report an initial successful reduction in subjective noise levels, few have demonstrated measurable or sustained reductions [1, 38, 41–44]. These studies suggest that strategies need to consider a range of approaches including sound elimination such as providing patients with earplugs and re-designing the environment rather than focusing solely on behaviour modification [29, 41, 44].

Research regarding environmental design indicates that it has the capacity to influence psychology, physiology and social behaviours, which may contribute to a reduction in noise [45].A landmark report published by Ulrich and colleagues [29] identified 600 studies which linked the clinical environment to positive or negative outcomes for patients and staff in four main areas: patient safety; staff stress and fatigue; increased effectiveness in care delivery; and improved overall healthcare quality. Specifically, these authors found that design features such as single-patient rooms, noise-absorbing materials and exposure to natural light to be useful in promoting appropriate circadian rhythms and reducing noise to facilitate sleep. Other authors have found that these design features were associated with a reduction in noise and improved sleep [4, 46–48], a reduction in medication errors [49, 50], improved communication [51] and reduced length of hospital stay [51–53]. However, despite the reported benefits, fiscal restraints imposed on healthcare organisations have resulted in selective implementation of recommendations [41].

Limitations

The findings of this study cannot be generalised to all ICU environments, as the study was conducted in a single Australian ICU, which may be unique in design and location. The noise levels recorded were recorded at night and are likely to be lower than the noise levels during the day. Further, the study did not undertake direct patient assessment regarding the impact of noise on ICU patients, and as a result, the impact of noise can only be postulated based on the current findings and

previous research. The presence of the observer and environmental-monitoring equipment in the clinical environment could have contributed to alterations in behaviour in order to conform to the presumed research objectives. If anything, this is likely to underestimate true noise levels. Despite these limitations, the study included the measurement of noise from multiple locations within the ICU, across three separate nights, and the identification of noise variability which may be an independent risk factor for noise-induced harm. The concurrent logging of noise sources during the monitoring period permitted the identification of primary noise sources rather than speculating on the primary contributing factors.

Conclusion

The occurrence of high mean noise levels in combination with the variability in noise levels and the frequency of peak noises may contribute to sleep disruption. Mean nocturnal noises in the ICU significantly exceeded those recommended by the WHO and demonstrated significant variability which is likely to result in substantial sleep disruption. The primary sources of noise were identified as staff conversations and monitor alarms. Single rooms had similar noise levels to those of two- and four-bedded bays. Further research into strategies to reduce noise, the physiological responses (e.g. heart rate, cortisol levels) and evaluation of interventions is required to enhance the therapeutic environment and understand their implications on patients. Providing patients with both relief from persistent exposure to noise and diurnal variation in noise levels have the potential to aid in their physiological and psychological recovery.

Abbreviations

ANOVA: Analysis of variance; dB (A): Decibels in A-weighted scale; ICU: Intensive care unit; $L_{A\ mean}$: Mean ambient noise; SD: Standard Deviation; SPSS: Statistical Package for Social Science; WHO: World Health Organization

Acknowledgements

The authors would like to acknowledge the funding support provided by the Canberra Hospital Foundation and the Office of the Chief Nurse in conducting the study.

Funding

This study was funded by the Canberra Hospital Foundation and the Office of the Chief Nurse, Australian Capital Territory Health.

Authors' contributions

LJD, MC, CH, VL, EL, and FvH did the literature review, data analysis and the development of the manuscript and its editing. All authors read and approved the final manuscript.

Competing interests

The authors declare that they have no competing interests.

Author details

[1]Faculty of Nursing, University of Canberra, Canberra, Australia. [2]College of Medicine, Biology and Environment, Australian National University, Canberra, Australia. [3]Respiratory and Sleep Medicine, Canberra Hospital, Canberra, Australia. [4]Alice Lee Centre for Nursing Studies, Yong Loo Lin School of Medicine, Singapore, Singapore. [5]St. John of God Hospital, Subiaco Perth Australia, Subiaco, Australia. [6]School of Medicine and Pharmacology, University of Western Australia, Perth 6009, Australia. [7]Intensive Care Unit, Canberra Hospital, Canberra, Australia. [8]Faculty of Health: Discipline of Nursing, University of Canberra, Canberra Act 2601, Australia.

References

1. Xie H, Kang J, Mills GH. Clinical review: the impact of noise on patients' sleep and the effectiveness of noise reduction strategies in intensive care units. Crit Care. 2009;13:209.
2. Beecroft JM, Ward M, Younes M, Crombach S, Smith O, Hanly PJ. Sleep monitoring in the intensive care unit: comparison of nursing assessment, actigraphy and polysomnography. Intensive Care Med. 2008;34(11):2076–83. doi:10.1007/s00134-008-1180-y.
3. Friese RS, Diaz-Arrastia R, McBride D, Frankel H, Gentilello LM. Quality and quantity of sleep in the surgical intensive care unit: are out patients sleeping? J Trauma. 2007;63:1210–4. doi:10.1097/TA.0b013e31815b83d7.
4. Gabor JY, Cooper AB, Crombach SA, Lee B, Kadikar N, Bettger HE, Hanly PJ. Contribution of the intensive care unit environmental to sleep disruption in mechanically ventilated patients and healthy subjects. Am J Respir Crit Care Med. 2003;167:708–15.
5. Tranmer JE, Minard J, Fox LA, Rebelo L. The sleep experience of medical and surgical patients. Clin Nurs Res. 2003;12(2):159–73. doi:10.1177/1054773803251163.
6. Honkus VL. Sleep deprivation in critical care units. J Crit Care Nurs. 2003;26(3):179–91.
7. Freedman NS, Gazendam J, Levan L, Pack AI, Schwab RJ. Abnormal sleep/wake cycles and the effect of environmental noise on sleep disruption in the intensive care unit. Am J Respir Crit Care Med. 2001;163:451–7.
8. Aurell J, Elmqvist D. Sleep in the surgical intensive care unit: continuous polygraphic recording of sleep in none patients receiving postoperative care. Br J Med. 1985;290:1029–32.
9. Elliott R, McKinley S, Cistulli P, Fien M. Characterisation of sleep in intensive care using 24-hour polysomnography: an observational study. Crit Care. 2013;17(2):R46.
10. Shipman JT, Wilson JD, Higgins CA. Chpater 6: Waves and Sounds. Boston: Introduction to physical Science. Cengage; 2013.
11. Stephens C, Daffurn K, Middleton S. A CQI approach to the investigation of noise levels within the intensive care unit environment. Aust Crit Care. 1995;8(1):20–6.
12. Grandner MA, Hale L, Moore M, Patel NP. Mortality associated with short sleep duration: the evidence, the possible mechanisms, and the future. Sleep Med Rev. 2010;14(3):191–203.
13. Gallicchio L, Kalesan B. Sleep duration and mortality: a systematic review and meta-analysis. J Sleep Res. 2009;18(2):148–58.
14. Weinhouse GL, Schwab RJ, Watson PL, Patil N, Vaccaro B, Pandharipande P, Ely EW. Bench-to-bedside review: delirium in ICU patients-importance of sleep deprivation. Crit Care. 2009;13(6):1.
15. Litton E, Carnegie V, Elliott R, Webb SA. The efficacy of earplugs as a sleep hygiene strategy for reducing delirium in the ICU: a systematic review and meta-analysis. Crit Care Med. 2016;44(5):992–9.
16. Berglund BL. Guidelines for community noise. Geneva: World Health Organization; 1999.
17. Topf M. Hospital noise pollution: an environmental stress model to guide research and clinical interventions. J Adv Nurs. 2000;31(3):520–9. doi:10.1046/j.1365-2648.2000.01307x.
18. Howard DM, Angus J. Acoustics and psychoacoustics. Taylor & Francis; 2009.
19. Stanchina ML, Abu-Hijleh M, Chaudhry BK, Carlisle CC, Millman RP. The influence of white noise on sleep in subjects exposed to ICU noise. Sleep Med. 2005;6(5):423–8.
20. Roth T, Kramer M, Trinder J. The effect of noise during sleep on the sleep patterns of different age groups. Can Psychiatr Assoc J. 1972;17(6_suppl2):197–201.
21. Muzet A. Environmental noise, sleep and health. Sleep Med Rev. 2007;11(2):135–42.
22. Wenham T, Pittard A. Intensive care unit environment. Contin Educ Anaesth Crit Care Pain. 2009;9(6):178–83.
23. Christensen M. Noise level in a general intensive care unit. A descriptive study. Nurs Crit Care. 2007;12(4):188–97. doi:10.1111/j.1478-5153.2007.00229.x.
24. Pereira RP, Toledo RN, Amaral JLG, Guilherme A. Qualification and quantification of ambient noise exposure in a general intensive care unit. Rev Bras Otorrinolaringol. 2003;69(6):766–71.
25. Elbaz M, Leger D, Sauvet F, Champignuelle B, Rio S, Strauss M, et al. Sound intensity severely disrupts sleep in ventilated ICU patient throughout a 24-h period: A preliminary 24-h study of sleep stages and associated sound levels. Ann Inten Care. 2017;7(25). doi: 10.1186/s13613-017-0248-7.
26. Aaron JN, Carlise CC, Carskado MA, Meyers TJ, Hill NS, Millman RP. Environmental noise as a cause of sleep disruption in an intermediate respiratory care unit. Sleep. 1996;19:707–10.
27. McCarthy DO, Ouimet ME, Daun JM. Shades of Florence Nightingale: potential impact of noise stress on wound healing. Holistic Nurs Prac. 1991;5(4):39–48.
28. Hweidi IM. Jordanian patients' perception of stressors in critical care units: a questionnaire survey. Int J Nurs Stud. 2007;44:227–35. doi:10.1016/j.ijnurstu.2005.11.025.
29. Ulrich RS, Zimring C, Joseph A, Quan X, Choudhary R. The role of the physical environment in the hospital of the 21stcentury. Center for Health Design website. https://www.healthdesign.org/sites/default/files/Role%20Physical%20Environ%20in%20the%2021st%20Century%20Hospital_0.pdf. Accessed 5 July 2017.
30. Sim CS, Sung JH, Cheon SH, Lee JM, Lee JW, Lee J. The effects of different noise types on heart rate variability in men. Yonsei Med J. 2015;56(1):235–43.
31. Lee GS, Chen ML, Wang GY. Evoked response of heart rate variability using short-duration white noise. Autonomic Neurosc. 2010;155(1):94–7.
32. Tzaneva L, Danev S, Nikolova R. Investigation of noise exposure effect on heart rate variability parameters. Central Eur J Pub Hlth. 2001;9(3):130–2.
33. Griefahn B, Spreng M. Disturbed sleep patterns and limitation of noise. Noise Hlth. 2004;6.27–33.
34. Hagerman I, Rasmanis G, Blomkvist V, Ulrich R, Eriksen CA, Theorell T. Influence of intensive coronary care acoustics on the quality of care and physiological state of patients. Int J Card. 2005;98(2):267–70.
35. Mazer S. Stop the noise: reduce errors by creating a quieter hospital environment. PSQH. 2005.
36. Sendelbach S, Funk M. Alarm fatigue: a patient safety concern. AACN Adv Crit Care. 2013;24(4):378–86.
37. Tegnestedt C, Günther A, Reichard A, Bjurström R, Alvarsson J, Martling CR, Sackey P. Levels and sources of sound in the intensive care unit—an observational study of three room types. Acta Anaes Scan. 2013;2013.57(8):1041–50.
38. Connor A, Ortiz E. Staff solutions for noise reduction in the workplace. Permanente J. 2009;13(4):23–7.
39. Call RB. Sound practices: noise control in the healthcare environment. Acad J. 2007.
40. Konkani A, Oakley B. Noise in hospital intensive care units—a critical review of a critical topic. J Crit Care. 2012;27(5):522–e1.
41. Trochelman K, Albert N, Spence J, Murray T, Slifeak E. Patient and their families weigh in on evidence-based hospital design. Crit Care Nur. 2012;32(1):e1–e10. Nurs, 2005;21(4); 208-219.
42. Padmakumar AD, Bhasin V, Wenham TN, Bodenham AR. Evaluation of noise levels in intensive care units in two large teaching hospitals—a prospective observational study. J Inten Care Soc. 2013;14(3):205–10.
43. Monsén MG, Edéll-Gustafsson UM. Noise and sleep disturbance factors before and after implementation of a behavioural modification programme. Intensive Crit Care Nurs. 2005;21(4):208–19.
44. Delaney LJ. Behavioral modification of healthcare professionals in an adult critical care unit to reduce nocturnal noise: An evidence based implementation project. JBI Database System Rev Implement Rep. 2014;12(7): 505–20.
45. Topf M. Hospital noise pollution: an environmental stress model to guide research and clinical interventions. J Adv Nurs. 2000;31(3):520–8.

46. Jiang XY, Zeng YM, Chen XY, Zhang YH. Effects of earplugs and eye masks on nocturnal sleep, melatonin and cortisol in a simulated intensive care unit environment. Crit Care. 2010;14(2):1.

47. Balogh D, Kittinger E, Benzer A, Hackl JM. Noise in the ICU. Intensive Care Med. 1993;19(6):343–6.

48. Parthasarathy S, Tobin MJ. Sleep in the intensive care unit. Intensive Care Med. 2004;30(2):197–206.

49. Durston P. Partners in caring: a partnership for healing. Nurs Adm Q. 2006; 30(2):105–11.

50. Hendrich A, Fay J, Sorrells A. Courage to heal: comprehensive cardiac critical care. J Healthc Des. 2002:11–13.

51. Hendrich A, Fay J, Sorrells A. Effects of acuity adaptable rooms on flow of patients and delivery of care. Am J Crit Care. 2004;13(1):35–45.

52. Benedetti F, Colombo C, Barbini B, Campori E, Smeraldi E. Morning sunlight reduces length of hospitalization in bipolar depression. J Affect Dis. 2001; 62(3):221–3.

53. Chaudhury H, Mahmood A, Valente M. Nurses' perception of single-occupancy versus multi-occupancy rooms in acute care environments: an exploratory comparative assessment. Applied Nurs Res. 2006;19(3):118–25.

Presence of chest tubes does not affect the hemodynamic efficacy of standard cardiopulmonary resuscitation

Gu Hyun Kang[1]*, Hyun Youk[2], Kyoung Chul Cha[2], Yoonsuk Lee[2], Hyung Il Kim[2], Yong Sung Cha[2], Oh Hyun Kim[2], Hyun Kim[2], Kang Hyun Lee[2] and Sung Oh Hwang[2]

Abstract

Background: During cardiopulmonary resuscitation (CPR), chest tubes can hinder increases in intrathoracic pressure by venting the pressure during chest compressions, thus reducing the blood flow generated by the thoracic pump effect. The aim of the present study was to investigate the effects of chest tubes on hemodynamic efficacy during standard CPR in a swine model of cardiac arrest.

Methods: Twelve domestic male pigs weighing 39.6 ± 8.4 kg underwent bilateral tube thoracostomy and received a total of 12 min of standard manual CPR, which comprised of two 6-min courses of CPR after 2 min of electrically induced ventricular fibrillation. Each 6-min set consisted of 3 min of CPR with clamped chest tubes (CCT-CPR) and 3 min of CPR with unclamped chest tubes (UCT-CPR). The sequence of CCT-CPR and UCT-CPR was randomized.

Results: Hemodynamic parameters including aortic pressure, left ventricular pressure, right ventricular pressure, right atrial pressure, and minimal and maximal dp/dt did not differ significantly between CCT-CPR and UCT-CPR. No significant differences were noted in carotid blood flow, end-tidal CO_2, or coronary perfusion pressure between CCT-CPR and UCT-CPR.

Conclusions: The presence of chest tubes did not affect the hemodynamic efficacy of standard CPR. There is no need to clamp chest tubes during standard CPR.

Keywords: Cardiopulmonary resuscitation, Thoracostomy, Cardiac arrest, External chest compression, Chest tube

Background

Closed-chest cardiopulmonary resuscitation (CPR), first introduced in 1960, is now used worldwide and has been documented as effective in resuscitating cardiac arrest patients [1]. However, the mechanism of blood flow during CPR in humans has not been clearly defined. The cardiac pump theory explains that direct compression of the cardiac structure is the basic mechanism of blood flow generated by chest compressions [2–4]. On the other hand, the thoracic pump theory postulates that fluctuations of the intrathoracic pressure, not direct cardiac compressions, cause blood flow by creating a pressure gradient between the intrathoracic and

extrathoracic vascular compartments [5–7]. The two mechanisms might generate blood flow with different magnitudes according to chest configuration or clinical conditions of the individual receiving CPR. The blood flow generated by standard CPR during cardiac arrest is known to be only 17–27% of the normal cardiac output [8–10]. Thus, there are concerns that any alteration of the mechanism generating blood flow during CPR could further reduce tissue perfusion.

It is not uncommon for patients to receive CPR in the presence of chest tubes due to cardiac arrest after cardiothoracic surgery or treatment of pleural diseases such as tension pneumothorax [11, 12]. The presence of chest tubes might alter the mechanism of blood flow generated by chest compressions. For instance, chest tubes might hinder increases in intrathoracic pressure by venting the pleural pressure during chest compressions, thus

* Correspondence: drkang9@hanmail.net
[1]Department of Emergency Medicine, Hallym University College of Medicine, Seoul, Republic of Korea
Full list of author information is available at the end of the article

reducing the blood flow generated by the thoracic pump mechanism. However, little is known about the hemodynamic effects of chest compressions in the presence of chest tubes during CPR. Furthermore, current CPR guidelines do not provide any recommendations about whether chest tubes should be clamped when chest compressions are performed [13, 14].

The aim of the present study was to investigate the effects of chest tubes on hemodynamic efficacy during standard CPR in a swine model of cardiac arrest.

Methods
Animals and ethics
Twelve domestic male pigs weighing 39.6 ± 8.4 kg from a single-source breeder were used in this study. The experimental procedures and protocols conformed to the institutional guidelines for the care and use of animals in research and were approved by the Institutional Animal Care and Use Committee of Wonju College of Medicine, Yonsei University (YWC-140408).

Animal preparation
The animals were fasted overnight but allowed free access to water. Anesthesia was initiated by the intramuscular injection of ketamine (20 mg/kg) and maintained by ear vein injection of ketamine (30 mg/kg). Body temperature was maintained between 36.5 and 37.5 °C during the procedures, using an incandescent heat lamp and electric heat pad. After anesthesia, endotracheal intubation was performed with a cuffed endotracheal tube. Intubation was confirmed based on the endotracheal end-tidal carbon dioxide concentration ($EtCO_2$) (CO2SMO, Phillips Respironics, Murrysville, PA, USA). After intubation, the pigs were placed in the supine position. The animals were ventilated with room air via a volume-controlled ventilator (MDS Matrix 3000, Orchard Park, NY, USA) during preparation. The tidal volume was set at 10 mL/kg, and the ventilation rate was set at 18 breaths per minute. Electrocardiography (ECG lead II) and $EtCO_2$ were monitored continuously.

Under aseptic conditions, the right femoral artery was cannulated with an introducer sheath (7.5 Fr, Arrow International Inc., Reading, PA, USA) by the Seldinger method, and the aortic blood pressure was recorded continuously with a micromanometer-tipped catheter (5 Fr., Millar Instruments, Inc., Houston, TX, USA) introduced into the femoral artery. After the right cervical dissection, the right carotid artery was cannulated with an introducer sheath (7.5 Fr) by the Seldinger method, and the left ventricle (LV) pressure was recorded continuously with a micromanometer-tipped catheter (5 Fr., Millar Instruments, Inc., Houston, TX, USA) introduced into the right carotid artery. Two introducer sheaths were placed in the right

external jugular vein—one recorded the right atrium (RA), and the other the right ventricle (RV) pressure via a micromanometer-tipped catheter (6 Fr., Millar Instruments, Inc., TX, USA). After the left cervical dissection, the left carotid artery was surgically exposed, and an ultrasonic flow probe (T106, Transonic Systems Inc., Ithaca, NY) was placed around it to quantify blood flow. The catheter position was confirmed by characteristic pressure tracing from the cardiac chamber and by postmortem examination. Once the catheters were in place, a heparin bolus (100 u/kg, IV) was administered to prevent thrombosis.

Chest tubes (16 Fr) were inserted in both the mid-lateral thoracic walls. A micromanometer-tipped catheter (5 Fr) was inserted into the thoracic space via the left chest tube to record the intrapleural pressure (IPP). The chest tubes were clamped with a curved hemostat without teeth after insertion.

Induction of ventricular fibrillation and CPR
After baseline data were collected, a pacing catheter (5 Fr, bipolar lead, Arrow International Inc., Reading, PA, USA) was positioned in the RV. For the induction of ventricular fibrillation (VF), an electrical current at 60 Hz was delivered to the endocardium. VF was confirmed by the ECG waveform and a decline in aortic pressure. Once VF was induced, the endotracheal tube was disconnected from the ventilator, and the pigs were observed for 2 min without any procedure or treatment.

After 2 min of VF, the animals received a total of 12 min of standard manual CPR. Chest compressions were performed by experienced emergency medical technicians who had passed the American Heart Association (AHA) Basic Life Support (BLS) Provider Course. Chest compressors were blinded to the study design. Two chest compressors performed chest compressions every 2 min according to BLS guidelines [15]. The compression and ventilation ratio was 30:2, and the compressors were switched every 2 min. Chest compressions were performed at a depth of 5 cm and a rate of 100/min. Positive pressure ventilations were delivered with a resuscitator bag (silicone resuscitator 870040, Laerdal Medical, Stavanger, Norway) every 30 chest compressions.

Experimental protocol
The animals received a total of 12 min of standard manual cardiopulmonary resuscitation (CPR), which comprised two 6-min courses of CPR. Each 6-min CPR set consisted of 3 min of CPR with clamped chest tubes (CCT-CPR) and 3 min of CPR with unclamped chest tubes (UCT-CPR). The experiment was designed as a crossover trial. The sequence of CCT-CPR and UCT-CPR was randomized according to a schedule enclosed

in a sealed envelope. For animals allocated to protocol A, both chest tubes were clamped (CCT-CPR) for the first 3 min and unclamped (UCT-CPR) for the next 3 min during CPR. For animals allocated to protocol B, both chest tubes were unclamped (UCT-CPR) during the first 3 min and clamped (CCT-CPR) for the next 3 min during CPR. Each sequence was performed twice, for a total of 12 min of CPR.

Data measurements
Data were digitized with a digital recording system (Powerlab, AD Instruments, Colorado Springs, CO, USA). All parameters (aortic, RV, RA, and LV systolic and diastolic pressures; left pleural pressure; carotid blood flow; and EtCO$_2$) were continuously recorded and analyzed at the baseline. The coronary perfusion pressure (CPP) during CPR was calculated as the difference between the aortic pressure and the RA pressure in the end-diastolic phase using an electronic subtraction unit. The rates of increase in LV and RV pressure were measured as the dp/dt (minimum and maximum). The dp/dt of the LV and RV was calculated from the pressure tracings with a program from a digital recording system.

Statistical analysis
For hemodynamic data analysis, the average value of each parameter measured during the data sampling period was used. Data are expressed according to the properties of the variables. Continuous variables are presented as the mean and standard deviation after normality assessment by the Shapiro-Wilk test. A two-sample t test or analysis of variance (ANOVA) was used to compare continuous variables as appropriate. Analyses were performed with SPSS V.23.0 software (IBM Corp., Chicago, IL, USA).

Differences were regarded as significant if the p values were less than 0.05.

Results
Baseline measurements of animals
Among the 12 animals initially included in the study, two suffered VF during catheterization. Therefore, ten animals were included in the final analysis. The mean body weight was 39 ± 8 kg, and the mean chest circumference was 69 ± 6 cm. No differences in baseline measurement (body weight, chest circumference, rectal temperature, and baseline oxygen saturation) were noted between the animals allocated to protocol A or B. There were no significant differences in baseline hemodynamic measurements between the animals allocated to protocol A or B (Table 1).

Effects of chest tubes on hemodynamic parameters during CPR
Chest tubes did not affect hemodynamic parameters during CPR. Systolic hemodynamic parameters including aortic systolic pressure, left ventricular systolic pressure, right ventricular systolic pressure, and right atrial systolic pressure did not differ significantly between CCT-CPR and UCT-CPR. No significant differences were noted in diastolic hemodynamic parameters including aortic diastolic pressure, left ventricular diastolic pressure, right ventricular diastolic pressure, and right atrial diastolic pressure between CCT-CPR and UCT-CPR. The rates of increase in LV and RV pressure (measured by the maximal dp/dt) did not differ between CCT-CPR and UCT-CPR. The rates of decrease in LV and RV pressure (measured by the minimal dp/dt) also did not differ between CCT-CPR and UCT-CPR (Table 2).

Table 1 Comparison of the baseline hemodynamic measurements between animals allocated to protocol A or B

Parameter	Animals of protocol A ($n = 5$)	Animals of protocol B ($n = 5$)	p value
Systolic aortic pressure (mmHg)	124 ± 4	120. ± 9	0.36
Diastolic aortic pressure (mmHg)	92 ± 8	82 ± 8	0.10
Systolic LV pressure (mmHg)	113 ± 9	116 ± 21	0.76
Diastolic LV pressure (mmHg)	7 ± 7	5 ± 4	0.46
Systolic RV pressure (mmHg)	21 ± 7	24 ± 20	0.80
Diastolic RV pressure (mmHg)	2 ± 1	2 ± 2	0.75
Mean RA pressure (mmHg)	3 ± 2	3 ± 3	0.93
dp/dt RV max. (mmHg/s)	143 ± 48	190 ± 102	0.38
dp/dt RV min. (mmHg/s)	− 135 ± 32	− 155 ± 37	0.40
dp/dt LV max. (mmHg/s)	435 ± 198	551 ± 343	0.54
dp/dt LV min. (mmHg/s)	− 445 ± 203	− 461 ± 154	0.89
CBF (mL/min)	232 ± 147	198 ± 83	0.67
EtCO$_2$ (mmHg)	45 ± 6	44 ± 5	0.66

All variables are shown as mean ± standard deviation. Baseline indicates measurements before induction of cardiac arrest
RA right atrium, *RV* right ventricle, *LV* left ventricle, *max.* maximum, *min.* minimum, *CBF* carotid blood flow, *EtCO$_2$* end-tidal CO$_2$ concentration

Table 2 Comparison of systolic and diastolic parameters between CCT-CPR and UCT-CPR

Parameter (mmHg)	CCT-CPR for 1st 3 min (n = 10)	UCT-CPR for 1st 3 min (n = 10)	p value	CCT-CPR for 2nd 3 min (n = 10)	UCT-CPR for 2nd 3 min (n = 10)	p value
Systolic aortic pressure (mmHg)	117 ± 69	105 ± 53	0.572	124 ± 161	104 ± 52	0.895
Diastolic aortic pressure (mmHg)	9 ± 8	11 ± 7	0.106	9 ± 8	11 ± 8	0.020
Systolic LV pressure (mmHg)	183 ± 72	164 ± 69	0.558	168 ± 77	162 ± 71	0.324
Diastolic LV pressure (mmHg)	9 ± 6	10.5 ± 7	0.102	8 ± 7	9 ± 7	0.229
Systolic RV pressure (mmHg)	184 ± 89	157 ± 83	0.075	171 ± 90	158 ± 85	0.032
Diastolic RV pressure (mmHg)	12 ± 7	12 ± 6	0.813	12 ± 6	12 ± 8	0.808
Systolic RA pressure (mmHg)	174 ± 87	149 ± 79	0.086	162 ± 91	151 ± 83	0.097
Diastolic RA pressure (mmHg)	11 ± 6	12 ± 6	0.658	11 ± 6	12 ± 6	0.333
dp/dt RV max. (mmHg/s)	747 ± 580	641 ± 500	0.544	698 ± 595	659 ± 545	0.162
dp/dt RV min. (mmHg/s)	− 657 ± 397	− 571 ± 354	0.781	− 603 ± 382	− 582 ± 370	0.313
dp/dt LV max. (mmHg/s)	751 ± 532	641 ± 500	0.813	687 ± 558	674 ± 508	0.808
dp/dt LV min. (mmHg/s)	− 681 ± 321	− 571 ± 354	0.453	−611 ± 325	− 615 ± 316	0.965

All variables are shown as mean ± standard deviation. Baseline indicates measurements before induction of cardiac arrest
CCT-CPR cardiopulmonary resuscitation with clamped chest tubes, *UCT-CPR* cardiopulmonary resuscitation with unclamped chest tubes, *RA* right atrium, *RV* right ventricle, *LV* left ventricle, *max.* maximum, *min.* minimum

Intrapleural pressure

The mean IPP was significantly lower during spontaneous circulation than during CCT-CPR and UCT-CPR ($p = 0.003$). However, chest tubes did not affect the IPP. No significant differences in the IPP variables were noted between CCT-CPR and UCT-CPR (Table 3).

Carotid blood flow, end-tidal carbon dioxide concentration, and coronary perfusion pressure

No significant differences were noted in the carotid blood flow, $EtCO_2$, or CPP between CCT-CPR and UCT-CPR (Table 4).

Discussion

Our study demonstrates that there are no differences in hemodynamic parameters including pressures and pressure changes rates of the ventricles, carotid blood flow, or coronary perfusion pressure between CPR with chest tubes and standard CPR (CPR with clamped chest tubes). This finding suggests that it is unnecessary to clamp the chest tubes when CPR is performed in cardiac

arrest patients with chest tubes. This is the first study to investigate the hemodynamic effects of chest tubes during CPR.

Chest tubes are inserted into the pleural cavity to drain air, blood, or fluid in patients who have pneumothorax or hemothorax or have undergone cardiothoracic surgery. Chest tubes should be connected to an underwater sealed drainage system to prevent backflow of air or fluid to the pleural cavity and thus maintain adequate respiratory function [16]. There is a high risk for cardiac arrest in a substantial proportion of patients with chest tubes. Perioperative cardiac arrest, which is associated with the high cardiac surgical mortality, occurs in 5.2–5.5% of patients undergoing cardiothoracic operations [17, 18]. When a patient with chest tubes is resuscitated, the presence of the chest tubes might alter the hemodynamic efficacy by exposing the intrapleural space to the atmosphere. The phasic rise of intrathoracic pressure or simultaneous lung inflation during chest compressions is known to augment cerebral and coronary perfusion [7, 19]. A chest tube might act as a vent that prevents this increase in

Table 3 Comparison of intrapleural pressure between CCT-CPR and UCT-CPR

Parameter	CCT-CPR for 1st 3 min (n = 10)	UCT-CPR for 1st 3 min (n = 10)	p value	CCT-CPR for 2nd 3 min (n = 10)	UCT-CPR for 2nd 3 min (n = 10)	p value
IPP max. (mmHg)	17 ± 22	12 ± 11	0.586	16 ± 23	10 ± 13	0.531
IPP min. (mmHg)	− 9 ± 6	− 6 ± 5	0.141	− 8 ± 6	− 13 ± 7	0.857
IPP mean (mmHg)	0 ± 4	1 ± 6	0.975	1 ± 5	1 ± 6	0.517
IPP gradient (mmHg)	26 ± 25	19 ± 9	0.441	24 ± 26	11 ± 8	0.15

All variables are shown as mean ± standard deviation
IPP intrapleural pressure, *CCT-CPR* cardiopulmonary resuscitation with clamped chest tubes, *UCT-CPR* cardiopulmonary resuscitation with unclamped chest tubes, *max.* maximum, *min.* minimum

Table 4 Comparison of coronary blood flow, end-tidal carbon dioxide concentration, and coronary perfusion pressure between CCT-CPR and UCT-CPR

Parameter	CCT-CPR for 1st 3 min (n = 10)	UCT-CPR for 1st 3 min (n = 10)	p value	CCT-CPR for 2nd 3 min (n = 10)	UCT-CPR for 2nd 3 min (n = 10)	p value
EtCO$_2$ (mmHg)	40 ± 10	34 ± 6	0.662	31 ± 5	38 ± 11	0.215
CBF (mL/min)	143 ± 151	158 ± 94	0.851	159 ± 107	103 ± 113	0.439
CPP (mmHg)	12 ± 5.2	16 ± 5	0.252	13 ± 7	9 ± 5	0.410

All variables are shown as mean ± standard deviation

EtCO$_2$ end-tidal carbon dioxide concentration, CBF carotid blood flow, CPP coronary perfusion pressure, CCT-CPR cardiopulmonary resuscitation with clamped chest tubes, UCT-CPR cardiopulmonary resuscitation with unclamped chest tubes

intrathoracic pressure and thus might reduce the thoracic pump effect that generates blood flow during chest compressions. If this is true, should chest tubes be clamped to maintain adequate hemodynamic effects during CPR? Our study provides the answer to this question.

In our study, unclamping the chest tubes during CPR did not alter hemodynamic parameters such as the systolic and diastolic pressures of the cardiac chambers, the coronary perfusion pressure, and the rates of pressure change measured by the dp/dt of the ventricles. Surrogates of blood flow to the brain and pulmonary circulation measured by carotid blood flow and end-tidal CO$_2$ tension were not altered when the chest tubes were unclamped. Unclamping the chest tubes during CPR also did not significantly alter the intrapleural pressure. This finding indicates that the chest tubes might be collapsed or sealed by the visceral pleura during the compression phase of CPR, thus preventing the venting of intrathoracic pressure. This needs to be investigated further. Unclamped chest tubes might produce a pneumothorax and thus reduce the venous return and blood flow generated by chest compressions. Exposure of the intrapleural space to the atmosphere through unclamped chest tubes would cause pneumothorax if spontaneous breathing were occurring. However, positive-pressure ventilation is performed during CPR so that persistent negative intrathoracic pressure does not develop. The maximal and minimal intrapleural pressure did not differ between UCT-CPR and CCT-CPR in this study. This demonstrates that the venting effect of unclamped chest tubes is negligible or minimal during CPR. Furthermore, the chest tubes are connected to an underwater sealed drainage system in clinical settings, so there is little possibility of hemodynamic alteration due to the chest tubes during CPR.

Chest compressions can cause parenchymal lung injuries including pneumothorax [20, 21]. Clamping of the chest tubes during CPR might increase the risk of tension pneumothorax when an unnoticed pneumothorax develops due to chest compressions. In this context, it is reasonable to keep the chest tubes unclamped during CPR.

Limitations
This study has some limitations. Our study protocol involved a crossover trial from UCT-CPR to CCT-CPR or vice versa every 3 min in each animal. Due to the nature of the study design, an order effect might have occurred. We randomized the order of CPR to minimize the order effect. Also, we placed a micromanometer-tipped catheter in the pleural cavity via the chest tube of the left thorax to measure the intrapleural pressure. These data might not have exactly matched the actual intrapleural pressures of both pleural spaces because we only measured the pleural pressure from the unilateral thorax. In this experiment, low CPP was observed because our experimental protocol did not include epinephrine administration to simulate BLS situation. However, maintaining adequate CPP over 20 mmHg is important to restore spontaneous circulation and cerebral oxygenation, so that low CPP observed in this experiment can be a limiting factor to apply our result to clinical setting [22]. Finally, this was an animal experimental study to simulate CPR in the presence of chest tubes. In the clinical setting, the patient with chest tubes might have additional clinical conditions which need thoracostomies such as pneumothorax, hemothorax, or surgical procedures of the thorax. Therefore, caution is needed when interpreting and applying these results in clinical settings.

Conclusion
The presence of chest tubes did not affect the hemodynamic efficacy of standard CPR in an animal model of cardiac arrest. There is no need to clamp the chest tubes during standard CPR.

Funding
This work was supported by a research grant from Yonsei University Wonju College of Medicine (YUWCM-2017-91).

Availability of data and materials
The datasets used and/or analyzed during the current study are available from the corresponding author on reasonable request.

Authors' contributions
IK, HY, YSL, OHK, YSC, and GHK performed the animal experiments. KCC and GHK contributed to the data analysis. KCC, GHK and SOH contributed to the

data interpretation. GHK, HY, YSL, OHK, and YSC contributed to the data collection. HIK contributed to the literature search. SOH designed and conceptualized the study. GHK and SOH completed the manuscript writing. KHK, HK, and KHL provided the critical revisions to the manuscript. All authors read and approved the final manuscript.

Competing interests
The authors declare that they have no competing interests.

Author details
[1]Department of Emergency Medicine, Hallym University College of Medicine, Seoul, Republic of Korea. [2]Department of Emergency Medicine, Yonsei University Wonju College of Medicine, 20 Ilsanro, Wonju, Republic of Korea.

References
1. Kouwenhoven WB, Jude JR, Knickerbocker GG. Closed-chest cardiac massage. JAMA. 1960;173:1064–7.
2. Hwang SO, Lee KH, Cho JH, Yoon J, Choe KH. Changes of aortic dimensions as evidence of cardiac pump mechanism during cardiopulmonary resuscitation in humans. Resuscitation. 2001;50:87–93.
3. Kim H, Hwang SO, Lee CC, et al. Direction of blood flow from the left ventricle during cardiopulmonary resuscitation in humans: its implications for mechanism of blood flow. Am Heart J. 2008;156:1222.e1–7.
4. Higano ST, Oh JK, Ewy GA, Seward JB. The mechanism of blood flow during closed chest cardiac massage in humans: transesophageal echocardiographic observations. Mayo Clin Proc. 1990;65:1432–40.
5. Guerci AD, Halperin HR, Beyar R, et al. Aortic diameter and pressure-flow sequence identify mechanism of blood flow during external chest compression in dogs. J Am Coll Cardiol. 1989;14:790–8.
6. Rudikoff MT, Maughan WL, Effron M, Freund P, Weisfeldt ML. Mechanisms of blood flow during cardiopulmonary resuscitation. Circulation. 1980;61:345–52.
7. Koehler RC, Chandra N, Guerci AD, et al. Augmentation of cerebral perfusion by simultaneous chest compression and lung inflation with abdominal binding after cardiac arrest in dogs. Circulation. 1983;67:266–75.
8. Fitzgerald KR, Babbs CF, Frissora HA, Davis RW, Silver DI. Cardiac output during cardiopulmonary resuscitation at various compression rates and durations. Am J Phys. 1981;241:H442–8.
9. Klouche K, Weil MH, Sun S, Tang W, Povoas H, Bisera J. Stroke volumes generated by precordial compression during cardiac resuscitation. Crit Care Med. 2002;30:2626–31.
10. Voorhees WD, Babbs CF, Tacker WA Jr. Regional blood flow during cardiopulmonary resuscitation in dogs. Crit Care Med. 1980;8:134–6.
11. Anthi A, Tzelepis GE, Alivizatos P, Michalis A, Palatianos GM, Geroulanos S. Unexpected cardiac arrest after cardiac surgery: incidence, predisposing causes, and outcome of open chest cardiopulmonary resuscitation. Chest. 1998;113:15–9.
12. Neumar RW, Otto CW, Link MS, et al. Part 8: adult advanced cardiovascular life support: 2010 American Heart Association Guidelines for Cardiopulmonary Resuscitation and Emergency Cardiovascular Care. Circulation. 2010;122:S729–67.
13. Dunning J, Fabbri A, Kolh PH, et al. Guideline for resuscitation in cardiac arrest after cardiac surgery. Eur J Cardiothorac Surg. 2009;36:3–28.
14. Perkins GD, Travers AH, Berg RA, et al. Part 3: adult basic life support and automated external defibrillation: 2015 International Consensus on Cardiopulmonary Resuscitation and Emergency Cardiovascular Care Science with Treatment Recommendations. Resuscitation. 2015;95:e43–69.
15. Sayre MR, Koster RW, Botha M, et al. Part 5: adult basic life support: 2010 International Consensus on Cardiopulmonary Resuscitation and Emergency Cardiovascular Care Science with Treatment Recommendations. Circulation. 2010;122:S298–324.
16. Laws D, Neville E, Duffy J, Pleural Diseases Group SoCCBTS. BTS guidelines for the insertion of a chest drain. Thorax. 2003;58 Suppl 2:ii53–9.
17. LaPar DJ, Ghanta RK, Kern JA, et al. Hospital variation in mortality from cardiac arrest after cardiac surgery: an opportunity for improvement? Ann Thorac Surg. 2014;98:534–9. discussion 9-40
18. Mackay JH, Powell SJ, Osgathorp J, Rozario CJ. Six-year prospective audit of chest reopening after cardiac arrest. Eur J Cardiothorac Surg. 2002;22:421–5.
19. Chandra N, Rudikoff M, Weisfeldt ML. Simultaneous chest compression and ventilation at high airway pressure during cardiopulmonary resuscitation. Lancet. 1980;1:175–8.
20. Buschmann CT, Tsokos M. Frequent and rare complications of resuscitation attempts. Intensive Care Med. 2009;35:397–404.
21. Krischer JP, Fine EG, Davis JH, Nagel EL. Complications of cardiac resuscitation. Chest. 1987;92:287–91.
22. Sutton RM, Friess SH, Maltese MR, et al. Hemodynamic-directed cardiopulmonary resuscitation during in-hospital cardiac arrest. Resuscitation. 2014;85:983–6.

Decreasing skeletal muscle as a risk factor for mortality in elderly patients with sepsis

Keita Shibahashi[*], Kazuhiro Sugiyama, Masahiro Kashiura and Yuichi Hamabe

Abstract

Background: Older patients account for the majority of patients with sepsis. The objective of this study was to determine if decreased skeletal muscle mass is associated with outcomes in elderly patients with sepsis.

Methods: Patients (60 years and older) who were admitted to a tertiary medical center intensive care unit with a primary diagnosis of sepsis between January 2012 and February 2016 were included. Patients who had not undergone abdominal computed tomography on the day of admission, had cardiopulmonary arrest on arrival, or had iliopsoas abscess were excluded from the analyses. Cross-sectional muscle area at the 3rd lumber vertebra was quantified, and the relation to in-hospital mortality was analyzed. Multivariable logistic regression analysis that included sex and APACHE II score as explanatory variables was performed. The optimal cutoff value to define decreased muscle mass (sarcopenia) was calculated using receiver operating characteristic curve analysis, and the odds ratio for in-hospital mortality was determined.

Results: There were 150 elderly patients with sepsis (median age, 75 years) enrolled; in-hospital mortality and median APACHE II score were 38.7 and 24%, respectively. The skeletal muscle area of deceased patients was significantly lower than that of the survival group ($P < 0.001$). The multivariable logistic regression analysis demonstrated that decreased muscle mass was significantly associated with increased mortality (odds ratio = 0.94, 95% confidence interval = 0.90 to 0.97, $P < 0.001$). The optimal cutoff value of skeletal muscle area to predict in-hospital mortality was 45.2 cm^2 for men and 39.0 cm^2 for women. With these cutoff values, the adjusted odds ratio for decreased muscle area was 3.27 (95% CI, 1.61 to 6.63, $P = 0.001$).

Conclusions: Less skeletal muscle mass is associated with higher in-hospital mortality in elderly patients with sepsis. The results of this study suggest that identifying patients with low muscularity contributes to better stratification in this population.

Keywords: Sepsis, Sarcopenia, Intensive care, Mortality

Background

Sepsis is a clinical syndrome characterized by physiologic, biologic, and biochemical abnormalities caused by a dysregulated inflammatory response to infection. It also includes organ dysfunction attributed to it and is a major public health concern. The reported incidence is disproportionately higher in older patients. Older patients account for the majority (60–85%) of all episodes, and this figure is likely to increase in the future [1–3].

Therefore, the importance of accurate stratification of elderly patients with sepsis is growing, as it can aid in developing a treatment strategy, allocating healthcare resources, and assessing the effectiveness of novel therapies. While chronologic age is an important element in assessing the anomaly in the host's inflammatory response, physiologic age is a more important determinant of outcomes. Recently, sarcopenia, which is defined as the loss of skeletal muscle mass and strength with advancing age [4], has increasingly been recognized as an important factor that can act as a marker of decreased physiologic reserve because it is highly important for

* Correspondence: kshibahashi@yahoo.co.jp
Department of Emergency and Intensive Care Center, Tokyo Metropolitan Bokutoh Hospital, 4-23-15, Kotobashi, Sumida-ku, Tokyo 130-8575, Japan

immune function, glucose disposal, protein synthesis, and mobility [5, 6].

We hypothesized that decreased skeletal muscle mass is a predictive marker for the outcome of elderly patients with sepsis. In this retrospective study, we investigated whether decreased skeletal muscle mass is associated with in-hospital mortality in elderly patients with sepsis.

Methods

Population cohort and data acquisition

Patients who were admitted to a tertiary medical center intensive care unit (ICU) with a primary diagnosis of sepsis between January 2012 and February 2016 were retrospectively identified. Our tertiary medical center admits only severe patients either directly transferred from the scene by an emergency response team or referred from another medical facility. We employ a strategy, wherein, we aggressively perform torso CT on almost all patients. This entails confirmation of the potential source of infection, assessment of anatomical structures of the lesion in detail, and identification of any coexisting lesions as reliably and immediately as possible. Elderly (60 years and older) patients were included in the analysis. Patients were excluded from the analysis who had not undergone abdominal computed tomography (CT) on the day of admission or had cardiopulmonary arrest on arrival (CPAOA). Because updated definitions of sepsis that offer greater consistency for clinical trials were released in 2016 [7], we determined whether the patients met the revised criteria for sepsis; otherwise, they were excluded from the study. Patients with iliopsoas abscess were also excluded from the analysis because of the possible confounding effect on skeletal muscle area.

Demographic and clinical data included age, sex, body weight, Glasgow coma scale (GCS) score, body temperature, mean arterial pressure, heart rate, respiratory rate, arterial oxygen partial pressure, fractional inspired oxygen, blood test results (platelets, bilirubin, creatinine, Na, K, hematocrit, white blood cell count, and lactate on admission), administration of vasopressors, length of stay (LOS) in the hospital, LOS in the ICU, in-hospital mortality, location of death, infection source, chronic health problems, and recent surgery. We calculated the Sepsis-related Organ Failure Assessment (SOFA) score [8], which determines the extent of a patient's organ failure based on the respiratory, cardiovascular, hepatic, coagulation, renal, and neurological systems, as well as the second version of the Acute Physiology and Chronic Health Evaluation (APACHE II) score [9], which determines the severity of disease based on a patient's age and physiological measurements.

Computed tomography measurement

Access to computed tomography (CT) images on the day of admission was available through the picture archiving

and communication system (PACS; SYNAPSE software, Fujifilm Medical Co., Tokyo, Japan). After the observer outlined the muscle, the range of the area of interest was calculated by the software. Muscle attenuation, a measure of muscle density and fatty infiltration, was quantified using Hounsfield units (HU) obtained from the CT image. Lean skeletal muscle mass was estimated by measuring the cross-sectional area of the psoas and paraspinal (quadratus lumborum, erector spinae) muscles at the third lumber vertebra (L3) as shown in Fig. 1. A strong correlation between the cross-sectional area of skeletal muscle at this landmark and whole-body muscle distribution has been reported, and the validity and reliability of this method to estimate lean skeletal muscle mass have been established [10–12]. HUs within the range of interest of each muscle were calculated, and the average value was used for the final muscle attenuation. The observer was blinded to patients' survival status.

Statistical analysis

Patients were grouped according to outcome (survival or deceased). For descriptive statistics, numeric or ordered variables are presented as medians with interquartile ranges and were compared using Mann–Whitney U tests. Categorical variables are presented as counts and percentages and were tested for significance using Fisher's exact tests. We used a multivariable logistic regression model to determine whether decreased skeletal muscle area is independently associated with in-hospital mortality in patients with sepsis. We also performed additional stratified analyses that divide patients into two groups of 60–80 years and over 80 years to adjust heterogeneity because muscle mass of over 80 years is lost at an accelerated rate (15%/year) compared to the rate of approximately 8% per decade from the age of 50 years [13]. To minimize the risk of falsely identifying

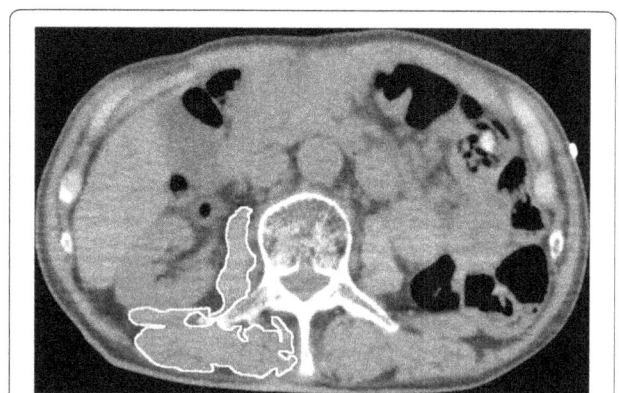

Fig. 1 CT image at the L3-sectional muscle. The right L3-sectional muscle area is outlined. Muscle area and mean muscle attenuation are calculated by the picture archiving and communication system (PACS) software

significant results, explanatory variables were predetermined before the analysis based on previous studies [9, 14–16]. In addition to the skeletal muscle area, the APACHE II score and sex were included in the model. To test multicollinearity, we evaluated the variance inflation factor. To determine the optimal cutoff value of skeletal muscle area for predicting in-hospital mortality and the area under the curve (AUC), we performed receiver operating characteristic (ROC) curve analysis. We defined the patients with a skeletal muscle area lower than the cutoff value as sarcopenic, and the odds ratio for mortality was determined. For each groups, event-time distributions were estimated with the use of the Kaplan–Meier method. The difference of estimated survival rate was tested using log-rank test. We performed an analysis using Cox

proportional hazards regression and taking time to in-hospital death as the dependent variable and sarcopenia as the main predictor variable. To adjust for potential confounders, APACHE II score and sex were included in a multivariable model. Hazard ratios and 95% confidence interval (CI) are given. All statistical tests were two-tailed, and P values <0.05 were considered significant.

All statistical analyses were performed with EZR (Saitama Medical Center, Jichi Medical University, Saitama, Japan), which is a graphical user interface for R (The R Foundation for Statistical Computing, Vienna, Austria). More precisely, it is a modified version of R commander designed to add statistical functions frequently used in biostatistics [17].

Table 1 Patient characteristics and radiological findings

| | All patients | Group | | P value |
		Survival	Deceased	
Number of patients	150	92	58	
Location of death				
ICU			44	
After transferred to general floor			14	
Age (years)	75 [68, 82]	74 [67, 81]	77 [71, 83]	0.13
Sex, men (%)	103 (69)	63 (69)	40 (69)	0.99
GCS	14 [9, 15]	14 [10, 15]	12 [7, 15]	0.21
Lactate on admission (mmol/L)	4.2 [2.3, 7.2]	3.9 [1.8, 6.3]	5.9 [2.4, 8.9]	0.053
Infection source (%)				0.33
Lung	45 (30)	23 (25)	22 (38)	
Urinary tract	32 (21)	24 (26)	8 (14)	
Peritonitis/abscess	16 (11)	8 (9)	8 (14)	
Perforated viscus	15 (10)	10 (11)	5 (9)	
Cholecystitis/cholangitis	10 (7)	8 (9)	2 (3)	
Unknown	9 (6)	4 (4)	5 (9)	
NecFas/decubitus ulcer	8 (5)	5 (5)	3 (5)	
Ischemic bowel	5 (3)	3 (3)	2 (3)	
Colitis	5 (3)	4 (4)	1 (2)	
Blood stream infection	3 (1)	1 (1)	2 (3)	
Bone/joint	1 (1)	1 (1)	0 (0)	
CNS	1 (1)	1 (1)	0 (0)	
SOFA score	9 [7, 12]	8 [7, 11]	10 [8, 12]	0.004
APACHE II score	24 [19, 30]	23 [18, 27]	26 [22, 34]	0.002
Body weight (kg)	54 [48, 60]	54 [48, 61]	54 [48, 58]	0.42
Skeletal muscle area (cm^2)	41.6 [34.0, 48.1]	43.3 [36.5, 50.9]	36.8 [30.1, 43.2]	<0.001
Muscle attenuation (HU)	32.6 [24.1, 39.9]	33.2 [24.2, 40.0]	31.0 [23.6, 39.8]	0.38
LOS in ICU	8 [4, 15]	9 [6, 15]	5 [2, 14]	
LOS in hospital	27 [7, 51]	40 [18, 62]	8 [3, 25]	

ICU intensive care unit, *GCS* Glasgow coma scale, *NecFas* necrotizing fasciitis, *CNS* central nervous system, *SOFA* Sepsis-related Organ Failure Assessment, *APACHE II* second version of the acute physiology and chronic health evaluation, *HU* Hounsfield unit, *LOS* length of stay

Results

During the study period, 168 patients met the inclusion criteria. Of those, patients were excluded for the following reasons: $n = 4$, no abdominal CT; $n = 10$, CPAOA; and $n = 1$, had an iliopsoas abscess. Of the remaining 153 patients, 3 patients who did not meet the recent criteria for sepsis were excluded, resulting in 150 patients (103 men, 47 women; age 75 [68, 82] years) in the analysis. All the predictors required to calculate the APACHE II and SOFA scores were present in the dataset.

The clinical characteristics and radiological features are summarized in Table 1. The overall APACHE II score was 24 [18, 19], and the in-hospital mortality rate was 38.7%. Lactate level on admission was 4.2 [2.3, 7.2], and that of 116 patients (77%) were higher than 2.0 mmol/L. The survival group included 92 patients, and the deceased group included 58 patients. Of the 58 deceased patients, 44 deceased at ICU and 14 deceased after transfer to general floor. The APACHE II score was significantly higher in the deceased group ($P = 0.002$).

The median skeletal muscle area in all patients was 41.6 [34.0, 48.1] cm^2. Those of the survival group was significantly larger than the deceased group (43.3 [36.5, 50.9] and 36.8 [30.1, 43.2] cm^2, $P < 0.001$; Fig. 2). The SOFA score of the deceased group was significantly higher than that of the survival group ($P = 0.004$).

The results of the multivariable regression analysis are shown in Table 2. The variance inflation factors for multicollinearity were lower than 1.06 among the predetermined explanatory variables. Among the variables, skeletal muscle area (cm^2) was an independent predictive parameter for in-hospital mortality, and the adjusted odds ratio was 0.94 (95% CI, 0.90 to 0.97, $P < 0.001$). In the stratified

Table 2 Results of multivariable logistic regression analysis to determine variables independently associated with in-hospital mortality of patients with sepsis

	Odds ratio (95% confidence interval)	P value
Overall analysis		
Skeletal muscle area (cm^2)	0.94 (0.90–0.97)	<0.001
APACHE II score	1.07 (1.02–1.12)	0.003
Sex, men	1.46 (0.67–3.22)	0.34
Stratified analysis		
60–80 years		
Skeletal muscle area (cm^2)	0.96 (0.92–0.99)	0.032
Over 80 years		
Skeletal muscle area (cm^2)	0.89 (0.81–0.98)	0.016

APACHE II second version of the Acute Physiology and Chronic Health Evaluation

analysis, the association between skeletal muscle area and in-hospital mortality was significant in both groups of 60–80 years and over 80 years, and the adjusted odds ratio was 0.96 (95% CI, 0.92 to 0.99, $P = 0.032$) and 0.89 (95% CI, 0.81 to 0.98, $P = 0.016$), respectively.

The cutoff value of skeletal muscle area to predict in-hospital mortality was calculated for each sex because the skeletal muscle area was significantly larger in men than in women (43.1 [35.5, 51.0] vs 39.0 [33.1, 43.0] cm^2, $P = 0.005$; Fig. 3). ROC curve analysis demonstrated that the optimal cutoff values were 45.2 cm^2 for men and 39.0 cm^2 for women, and the AUCs were 0.65 (95% CI, 0.54 to 0.76) and 0.72 (95% CI, 0.58 to 0.88), respectively. Based on our definition of sarcopenia (using the cutoff value), in-hospital mortality was significantly higher for patients with sarcopenia, and the adjusted odds ratio was 3.27 (95% CI, 1.61 to 6.63, $P = 0.001$). Kaplan–Meier estimates of mortality were drown for each group (Fig. 4). The estimated survival rate 100 days after admission was 0.70 (95% CI, 0.54 to 0.81) for not sarcopenic patients and 0.37 (95% CI, 0.23 to 0.50) for sarcopenic patients, and the difference was significant ($P < 0.001$). Cox proportional hazards regression analysis showed a higher risk of in-hospital mortality for sarcopenic patients even when adjusted for APACHE II score and sex, and the hazard ratio was 2.55 (95% CI, 1.43 to 4.56, $P = 0.001$).

Discussion

Sarcopenia is important as an independent predictor of falls, disability, loss of independence, and increased mortality. While the prognostic value of sarcopenia has been determined for patients after surgery, trauma, or with cancer [9–12, 18, 20–25], its importance for patients with sepsis has not been evaluated. In the present sample of elderly patients with sepsis admitted to a tertiary medical

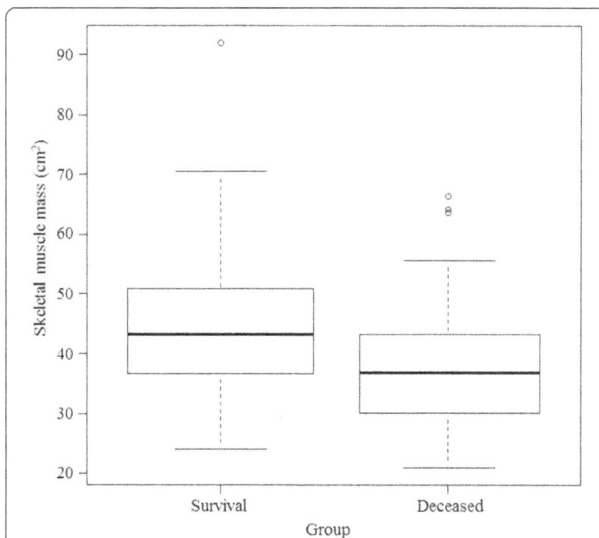

Fig. 2 Comparison of the skeletal muscle area between survival group and deceased group. Skeletal muscle area was significantly larger in survival group (43.3 [36.5, 50.9] vs 36.8 [30.1, 43.2], P < 0.001)

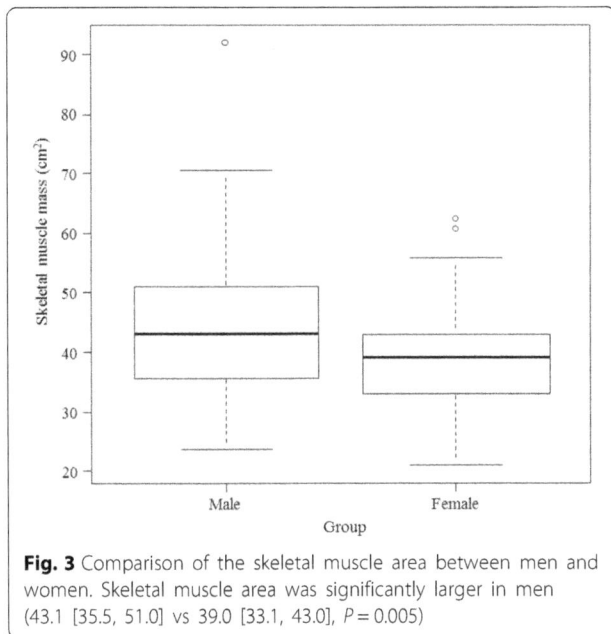

Fig. 3 Comparison of the skeletal muscle area between men and women. Skeletal muscle area was significantly larger in men (43.1 [35.5, 51.0] vs 39.0 [33.1, 43.0], $P = 0.005$)

center ICU, decreased skeletal muscle mass was a significant predictor of in-hospital mortality. This is the first study, to the best of our knowledge, to examine the implications of sarcopenia in elderly patients with sepsis.

A wide range of techniques can be used to assess muscle mass. CT and magnetic resonance imaging (MRI) are considered to be very precise imaging systems and as gold standards for estimating muscle mass. In this study, we used the cross-sectional area of the muscle determined using CT; this provides an estimation of the overall muscle mass and has been used in a variety of studies to predict lean muscle mass [10–12]. While it is difficult to perform these measurements for

the sole purpose of estimating skeletal muscle mass, CT is frequently required in patients with sepsis as a part of the initial work up; therefore, an early assessment of muscularity in this patient population is possible, and the cross-sectional view of the muscle provides an easily obtained objective method for estimating lean muscle mass in these patients. Because it takes only a few minutes, it can be easily performed in most clinical scenarios. A strength of this study is the ease of incorporating our findings into practice.

Clinical characteristics that impact the severity of sepsis and outcome include the host's response to infection, site and type of infection, and therapeutic strategy. The therapeutic strategy for sepsis has been standardized in practice guidelines; several studies have reported decreasing sepsis-related mortality rates over time with the implementation of therapeutic strategies, after adjusting for multiple variables, suggesting improvement owing not only to sepsis criteria and to the progress in medicine in general but also to these strategies [26, 27]. Furthermore, the importance of the host response as a prognostic factor for patients with sepsis is growing. Among the factors related with host response, age is reportedly a primary risk factor for mortality because of its association with comorbid illnesses, impaired immunologic responses, malnutrition, and increased exposure to potentially resistant pathogens. Although chronologic age is a good objective marker of the anomaly in the host response and included in scoring models of prognosis for patients in the ICU, considerable individual variation in physical condition exists among the elderly. While muscle mass is generally lost with aging and the prevalence of sarcopenia ranges between 5 and 13% in older people, the severity of muscle loss significantly varies in this population. In the current

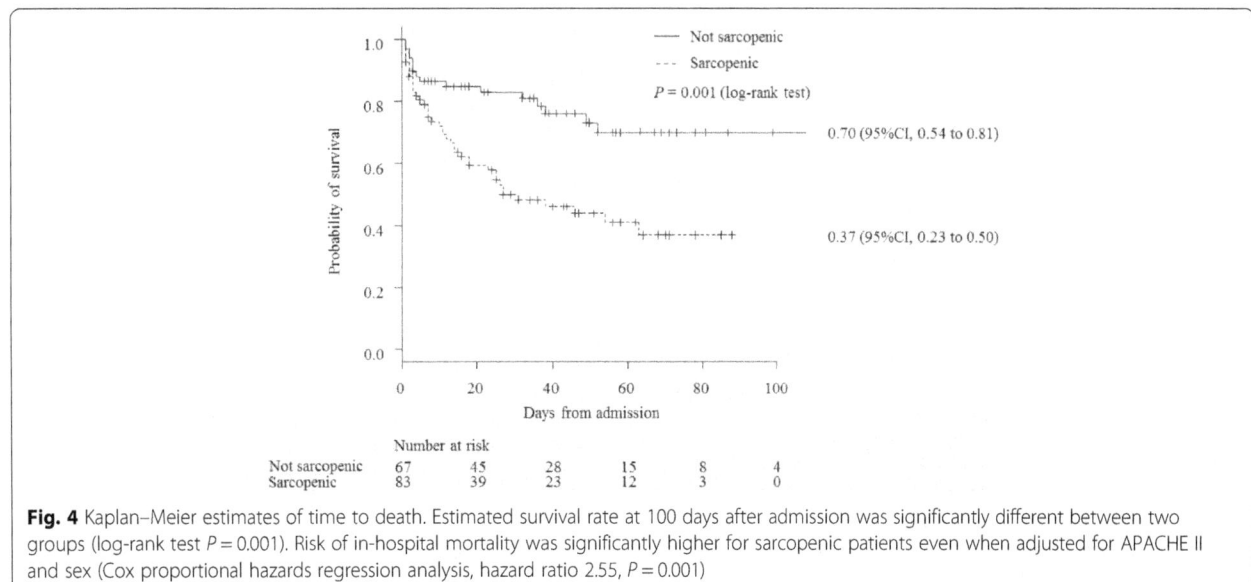

Fig. 4 Kaplan–Meier estimates of time to death. Estimated survival rate at 100 days after admission was significantly different between two groups (log-rank test $P = 0.001$). Risk of in-hospital mortality was significantly higher for sarcopenic patients even when adjusted for APACHE II and sex (Cox proportional hazards regression analysis, hazard ratio 2.55, $P = 0.001$)

study, we confirmed associations between decreasing muscle mass and sepsis related mortality. Because skeletal muscle atrophy can cause physical decline such as impaired cytokine [28] and insulin signaling [19, 29] that may result in glucose intolerance, we speculate that stratification by muscle mass may reflect physical age and help circumvent the difficulties associated with prognostication and classification of elderly patients with sepsis by chronologic age. The mechanisms for the relationship between sarcopenia and poor prognosis cannot be definitively determined because of the study design. However, the results of the current study highlight the need to prevent progressive loss of skeletal muscle mass and function in the elderly.

The literature suggests that the combination of exercise and nutrition is the key intervention for preventing, treating, and slowing down the progress of sarcopenia [30, 31]. Resistance exercise combined with protein supplementation at higher protein doses of 40 g leads to greater muscle gain than exercise or protein supplementation alone in the elderly [31, 32]. The awareness of the benefits of exercise and diet is not enough in older people. Enhancing participation in exercise for older patients might prevent sarcopenia and improve sepsis outcomes in the elderly population. Rehabilitation and nutritional strategies that focus on preventing muscle loss may also contribute to better outcomes. Further research is required to test these hypotheses; however, the results of the present study highlight the importance of muscle mass in patients with sepsis.

Limitations
Owing to the retrospective design, biases and confounding are major concern. We tried to adjust for possible confounders such as age, comorbidity, recent surgery, and sex by performing multivariable regression analysis using the APACHE II score, which is calculated with these variables, and sex as explanatory variables. This study was performed at a single center with a small sample. Because it is our strategy to aggressively perform torso CT for patients with sepsis, almost all patients including those with lung infection, CNS infection, and necrotizing fasciitis/decubitus ulcer undergo abdominal CT at our ICU. Some institutes may not perform abdominal CT for such cases. Hence, the infection source of patients with abdominal CT may differ between other studies and the present study, limiting external validity of our results. We expect similar associations between muscle mass and in-hospital mortality in other cohorts; however, the optimal cutoff value should be validated. We report that the odds ratio for in-hospital mortality was 3.27, but the 95% CI was wide, with a minimum value of 1.61. Further research with a larger sample is necessary to establish the clinical significance of sarcopenia.

Conclusions
We found that less skeletal muscle mass is associated with higher in-hospital mortality of elderly patients with sepsis. The results of this study suggest that identifying patients with low muscularity may contribute to better stratification of elderly patients.

Abbreviations
APACHE II: Second version of the Acute Physiology and Chronic Health Evaluation; AUC: Area under the curve; CPAOA: Cardiopulmonary arrest on arrival; CT: Computed tomography; GCS: Glasgow coma scale; HU: Hounsfield unit; ICU: Intensive care unit; LOS: Length of stay; MRI: Magnetic resonance imaging; ROC: Receiver operating characteristic; SOFA: Sepsis-related Organ Failure Assessment

Acknowledgements
Not applicable.

Authors' contributions
K. Shibahashi designed this study. K. Shibahashi conducted the literature search and data collection. K. Shibahashi, K. Sugiyama, and MK performed the data analysis and interpreted the data. K. Shibahashi wrote the manuscript, and K. Sugiyama, MK, and YH critically revised the final manuscript. All authors read and approved the final manuscript.

Competing interests
The authors declare that they have no competing interests.

References
1. Kaukonen KM, Bailey M, Suzuki S, Pilcher D, Bellomo R. Mortality related to severe sepsis and septic shock among critically ill patients in Australia and New Zealand, 2000-2012. JAMA. 2014;311(13):1308–16.
2. Angus DC, Linde-Zwirble WT, Lidicker J, Clermont G, Carcillo J, Pinsky MR. Epidemiology of severe sepsis in the United States: analysis of incidence, outcome, and associated costs of care. Crit Care Med. 2001;29(7):1303–10.
3. Angus DC, Kelley MA, Schmitz RJ, White A, Popovich Jr J, Committee on Manpower for Pulmonary and Critical Care Societies (COMPACCS). Caring for the critically ill patient. Current and projected workforce requirements for care of the critically ill and patients with pulmonary disease: can we meet the requirements of an aging population? JAMA. 2000;284(21):2762–70.
4. Morley JE, Baumgartner RN, Roubenoff R, Mayer J, Nair KS. Sarcopenia. J Lab Clin Med. 2001;137(4):231–43.
5. Kemeny MM, Peterson BL, Kornblith AB, Muss HB, Wheeler J, Levine E, et al. Barriers to clinical trial participation by older women with breast cancer. J Clin Oncol. 2003;21(12):2268–75.
6. McCleary NJ, Dotan E, Browner I. Refining the chemotherapy approach for older patients with colon cancer. J Clin Oncol. 2014;32(24):2570–80.
7. Singer M, Deutschman CS, Seymour CW, Shankar-Hari M, Annane D, Bauer M, et al. The third international consensus definitions for sepsis and septic shock (sepsis-3). JAMA. 2016;315(8):801–10.
8. Vincent JL, Moreno R, Takala J, Willatts S, De Mendonca A, Bruining H, et al. The SOFA (Sepsis-related Organ Failure Assessment) score to describe organ dysfunction/failure. On behalf of the Working Group on Sepsis-Related

Problems of the European Society of Intensive Care Medicine. Intensive Care Med. 1996;22(7):707–10.

9   Knaus WA, Draper EA, Wagner DP, Zimmerman JE. APACHE II: a severity of disease classification system. Crit Care Med. 1985;13(10):818–29.

10 Mourtzakis M, Prado CM, Lieffers JR, Reiman T, McCargar LJ, Baracos VE. A practical and precise approach to quantification of body composition in cancer patients using computed tomography images acquired during routine care. Appl Physiol Nutr Metab. 2008;33(5):997–1006.

11 Shen W, Punyanitya M, Wang Z, Gallagher D, St-Onge MP, Albu J, et al. Total body skeletal muscle and adipose tissue volumes: estimation from a single abdominal cross-sectional image. J Appl Physiol (1985). 2004;97(6):2333–8.

12 Martin L, Birdsell L, Macdonald N, Reiman T, Clandinin MT, McCargar LJ, et al. Cancer cachexia in the age of obesity: skeletal muscle depletion is a powerful prognostic factor, independent of body mass index. J Clin Oncol. 2013;31(12):1539–47.

13 Grimby G, Saltin B. The ageing muscle. Clin Physiol. 1983;3(3):209–18.

14 Schröder J, Kahlke V, Staubach KH, Zabel P, Stüber F. Gender differences in human sepsis. Arch Surg. 1998;133:1200–5.

15 Kisat M, Villegas CV, Onguti S, Zafar SN, Latif A, Efron DT, et al. Predictors of sepsis in moderately severely injured patients: an analysis of the National Trauma Data Bank. Surg Infect (Larchmt). 2013;14:62–8.

16 Kisat M, Villegas CV, Onguti S, Zafar SN, Latif A, Efron DT, et al. Skeletal muscle predicts ventilator-free days, ICU-free days, and mortality in elderly ICU patients. Crit Care. 2013;17(5):R206.

17 Kanda Y. Investigation of the freely available easy-to-use software 'EZR' for medical statistics. Bone Marrow Transplant. 2013;48(3):452–8.

18 Danai PA, Moss M, Mannino DM, Martin GS. The epidemiology of sepsis in patients with malignancy. Chest. 2006;129(6):1432–40.

19 Mikines KJ, Richter EA, Dela F, Galbo H. Seven days of bed rest decrease insulin action on glucose uptake in leg and whole body. J Appl Physiol (1985). 1991;70(3):1245–54.

20 Peng PD, van Vledder MG, Tsai S, de Jong MC, Makary M, Ng J, et al. Sarcopenia negatively impacts short-term outcomes in patients undergoing hepatic resection for colorectal liver metastasis. HPB (Oxford). 2011;13(7):439–46.

21 Itoh S, Shirabe K, Matsumoto Y, Yoshiya S, Muto J, Harimoto N, et al. Effect of body composition on outcomes after hepatic resection for hepatocellular carcinoma. Ann Surg Oncol. 2014;21(9):3063–8.

22 Reisinger KW, van Vugt JL, Tegels JJ, Snijders C, Hulsewe KW, Hoofwijk AG, et al. Functional compromise reflected by sarcopenia, frailty, and nutritional depletion predicts adverse postoperative outcome after colorectal cancer surgery. Ann Surg. 2015;261(2):345–52.

23 Peng P, Hyder O, Firoozmand A, Kneuertz P, Schulick RD, Huang D, et al. Impact of sarcopenia on outcomes following resection of pancreatic adenocarcinoma. J Gastrointest Surg. 2012;16(8):1478–86.

24 Shachar SS, Williams GR, Muss HB, Nishijima TF. Prognostic value of sarcopenia in adults with solid tumours: a meta-analysis and systematic review. Eur J Cancer. 2016;57:58–67.

25 Kim TN, Choi KM. Sarcopenia: definition, epidemiology, and pathophysiology. J Bone Metab. 2013;20(1):1–10.

26 Martin GS, Mannino DM, Eaton S, Moss M. The epidemiology of sepsis in the United States from 1979 through 2000. N Engl J Med. 2003;348(16):1546–54.

27 Stevenson EK, Rubenstein AR, Radin GT, Wiener RS, Walkey AJ. Two decades of mortality trends among patients with severe sepsis: a comparative meta-analysis*. Crit Care Med. 2014;42(3):625–31.

28 Brandt C, Pedersen BK. The role of exercise-induced myokines in muscle homeostasis and the defense against chronic diseases. J Biomed Biotechnol. 2010;2010:520258.

29 Blanc S, Normand S, Pachiaudi C, Fortrat JO, Laville M, Gharib C. Fuel homeostasis during physical inactivity induced by bed rest. J Clin Endocrinol Metab. 2000;85(6):2223–33.

30 Deutz NE, Bauer JM, Barazzoni R, Biolo G, Boirie Y, Bosy-Westphal A, et al. Protein intake and exercise for optimal muscle function with aging: recommendations from the ESPEN Expert Group. Clin Nutr. 2014;33(6):929–36.

31 Kim HK, Suzuki T, Saito K, Yoshida H, Kobayashi H, Kato H, et al. Effects of exercise and amino acid supplementation on body composition and physical function in community-dwelling elderly Japanese sarcopenic women: a randomized controlled trial. J Am Geriatr Soc. 2012;60(1):16–23.

32 Kim HK, Suzuki T, Saito K, Yoshida H, Kobayashi H, Kato H, et al. Resistance exercise enhances myofibrillar protein synthesis with graded intakes of whey protein in older men. Br J Nutr. 2012;108(10):1780–8.

Clinically integrated multi-organ point-of-care ultrasound for undifferentiated respiratory difficulty, chest pain, or shock

Young-Rock Ha[1]* and Hong-Chuen Toh[2]

Abstract

Rapid and accurate diagnosis and treatment are paramount in the management of the critically ill. Critical care ultrasound has been widely used as an adjunct to standard clinical examination, an invaluable extension of physical examination to guide clinical decision-making at bedside. Recently, there is growing interest in the use of multi-organ point-of-care ultrasound (MOPOCUS) for the management of the critically ill, especially in the early phase of resuscitation. This article will review the role and utility of symptom-based and sign-oriented MOPOCUS in patients with undifferentiated respiratory difficulty, chest pain, or shock and how it can be performed in a timely, effective, and efficient manner.

Keywords: Multi-organ point-of-care ultrasound, Respiratory difficulty, Chest pain, Shock

Background

The capability to recognize and resuscitate the critically ill, or peri-cardiac arrest patients, is one of the defining traits of critical care and emergency medicine. These patients can be categorized into three groups: pre-arrest, intra-arrest, and post-arrest with return of spontaneous circulation (ROSC). For all three groups, and especially the pre-arrest patients, rapid diagnosis of the underlying physiology and etiology and timely intervention are essential for effective management and stabilization. Speedy and accurate clinical decisions can be lifesaving. Traditionally, acute care physicians evaluate patients based on history and physical examinations. For those presenting with respiratory difficulty, chest pain, shock, or shock-related symptoms or signs, the assessment has to be performed in a focused and time-sensitive manner. Now, bedside multi-organ point-of-care ultrasound (MOPOCUS) and MOPOCUS-guided protocols can be used as an adjunct to standard clinical examination, especially during the initial and undifferentiated phase.

MOPOCUS can provide many critical pieces of information to guide clinical decision-making, while waiting for laboratory and imaging results.

According to the consensus statement of the American Society of Echocardiography and the American College of Emergency Medicine [1], respiratory difficulty, chest pain, or shock are recommended indications of the focused cardiac ultrasound in an emergency setting. A growing body of evidence also supports the use of MOPOCUS of the critically ill to evaluate cause of shock or dyspnea [2–15]. Although there are only few studies reporting the utility of MOPOCUS using chest pain alone as the primary indication, the astute clinician is cognizant that etiologies classically associated with chest pain, such as acute coronary syndrome and aortic dissection, can be associated with dyspnea or hypotension or even presents atypically with these two "non-cardiac" presentations alone in the absence of chest pain. A patient with pneumothorax can present with shortness of breath and chest pain and develop hypotension when it becomes a tension pneumothorax. Acute myocardial infarction complicated with cardiogenic shock and pulmonary edema can produce dyspnea, chest pain, and shock concurrently. Indeed, the patient's signs and

* Correspondence: youngrock.ha@gmail.com
[1]Emergency Department, Bundang Jesaeng Hospital, 20 Seohyeon-ro 180beongil, Bundang-gu, Seongnam-si, Gyeonggi-do, South Korea
Full list of author information is available at the end of the article

symptoms can vary depending on the severity of disease and presence of complications. Therefore, it is prudent for acute care physicians to perform a symptom- or sign-based MOPOCUS for any combination of the three indications listed above.

MOPOCUS is a powerful adjunct to clinical assessment. The certainty of presumptive diagnosis derived from history-taking and physical examination can be validated, or occasionally refuted, by information provided by MOPOCUS. In this article, we will appraise the utility of an integrated MOPOCUS, focusing on the differential diagnostic process in pre-cardiac arrest situation and the sequence of scanning. A detailed review of each organ, especially the abdomen, using point-of-care ultrasound (POCUS) will be covered subsequently in this thematic series.

The sequence of MOPOCUS scanning

There is no universally accepted sequence of scanning using MOPOCUS. In this review, we advocate that the physician begin by assessing the lung and inferior vena cava (IVC), with the abdominal aorta, followed by the heart (including the thoracic aorta in case of chest pain) and, lastly, the abdomen for evaluation of the source of intra-abdominal sepsis or blood loss (Fig. 1). Although all the organs can be scanned with either an abdominal convex (2–6 MHz) or cardiac sector (2–4 MHz) transducer, we can change the transducers for a detailed evaluation if time permits. This sequence is both practical and time-efficient. Firstly, ultrasound findings from the lung and IVC allow rapid categorization of the causes of dyspnea or shock. Secondly, the critically ill are most often supine, a position that is conducive for scanning these two systems. Lastly, from the same site for IVC evaluation, the physician can easily tilt the probe into the subxiphoid plane to evaluate the heart and integrate the focused cardiac ultrasound findings with those from the lung and IVC to elucidate the pathophysiology of shock. In this review, we formulated these MOPOCUS findings into several structured algorithmic approaches. While these are not exhaustive, the underlying pathophysiology and hemodynamics can be systematically categorized and subsequently narrowed to those that are critical, commonly encountered, and warrant timely diagnosis and intervention. The legends used in the algorithms (Fig. 2, 7, 8, 12, 14, 16, and 19) are detailed in Fig. 2.

Lung ultrasound

The first and most important ultrasound sign to recognize in the lung is the "bat sign." The bat sign is essential for the accurate identification of the pleural line. Conceptually, the lung should be interrogated in three zones: the chest wall, pleural line, and subpleural space. Sonographic findings and their definitions at each part are summarized in Table 1.

Do we need to scan the entire lung when performing lung ultrasound? On the one hand, in the interest of rapid assessment, many favor the BLUE protocol

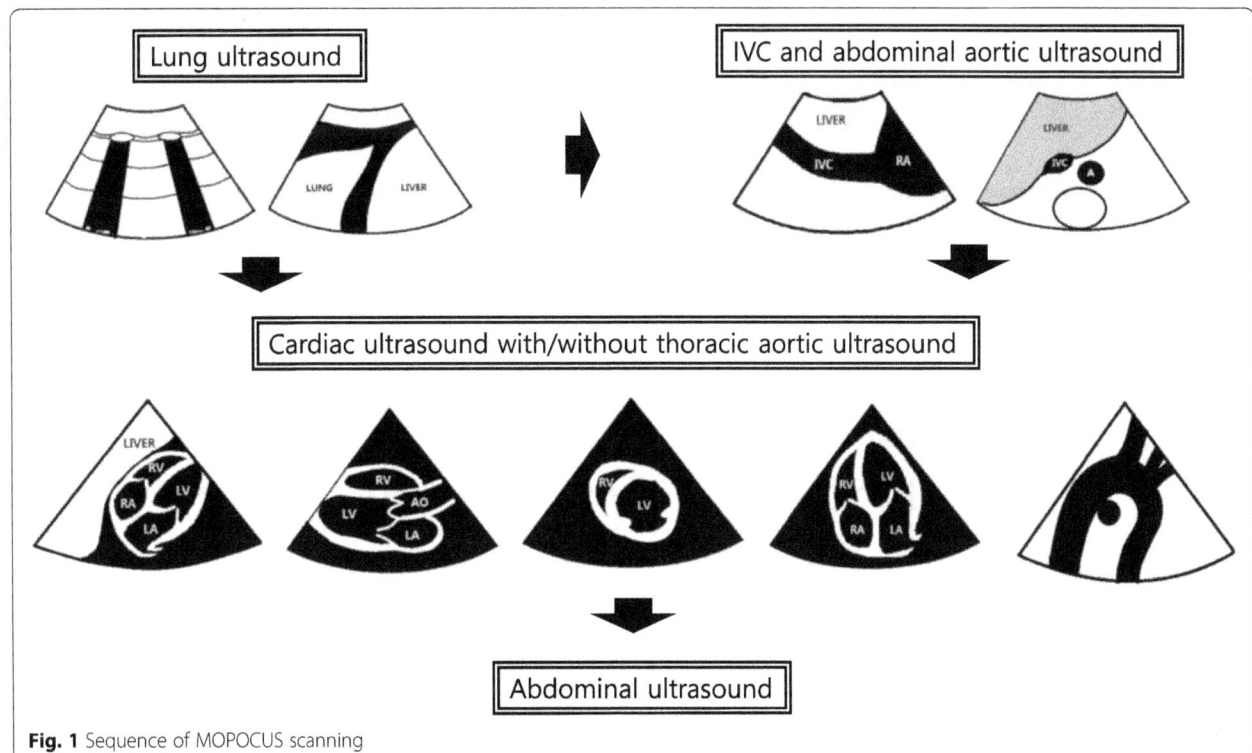

Fig. 1 Sequence of MOPOCUS scanning

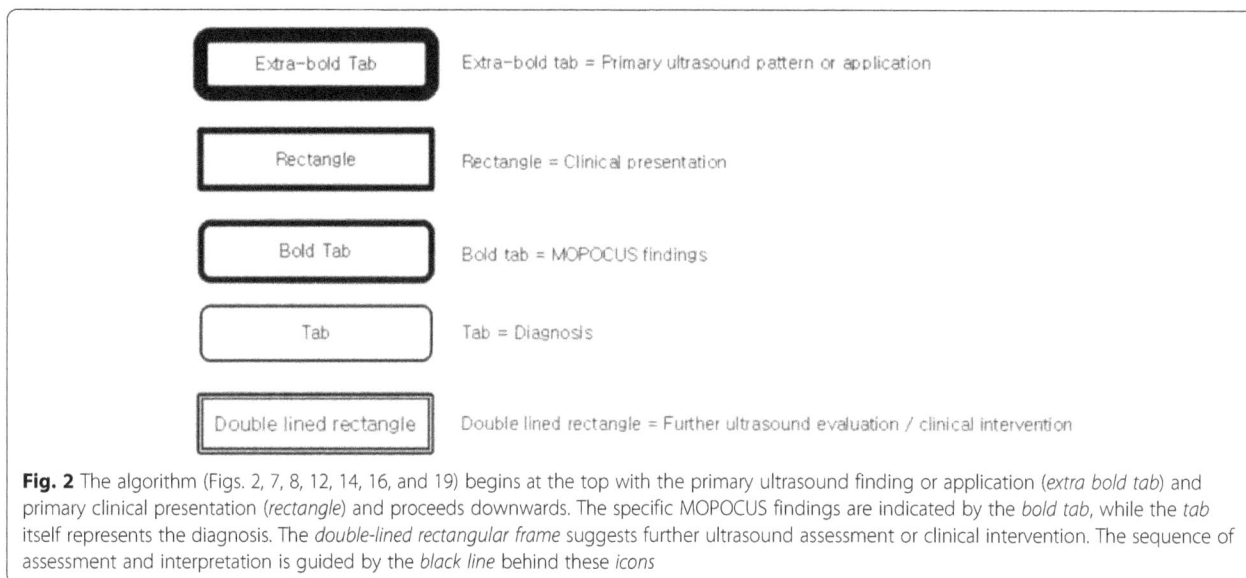

Fig. 2 The algorithm (Figs. 2, 7, 8, 12, 14, 16, and 19) begins at the top with the primary ultrasound finding or application (*extra bold tab*) and primary clinical presentation (*rectangle*) and proceeds downwards. The specific MOPOCUS findings are indicated by the *bold tab*, while the *tab* itself represents the diagnosis. The *double-lined rectangular frame* suggests further ultrasound assessment or clinical intervention. The sequence of assessment and interpretation is guided by the *black line* behind these *icons*

described by Dr. Lichtenstein which uses only three points on each chest [16]. Some sampled five to seven points, taken to be representative of the areas covered [12, 17]. In the comprehensive lung ultrasound, all intercostal spaces are scanned. Regardless of the number of sites scanned, five sonographic lung patterns can be distinguished: normal lung pattern, pneumothorax, interstitial syndrome, alveolar consolidation, and pleural effusion. For practical purposes, we can categorize them into "non-diffuse interstitial pattern" (subdivided into normal lung pattern and abnormal non-diffuse interstitial pattern) and "diffuse interstitial pattern." This review will describe these lung patterns in the context of different clinical situations and integrate them using the concept of MOPOCUS.

Normal lung pattern

Normal lung pattern is defined as A-lines with the lung sliding on the anterolateral chest examination bilaterally, without alveolar consolidation or pleural effusion on posterior examination (Figs. 3 and 4). It is important to recognize that a normal lung pattern does not equate a normal lung. Acute dyspnea and a normal lung pattern can be seen in acute exacerbation of chronic obstructive pulmonary disease (COPD) or asthma attack [16]. Pulmonary embolism (PE) can also have normal lung ultrasound findings, especially in the absence of peripheral lung infarction. In a recent systematic review, the accuracy of lung ultrasound alone to detect PE has an estimated sensitivity of 87.0 % and a specificity of 81.8 % [18]. Lichtenstein added a venous analysis right after

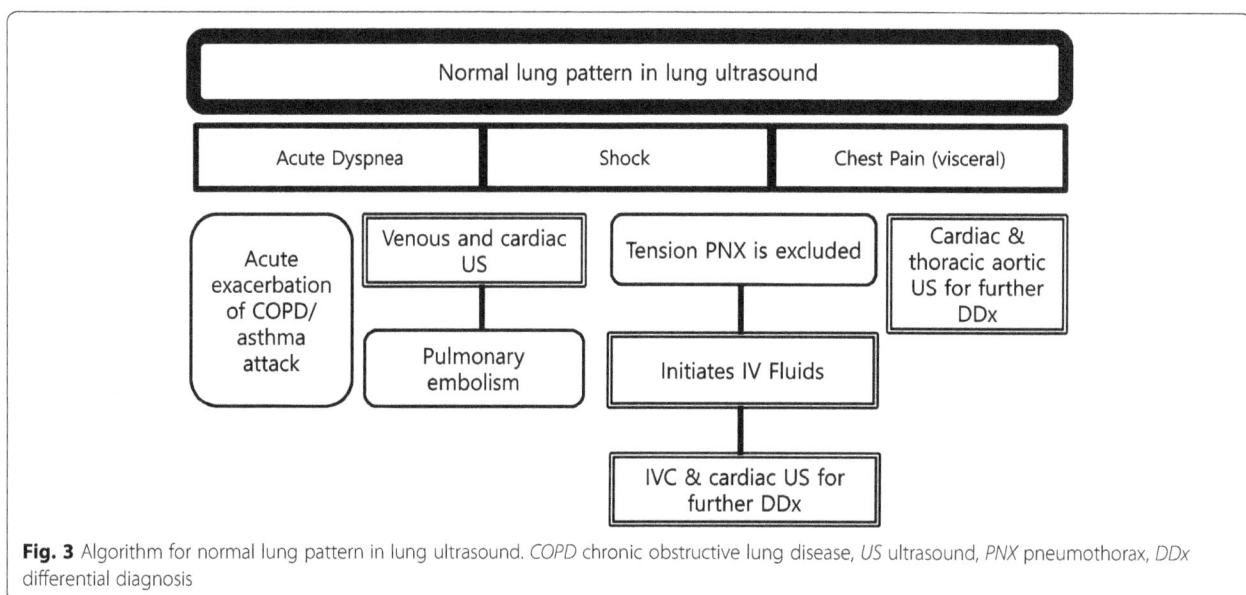

Fig. 3 Algorithm for normal lung pattern in lung ultrasound. *COPD* chronic obstructive lung disease, *US* ultrasound, *PNX* pneumothorax, *DDx* differential diagnosis

Table 1 Interpretation of lung ultrasound

Location	Normal findings	Abnormal findings
Chest wall	Hypoechoic intercostal muscle and echoic ribs with acoustic shadow	Subcutaneous emphysema (E-lines)
Pleural line	Lung sliding	Lung point
	Lung pulse	Pleural line abnormalities
		• Irregular
		• Thickened
		• Fragmented
Supleural space	A-lines[a]	Multiple B-lines (3 or more per intercostal space) consolidation pleural effusion
	Few or no B-lines (2 or less per intercostal space)	

[a]A-lines can also be seen in pathologic situation, such as a pneumothorax, though without lung sliding in this case

identifying an A-pattern on anterior chest examination: the A-pattern plus deep vein thrombosis in the venous analysis has a sensitivity of 81 % and a specificity of 99 % for PE [16, 19]. Nazerian et al. reported that MOPOCUS yielded a sensitivity of 90 % and a specificity of 86.2 % for the diagnosis of PE, comparing that with respective test characteristics of isolated system evaluation: lung ultrasound (60.9 and 95.9 %), cardiac ultrasound (32.7 and 90.9 %), and venous analysis (52.7 and 97.6 %) [20]. This supports the rationale of using an integrated, rather than isolated, approach when performing POCUS.

A normal lung pattern in patients with shock warrants two immediate follow-up actions: the first is to rule out tension pneumothorax and, secondly, to initiate fluid resuscitation based on the Fluid Administration Limited by Lung Sonography (FALLS) protocol [21–23]. Although it has not been validated in shock, non-diffuse interstitial pattern in critically ill patients had a 97 % positive predictive value for a pulmonary artery occlusion pressure of 18 mmHg or less [24]. Apart from tension pneumothorax, a caval and cardiac ultrasound following lung examination will help define the remaining causes of obstructive shock.

The last pearl to note is that chest pain in patients with a normal lung pattern is mostly visceral in nature. The physician should focus the search for the etiology using cardiac and aortic ultrasound.

Pleural diseases
Pneumothorax
Patients with pneumothorax present with shortness of breath and pleuritic chest pain. The absence of lung sliding does not have adequate specificity to rule in the disease, as this absence can be observed in severe emphysema, adult respiratory distress syndrome (ARDS), and atelectasis [25, 26]. The lung point is highly specific for and thus rules in pneumothorax (Fig. 5) [27]. The presence of lung sliding, B-line, or lung pulse rules out pneumothorax, as all of them require the apposition of the parietal and visceral pleura [21].

When the size of the pneumothorax becomes large enough to surround the entire lung surface, the lung point will disappear. Consequently, the acute care physician should not waste time looking for the lung point and thus delay a chest tube insertion, especially when

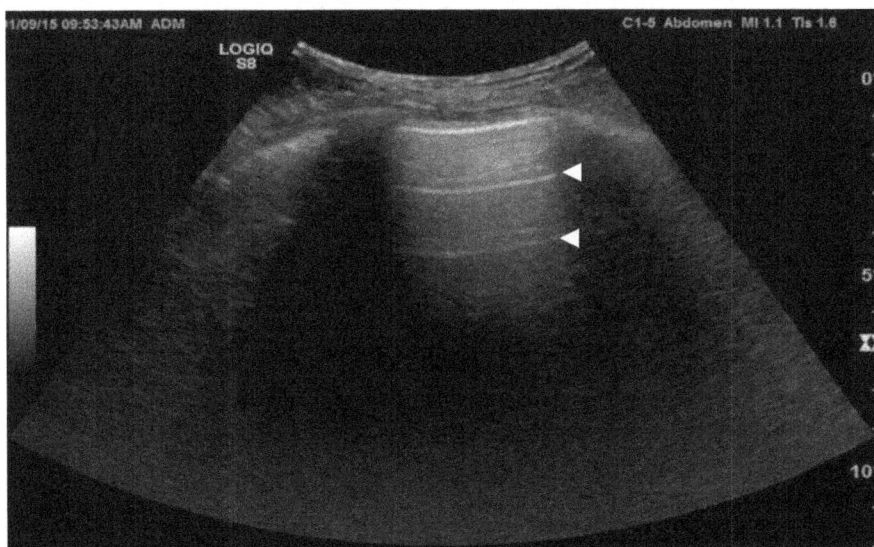

Fig. 4 A-lines. A-lines (*arrowheads*) are horizontal artifacts generated by the repeated reflection of the ultrasound beam between the pleural line and the probe surface

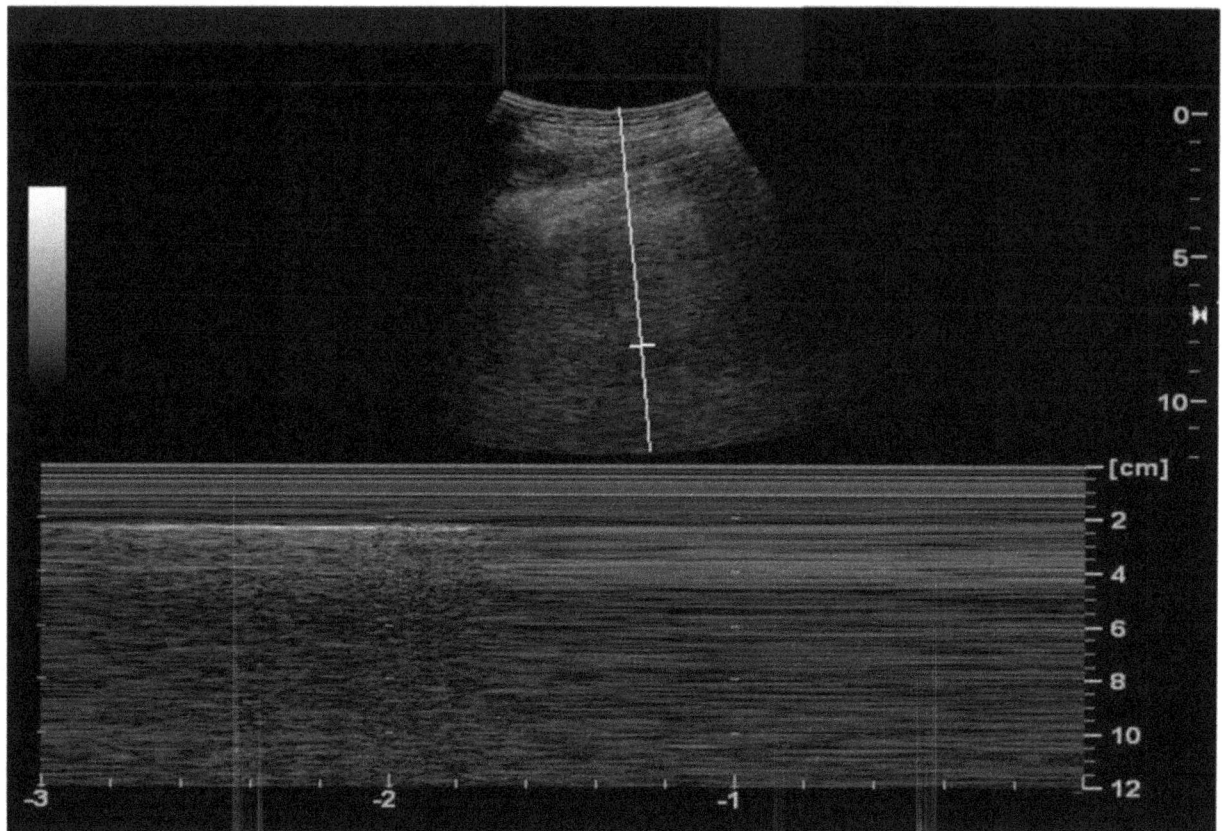

Fig. 5 Lung point. Alternating seashore sign (*left*) and stratosphere sign (*right*) on M mode is pathognomonic for pneumothorax

the patient is in shock. In this case, one would expect to find a plethoric IVC on the subxiphoid view, with the heart displaced to the contralateral side. Tension pneumothorax is the first etiology to rule out among the other causes of obstructive shocks.

Pleural effusion

Pleural effusion can be identified in posterolateral lung examination (Fig. 6). It can cause respiratory difficulty, pleural chest pain, or both. The amount and nature of pleural effusion can be estimated by using an inter-pleural distance or area and sonographic appearances [28–30].

A large pleural effusion can cause respiratory embarrassment, hypovolemic shock (especially in a large hemothorax), or even obstructive shock due to compression of the IVC and heart, which induces the diastolic failure [31]. In patients who required mechanical ventilation and had a significant transudate pleural effusion, chest tube drainage in addition to standard therapy was reported to result in more rapid discontinuation from mechanical ventilation [32]. Occasionally, increased resistance of venous return due to a large pleural effusion itself can result in IVC dilation.

Parenchymal disease

Interstitial syndrome

Interstitial syndrome (IS) is divided into diffuse and focal patterns (Figs. 7 and 8). In diffuse IS, the posterior chest is not evaluated—only the eight anterolateral regions are examined [21]. Four regions per side (two anterior and two lateral) are evaluated. The anterior chest wall was delineated from the sternum to the anterior axillary line and was subdivided into upper and lower halves. The lateral zone was delineated from the anterior to the posterior axillary line and also was subdivided into upper and lower halves.

Diffuse IS is defined as the presence of multiple diffuse bilateral B-lines with at least two positive scans on each side of the thorax (Fig. 9) [33]. Causes of diffuse IS include pulmonary edema of various causes, diffuse parenchymal lung disease (pulmonary fibrosis), or interstitial pneumonia [21]. The presence of diffuse bilateral B-lines has an 86–93 % sensitivity and 93–98 % specificity in the diagnosis of IS [33, 34]. Note that diffuse IS alone does not rule in any specific etiology: it could be detected in many dyspneic patients, as well as those presenting with shock and/or chest pain. As the circulatory and pulmonary systems are interconnected, an

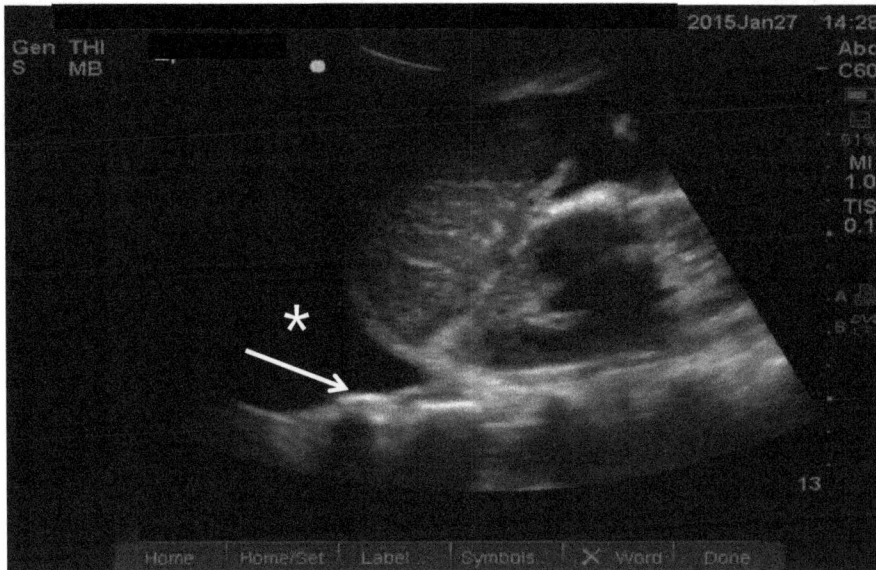

Fig. 6 Pleural effusion. Pleural effusion (*asterisk*) permits the ultrasound beam to penetrate deeply to reveal the vertebral stripe (*arrow*). The vertebral stripe will not be visible above the diaphragm if the lung is aerated

integrated MOPOCUS is mandatory. The presence of diffuse IS associated with either left ventricular (LV) systolic and/or diastolic dysfunction or valvular heart disease is highly indicative of cardiogenic pulmonary congestion [35]. Many recent studies have demonstrated the reliability of MOPOCUS as an approach to distinguish cardiogenic pulmonary edema from non-cardiogenic etiologies [2, 4, 5, 8, 9, 11, 14, 36]. Kajimoto et al. demonstrated that lung ultrasound alone showed a sensitivity and specificity of 96.0 and 54.0 %, respectively, for differentiating acute cardiogenic pulmonary edema from pulmonary disease, while lung-heart-IVC integrated ultrasound

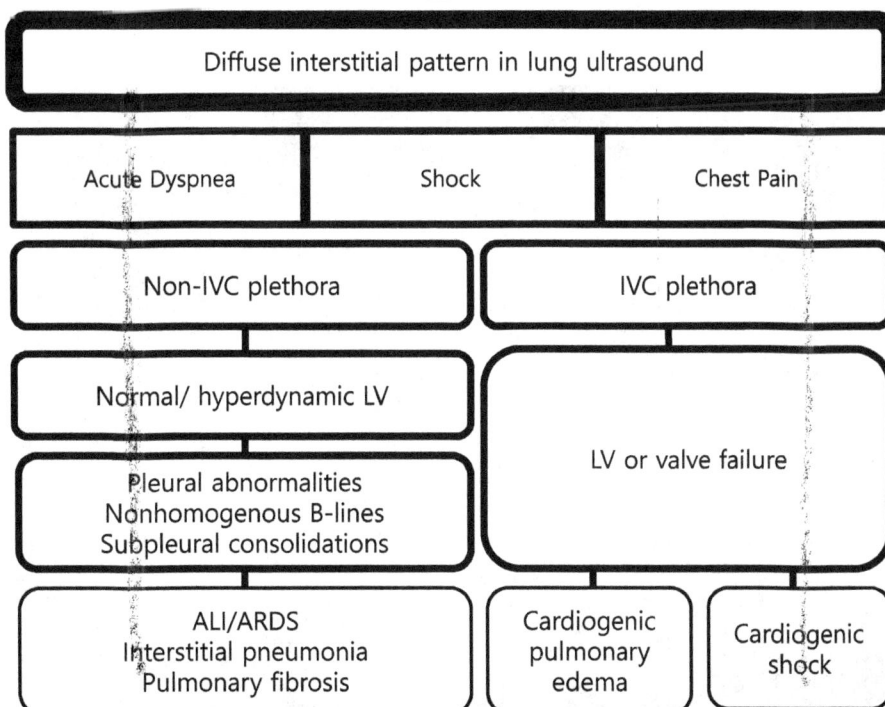

Fig. 7 Algorithm for diffuse interstitial pattern in lung ultrasound. *IVC* inferior vena cava, *LV* left ventricle, *ALI* acute lung injury, *ARDS* acute respiratory distress syndrome

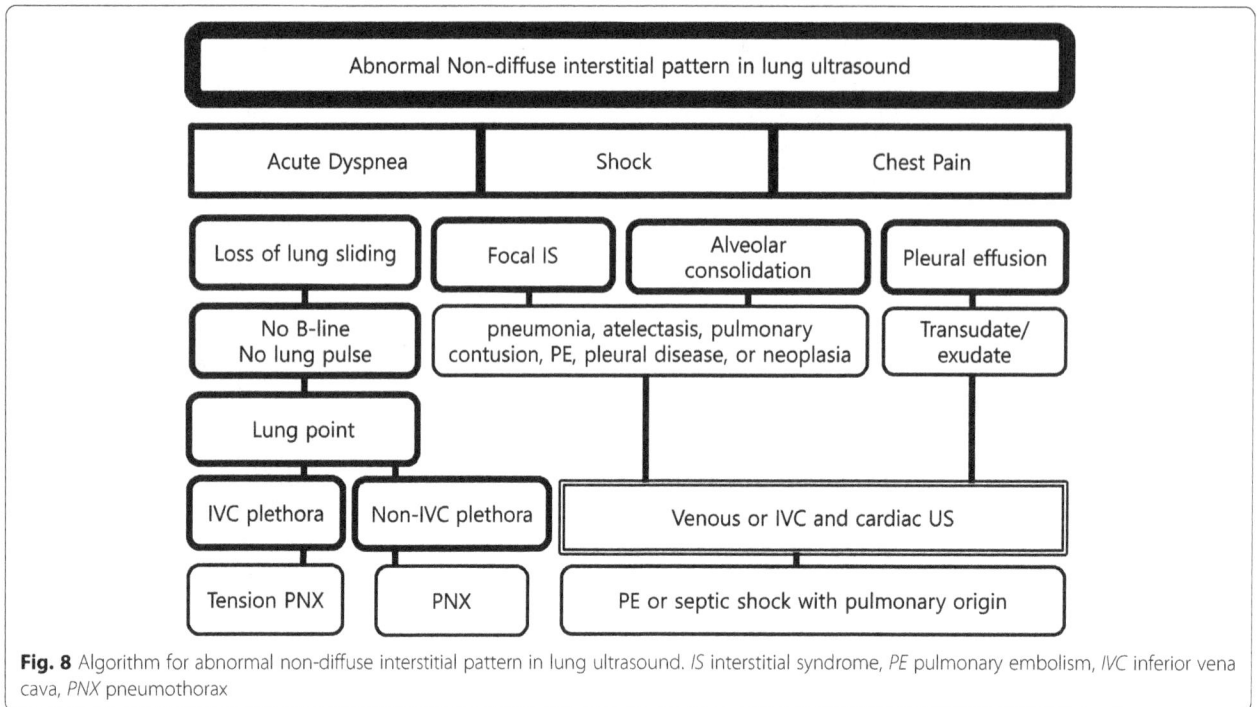

Fig. 8 Algorithm for abnormal non-diffuse interstitial pattern in lung ultrasound. *IS* interstitial syndrome, *PE* pulmonary embolism, *IVC* inferior vena cava, *PNX* pneumothorax

had a sensitivity and specificity of 94.3 and 91.9 %, respectively [2]. Generally, isolated ultrasonography of a single organ itself has low accuracy in differentiating acute heart failure from other causes of acute dyspnea. Acute dyspnea (clinical congestion) results from the failure of alveolar-capillary membrane (pulmonary congestion), which is induced by more stress, following the increase of LV-filling pressure (hemodynamic congestion) [35]. This is one good reason why lung ultrasound should be added to cardiac ultrasound. The presence of diffuse interstitial pattern associated to a normal heart indicates a non-cardiac cause of pulmonary edema, as acute lung injury (ALI)/ARDS,

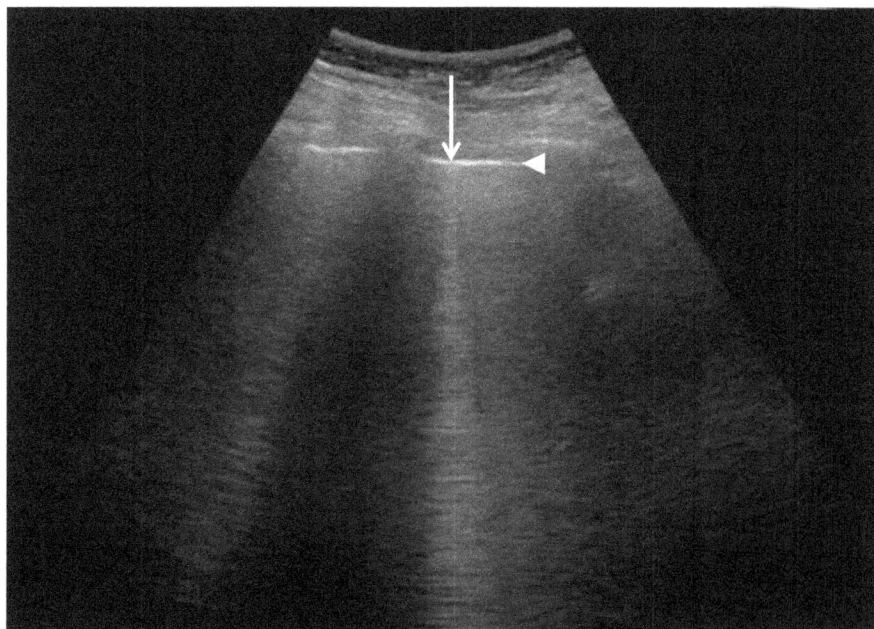

Fig. 9 B-lines. B-line (*arrow*) is a bright comet-tail artifact that arises from the pleural line (*arrowhead*). It will move with lung sliding, if the sliding is present, and extends to the end of the screen without fading

interstitial pneumonia, and diffuse parenchymal lung disease (pulmonary fibrosis, in a chronic setting). Unlike cardiogenic pulmonary edema, the associated lung findings for non-cardiac causes include pleural line abnormalities, non-homogenous distribution of B-lines, and subpleural echo-poor area (or consolidation) [21]. ARDS, in addition, has findings of spared area, loss, or reduced lung sliding and various consolidations [37].

If diffuse IS accompanies shock, the presumptive shock physiology is likely cardiogenic. The physician should try to elucidate the cause using IVC and cardiac ultrasound.

Focal (localized) interstitial sonographic pattern is seen in a variety of pathologies of pulmonary origin, such as pneumonia, atelectasis, pulmonary contusion, pulmonary infarction, pleural disease, or neoplasia [21]. Note that the main difference between diffuse and focal interstitial patterns on ultrasound is that the lung findings on the latter are asymmetrical. In itself, focal IS is not specific for an etiology: physicians need to integrate it in the entire clinical context, including other sonographic findings.

Alveolar consolidation

The consolidated region of the lung is visualized as an echo-poor or tissue-like pattern, depending on the extent of aeration loss and fluid predominance (Fig. 10). A dynamic air bronchogram (Fig. 11) showing inspiratory centrifugal movement is a highly specific sign of pneumonia and is the most important sign to differentiate it from other causes of consolidation (atelectasis, pulmonary infarction, lung cancer) [38]. The alveolar consolidation pattern is usually associated with dyspnea or pleuritic chest pain [39]. In patients with hemodynamic instability, additional findings in MOPOCUS are needed to determine if the alveolar consolidation pattern results from pneumonia (septic shock) or PE.

Inferior vena cava

IVC ultrasound is particularly useful in shock assessment (Figs. 12 and 13). IVC is easily evaluated sonographically, using the liver as a window. Studies have examined the ability of IVC assessment to predict preload or volume responsibility: using IVC distensibility in patients with passive mechanical ventilation and maximal diameter of IVC or collapsibility in spontaneous breathing patients. Previous data on IVC distensibility in mechanically ventilated patients with sepsis provided encouraging results, being able to accurately predict volume responsiveness in sepsis or septic shock [40, 41]. However, recent studies, particularly those recruiting spontaneously breathing patients, have failed to show the same predictive value. Corl et al. found the collapsibility of IVC could not predict fluid responsiveness in a heterogeneous emergency department patient population with suspected hypovolemia [42]. In a practically time-limited clinical situation, the physician can evaluate this using other modalities. Most recent studies evaluating the effectiveness of MOPOCUS in undifferentiated shock use IVC size and respiratory variation as an indicator for fluid resuscitation [7, 10, 13]. While IVC size and variation in spontaneous breathing patients may serve as a surrogate for central venous pressure, it has not been proven a credible indicator of volume responsiveness on its own [43]. The approach using an integrated MOPOCUS assessment to guide fluid therapy needs further evidence. Combining lung ultrasound findings with IVC assessment, however, has a great potential

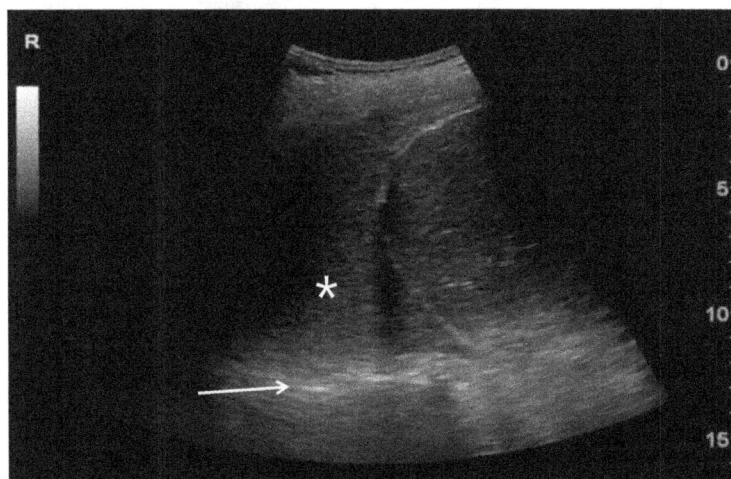

Fig. 10 Lung consolidation. When the lung is consolidated (*asterisk*), it has a tissue-like appearance. The consolidation also allows penetration of the ultrasound beam, revealing the vertebral stripe (*arrow*)

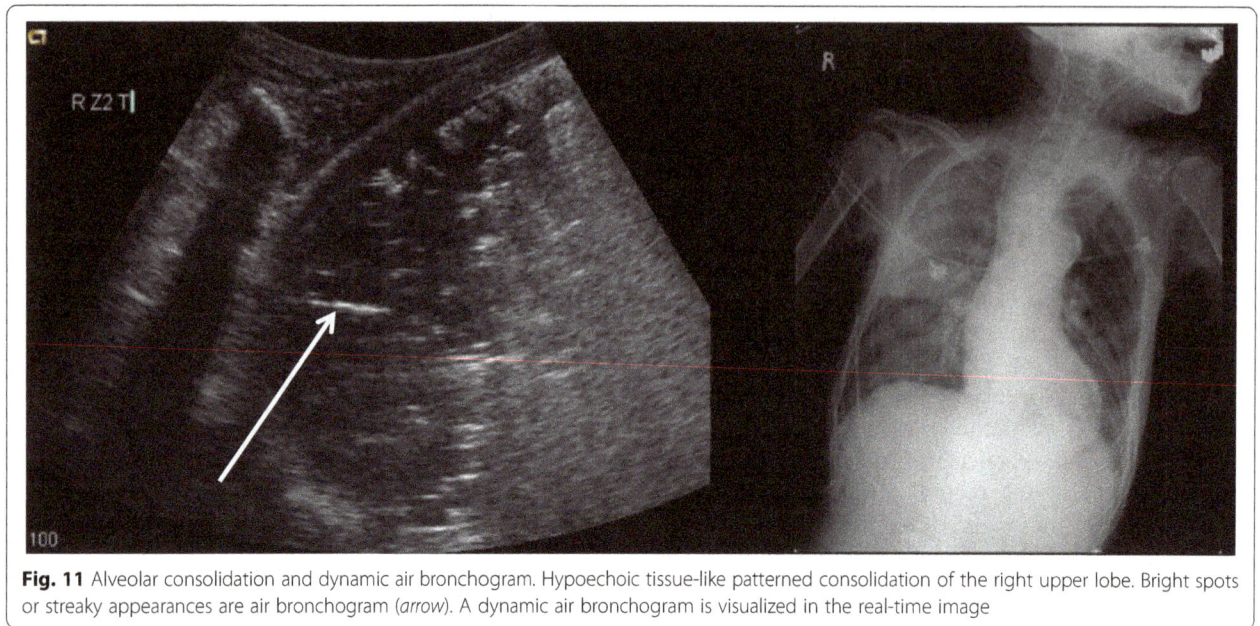

Fig. 11 Alveolar consolidation and dynamic air bronchogram. Hypoechoic tissue-like patterned consolidation of the right upper lobe. Bright spots or streaky appearances are air bronchogram (*arrow*). A dynamic air bronchogram is visualized in the real-time image

to better inform fluid resuscitation decisions [44, 45]. Ultrasound findings of the absence of a diffuse interstitial pattern plus a small IVC diameter with high collapsibility of IVC indicate a fluid-tolerant state [22, 46]. If cardiac function is normal or hyperdynamic, as assessed using additional cardiac ultrasound, fluid boluses can be given, with serial clinical and sonographic reassessment [44, 45]. It is a decision-making process based on the concept of MOPOCUS and fluid tolerance. Furthermore, Caltabeloti et al. demonstrated the ability of lung ultrasound to define a fluid-tolerant state. In their study of

patients with septic shock and ARDS whose LV ejection fraction (EF) was more than 50 % and pulmonary wedge pressure less than 18 mmHg, fluid loading produced only a transient improvement in hemodynamics and oxygenation, but aeration changes can be detected at the bedside lung ultrasound, which may serve as a safeguard against fluid over-resuscitation [47].

The presence of diffuse interstitial pattern with dilated and fixed IVC in shock patients prompts the physician to scan the heart, because the cause of shock is likely cardiogenic. Causes of obstructive shock (cardiac tamponade,

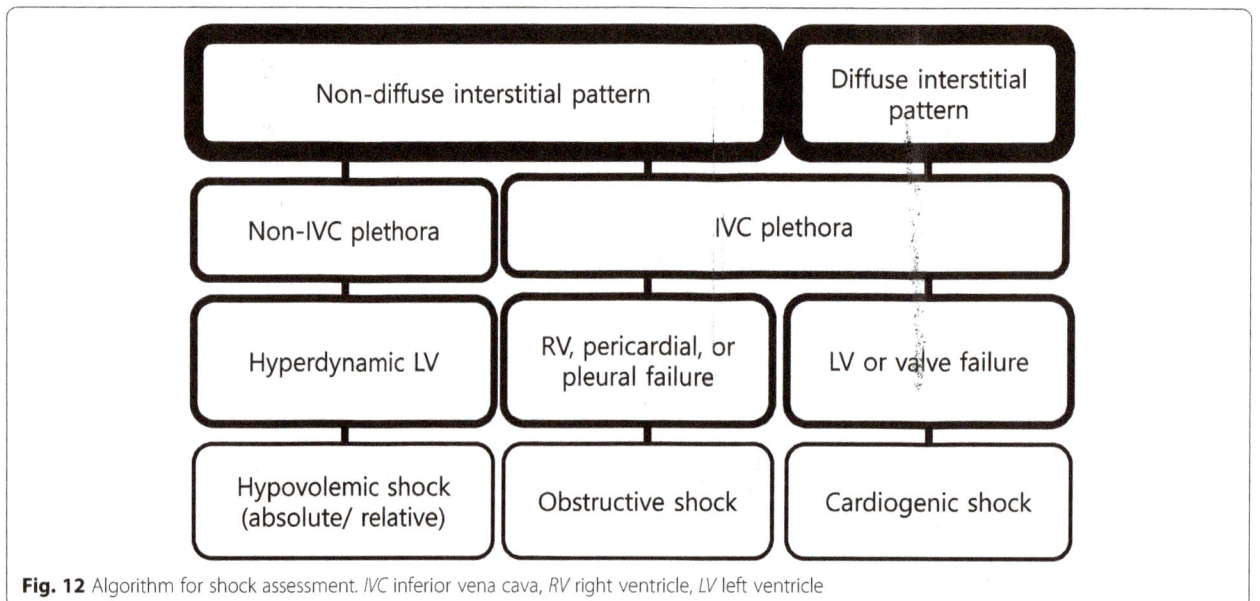

Fig. 12 Algorithm for shock assessment. *IVC* inferior vena cava, *RV* right ventricle, *LV* left ventricle

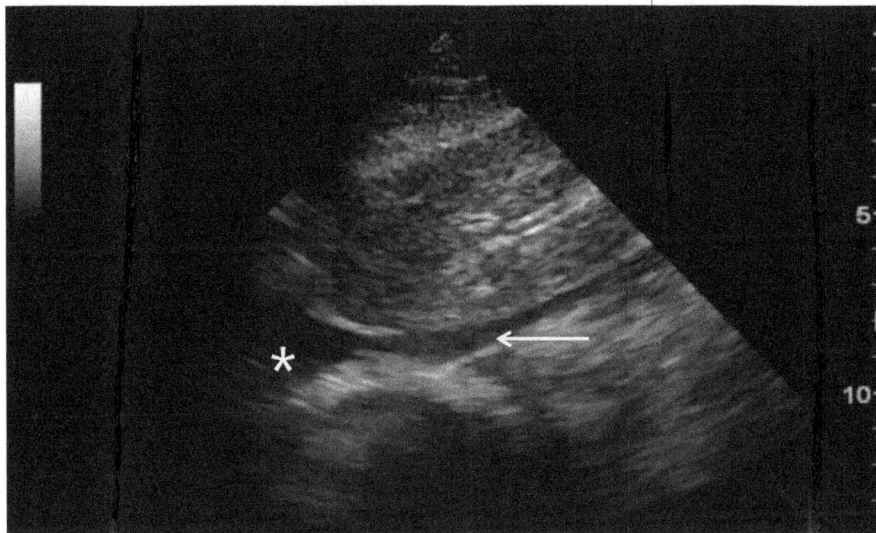

Fig. 13 Inferior vena cava (IVC). IVC (*arrow*) draining into the right atrium (*asterisk*)

tension pneumothorax, and PE) resulted in dilated IVC and non-diffuse interstitial pattern of the lung. A large pleural effusion resulting in diastolic failure or pulmonary hypertension caused by hypoxemia/hypercarbia also can lead to IVC plethora [31].

The key decisions for an acute care physician to make in undifferentiated shock depend on the categorization among three fluid management states: fluid resuscitate, fluid challenge, or fluid restrict. Using information from lung and IVC ultrasound, the physician can embark on an action and guide subsequent decision by cardiac ultrasound [46].

Cardiac ultrasound

With information integrated from the preceding lung and IVC assessment, cardiac ultrasound can readily define the etiology of acute dyspnea and shock. It also plays a pivotal role in the case of visceral chest pain. This section describes the utility of cardiac ultrasound in the context of MOPOCUS for dyspnea, chest pain, and shock in turn.

Acute dyspnea

Patient with diffuse interstitial pattern should have a focused cardiac ultrasound evaluation to determine the etiology, such as acute cardiogenic pulmonary edema, ARDS, or pulmonary fibrosis (Fig. 14). If LV systolic function is impaired, the most likely cause is cardiogenic pulmonary edema [2, 5, 9]. In the absence of gross signs of preexisting cardiac disease (i.e., LV enlargement or hypertrophy, right ventricular (RV) hypertrophy, or atrial dilation) (Fig. 15), the differentials can be narrowed

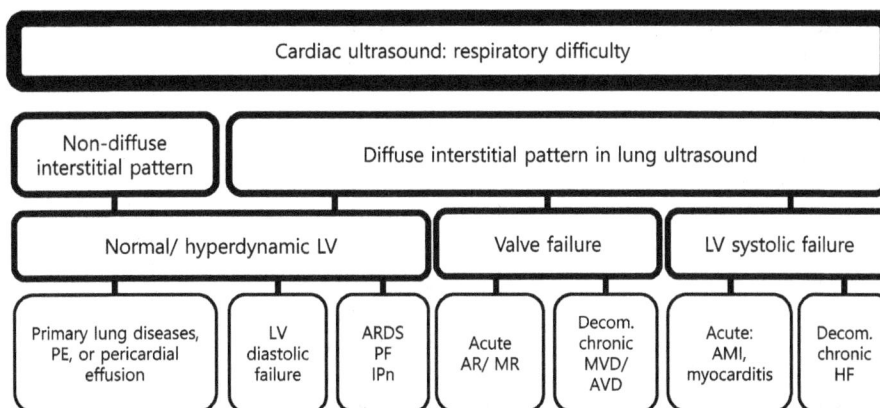

Fig. 14 Cardiac ultrasound in respiratory difficulty. *PE* pulmonary embolism, *LV* left ventricle, *ARDS* acute respiratory distress syndrome, *PF* pulmonary fibrosis, *IPn* interstitial pneumonia, *AR* aortic regurgitation, *MR* mitral regurgitation, *Decom.* decompensated, *MVD* mitral valve disease, *AVD* aortic valve disease, *AMI* acute myocardial infarction, *HF* heart failure

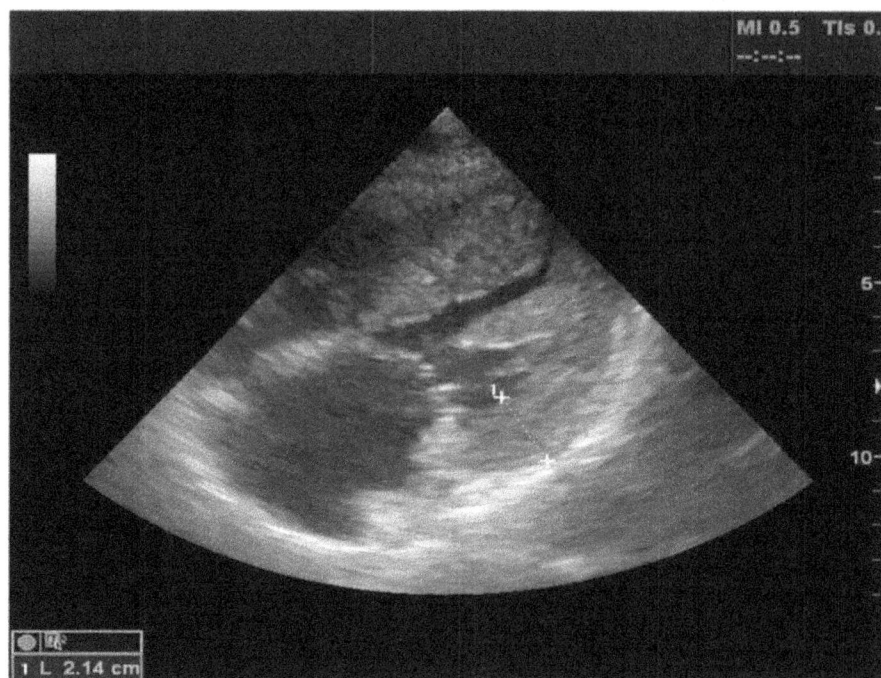

Fig. 15 Left ventricular hypertrophy. Left ventricular hypertrophy involving both septal and lateral walls (2.14 cm). The left atrial appeared enlarged

down to acute processes, such as acute myocardial infarction or myocarditis [48]. Signs of preexisting cardiac disease are usually apparent in acute decompensation. If LV systolic function is normal, non-cardiogenic origin such as ARDS, interstitial pneumonia, or pulmonary fibrosis should be suspected, though cardiac pathologies such as significant mitral regurgitation (MR) or diastolic dysfunction are possible [2]. Significant valvulopathies can lead to cardiogenic pulmonary edema. The first task in valve evaluation is to exclude acute severe aortic or MR. Subsequently, the possibility of decompensated chronic severe aortic or MR/stenosis should be entertained [49]. Full evaluation with a comprehensive echocardiography is recommended for the quantitative analysis.

A non-diffuse interstitial pattern typically points to a pulmonary origin as a cause of dyspnea, in which lung ultrasound alone is usually sufficient.

Chest pain

Pleural (pleuritic) chest pain results from lung pathologies such as pneumonia, pulmonary infarction, exudative pleural effusion, or pneumothorax (Fig. 16). These are readily diagnosed by lung ultrasound. On the other hand, visceral chest pain should prompt evaluation for acute coronary syndrome (ACS), pericarditis, or aortic dissection [50]. Following an initial electrocardiography (ECG), the presence of pericardial effusion, RV enlargement, or

regional wall motion abnormality (RWMA) compatible to coronary artery distribution should be evaluated on cardiac ultrasound. Attempt should be made to visualize the thoracic aorta, starting from the aortic root, arch, and parts of the descending thoracic aorta behind the heart (Fig. 17). The abdominal aorta needs to be scanned when a dissection flap is visualized in the thorax above (Fig. 18). Note the multi-detector computerized tomography (CT) is the current gold standard in the evaluation for an aortic dissection. While the presence of RWMA in patients with ongoing chest pain without the previous history prompts appropriate management including percutaneous coronary intervention, absence of RWMA in patients with ongoing chest pain excludes a significant ACS [51]. Pericarditis is not always distinguished by clinical feature and ECG [52]. Cardiac ultrasound can be used as an adjunct, with supporting features such as the presence of a pericardial effusion and absence of RWMA. A flap in the aorta or a crescent shape of the aortic wall (direct sign) and aortic regurgitation, ascending aortic dilation, or pericardial effusion (indirect signs) suggest aortic dissection. They showed 98 % specificity for identifying patients with suspected type A aortic dissection combining aortic dissection risk score [53, 54].

Shock or shock-related symptoms or signs

Cardiac ultrasound in a shock patient provides critical information about the pericardium, bilateral chamber size and function, and valvular competency (Fig. 19). We

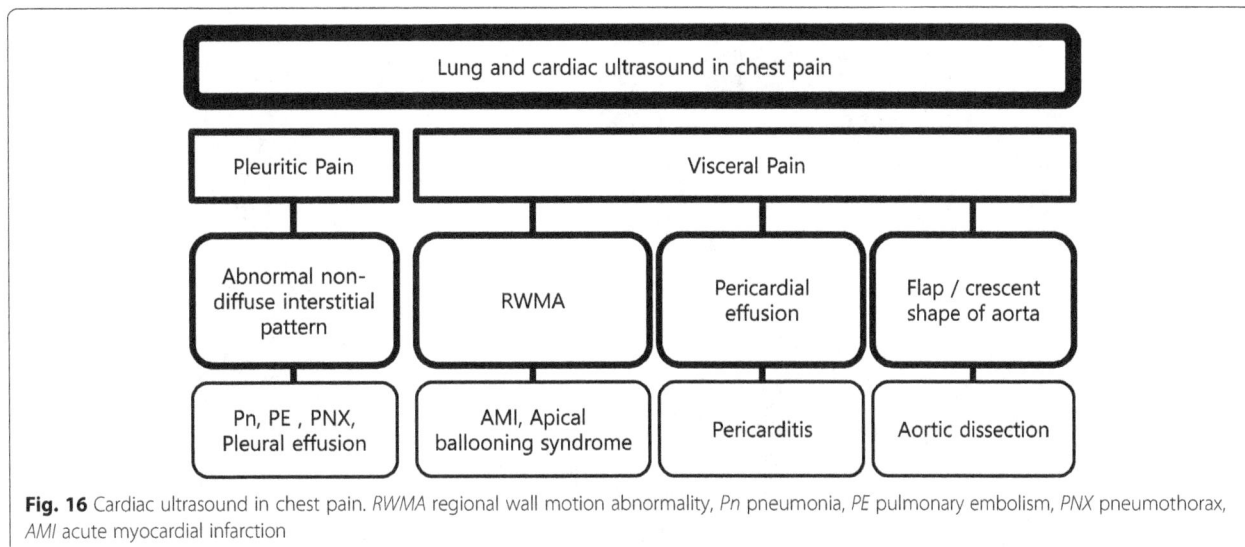

Fig. 16 Cardiac ultrasound in chest pain. *RWMA* regional wall motion abnormality, *Pn* pneumonia, *PE* pulmonary embolism, *PNX* pneumothorax, *AMI* acute myocardial infarction

emphasize that the priority is to rule out obstructive shock first, followed by cardiogenic shock, and then finally absolute or relative (distributive) hypovolemic shocks [49]. An approach based on the previous lung ultrasound pattern, diffuse interstitial pattern vs. non-diffuse interstitial pattern, is described here.

Non-diffuse interstitial pattern It is suggestive of obstructive or hypovolemic shock: IVC plethora indicates obstructive shock, while a small non-plethoric IVC is usually associated with hypovolemic shock.

Pericardial failure (cardiac tamponade) The sonographic signs of tamponade in the setting of a pericardial effusion include end-diastolic right atrium collapse (a highly sensitive sign) and RV collapse (less sensitive but

more specific), IVC dilation, and greater than 25 % inspiratory variation in mitral inflow velocity measured by pulse-wave Doppler (Figs. 20 and 21) [55, 56]. In particular, IVC plethora (defined as a decrease in the proximal IVC diameter by <50 % during deep inspiration) has been described as the most sensitive (97 %) although least specific (40 %), while RV diastolic collapse is 48 % sensitive and 95 % specific [57]. It is important to remember that cardiac tamponade can complicate an aortic dissection or ACS (ventricular rupture); therefore, a high index of suspicion for two concurrent etiologies must be maintained [58].

RV failure (PE) Acute PE may lead to RV pressure overload and dysfunction (Fig. 22), which can be visualized by cardiac ultrasound. An RV-to-LV end-

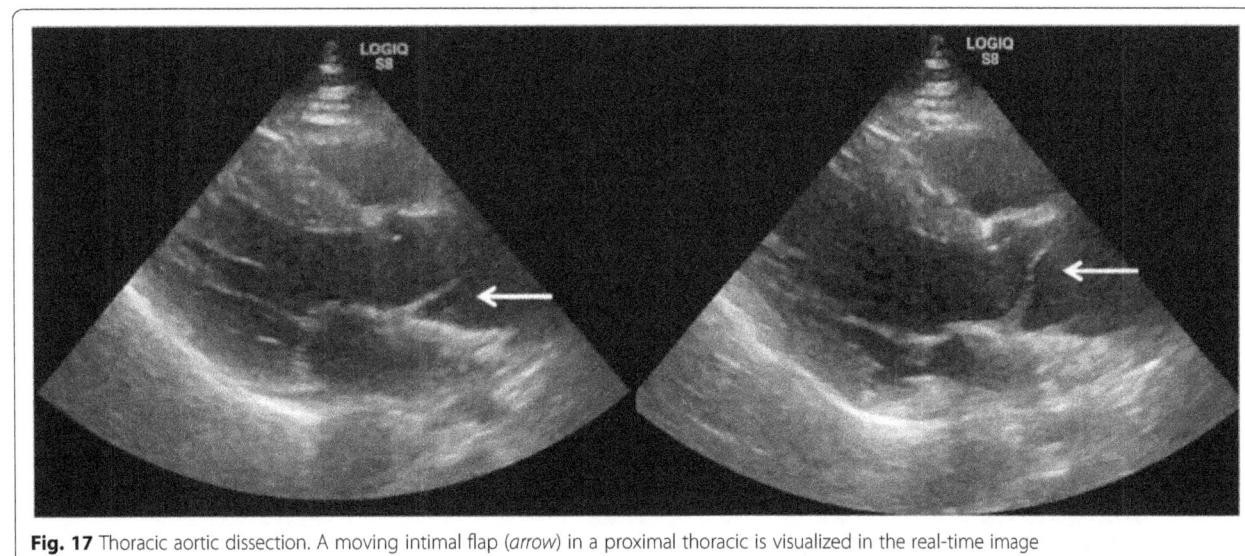

Fig. 17 Thoracic aortic dissection. A moving intimal flap (*arrow*) in a proximal thoracic is visualized in the real-time image

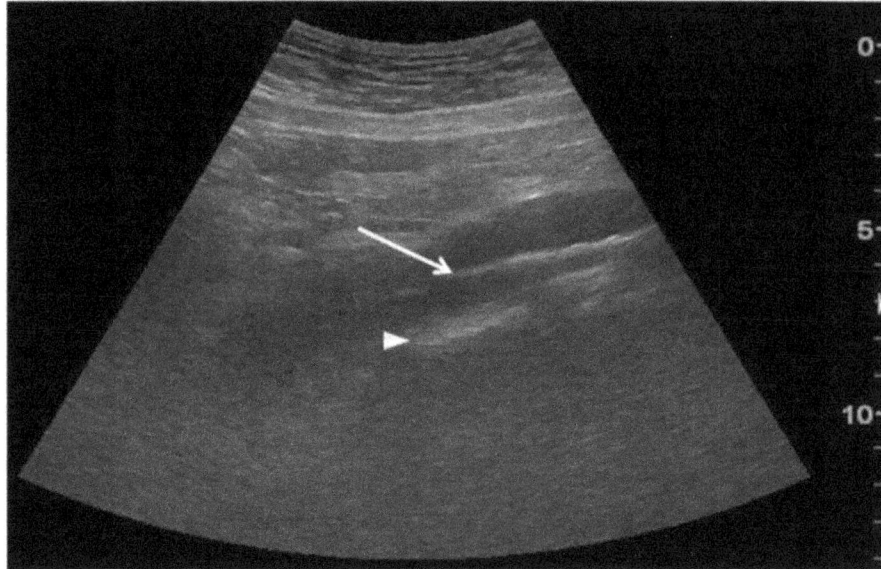

Fig. 18 Abdominal aortic dissection. An intimal flap (*arrow*) dissecting into the lumen of the abdominal aorta. The *arrowhead* points to the vertebral stripe, on which the aorta lies

diastolic diameter ratio >0.9 was reported to indicate critical PE (Fig. 23) [59]. The absence of sonographic signs of RV overload or dysfunction practically excludes PE as the cause of hemodynamic instability [60]. Therefore, in a hemodynamically unstable patient with suspected PE, definite signs of RV pressure overload and dysfunction support emergency reperfusion treatment if immediate CT angiography is not feasible [61]. The potential pitfall in this setting is discriminating acute vs. chronic cor pulmonale. Chronic etiologies (COPD, chronic PE) can cause RV hypertrophy (diastolic RV thickness >6 mm) and

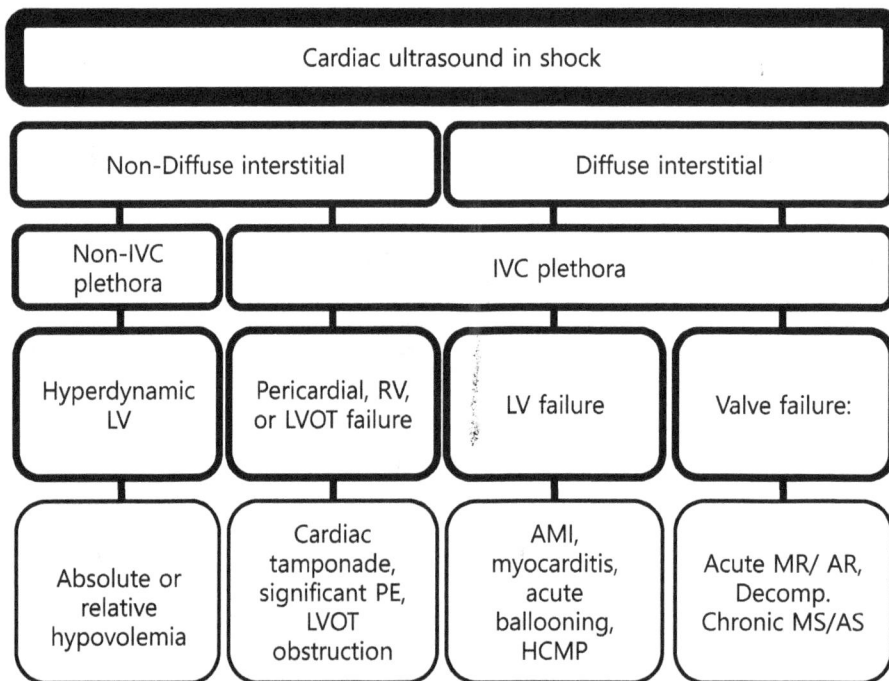

Fig. 19 Cardiac ultrasound in shock. *IVC* inferior vena cava, *LV* left ventricle, *RV* right ventricle, *LVOT* left ventricular outflow tract, *PE* pulmonary embolism, *AMI* acute myocardial infarction, *HCMP* hypertrophic cardiomyopathy, *MR* mitral regurgitation, *AR* aortic regurgitation, *Decomp.* decompensated, *MS* mitral stenosis, *AS* aortic stenosis

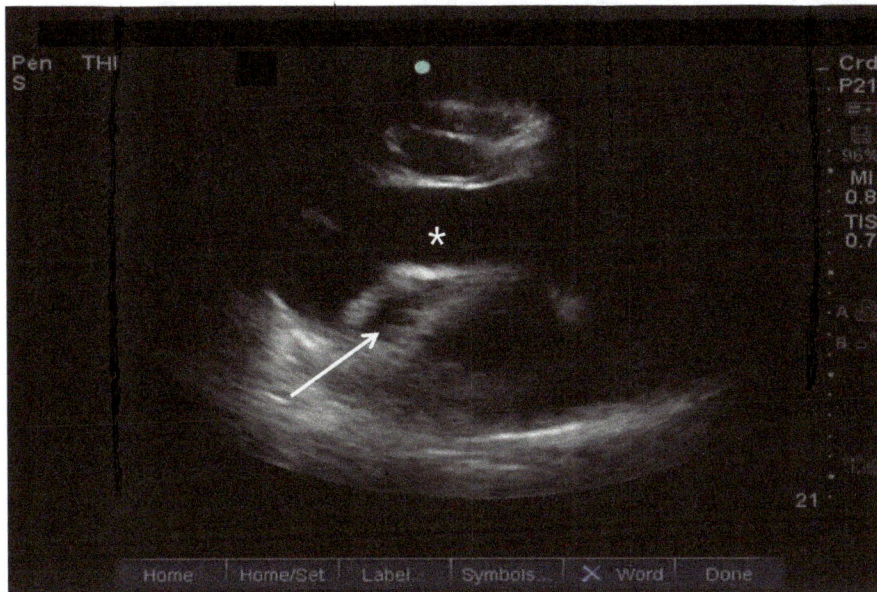

Fig. 20 Cardiac tamponade. Right-sided heart chambers collapsed (*arrow*), due to increased intrapericardial pressure from a large pericardial effusion (*asterisk*)

beyond the values compatible with acute etiology (so-called 60/60 sign defined as RV acceleration time of <60 ms in the presence of tricuspid insufficiency pressure gradient <60 mmHg) [62, 63]. The physician keeps in mind that RV overload sometimes results from ARDS or RV infarction [64].

LV outflow tract failure Dynamic LV outflow tract obstruction causing obstructive shock can be easily missed if cardiac ultrasound is not performed. Diagnosis of this is critical for the patient because the hemodynamic management is opposite to that of cardiogenic shock. Cardiac ultrasound generally shows hyperdynamic ventricular function with near complete or partial obliteration of the ventricular cavities. Additional sonographic signs include systolic anterior motion of the mitral valve, high ejection flow velocity in the LV outflow tract, and MR in the color Doppler image. LV outflow tract obstruction has been reported with LV hypertrophy, profound dehydration, excessive sympathetic stimulation, apical ballooning syndrome (i.e., takotsubo cardiomyopathy, Fig. 24), and acute myocardial infarction [65, 66].

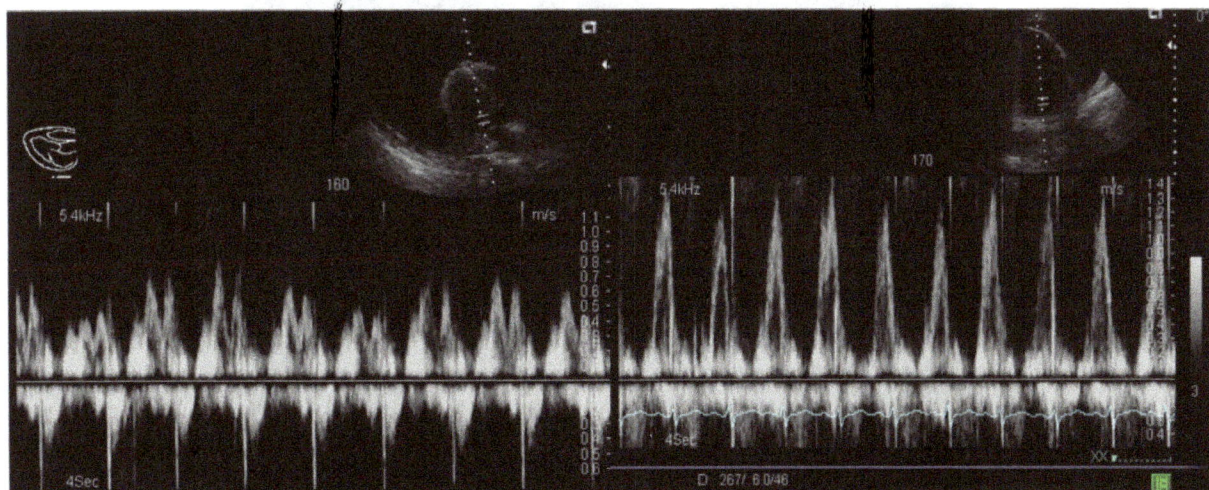

Fig. 21 Cardiac tamponade physiology. (*Left*) Cardiac tamponade physiology, demonstrating reduced and aggravated variation of mitral valve inflow velocity. (*Right*) Post-pericardiocentesis: significant improvement in mitral valve inflow velocity

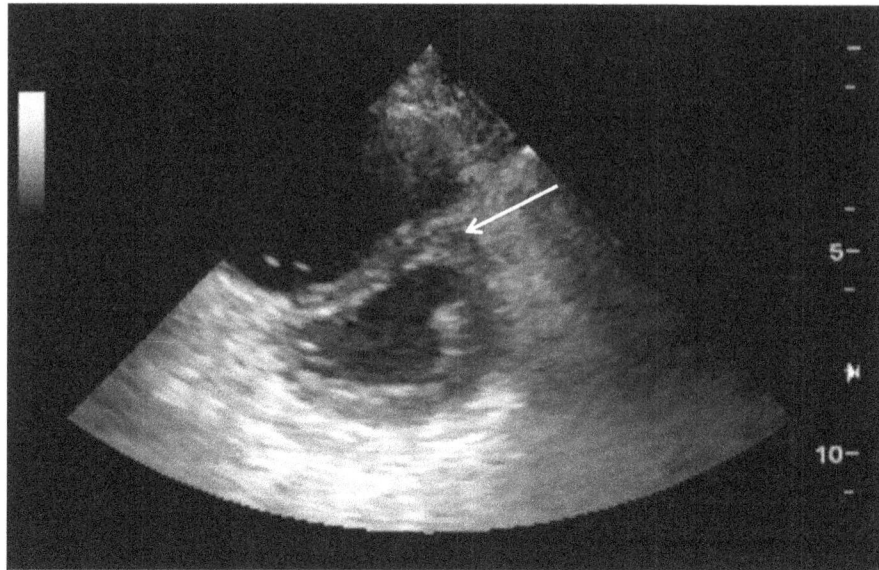

Fig. 22 D-shaped left ventricle. The interventricular septum is normally round and bulges into the right ventricle (RV) throughout the cardiac cycle. Increased RV pressure causes the septum to be deformed to assume a "D"-shaped left ventricle (*arrow*)

Apical ballooning syndrome is reported to cause LV outflow tract obstruction in up to 25 % [67].

Other useful LV findings in shock states not caused by LV itself After excluding obstructive shocks by information from sonographic findings of the lung, IVC, pericardium, and RV, the physician then needs to pay attention to the LV. Hyperdynamic LV without other abnormalities including significant valvular pathology suggests either distributive or hypovolemic shock. Distributive shock and hypovolemic shock commonly coexist in the critically ill, and early recognition and treatment with fluid resuscitation are paramount to manage these patients [49]. Therefore, we can practically categorize both as hypovolemic shock. It can be subdivided into absolute (hypovolemic) and relative (distributive) hypovolemic shock. Absolute hypovolemic shock has small-sized LV, while relative hypovolemic shock has normal-sized LV [31]. Jones et al. reported the presence of hyperdynamic left

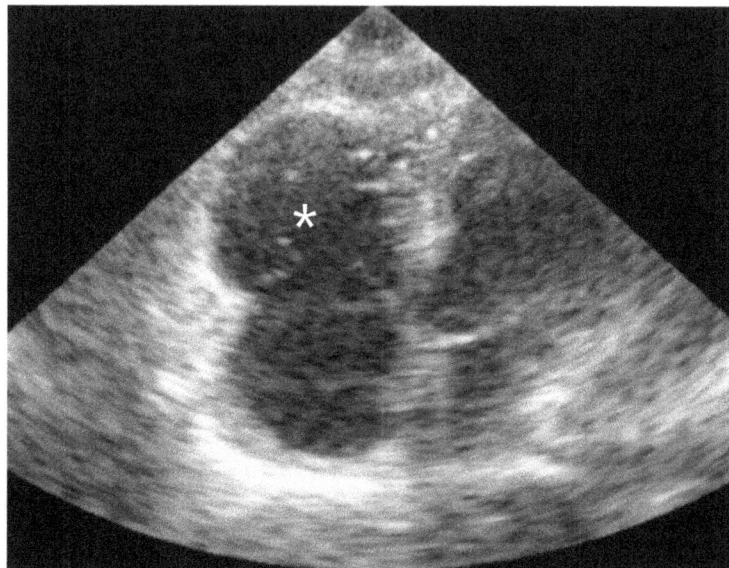

Fig. 23 Pulmonary embolism, severe. Right ventricular enlargement (more than 0.9 of left ventricular size) is demonstrated (*white asterisk*). The RV free wall does not appear thickened, indicating an acute RV failure

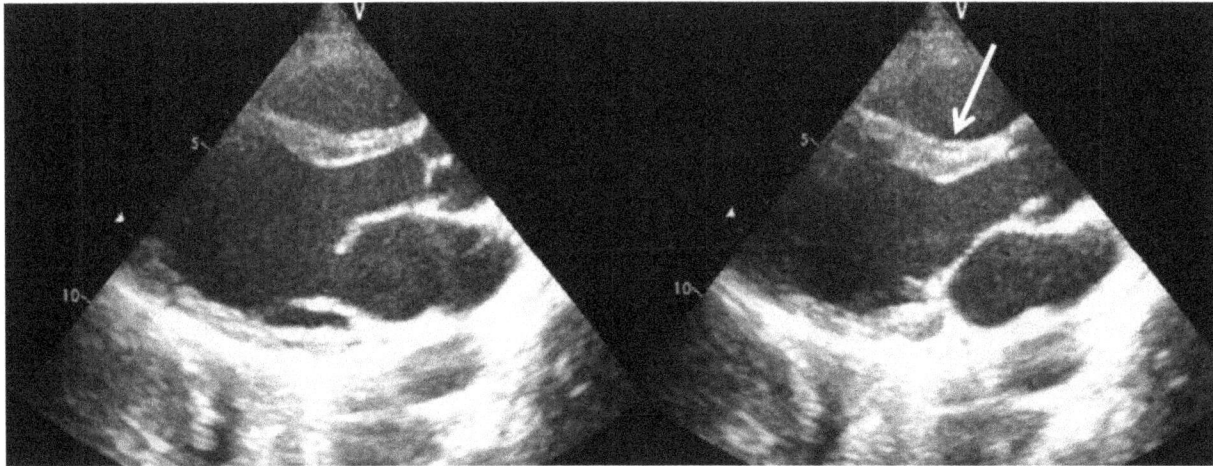

Fig. 24 Apical ballooning syndrome. Severe hypokinesia of mid-ventricle sparing the basal segments (*arrow*). This is better appreciated during real-time scanning. Courtesy of Dr. Seong-Beom Oh

ventricular function (EF > 55 %) in emergency department patients with non-traumatic shock is highly specific for sepsis as the etiology of shock [68].

Diffuse interstitial pattern Cardiogenic shock is most likely.

LV failure MI with LV failure remains the most common cause of cardiogenic shock. The SHOCK trial registry demonstrated that predominant LV failure was the most common cause of cardiogenic shock, occurring in 78.5 % of patients. Patients with predominant LV failure

complicating acute MI were more likely to have an anterior MI. Inferior MI was less often associated with LV failure but associated with a greater risk of mechanical complications [69]. Therefore, the presence of an extensive anterior MI or mechanical complications (severe MR due to papillary muscle rupture, ventricular septal defect, tamponade secondary to cardiac rupture, etc.) is a major concern in this setting [70]. In these settings, cardiac ultrasound is the investigation of choice. The clinical presentations of myopericarditis, apical ballooning syndrome, and hypertrophic cardiomyopathy can be similar to ACS and even cardiogenic shock. Sonographic

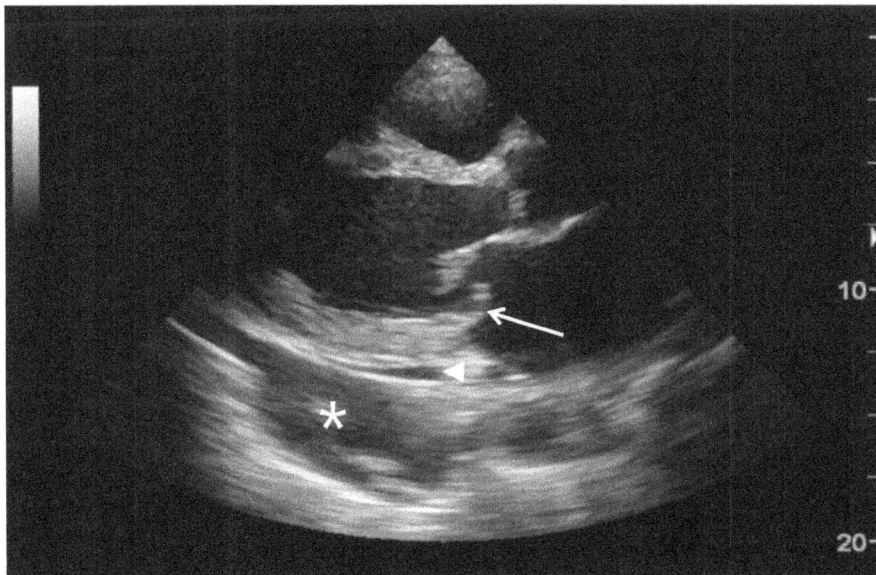

Fig. 25 Flailed mitral valve. Flailed posterior mitral leaflet (*arrow*). Note the presence of a small pericardial effusion (*arrowhead*) and larger left pleural effusion (*asterisk*)

findings of apical ballooning syndrome is a moderate-to-severe mid-ventricular dysfunction and apical akinesia with preserved basal function [71].

Valve failure Valvular pathologies also are potential causes of cardiogenic shock (Fig. 25). The life-threatening acute severe regurgitation resulting from infectious endocarditis, acute myocardial infarction, or aortic dissection should be placed at the top of the list to be screened, as it prompts an emergent operation [70, 72]. Then hemodynamically compromised decompensation of preexisting aortic or mitral stenosis should be identified. In a patient suspected with aortic dissection complicating shock, not only severe acute aortic regurgitation but also pericardial effusion causing tamponade and acute myocardial infarction secondary to coronary artery involvement should be taken into account [73].

Abdominal ultrasound

Abdominal ultrasound can help to determine the cause of hypovolemic (both absolute and relative) shock. Intra-abdominal source of blood loss or infection such as peritoneal effusion, ruptured abdominal aortic aneurysm or ectopic pregnancy, liver/spleen abscess, cholecystitis, cholangitis, or pyonephritis can be visualized [74].

Conclusions

Multi-organ point-of-care ultrasound is a powerful adjunct to standard clinical assessment. It provides critical and timely information in the evaluation of patients presenting with acute dyspnea, chest pain, or shock: when and where it matters most, right at the bedside. It has become an indispensable part of the acute care physician's armamentarium, in the battle for our patients' lives.

Abbreviations
ACS, acute coronary syndrome; ARDS, adult respiratory distress syndrome; COPD, chronic obstructive pulmonary disease; CT, computerized tomography; ECG, electrocardiography; FALLS, Fluid Administration Limited by Lung Sonography; IS, interstitial syndrome; IVC, inferior vena cava; LV, left ventricle or left ventricular; MOPOCUS, multi-organ point-of-care ultrasound; MR, mitral regurgitation; PE, pulmonary embolism; POCUS, point-of-care ultrasound; ROSC, return of spontaneous circulation; RV, right ventricle or right ventricular; RWMA, regional wall motion abnormality

Acknowledgements
The authors would like to acknowledge Dr. Seong-Beom Oh for contributing Fig. 24: apical ballooning syndrome.

Funding
No funding to declare.

Authors' contributions
YRH conceived the review, performed the literature search, and wrote the first draft of this paper. HCT revised the manuscript. Both authors contributed to the figures, read, and approved the final manuscript.

Competing interests
The authors declare that they have no competing interests.

Author details
[1]Emergency Department, Bundang Jesaeng Hospital, 20 Seohyeon-ro 180beongil, Bundang-gu, Seongnam-si, Gyeonggi-do, South Korea. [2]Acute and Emergency Care Centre, Khoo Teck Puat Hospital, 90 Yishun Central, S768828 Singapore, Singapore.

References

1. Labovitz AJ, Noble VE, Bierig M, Goldstein SA, Jones R, Kort S, et al. Focused cardiac ultrasound in the emergent setting: a consensus statement of the American Society of Echocardiography and American College of Emergency Physicians. J Am Soc Echocardiogr. 2010;23(12):1225–30.
2. Kajimoto K, Madeen K, Nakayama T, Tsudo H, Kuroda T, Abe T. Rapid evaluation by lung-cardiac-inferior vena cava (LCI) integrated ultrasound for differentiating heart failure from pulmonary disease as the cause of acute dyspnea in the emergency setting. Cardiovasc Ultrasound. 2012;10(1):49. Pubmed Central PMCID: 3527194.
3. Laursen CB, Sloth E, Lassen AT, Christensen RD, Lambrechtsen J, Madsen PH, et al. Focused sonographic examination of the heart, lungs and deep veins in an unselected population of acute admitted patients with respiratory symptoms: a protocol for a prospective, blinded, randomised controlled trial. BMJ open. 2012; 2(3). Pubmed Central PMCID: PMC3367153. Epub 2012/06/01. eng
4. Mantuani D, Nagdev A, Stone M. Three-view bedside ultrasound for the differentiation of acute respiratory distress syndrome from cardiogenic pulmonary edema. Am J Emerg Med. 2012;30(7):1324. e1-4.
5. Anderson KL, Jenq KY, Fields JM, Panebianco NL, Dean AJ. Diagnosing heart failure among acutely dyspneic patients with cardiac, inferior vena cava, and lung ultrasonography. Am J Emerg Med. 2013;31(8):1208–14.
6. Laursen CB, Sloth E, Lambrechtsen J, Lassen AT, Madsen PH, Henriksen DP, et al. Focused sonography of the heart, lungs, and deep veins identifies missed life-threatening conditions in admitted patients with acute respiratory symptoms. Chest. 2013;144(6):1868–75.
7. Volpicelli G, Lamorte A, Tullio M, Cardinale L, Giraudo M, Stefanone V, et al. Point-of-care multiorgan ultrasonography for the evaluation of undifferentiated hypotension in the emergency department. Intensive Care Med. 2013;39(7):1290–8.
8. Pirozzi C, Numis FG, Pagano A, Melillo P, Copetti R, Schiraldi F. Immediate versus delayed integrated point-of-care-ultrasonography to manage acute dyspnea in the emergency department. Crit Ultrasound J. 2014;6(1):5. Pubmed Central PMCID: 4039047.
9. Wang XT, Liu DW, Zhang HM, Chai WZ. Integrated cardiopulmonary sonography: a useful tool for assessment of acute pulmonary edema in the intensive care unit. J Ultrasound Med. 2014;33(7):1231–9.
10. Bagheri-Hariri S, Yekesadat M, Farahmand S, Arbab M, Sedaghat M, Shahlafar N, et al. The impact of using RUSH protocol for diagnosing the type of unknown shock in the emergency department. Emerg Radiol. 2015;22(5): 517–20. Epub 2015/03/22. eng.
11. Russell FM, Ehrman RR, Cosby K, Ansari A, Tseeng S, Christain E, et al. Diagnosing acute heart failure in patients with undifferentiated dyspnea: a lung and cardiac ultrasound (LuCUS) protocol. Acad Emerg Med Off J Soc Acad Emerg Med. 2015;22(2):182–91. Epub 2015/02/03. eng.
12. Sekiguchi H, Schenck LA, Horie R, Suzuki J, Lee EH, McMenomy BP, et al. Critical care ultrasonography differentiates ARDS, pulmonary edema, and other causes in the early course of acute hypoxemic respiratory failure. Chest. 2015;148(4):912–8.
13. Shokoohi H, Boniface KS, Pourmand A, Liu YT, Davison DL, Hawkins KD, et al. Bedside ultrasound reduces diagnostic uncertainty and guides resuscitation in patients with undifferentiated hypotension. Crit Care Med. 2015;43(12):2562–9. Epub 2015/11/18. eng.
14. Mantuani D, Frazee BW, Fahimi J, Nagdev A. Point-of-care multi-organ ultrasound improves diagnostic accuracy in adults presenting to the emergency department with acute dyspnea. West J Emerg Med. 2016;17(1): 46–53. Pubmed Central PMCID: PMC4729418, Epub 2016/01/30. eng.
15. Stewart VM, Bjornsson HM, Clinton M, Byars DV. BRIPPED scan for evaluation of ED patients with shortness of breath. Am J Emerg Med. 2016;34(3):386–91.

16. Lichtenstein DA, Meziere GA. Relevance of lung ultrasound in the diagnosis of acute respiratory failure: the BLUE protocol. Chest. 2008;134(1):117–25. Pubmed Central PMCID: 3734893.

17. Kristensen MS, Teoh WH, Graumann O, Laursen CB. Ultrasonography for clinical decision-making and intervention in airway management: from the mouth to the lungs and pleurae. Insights Imaging. 2014;5(2):253–79. Pubmed Central PMCID: 3999368.

18. Squizzato A, Rancan E, Dentali F, Bonzini M, Guasti L, Steidl L, et al. Diagnostic accuracy of lung ultrasound for pulmonary embolism: a systematic review and meta-analysis. J Thromb Haemost. 2013;11(7):1269–78.

19. Lichtenstein DA. BLUE-protocol and FALLS-protocol: two applications of lung ultrasound in the critically ill. Chest. 2015;147(6):1659–70.

20. Nazerian P, Vanni S, Volpicelli G, Gigli C, Zanobetti M, Bartolucci M, et al. Accuracy of point-of-care multiorgan ultrasonography for the diagnosis of pulmonary embolism. Chest. 2014;145(5):950–7.

21. Volpicelli G, Elbarbary M, Blaivas M, Lichtenstein DA, Mathis G, Kirkpatrick AW, et al. International evidence-based recommendations for point-of-care lung ultrasound. Intensive Care Med. 2012;38(4):577–91.

22. Lichtenstein D. Fluid administration limited by lung sonography: the place of lung ultrasound in assessment of acute circulatory failure (the FALLS-protocol). Expert Rev Respir Med. 2012;6(2):155–62.

23. Lichtenstein D, Malbrain ML. Critical care ultrasound in cardiac arrest. Technological requirements for performing the SESAME-protocol—a holistic approach. Anaesthesiol Intensive Ther. 2015;47(5):471–81.

24. Lichtenstein DA, Meziere GA, Lagoueyte JF, Biderman P, Goldstein I, Gepner A. A-lines and B-lines: lung ultrasound as a bedside tool for predicting pulmonary artery occlusion pressure in the critically ill. Chest. 2009;136(4):1014–20.

25. Lichtenstein DA, Menu Y. A bedside ultrasound sign ruling out pneumothorax in the critically ill. Lung Sliding Chest. 1995;108(5):1345–8.

26. Ding W, Shen Y, Yang J, He X, Zhang M. Diagnosis of pneumothorax by radiography and ultrasonography: a meta-analysis. Chest. 2011;140(4):859–66.

27. Lichtenstein D, Meziere G, Biderman P, Gepner A. The "lung point": an ultrasound sign specific to pneumothorax. Intensive Care Med. 2000;26(10):1434–40.

28. Remerand F, Dellamonica J, Mao Z, Ferrari F, Bouhemad B, Jianxin Y, et al. Multiplane ultrasound approach to quantify pleural effusion at the bedside. Intensive Care Med. 2010;36(4):656–64.

29. Vignon P, Chastagner C, Berkane V, Chardac E, Francois B, Normand S, et al. Quantitative assessment of pleural effusion in critically ill patients by means of ultrasonography. Crit Care Med. 2005;33(8):1757–63.

30. Yang PC, Luh KT, Chang DB, Wu HD, Yu CJ, Kuo SH. Value of sonography in determining the nature of pleural effusion: analysis of 320 cases. AJR Am J Roentgenol. 1992;159(1):29–33.

31. Vegas A, Denault A, Royse C. A bedside clinical and ultrasound-based approach to hemodynamic instability—part II: bedside ultrasound in hemodynamic shock: continuing professional development. Can J Anaesth. 2014;61(11):1008–27. Epub 2014/10/03. eng.

32. Kupfer Y, Seneviratne C, Chawla K, Ramachandran K, Tessler S. Chest tube drainage of transudative pleural effusions hastens liberation from mechanical ventilation. Chest. 2011;139(3):519–23.

33. Volpicelli G, Mussa A, Garofalo G, Cardinale L, Casoli G, Perotto F, et al. Bedside lung ultrasound in the assessment of alveolar-interstitial syndrome. Am J Emerg Med. 2006;24(6):689–96.

34. Lichtenstein D, Meziere G, Biderman P, Gepner A, Barre O. The comet-tail artifact. An ultrasound sign of alveolar-interstitial syndrome. Am J Respir Crit Care Med. 1997;156(5):1640–6.

35. Gargani L. Lung ultrasound: a new tool for the cardiologist. Cardiovasc Ultrasound. 2011;9:6. Pubmed Central PMCID: 3059291.

36. Gallard E, Redonnet JP, Bourcier JE, Deshaies D, Largeteau N, Amalric JM, et al. Diagnostic performance of cardiopulmonary ultrasound performed by the emergency physician in the management of acute dyspnea. Am J Emerg Med. 2015;33(3):352–8. Epub 2015/01/13. eng.

37. Copetti R, Soldati G, Copetti P. Chest sonography: a useful tool to differentiate acute cardiogenic pulmonary edema from acute respiratory distress syndrome. Cardiovasc Ultrasound. 2008;6:16. Pubmed Central PMCID: 2386861.

38. Lichtenstein D, Meziere G, Seitz J. The dynamic air bronchogram. A lung ultrasound sign of alveolar consolidation ruling out atelectasis. Chest. 2009;135(6):1421–5.

39. Volpicelli G, Cardinale L, Berchialla P, Mussa A, Bar F, Frascisco MF. A comparison of different diagnostic tests in the bedside evaluation of pleuritic pain in the ED. Am J Emerg Med. 2012;30(2):317–24. Epub 2011/02/01. eng.

40. Feissel M, Michard F, Faller JP, Teboul JL. The respiratory variation in inferior vena cava diameter as a guide to fluid therapy. Intensive Care Med. 2004;30(9):1834–7.

41. Barbier C, Loubieres Y, Schmit C, Hayon J, Ricome JL, Jardin F, et al. Respiratory changes in inferior vena cava diameter are helpful in predicting fluid responsiveness in ventilated septic patients. Intensive Care Med. 2004;30(9):1740–6.

42. Corl K, Napoli AM, Gardiner F. Bedside sonographic measurement of the inferior vena cava caval index is a poor predictor of fluid responsiveness in emergency department patients. Emerg Med Australas. 2012;24(5):534–9.

43. Dipti A, Soucy Z, Surana A, Chandra S. Role of inferior vena cava diameter in assessment of volume status: a meta-analysis. Am J Emerg Med. 2012;30(8):1414–9. e1.

44. Kanji HD, McCallum J, Sirounis D, MacRedmond R, Moss R, Boyd JH. Limited echocardiography-guided therapy in subacute shock is associated with change in management and improved outcomes. J Crit Care. 2014;29(5):700–5.

45. Haydar SA, Moore ET, Higgins 3rd GL, Irish CB, Owens WB, Strout TD. Effect of bedside ultrasonography on the certainty of physician clinical decisionmaking for septic patients in the emergency department. Ann Emerg Med. 2012;60(3):346–58. e4. Epub 2012/05/29. eng.

46. Lee CW, Kory PD, Arntfield RT. Development of a fluid resuscitation protocol using inferior vena cava and lung ultrasound. J Crit Care. 2016;31(1):96–100.

47. Caltabeloti F, Monsel A, Arbelot C, Brisson H, Lu Q, Gu WJ, et al. Early fluid loading in acute respiratory distress syndrome with septic shock deteriorates lung aeration without impairing arterial oxygenation: a lung ultrasound observational study. Crit Care. 2014;18(3):R91. Pubmed Central PMCID: 4055974.

48. Via G, Hussain A, Wells M, Reardon R, ElBarbary M, Noble VE, et al. International evidence-based recommendations for focused cardiac ultrasound. J Am Soc Echocardiogr. 2014;27(7):683. e1- e33.

49. Sekiguchi H. Tools of the trade: point-of-care ultrasonography as a stethoscope. Semin Respir Crit Care Med. 2016;37(1):68–87. Epub 2016/02/06. eng.

50. Kienzl D, Prosch H, Topker M, Herold C. Imaging of non-cardiac, non-traumatic causes of acute chest pain. Eur J Radiol. 2012;81(12):3669–74.

51. Nanuwa K, Chambers J, Senior R. Echocardiography for chest pain in the emergency department. Int J Clin Pract. 2005;59(12):1374–6.

52. Spodick DH, Greene TO, Saperia G. Images in cardiovascular medicine. Acute myocarditis masquerading as acute myocardial infarction. Circulation. 1995;91(6):1886–7.

53. Nazerian P, Vanni S, Castelli M, Morello F, Tozzetti C, Zagli G, et al. Diagnostic performance of emergency transthoracic focus cardiac ultrasound in suspected acute type A aortic dissection. Intern Emerg Med. 2014;9(6):665–70.

54. Hiratzka LF, Bakris GL, Beckman JA, Bersin RM, Carr VF, Casey Jr DE, et al. 2010 ACCF/AHA/AATS/ACR/ASA/SCA/SCAI/SIR/STS/SVM guidelines for the diagnosis and management of patients with thoracic aortic disease: a report of the American College of Cardiology Foundation/American Heart Association Task Force on Practice Guidelines, American Association for Thoracic Surgery, American College of Radiology, American Stroke Association, Society of Cardiovascular Anesthesiologists, Society for Cardiovascular Angiography and Interventions, Society of Interventional Radiology, Society of Thoracic Surgeons, and Society for Vascular Medicine. Circulation. 2010;121(13):e266–369.

55. Reydel B, Spodick DH. Frequency and significance of chamber collapses during cardiac tamponade. Am Heart J. 1990;119(5):1160–3.

56. Zhang S, Kerins DM, Byrd 3rd BF. Doppler echocardiography in cardiac tamponade and constrictive pericarditis. Echocardiography. 1994;11(5):507–21.

57. Himelman RB, Kircher B, Rockey DC, Schiller NB. Inferior vena cava plethora with blunted respiratory response: a sensitive echocardiographic sign of cardiac tamponade. J Am Coll Cardiol. 1988;12(6):1470–7.

58. Gilon D, Mehta RH, Oh JK, Januzzi Jr JL, Bossone E, Cooper JV, et al. Characteristics and in-hospital outcomes of patients with cardiac tamponade complicating type A acute aortic dissection. Am J Cardiol. 2009;103(7):1029–31.

59. Fremont B, Pacouret G, Jacobi D, Puglisi R, Charbonnier B, de Labriolle A. Prognostic value of echocardiographic right/left ventricular end-diastolic diameter ratio in patients with acute pulmonary embolism: results from a monocenter registry of 1,416 patients. Chest. 2008;133(2):358–62.

60. Konstantinides SV, Torbicki A, Agnelli G, Danchin N, Fitzmaurice D, Galie N, et al. 2014 ESC guidelines on the diagnosis and management of acute pulmonary embolism. Eur Heart J. 2014;35(43):3033–69. 69a-69k.

61. Kucher N, Luder CM, Dornhofer T, Windecker S, Meier B, Hess OM. Novel management strategy for patients with suspected pulmonary embolism. Eur Heart J. 2003;24(4):366–76.

62. Jardin F, Dubourg O, Bourdarias JP. Echocardiographic pattern of acute cor pulmonale. Chest. 1997;111(1):209–17.

63. Kurzyna M, Torbicki A, Pruszczyk P, Burakowska B, Fijalkowska A, Kober J, et al. Disturbed right ventricular ejection pattern as a new Doppler echocardiographic sign of acute pulmonary embolism. Am J Cardiol. 2002; 90(5):507–11.

64. Harjola VP, Mebazaa A, Celutkiene J, Bettex D, Bueno H, Chioncel O, et al. Contemporary management of acute right ventricular failure: a statement from the Heart Failure Association and the Working Group on Pulmonary Circulation and Right Ventricular Function of the European Society of Cardiology. Eur J Heart Fail. 2016;18(3):226–41.

65. Haley JH, Sinak LJ, Tajik AJ, Ommen SR, Oh JK. Dynamic left ventricular outflow tract obstruction in acute coronary syndromes: an important cause of new systolic murmur and cardiogenic shock. Mayo Clin Proc. 1999;74(9):901–6.

66. Kim D, Mun JB, Kim EY, Moon J. Paradoxical heart failure precipitated by profound dehydration: intraventricular dynamic obstruction and significant mitral regurgitation in a volume-depleted heart. Yonsei Med J. 2013;54(4): 1058–61. Pubmed Central PMCID: 3663219.

67. El Mahmoud R, Mansencal N, Pilliere R, Leyer F, Abbou N, Michaud P, et al. Prevalence and characteristics of left ventricular outflow tract obstruction in Tako-Tsubo syndrome. Am Heart J. 2008;156(3):543–8.

68. Jones AE, Craddock PA, Tayal VS, Kline JA. Diagnostic accuracy of left ventricular function for identifying sepsis among emergency department patients with nontraumatic symptomatic undifferentiated hypotension. Shock. 2005;24(6):513–7.

69. Hochman JS, Buller CE, Sleeper LA, Boland J, Dzavik V, Sanborn TA, et al. Cardiogenic shock complicating acute myocardial infarction—etiologies, management and outcome: a report from the SHOCK Trial Registry. SHould we emergently revascularize Occluded Coronaries for cardiogenic shocK? J Am Coll Cardiol. 2000;36(3 Suppl A):1063–70.

70. Reynolds HR, Hochman JS. Cardiogenic shock: current concepts and improving outcomes. Circulation. 2008;117(5):686–97.

71. Gianni M, Dentali F, Grandi AM, Sumner G, Hiralal R, Lonn E. Apical ballooning syndrome or takotsubo cardiomyopathy: a systematic review. Eur Heart J. 2006;27(13):1523–9.

72. Vahanian A, Ducrocq G. Emergencies in valve disease. Curr Opin Crit Care. 2008;14(5):555–60.

73. Baliga RR, Nienaber CA, Bossone E, Oh JK, Isselbacher EM, Sechtem U, et al. The role of imaging in aortic dissection and related syndromes. J Am Coll Cardiol Img. 2014;7(4):406–24.

74. Copetti R, Copetti P, Reissig A. Clinical integrated ultrasound of the thorax including causes of shock in nontraumatic critically ill patients. A practical approach. Ultrasound Med Biol. 2012;38(3):349–59. Epub 2012/01/24. eng.

Clinical outcomes of patients undergoing primary percutaneous coronary intervention for acute myocardial infarction requiring the intensive care unit

Ken Parhar[1,3]* [iD], Victoria Millar[1], Vasileios Zochios[1,4], Emilia Bruton[1], Catherine Jaworksi[2], Nick West[2] and Alain Vuylsteke[1]

Abstract

Background: Outcomes for patients with ST-segment elevation myocardial infarction continue to improve, largely due to timely provision of reperfusion by primary percutaneous coronary intervention (PPCI). However, despite prompt and successful PPCI, a small proportion of patients require ventilatory and hemodynamic support in an intensive care unit (ICU). The outcome of these patients remains poorly defined.

Methods: A retrospective review of all consecutive admissions post-PPCI pathway to a single ICU between January 2009 and May 2014 was performed. Patients were analysed based on survival and indication for admission. Preadmission characteristics and ICU course were reviewed. Univariate and multivariable regression analysis was performed to determine predictors of outcome.

Results: During the study period 2902 PPCI were performed and 101 patients were admitted to ICU following PPCI (incidence 3.5%). ICU mortality post-PPCI was 33.7%. Pre-ICU admission factors in a multivariable logistic regression analysis associated with increased mortality included requirement for an intra-aortic balloon pump and a high SOFA score.

Conclusions: ICU admission post PPCI is associated with significant mortality. Mortality was related to high presenting SOFA score and need for IABP. These results provide important prognostic information and an acceptable method for risk-stratifying patients with acute myocardial infarction requiring intensive care.

Keywords: Acute myocardial infarction, Primary percutaneous coronary intervention, Mechanical ventilation, Intensive care unit

Background

Acute myocardial infarction, in particular ST-segment elevation myocardial infarction (STEMI) remains a time-sensitive medical emergency associated with significant morbidity and mortality [1]. In recent years, the widespread recognition of primary percutaneous coronary intervention (PPCI) as an evidence-based treatment strategy that can improve outcomes has led to both an increase in PPCI volume and a reduction in hospital mortality associated with STEMI [2, 3]. A major driver to facilitate this has been the creation and implementation of organised PPCI networks that are able to triage and deliver patients directly to centres able to routinely provide this service both in- and out-of-hours [4, 5]. Patients are subsequently generally cared for in a coronary-care unit (CCU), which has been shown to reduce mortality [6].

The National Infarct Angioplasty Project has demonstrated the benefits of PPCI over thrombolysis for treatment of STEMI patients [7] and has led to the creation of PPCI centres across England. By 2013, some regions demonstrated that more than 95% of patients treated for

* Correspondence: ken.parhar@albertahealthservices.ca
[1]Department of Anesthesia and Intensive Care, Papworth Hospital, Cambridge, England
[3]Department of Critical Care Medicine, University of Calgary, ICU Administration - Ground Floor - McCaig Tower, Foothills Medical Center, 3134 Hospital Drive NW, Calgary, AB T2N 5A1, Canada
Full list of author information is available at the end of the article

STEMI received PPCI, compared with only 30% in the third quarter of 2008 [5].

Despite the pervasiveness of PPCI in the management of STEMI and the appropriate use of CCU care, there remains a small proportion of patients that become critically ill and require advanced life support modalities post-PPCI, such as mechanical ventilation or vasoactive therapy that may only be provided within the intensive care unit (ICU). Historically, patients with a complicated myocardial infarction requiring mechanical ventilation have been associated with high rates of morbidity and mortality [8–13].

Patients that may require ICU post-PPCI remain poorly defined. This retrospective single-centre cohort review aims to describe the incidence of admission to ICU, indication for ICU admission, and quantify the morbidity and mortality associated with ICU admission. In addition, factors associated with survival are assessed.

Methods
Patient population
We undertook a retrospective review of all consecutive patients admitted to a single tertiary cardiothoracic ICU post-PPCI between January 2009 and May 2014. The unit is the sole provider of intensive care in a subspecialty cardiothoracic hospital serving an English region with a catchment area of approximately three million. All patients requiring PPCI in this region are transferred to this institution.

The search was performed via the electronic Clinical Information System (CIS), which maintains the electronic medical record of all patients admitted to ICU. The initial search yielded 191 patients. Patients were excluded if not admitted directly post-PPCI. Ninety patients were excluded including: patients admitted immediately before or after cardiac surgery or cardiac procedures other than PPCI ($n = 78$), post respiratory medicine procedures ($n = 2$), patients admitted due to lack of beds in CCU ($n = 9$), and patients admitted for end of life care ($n = 1$). A total of 101 patients post-PPCI were appropriate for detailed chart review and analysis (Fig. 1).

Clinical data
Demographic data (including age, gender, past medical history, and cardiovascular risk factors) were extracted from case-notes and the electronic CIS. Baseline physiological characteristics (vital signs, Glasgow coma scale (GCS), laboratory values) were extracted from the electronic CIS. Details related to PPCI admission, echocardiograms, and cardiac catheterization (downtime, location of infarction, procedures performed, anatomy of coronary disease, complications, door-to-balloon time, pre-PCI interventions) were extracted from a dedicated

local database (Philips CVIS, Netherlands), routinely collected for national audits, and patient case-notes where appropriate. ICU interventions, length of stay, and complications were extracted from CIS. Survival data including the ICU and 28 day/hospital outcome was derived from both CIS, case notes and local databases linked to national outcome data.

Vital signs on admission (including heart rate, blood pressure and mean arterial pressure) are reported as mean over the first 24 h of ICU admission. The admission PaO2 to FiO2 (PF) ratio, creatinine, platelets, bilirubin were the worst value measured over the first 24 h. Pulmonary edema was defined as hypoxemia with associated radiographic evidence of interstitial and/or alveolar edema. Cardiogenic shock was defined as a systolic blood pressure < 90 mmHg with clinical evidence of hypoperfusion (cyanosis, mottling, oliguria, cold extremities) or the requirement for an inotrope. New onset renal dysfunction was defined as a 25% rise in serum creatinine or the requirement for renal replacement therapy. The initiation of renal replacement therapy was based on refractory hyperkalemia, refractory acidosis, or volume overload despite medical management. Major hemorrhage was clinical evidence of bleeding with the requirement for four or more units of red blood cells. Infection was a positive culture result, or clinical syndrome consistent with infection such as pneumonia (fever, elevated white cell count, purulent sputum, hypoxemia). Sequential organ function failure assessment (SOFA) score was calculated as previously described [14, 15].

Groups
Patient outcomes were analysed based on ICU survival. Patient were stratified and analysed based on one of four indications for ICU admission including out-of-hospital cardiac arrest (OHCA), in-hospital cardiac arrest (IHCA), cardiogenic shock, or pulmonary edema. IHCA was defined as a cardiac arrest occurring following arrival to hospital (most commonly during cardiac catheterization), but prior to admission to ICU. Cardiac arrests occurring while in ICU were listed as an ICU complication.

Statistical analysis
The Shapiro-Wilks test for normality was performed on all continuous variables. Continuous variables with normal distribution were reported as means with standard deviation and analysed by unpaired student's two-tailed t test or one-way analysis of variance (ANOVA) where appropriate. Non-normally-distributed data were reported as median with interquartile range and analysed with the Mann-Whitney U test or the Kruskal-Wallis test where appropriate. Categorical variables were analysed with the chi-squared test or Fisher's exact test where appropriate. A p value of < 0.05 was considered statistically significant.

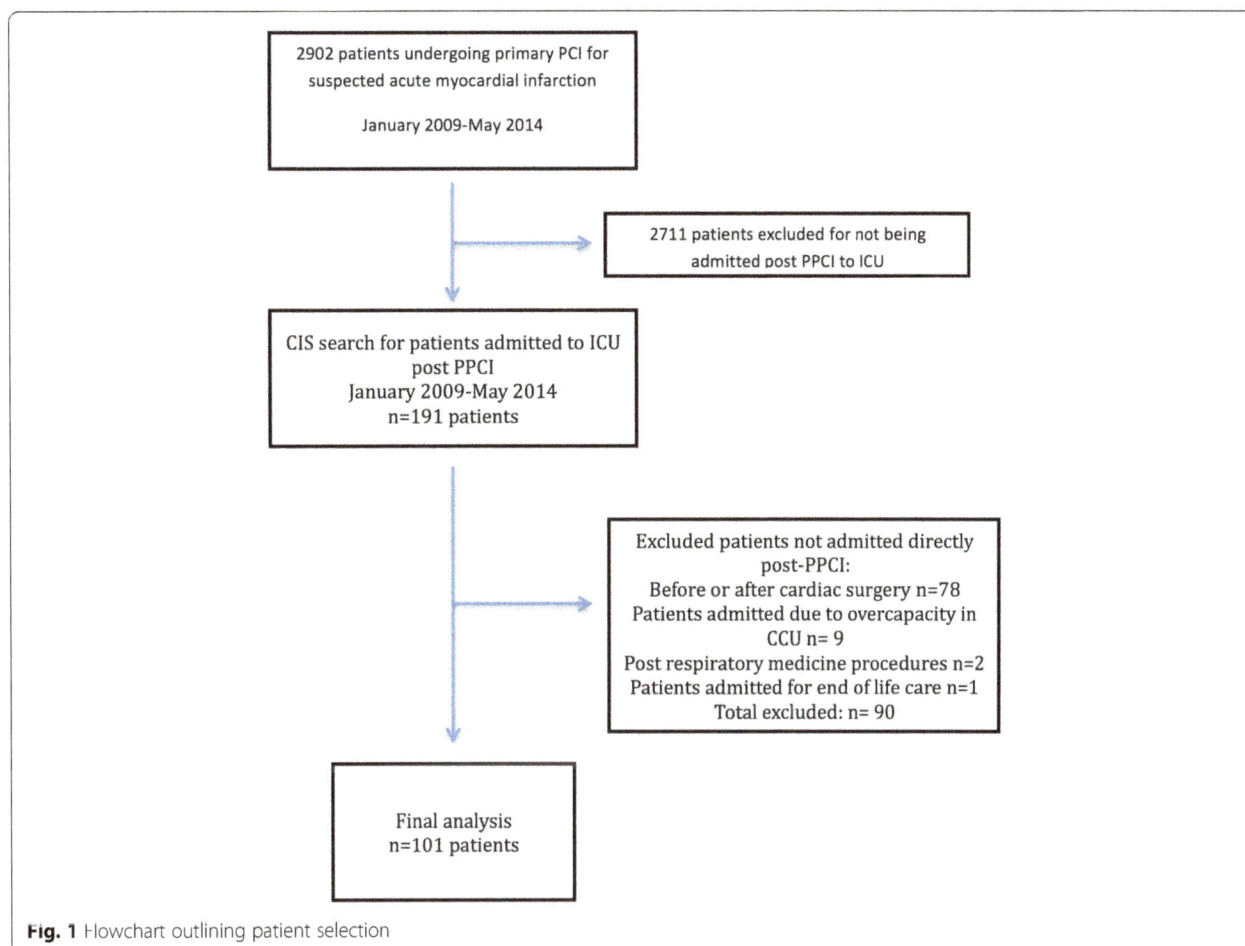

Fig. 1 Flowchart outlining patient selection

Variables that were statistically significant in the univariate analysis (with a p value < 0.10) were considered for inclusion in the multivariable logistic regression model. ICU mortality was defined as the dependant variable. Backward stepwise variable elimination was performed (with a variable exit threshold set at $p > 0.05$). The performance of the final model was assessed using the area under the receiver-operating characteristic (AUROC) curve.

Statistical analysis was performed using Stata Version 13.1 (StataCorp, USA).

Ethics

Ethical approval was obtained from the Papworth Hospital NHS Foundation Trust research and development board for the completion of this study.

Results

One-hundred one patients met the inclusion criteria for this retrospective observational study (Fig. 1). During this time, a total of 2902 PPCI were performed, resulting in a post-PPCI incidence of admission to ICU post PPCI of 3.5%.

Of the 101 patients who were admitted to ICU, the majority were male (69%), with a mean age of 65 years (Table 1). Out of hospital cardiac arrest (OHCA) was the most common indication for admission to ICU (36.6%). A significant proportion of patients were admitted for in-hospital cardiac arrest (IHCA; 31.7%) and cardiogenic shock (22.8%). The least common indication for admission to ICU post-PPCI was pulmonary edema (8.9%). Overall ICU mortality was 33.7% for the entire cohort.

Univariate factors that demonstrated a statistically significant difference between survivors and non-survivors included age, low blood pressure on admission (both systolic and mean arterial pressure), low PF ratio, low GCS, high creatinine, and high SOFA scores. In the subgroup of patients suffering from an OHCA, downtime before return of spontaneous circulation (ROSC) was statistically different between survivors and non-survivors. Survivors of ICU post PPCI were associated with a shorter downtime in comparison to non-survivors (Fig. 2). Patients who suffered a witnessed IHCA did not demonstrate a difference in time to ROSC between survivors and non-survivors. When patients were stratified based on their indication for admission (OHCA, IHCA, shock, or pulmonary edema) to ICU

Table 1 Patient demographic factors for patients admitted to ICU post PPCI. Results are expressed as mean (SD) unless otherwise denoted

	All patients	Outcome			Indication for ICU				
		Survivor	Non-survivor	Sign	OHCA	IHCA	Card shock	Pulm edema	Sign
Total no of patients (%)	101 (100)	67 (66.3)	34 (33.7)		37 (36.6)	32 (31.7)	23 (22.8)	9 (8.9)	
Gender Male, no (%)	70 (69.3)	48 (47.5)	22 (21.8)	0.500	29 (28.7)	20 (19.8)	15 (14.9)	6 (5.9)	0.505
Age, years	65.3 (12.8)	63.8 (11.5)	68.3 (14.8)	0.047	60.2 (12.8)	66.8 (12.6)	71.2 (10.7)	66.0 (11.8)	0.009
Cardiovascular risk factors									
Smoking, no (%)	28 (27.7)	19 (18.8)	9 (8.91)	1.000	11 (10.9)	11 (10.9)	3 (3.0)	3 (3.0)	0.335
Diabetes mellitus, no (%)	21 (20.8)	10 (9.9)	11(10.9)	0.067	4 (4.0)	7 (6.9)	8 (7.9)	2 (2.0)	0.171
Dyslipidaemia, no (%)	30 (29.7)	22 (21.8)	8 (7.9)	0.367	8 (7.9)	10 (9.9)	9 (8.9)	3 (3.0)	0.526
Hypertension, no (%)	58 (57.4)	40 (39.6)	18 (17.8)	0.531	18 (17.8)	17 (16.8)	16 (15.8)	7 (6.9)	0.229
Past medical history									
Previous MI, no (%)	20 (19.8)	15 (14.9)	5 (5.0)	0.436	3 (3.0)	4 (4.0)	8 (7.9)	5 (5.0)	0.002
Previous CAD, no (%)	29 (28.7)	21 (20.8)	8 (7.9)	0.490	4 (4.0)	9 (8.9)	10 (9.9)	6 (5.9)	0.002
Previous CHF, no (%)	3 (3.0)	2 (2.0)	1 (1.0)	1.000	0 (0.0)	1 (1.0)	1 (1.0)	1 (1.0)	0.340
Renal failure, no (%)	12 (11.9)	8 (7.9)	4 (4.0)	1.000	3 (3.0)	2 (2.0)	5 (5.0)	2 (2.0)	0.210
COPD no, no (%)	11 (10.9)	9 (8.9)	2 (2.0)	0.326	3 (3.0)	6 (5.9)	0 (0.0)	2 (2.0)	0.096
Baseline characteristics on admission									
HR (bpm)	79.7 (15.6)	78.5 (16.0)	82.0 (14.5)	0.297	70.6 (15)	80.4 (12.3)	87.8 (13.4)	93.8 (11.7)	< 0.001
Systolic BP (mmHg)	106.8 (19.5)	111.8 (17.9)	96.3 (18.7)	< 0.001	106.9 (16.4)	103.16 (20.7)	108.9 (21.2)	114.0 (22.2)	0.462
MAP (mmHg)	73.0 (13.0)	77.7 (10.3)	63.7 (12.9)	< 0.001	72.5 (12.4)	73.7 (15.3)	71.4 (9.5)	77.0 (15.0)	0.720
PaO2/FiO2 ratio, med (IQR)	143 (98–233)	154 (98–271)	105 (83–173)	0.036	157.9 (105–241)	165 (83–286)	105 (83–143)	128 (75–278)	0.138
GCS, med (IQR)	3 (3–15)	11 (3–15)	3 (3–3)	< 0.001	3 (3–4)	3 (3–14.5)	14 (3–15)	3 (3–15)	0.071
Serum creatinine (µmol/L), med (IQR)	116 (87–157)	102 (84–129)	156 (115–203)	< 0.001	101 (71–126)	116 (95–155)	140 (112–191)	135 (117–144)	0.012
SOFA score	8.4 (3.3)	7.4 (2.9)	10.4 (3.1)	< 0.001	8.6 (2.6)	8.5 (3.5)	8.3 (3.4)	8.0 (5.2)	0.953
Indication for ICU admission									
OHCA, no (%)	37 (36.6)	26 (25.7)	11 (10.9)	0.663					
Downtime before ROSC (min), (IQR)	20 (15–30)	15 (10–20)	35 (30–40)	< 0.001					
IHCA, no (%)	32 (31.7)	19 (18.8)	13 (12.7)	0.368					
Downtime before ROSC (min), (IQR)	10 (5–20)	9 (5–14)	15 (5–42)	0.214					
Cardiogenic shock, no (%)	23 (22.8)	14 (13.9)	9 (8.9)	0.617					
Acute pulmonary oedema, no (%)	9 (8.9)	8 (7.9)	1 (1.0)	0.266					

post PPCI, there was no difference in mortality amongst the four groups.

STEMI was the most common type of presenting acute coronary syndrome (91%) (Table 2). Other patients who underwent PPCI had either indeterminate ACS (due to a left bundle branch block) or a high suspicion of an evolving transmural infarct. The majority were in the anterior territory (61%) and uncommonly involved the right ventricle (5.0%). Left ventricular (LV) systolic function was depressed in the majority of patients with over 50% of patients having either moderate or severe LV dysfunction as determined by echocardiography during admission. Only one patient received thrombolytics prior to PPCI. Angiogram was successfully performed in the majority of patients (98.0%) with the exception of two patients in whom it was attempted but aborted due to cardiac arrest. There was a high rate of PCI performed (90.1%). Factors that were statistically associated

with reduced survival included severe LV dysfunction, right ventricle (RV) involvement, and the need for intra-aortic balloon pump (IABP) insertion in the cath lab. The indications for IABP insertion in the cath lab included cardiogenic shock, bridge for high risk PCI, and ongoing chest pain. IABP were all inserted prior to admission to ICU. The cardiologic factors did not influence the indication for admission to ICU (Additional file 1: Table S1).

The median duration of stay in the ICU was 3 days (Table 3). Most patients required invasive mechanical ventilation (IMV) (86.1%) with median duration of IMV being 2 days. The majority of the mortality occurred within the ICU (34 of 37 patients). Significant complications were common with patients suffering major bleeding (9.9%), infections (31.7%), acute kidney injury (33.7%), or in ICU cardiac arrest (6.9%). Factors that statistically associated with reduced survival included the lack of use of non-invasive ventilation (NIV), inotropes and vasopressor

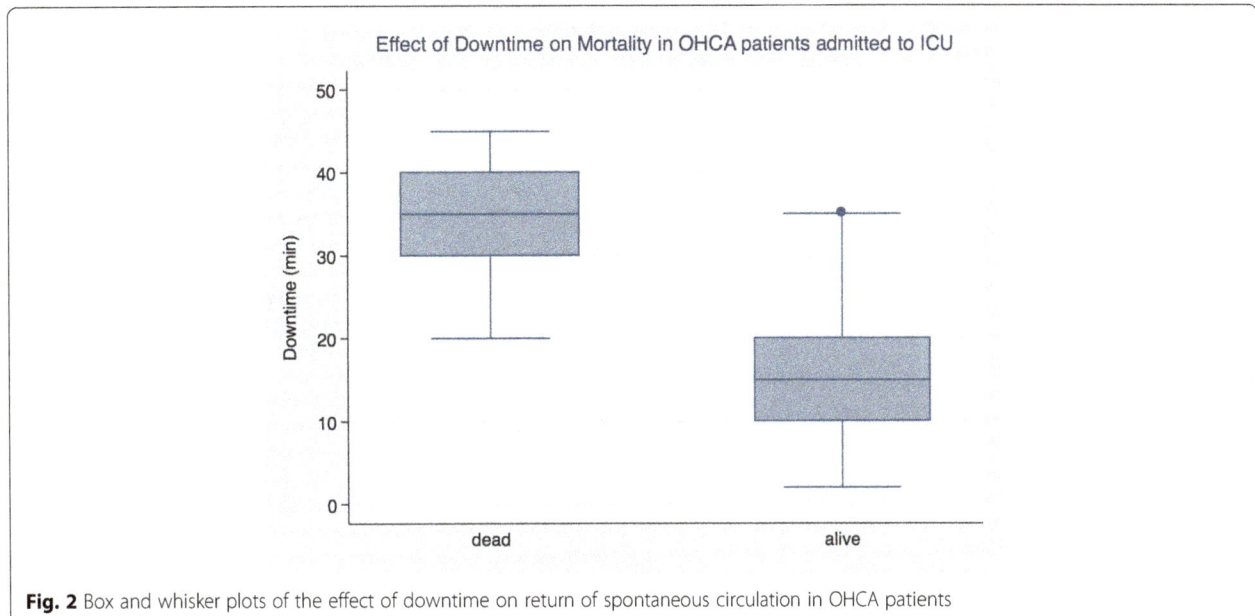

Fig. 2 Box and whisker plots of the effect of downtime on return of spontaneous circulation in OHCA patients

Table 2 Cardiac characteristics of patients admitted to ICU post PPCI. Results are expressed as mean (SD) unless otherwise denoted

	All Patients	Outcome		
		Survivor	Non-survivor	Sign
Total number of patients (%)	101 (100)	67 (66.3)	34 (33.7)	
STEMI, no (%)	91 (90.1)	58 (57.4)	33 (32.7)	0.158
MI territory				
Anterior, no (%)	61 (61.0)	42 (42.0)	19 (19.0)	0.667
Inferior, no (%)	38 (38.0)	26 (26.0)	12 (12.0)	1.000
Lateral, no (%)	32 (32.0)	22 (22.0)	10 (10.0)	1.000
RV involvement, no (%)	5 (5.0)	1 (1.0)	4 (4.0)	0.040
Peak troponin, ng/L med (IQR)	38.9 (13.7–40.0)	26.8 (10.9–40.0)	40.0 (19.1–626.0)	0.146
LV systolic function				
Normal, no (%)	10 (11.6)	8 (9.3)	2 (2.3)	0.488
Mild dysfunction, no (%)	26 (30.2)	21 (24.4)	5 (5.8)	0.093
Moderate dysfunction, no (%)	22 (25.6)	17 (19.8)	5 (5.8)	0.309
Severe dysfunction, no (%)	28 (32.6)	14 (16.3)	14 (16.3)	0.037
Thrombolysis pre-PPCI, no (%)	1 (1.0)	1 (1.0)	0 (0.0)	1.000
Angiogram, (successful completion) no (%)	99 (98.0)	67 (66.3)	32 (31.7)	0.111
PCI performed (successful completion), no (%)	91 (90.1)	62 (61.4)	29 (28.7)	0.298
IABP in cath lab, no (%)	50 (49.5)	28 (27.7)	22 (21.8)	0.036
Number of diseased vessels, med (IQR)	2 (1–3)	2 (1–3)	2 (2–3)	0.514
Left main stem disease, no (%)	14 (14.1)	8 (8.1)	6 (6.1)	0.371
TIMI flow, med (IQR)	3 (2–3)	3 (2–3)	3 (2–3)	0.862
Symptom onset to device time (min, med (IQR)	210 (155–332)	219 (159–328)	200 (150–350)	0.665

Table 3 Intensive care characteristics and complications of patients admitted to ICU post PPCI. Results are expressed as mean (SD) unless otherwise denoted

	All patients	Outcome			Indication for ICU				
		Survivor	Non-survivor	Sign	OHCA	IHCA	Card shock	Pulm edema	Sign
Total number of patients (%)	101 (100)	67 (66.3)	34 (33.7)		37 (36.6)	32 (31.7)	23 (22.8)	9 (8.9)	
ICU interventions									
Invasive mechanical ventilation, no (%)	87 (86.1)	56 (55.5)	31 (30.7)	0.373	37 (36.6)	31 (30.7)	12 (11.9)	7 (6.9)	< 0.001
Duration of IMV, median days (IQR)	2 (1–3)	2 (1–2)	2 (1–6)	0.314	2 (2–4)	1 (1–2)	2 (1–5)	1 (1–1)	0.011
Non-invasive ventilation, no (%)	25 (24.8)	21 (20.8)	4 (4.0)	0.049	7 (6.9)	5 (5.0)	8 (7.9)	5 (5.0)	0.047
Duration of NIV, median days (IQR)	1 (1–2)	1 (1–2)	2.5 (1.5–3)	0.075	1 (1–1)	2 (1–2)	2 (1.5–3)	1 (1–1)	0.032
Inotropes, median number (IQR)	1 (0–1)	0 (0–1)	1 (0–2)	0.005	1 (0–1)	1 (0–2)	0 (0–1)	0 (0–1)	0.617
Vasopressors, median number (IQR)	0 (0–1)	0 (0–1)	1 (0–1)	0.001	0 (0–1)	0 (0–1)	0 (0–1)	0 (0–1)	0.971
ECMO, no (%)	7 (6.9)	1 (1.0)	6 (5.9)	0.006	0 (0.0)	7 (6.9)	0 (0.0)	0 (0.0)	0.001
Therapeutic hypothermia, no (%)	48 (47.5)	33 (32.7)	15 (14.9)	0.677	32 (31.7)	14 (13.9)	0 (0.0)	2 (2.0)	< 0.001
IABP, no (%)	59 (58.4)	35 (34.7)	24 (23.8)	0.090	15 (14.9)	23 (22.8)	18 (17.8)	3 (3.0)	0.004
Renal repl therapy, no (%)	27 (26.7)	10 (9.9)	17 (16.8)	< 0.001	6 (5.9)	11 (10.9)	8 (7.9)	2 (2.0)	0.273
In-hospital complications									
Major bleeding, no (%)	10 (9.9)	6 (5.9)	4 (4.0)	0.082	0 (0.0)	7 (6.9)	2 (2.0)	1 (1.0)	0.026
Infections, no (%)	32 (31.7)	21 (20.8)	11 (10.9)	1.000	13 (12.9)	9 (8.9)	7 (6.9)	3 (3.0)	0.936
Renal dysfunction (new onset), no (%)	34 (33.7)	18 (17.8)	16 (15.8)	0.048	12 (11.9)	11 (10.9)	9 (8.9)	2 (2.0)	0.833
In ICU Cardiopulmonary arrest, no (%)	7 (6.9)	0 (0.0)	7 (6.9)	< 0.001	3 (3.0)	4 (4.0)	0 (0.0)	0 (0.0)	0.261
Outcomes									
Duration of ICU stay, median days (IQR)	3 (1–5)	3 (1–4)	2 (0.5–7)	0.389	3 (2–7)	2 (1–5)	3 (0.5–5)	1 (0.5–2)	0.095
ICU mortality, no (%)	34 (33.7)				11 (10.9)	13 (12.9)	9 (8.9)	1 (1.0)	0.346
Hospital / 28-day mortality, no (%)	37 (36.6)				12 (11.9)	14 (13.9)	10 (9.9)	1 (1.0)	0.265
Cause of death (of 37 patients)									
Treatment withdrawn, no (%)	25 (67.6)				7 (18.9)	9 (24.3)	8 (21.6)	1 (2.7)	0.632
Cardiac Arrest, no (%)	7 (18.9)				3 (8.1)	2 (5.4)	2 (5.4)	0 (0.0)	0.867
Other	5 (13.5)				2 (5.4)	3 (8.1)	0 (0.0)	0 (0.0)	0.463

use, transfusion of blood products including red blood cells (RBCs) and nonRBCs, as well as need for extracorporeal membrane oxygenation (ECMO) or renal replacement therapy (RRT). ECMO was used exclusively in patients who suffered IHCA at any point during the ICU admission. Therapeutic hypothermia was used in patients who suffered either OHCA or IHCA in patients with an initial rhythm of ventricular tachycardia or ventricular fibrillation, but was not associated with a statistically significant increase in survival. There were higher than expected rates of bleeding and transfusions (RBC) in the IHCA group.

Twenty-eight-day mortality was similar to ICU mortality (Table 3, 36.6 vs 33.7%). The cause of death in most patients was withdrawal of care (67.6%). Post ICU admission cardiac arrest occurred in seven patients (18.9%), none of whom survived.

Pre-ICU admission factors that demonstrated a statistically significant difference between survivors and non-survivors in univariate analysis were selected for inclusion in multivariable regression analysis. Factors that were independently associated with ICU mortality included high SOFA score and pre-ICU insertion of an IABP (Table 4). Notable factors that were not independently associate with mortality included age, presence of RV dysfunction, and presence of severe LV dysfunction. The odds ratio (OR) for increased mortality for each point increase in SOFA was 1.43 (95% CI 1.2–1.7). The OR for increased mortality when an IABP was inserted pre-ICU admission (during cardiac catheterization) was 3.38 (95% CI 1.27–9.03). The sensitivity and specificity of this model was 50 and 91% respectively with a positive predictive value (PPV) of 73.9%

Table 4 Multivariable logistic regression analysis of factors associated with ICU mortality

	Odds ratio	Standard error	z	P value	95% CI
SOFA	1.43	0.127	4.01	0.000	1.200–1.700
IABP	3.38	1.695	2.43	0.015	1.266–9.030

and a negative predictive value (NPV) of 78.2%. This model correctly classified 77.2% of patients in this series and had an AUROC curve of 0.7842 (Fig. 3). When using a model with only SOFA and without IABP, the AUROC was slightly lower (0.75 CI 0.65–0.85) in comparison to the model with SOFA and IABP (0.78 CI 0.68–0.89).

Discussion

In this retrospective observational study, we present a series of consecutive patients post-PPCI pathway that are critically ill and require admission to the ICU for advanced therapies that may only be provided in ICU such as invasive mechanical ventilation or vasoactive support. There is a significant mortality amongst these patients (33.6%), which is significantly higher than the general PPCI population. Indication for admission (cardiac arrest, pulmonary edema, cardiogenic shock) does not statistically influence mortality and all groups were similar despite their indication. Those patients presenting with higher SOFA scores (reflecting a higher degree of multiple-organ dysfunction), or requiring an IABP during cardiac catheterization were independently associated with higher mortality.

Despite an era of appropriate anti-ischemic therapy post-STEMI and provision of organised and timely reperfusion via PPCI, there remain a proportion of patients who become critically ill and require admission to ICU for invasive monitoring, mechanical ventilation or vasoactive therapy. Patient mortality in this group remains high despite improving outcome for all patients with STEMI presenting for PPCI [3].

In contrast to previous studies of patients requiring mechanical ventilation or suffering from cardiogenic shock following complicated myocardial infarction, our study reviewed consecutive patients admitted to ICU exclusively via the PPCI pathway [8–13, 16, 17]. This included both patients who required mechanical ventilation and those who did not.

A higher SOFA score was associated with increased mortality (Table 4). This suggests that degree of organ dysfunction in patients with complicated myocardial infarction, as with many other critical illnesses, is a major determinant of survival. Surprisingly, neither the requirement for mechanical ventilation nor the indication for admission were independently associated with mortality. To date, no study has described this relationship exclusively in the post-PPCI patient population. A previous study looking at traditional risks scores used in the myocardial infarction population such as the Global Registry of Acute Coronary Events (GRACE) risk score or the Thrombolysis in Myocardial Infarction (TIMI) risk score in comparison with SOFA demonstrated that SOFA provided reasonable discrimination of prognosis [18]. This study was limited, as it did not focus on the post-PPCI population or those patients specifically who were admitted to ICU, which are most likely to be critically ill and potentially benefit from prognostication. Our study is novel as we demonstrate that the SOFA score does predict mortality in this high-risk group of patients admitted to the ICU who require mechanical ventilation and vasopressors. Previous studies looking specifically at patients admitted to ICU with cardiogenic shock demonstrated that there was an association between scores such as Acute Physiology and Chronic Health II/III (APACHE II/III), Simplified Acute Physiology Score II (SAPSII), SOFA and survival outcome [16, 17]. The specific organ

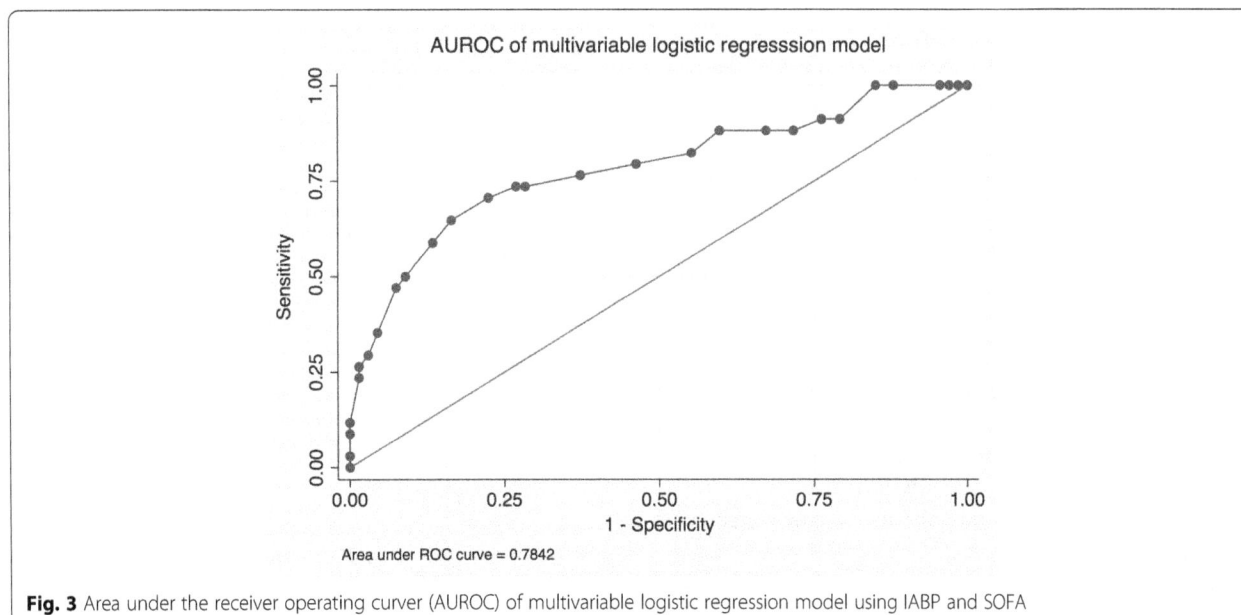

Fig. 3 Area under the receiver operating curver (AUROC) of multivariable logistic regression model using IABP and SOFA

systems within the SOFA score that were responsible for the higher scores included increased renal dysfunction, lower admission GCS, as well as worse hypoxemia (lower PaO2/FiO2 ratio (Table 1). The benefit of using SOFA scores and the presence or absence of IABP to prognosticate patients is that it can be easily calculated upon admission to ICU with information routinely available. This is the drawback of scores such as APACHE II/III and SAPSII as they are more complex and time consuming to calculate when compared to SOFA [19]. SOFA was used as a prognostic score due to its simplicity and ability to be calculated with very routine and objective patient data. Retrospective data collection made it difficult to use alternate scores such as APACHE II due to the high number of variables required in these scores including patient historical factors and the risk of missing data [19]. For example, any missing data precluded patients from being included in APACHE II score calculation as per the original description of APACHE II [20]. In addition, it has been demonstrated that there are significant differences in the ability of APACHE II to be calculated accurately when comparing prospective and retrospective collection of data [21]. This further highlights the strength of the SOFA score as it is quick and easy to calculate using commonly available objective clinical data.

We demonstrated that use of IABP was independently associated with mortality which is in keeping with previously reported observational data [22, 23]. The cohort of the study patients who required mechanical circulatory support with IABP and ICU admission was representative of the higher risk patient population and therefore IABP support may have been given to the sicker patients which would induce bias towards poor outcomes in that group. A meta-analysis of cohort studies in the context of STEMI leading to cardiogenic shock supported the use of IABP adjunctive to fibrinolysis [24]. It remains unknown whether early IABP placement can improve clinically important outcomes in patients with STEMI requiring ICU admission.

In the subgroup of patients with an OHCA, a longer down time before ROSC was associated with higher mortality; however, in the multivariable analysis, this was not an independent predictor for increased mortality. The association between prompt ROSC and outcome has been well described previously [25]. Similarly age was a univariate factor associated with increased mortality however was not an independent predictor in the multivariable analysis. It may be that increased age and longer downtimes before ROSC are all reflective of increased likelihood of organ dysfunction and a higher SOFA score, thus not independently associated with mortality.

In the IHCA group, there were five patients who were supported with ECMO under cardiac arrest conditions

(E-CPR). The IHCA group had a high rate of major bleeding most likely associated with the use of E-CPR, as this association is a well described in other ECMO populations [26]. Survival in this group was low which is consistent with previously published reviews on the use of E-CPR in this age demographic [27].

This study had several limitations. It was performed at a single tertiary PPCI referral centre and is retrospective in nature and thus data collection was based on review of the CIS and paper charts. The multivariable logistic regression model was not externally validated in an alternate population or in patients not admitted to ICU. Furthermore, there may be selection bias for patients requiring mechanical circulatory support with IABP due to differences in individual clinical practice patterns.

This study provides a rationale for a future prospective observational study and validation of the multivariable model to determine if this may help triage and prognosticate patients who are not likely to survive post complicated acute myocardial infarction. Potential uses for this type of model include being able to provide prognostic information for care providers and patient family members. It may also help identify patients in whom aggressive care may be deemed unlikely to succeed. Alternatively, if these patients are identified correctly a priori, it may allow a targeted intervention to improve outcomes in this cohort of patients who continue to have an extremely poor outcome.

Conclusions

Despite only requiring admission 3.5% of the time to ICU (101 of 2902 patients), those patients suffering an MI that do require ICU post PPCI are very critically ill and have a mortality of 33.7%. The most effective way to prognosticate survival in this cohort of patients is by using the SOFA score, in addition to the requirement for an intra-aortic balloon pump.

Additional file

Additional file 1: Table S1. Cardiac characteristics of patients admitted to ICU post PPCI by indication. Results are expressed as mean (SD) unless otherwise denoted. (DOCX 17 kb)

Abbreviations
ANOVA: Analysis of variance; APACHE: Acute physiology and chronic health; AUROC: Area under the receiver operating curve; CAD: Coronary artery disease; CCU: Coronary care unit; CIS: Clinical information system; ECMO: Extracorporeal membrane oxygenation; E-CPR: Ecmo during cardio-pulmonary resuscitation; GCS: Glasgow coma scale; IABP: Intra-aortic balloon pump; ICU: Intensive care unit; IHCA: In-hospital cardiac arrest; IMV: Invasive mechanical ventilation; LV: Left ventricle; NIV: Non-invasive mechanical ventilation; NPV: Negative predictive value; OHCA: Out of hospital cardiac arrest; OR: Odds ratio; PF: PaO2:FiO2; PPCI: Primary percutaneous coronary intervention; PPV: Positive predictive value; RBC: Red blood cells; ROSC: Return of spontaneous circulation; RRT: Renal replacement therapy; RV: Right ventricle; SAPSII: Simplified acute

physiology score II; SOFA: Sequential organ failure assessment; STEMI: ST-segment elevation myocardial infarction

Acknowledgements
Thank Dr. Dan Niven with advice on statistical analysis with this manuscript.

Funding
This research did not receive any specific grant from funding agencies in the public, commercial, or not-for-profit sectors.

Author's contributions
KP, KJ, VM, EB, and VZ contributed to data collection. KP, VZ, NW, and AV were involved in the study design, statistical methodology, interpretation of results, and writing of the manuscript. All authors read and approved the final manuscript.

Competing interests
The authors declare that they have no competing interests.

Author details
[1]Department of Anesthesia and Intensive Care, Papworth Hospital, Cambridge, England. [2]Department of Interventional Cardiology, Papworth Hospital, Cambridge, England. [3]Department of Critical Care Medicine, University of Calgary, ICU Administration - Ground Floor - McCaig Tower, Foothills Medical Center, 3134 Hospital Drive NW, Calgary, AB T2N 5A1, Canada. [4]Department of Critical Care Medicine, University Hospitals of Birmingham NHS Foundation Trust, Queen Elizabeth Hospital, Birmingham, England.

References
1. Nallamothu BK, Normand SL, Wang Y, Hofer TP, Brush JE Jr, Messenger JC, Bradley EH, Rumsfeld JS, Krumholz HM. Relation between door-to-balloon times and mortality after primary percutaneous coronary intervention over time: a retrospective study. Lancet. 2015;385:1114–22.
2. Keeley EC, Boura JA, Grines CL. Primary angioplasty versus intravenous thrombolytic therapy for acute myocardial infarction: a quantitative review of 23 randomised trials. Lancet. 2003;361:13–20.
3. Shah RU, Henry TD, Rutten-Ramos S, Garberich RF, Tighiouart M, Bairey Merz CN. Increasing percutaneous coronary interventions for ST-segment elevation myocardial infarction in the United States: progress and opportunity. JACC Cardiovasc Interv. 2015;8:139–46.
4. O'Gara PT, Kushner FG, Ascheim DD, Casey DE Jr, Chung MK, de Lemos JA, Ettinger SM, Fang JC, Fesmire FM, Franklin BA, et al. 2013 ACCF/AHA guideline for the management of ST-elevation myocardial infarction: executive summary: a report of the American College of Cardiology Foundation/American Heart Association task force on practice guidelines. Circulation. 2013;127:529–55.
5. de Belder MA, Ludman PF, McLenachan JM, Weston CF, Cunningham D, Lazaridis EN, Gray HH. The national infarct angioplasty project: UK experience and subsequent developments. EuroIntervention. 2014; 10(Suppl T):T96–T104.
6. Rotstein Z, Mandelzweig L, Lavi B, Eldar M, Gottlieb S, Hod H. Does the coronary care unit improve prognosis of patients with acute myocardial infarction? A thrombolytic era study. Eur Heart J. 1999;20:813–8.
7. McLenachan JM, Gray HH, de Belder MA, Ludman PF, Cunningham D, Birkhead J. Developing primary PCI as a national reperfusion strategy for patients with ST-elevation myocardial infarction: the UK experience. EuroIntervention. 2012;8(Suppl P):P99–107.
8. Ariza Sole A, Salazar-Mendiguchia J, Lorente-Tordera V, Sanchez-Salado JC, Gonzalez-Costello J, Moliner-Borja P, Gomez-Hospital JA, Manito-Lorite N, Cequier-Fillat A. Invasive mechanical ventilation in acute coronary syndromes in the era of percutaneous coronary intervention. Eur Heart J Acute Cardiovasc Care. 2013;2:109–17.
9. Lopez Messa JB, Andres De Llano JM, Berrocal De La Fuente CA, Pascual Palacin R, Analisis Retraso Infarto Agudo M. Characteristics of acute myocardial infarction patients treated with mechanical ventilation. Data from the ARIAM registry. Rev Esp Cardiol. 2001;54:851 9.
10. Kouraki K, Schneider S, Uebis R, Tebbe U, Klein HH, Janssens U, Zahn R, Senges J, Zeymer U. Characteristics and clinical outcome of 458 patients with acute myocardial infarction requiring mechanical ventilation. Results of the BEAT registry of the ALKK-study group. Clin Res Cardiol. 2011;100:235–9.
11. Zahger D, Maimon N, Novack V, Wolak A, Friger M, Gilutz H, Ilia R, Almog Y. Clinical characteristics and prognostic factors in patients with complicated acute coronary syndromes requiring prolonged mechanical ventilation. Am J Cardiol. 2005;96:1644–8.
12. Lesage A, Ramakers M, Daubin C, Verrier V, Beynier D, Charbonneau P, du Cheyron D. Complicated acute myocardial infarction requiring mechanical ventilation in the intensive care unit: prognostic factors of clinical outcome in a series of 157 patients. Crit Care Med. 2004;32:100–5.
13. Eran O, Novack V, Gilutz H, Zahger D. Comparison of thrombolysis in myocardial infarction, global registry of acute coronary events, and acute physiology and chronic health evaluation II risk scores in patients with acute myocardial infarction who require mechanical ventilation for more than 24 hours. Am J Cardiol. 2011;107:343–6.
14. Vincent JL, Moreno R, Takala J, Willatts S, De Mendonca A, Bruining H, Reinhart CK, Suter PM, Thijs LG. The SOFA (sepsis-related organ failure assessment) score to describe organ dysfunction/failure. On behalf of the working group on sepsis-related problems of the European Society of Intensive Care Medicine. Intensive Care Med. 1996;22:707–10.
15. Vincent JL, de Mendonca A, Cantraine F, Moreno R, Takala J, Suter PM, Sprung CL, Colardyn F, Blecher S. Use of the SOFA score to assess the incidence of organ dysfunction/failure in intensive care units: results of a multicenter, prospective study. Working group on "sepsis-related problems" of the European Society of Intensive Care Medicine. Crit Care Med. 1998;26:1793–800.
16. Kellner P, Prondzinsky R, Pallmann L, Siegmann S, Unverzagt S, Lemm H, Dietz S, Soukup J, Werdan K, Buerke M. Predictive value of outcome scores in patients suffering from cardiogenic shock complicating AMI: APACHE II, APACHE III, Elebute-stoner, SOFA, and SAPS II. Med Klin Intensivmed Notfmed. 2013;108:666–74.
17. Popovic B, Fay R, Cravoisy-Popovic A, Levy B. Cardiac power index, mean arterial pressure, and simplified acute physiology score II are strong predictors of survival and response to revascularization in cardiogenic shock. Shock. 2014;42:22–6.
18. Huang SS, Chen YH, Lu TM, Chen LC, Chen JW, Lin SJ. Application of the sequential organ failure assessment score for predicting mortality in patients with acute myocardial infarction. Resuscitation. 2012;83:591–5.
19. Vincent JL, Moreno R. Clinical review: scoring systems in the critically ill. Crit Care. 2010;14:207.
20. Knaus WA, Draper EA, Wagner DP, Zimmerman JE. APACHE II: a severity of disease classification system. Crit Care Med. 1985;13:818–29.
21. Polderman KH, Girbes AR, Thijs LG, Strack van Schijndel RJ. Accuracy and reliability of APACHE II scoring in two intensive care units problems and pitfalls in the use of APACHE II and suggestions for improvement. Anaesthesia. 2001;56:47–50.
22. Zeymer U, Bauer T, Hamm C, Zahn R, Weidinger F, Seabra-Gomes R, Hochadel M, Marco J, Gitt A. Use and impact of intra-aortic balloon pump on mortality in patients with acute myocardial infarction complicated by cardiogenic shock: results of the euro heart survey on PCI. EuroIntervention. 2011;7:437–41.
23. Zeymer U, Hochadel M, Hauptmann KE, Wiegand K, Schuhmacher B, Brachmann J, Gitt A, Zahn R. Intra-aortic balloon pump in patients with acute myocardial infarction complicated by cardiogenic shock: results of the ALKK-PCI registry. Clin Res Cardiol. 2013;102:223–7.
24. Sjauw KD, Engstrom AE, Vis MM, van der Schaaf RJ, Baan J Jr, Koch KT, de Winter RJ, Piek JJ, Tijssen JG, Henriques JP. A systematic review and meta-analysis of intra-aortic balloon pump therapy in ST-elevation myocardial infarction: should we change the guidelines? Eur Heart J. 2009;30:459–68.
25. Sasson C, Rogers MA, Dahl J, Kellermann AL. Predictors of survival from out-of-hospital cardiac arrest: a systematic review and meta-analysis. Circ Cardiovasc Qual Outcomes. 2010;3:63–81.
26. Cheng R, Hachamovitch R, Kittleson M, Patel J, Arabia F, Moriguchi J, Esmailian F, Azarbal B. Complications of extracorporeal membrane oxygenation for treatment of cardiogenic shock and cardiac arrest: a meta-analysis of 1,866 adult patients. Ann Thorac Surg. 2014;97:610–6.
27. Menditta P, Tang X, Collins RT 2nd, Rycus P, Brogan TV, Prodhan P. Extracorporeal membrane oxygenation for respiratory failure in the elderly: a review of the extracorporeal life support organization registry. ASAIO J. 2014; 60(4):385–90.

Sepsis-induced cardiac dysfunction and β-adrenergic blockade therapy for sepsis

Takeshi Suzuki*[ID], Yuta Suzuki, Jun Okuda, Takuya Kurazumi, Tomohiro Suhara, Tomomi Ueda, Hiromasa Nagata and Hiroshi Morisaki

Abstract

Despite recent advances in medical care, mortality due to sepsis, defined as life-threatening organ dysfunction caused by a dysregulated host response to infection, remains high. Fluid resuscitation and vasopressors are the first-line treatment for sepsis in order to optimize hemodynamic instability caused by vasodilation and increased vascular permeability. However, these therapies, aimed at maintaining blood pressure and blood flow to vital organs, could have deleterious cardiac effects, as cardiomyocyte damage occurs in the early stages of sepsis. Recent experimental and clinical studies have demonstrated that a number of factors contribute to sepsis-induced cardiac dysfunction and the degree of cardiac dysfunction is one of the major prognostic factors of sepsis. Therefore, strategies to prevent further cardiomyocyte damage could be of crucial importance in improving the outcome of sepsis.

Among many factors causing sepsis-induced cardiac dysfunction, sympathetic nerve overstimulation, due to endogenous elevated catecholamine levels and exogenous catecholamine administration, is thought to play a major role. β-adrenergic blockade therapy is widely used for ischemic heart disease and chronic heart failure and in the prevention of cardiovascular events in high-risk perioperative patients undergoing major surgery. It has also been shown to restore cardiac function in experimental septic animal models. In a single-center randomized controlled trial, esmolol infusion in patients with septic shock with persistent tachycardia reduced the 28-day mortality. Furthermore, it is likely that β-adrenergic blockade therapy may result in further beneficial effects in patients with sepsis, such as the reduction of inflammatory cytokine production, suppression of hypermetabolic status, maintenance of glucose homeostasis, and improvement of coagulation disorders.

Recent accumulating evidence suggests that β-adrenergic blockade could be an attractive therapy to improve the prognosis of sepsis. We await a large multicenter randomized clinical trial to confirm the beneficial effects of β-adrenergic blockade therapy in sepsis, of which mortality is still high.

Keywords: Sepsis, Sepsis-induced cardiac dysfunction, β-adrenergic blockade therapy

Background

Sepsis, defined as a life-threatening organ dysfunction caused by a dysregulated host response to infection, according to the third international consensus definitions for sepsis and septic shock [1], is one of the leading causes of death in the intensive care unit (ICU), despite significant recent advances in intensive care medicine [2, 3]. It is estimated that from 56 to 91 per 100,000 adults experience severe sepsis and septic shock worldwide each year [4], and the mortality rates from septic shock, a refractory severe hypotensive state, have ranged from 40 to 50% over the past decades [5]. It has been estimated that worldwide, one patient dies due to sepsis every few seconds and sepsis-related mortality has exceeded mortality due to acute myocardial infarction. Therefore, improving the prognosis in patients with sepsis remains a challenging area for clinicians working in the ICU.

Although the hemodynamic response to sepsis has been characterized as a hyperdynamic state, typically characterized by an increased cardiac output due to fluid resuscitation and decreased systemic vascular resistance, cardiac dysfunction occurs during the early stages of sepsis [6].

* Correspondence: takeshi-su@a7.keio.jp
Department of Anesthesiology and General Intensive Care Unit, Keio University School of Medicine, 35 Shinanomachi, Shinjuku-ku, Tokyo 160-8582, Japan

On echocardiography examination, sepsis-induced cardiac dysfunction is identifiable as a reduction in stroke volume and ejection fraction [6, 7]. Many factors have been shown to contribute to sepsis-induced cardiac dysfunction [8], and adrenergic overstimulation may exacerbate myocardial dysfunction during sepsis [9, 10]. Over recent decades, a growing body of experimental and clinical studies has focused on the beneficial effects of β-adrenergic blocker therapy for treating sepsis [9, 11], suggesting that this may be a promising therapeutic intervention.

In this review article, we summarize the pathophysiology of sepsis-induced cardiac dysfunction and discuss the potentially therapeutic effects of β-adrenergic blockade on sepsis-induced cardiac dysfunction and other damaged organs during sepsis.

Review

Hemodynamic management in septic shock

Sepsis is characterized by a dysregulated systemic inflammatory response caused by infection, leading to multiple organ injury and shock [1, 12]. Many mediators, such as pro-inflammatory cytokines, including tumor necrosis factor-α (TNF-α) and interleukin (IL-1β), nitric oxide, and reactive oxygen species, have been shown to cause cardiac dysfunction, increased vascular permeability, and reduced peripheral vascular resistance [8, 13], which can induce hemodynamic instability and multiple organ injury.

In 2001, Rivers et al. reported the findings of a single-center trial and concluded that early goal-directed therapy (EGDT), targeting mean blood pressure over 65 mmHg and oxygen saturation of central venous blood (ScVO₂) over 70% within 6 h of the onset of severe sepsis, significantly reduced mortality rates [14]. Although, recently, three multicenter randomized trials have demonstrated that EGDT did not improve the outcome in patients with severe sepsis [15–17], it is clear that stabilizing hemodynamics at the early stages of sepsis is crucial for the management of septic patients, as the degree of lactate clearance has been shown to reflect the prognosis in critically ill patients [18].

During the early stages of sepsis, particularly in patients with septic shock, the primary aim of treatment is optimization of the hemodynamic status by adequate fluid resuscitation and vasopressors, in order to meet the oxygen demands of peripheral tissues and prevent organ injury [19]. However, excessive fluid and adrenergic overstimulation could be detrimental to the heart, which has already sustained injury during the early stages of sepsis. Previous studies have demonstrated that the mortality rate of patients developing cardiac dysfunction during the early stages of sepsis was higher than that of patients without cardiac dysfunction [20,

21], which implies that reducing cardiomyocyte damage is a very important strategy in the management of patients with sepsis in order to improve the prognosis.

Sepsis-induced cardiac dysfunction

Calvin et al. first described myocardial dysfunction in adequately volume-resuscitated patients with septic shock in 1981, reporting a reduced ejection fraction and enlarged end-diastolic volume index [22]. Packer et al. demonstrated that surviving patients with sepsis had a decreased ejection fraction and increased end-diastolic volume index, which recovered between 7 and 10 days after the onset of sepsis; however, non-survivors maintained a normal ejection fraction and end-diastolic volume [6, 23], suggesting that cardiac dysfunction in sepsis is a compensatory mechanism to confer a protective effect against myocardial dysfunction.

Experimental studies have also identified sepsis-induced morphological and functional damage to the heart. A study examining cardiac morphological changes evoked by cecum ligation and puncture (CLP)-induced abdominal peritonitis in a sheep model described damage to the mitochondrial structure and impaired microcirculation, due to myocardial and vascular endothelial cell edema [24], which could contribute to cardiac dysfunction during the early stages of sepsis. In an ex vivo study, evaluating cardiac function in the working heart model 24 h after CLP in a rat model, dP/dt max, an indicator of cardiac systolic function, cardiac work, and cardiac efficiency, was impaired in a CLP rat, compared with a sham rat [25]. These experimental studies demonstrated structural and functional cardiac injuries, even though cardiac function could be modulated by the change of preload and afterload in clinical situations.

Recent clinical studies evaluating cardiac function of patients with sepsis by echocardiography also showed a reduced ejection fraction, followed by both systolic and diastolic dysfunction [21, 26, 27]. However, a number of studies did not find an increased left ventricular end-diastolic volume index, which was shown in the previous study [28–30]. Furthermore, it has been reported that impaired ejection fraction was associated with a poor prognosis [21], contrary to an earlier study by Packer et al. [23], which found that a reduced ejection fraction was associated with improved outcome. While there are some discrepancies among studies regarding the association between reduced ejection fraction and prognosis, there is clear evidence of an association between sepsis-induced cardiac morphological changes and the resulting myocardial dysfunction, manifested as decreased contractility and impaired myocardial compliance [31]. This progressive dysfunction develops during the early stages of sepsis and can affect prognosis.

Mechanisms of sepsis-induced cardiac dysfunction

Despite advances in our understanding of the patho-physiology of sepsis, the mechanisms of sepsis-induced cardiomyopathy have not been fully elucidated. Over recent decades, a number of experimental and clinical studies have suggested possible causative mechanisms for the progressive cardiac dysfunction observed in patients with sepsis (Fig. 1).

Disturbed coronary blood flow   In the 1970s, it was postulated that inadequate coronary blood flow, due to intravascular volume depletion, myocardial and endo-thelial cell edema, and vasodilation, was a major cause of sepsis-induced myocardial dysfunction [32, 33]. However, further human studies rejected the myocar-dial ischemia theory, demonstrating that coronary flow in patients with sepsis with cardiac dysfunction was comparable to, or greater, than coronary flow in con-trols [34, 35]. Furthermore, postmortem studies have found no myocardial necrosis in patients with septic shock [36]. While there may be changes in cardiac microcirculation in sepsis, caused by endothelial cell disruption and maldistribution of coronary blood flow, it is not obvious that myocardial ischemia contributes to the pathogenesis of sepsis-induced cardiomyopathy [8, 28].

Myocardial depressant factor and inflammatory cytokines   In an in vitro study conducted in 1985, Parrillo et al. found that serum from patients with sepsis depressed myocardial cell performance, unlike serum from critically ill patients without sepsis [37], and sug-gested that a circulating myocardial depressant factor (MDF) was the main cause of cardiac dysfunction in sep-sis. Researchers subsequently investigated the molecular

structure of MDF and concluded that MDF was likely to be an endotoxin and cell wall component of gram-negative bacteria. However, further studies revealed that the characteristics of inflammatory cytokines were comparable to those of MDF. Of these cytokines, tumor necrosis factor-α (TNF-α) and interleukin-1β (IL-1β), which are produced excessively at the early stages of sepsis, have been found to depress cardiac function synergistically [13, 38].

Nitric oxide and reactive oxygen species   TNF-α and IL-1β are major mediators causing myocardial dysfunction in sepsis. However, these cytokines have short half-lives, and studies have shown that their concentrations decrease in the early stages of sepsis. Therefore, other mediators, such as nitric oxide (NO) and reactive oxygen species (ROS), have been considered to be secondary effectors in sepsis-induced cardiac dysfunction [13, 39]. Excessive inducible NO synthase (iNOS), and specifically iNOS-2, induced in the myocardium by pro-inflammatory cyto-kines, results in a significant amount of NO production. This contributes to myocardial dysfunction through reduced sensitivity of myofibril response to calcium, inhibition of β-adrenergic signaling, downregulation of β-adrenergic receptor, and mitochondrial dysfunction [8, 28]. Peroxynitrite, produced by NO reaction with ROS, has a strong myocardial depressant effect with high cytotoxicity [40]. Reports indicate that NO and ROS cause mitochondrial dysfunction, as described in the following section.

Mitochondrial dysfunction   Mitochondrial dysfunction plays a key role in the pathogenesis of sepsis-induced cardiac dysfunction, leading to the so-called cytopathic hypoxia, which may contribute to multiple organ injury.

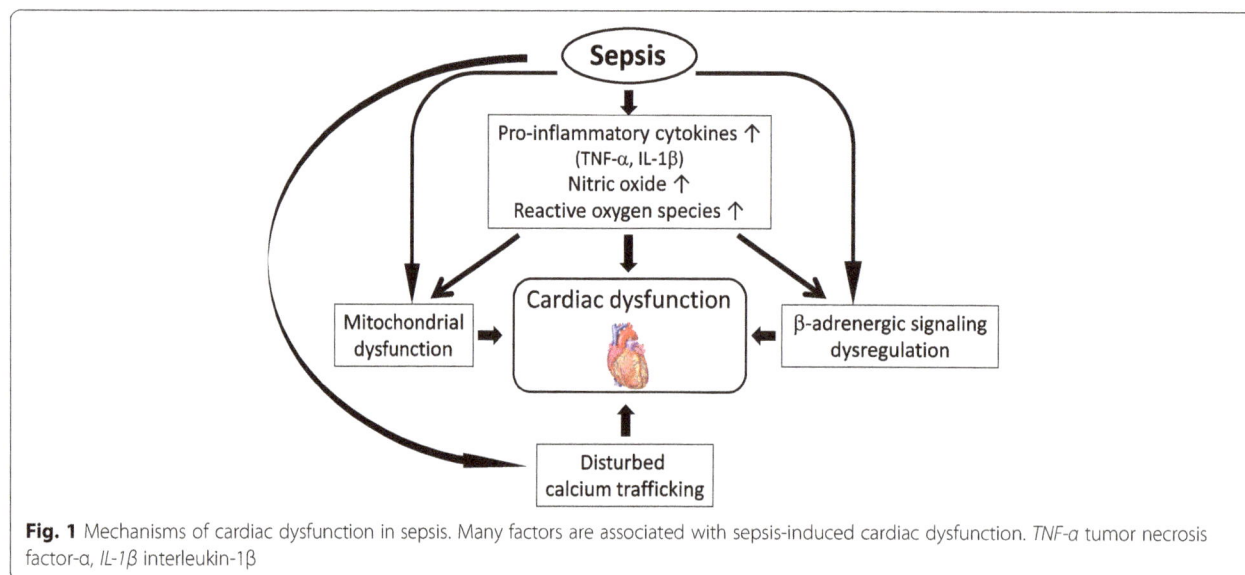

Fig. 1 Mechanisms of cardiac dysfunction in sepsis. Many factors are associated with sepsis-induced cardiac dysfunction. *TNF-α* tumor necrosis factor-α, *IL-1β* interleukin-1β

NO and ROS contribute significantly to disturbed mitochondrial respiratory function, caused by inhibition of oxidative phosphorylation and adenosine triphosphate (ATP) production in the respiratory chain complex [8, 41]. Recent studies have demonstrated that mediators, including ROS and cytochrome C, released from mitochondria during cell death, could induce further inflammation [13].

β-Adrenergic signaling dysregulation   In patients with sepsis, adrenergic signaling dysregulation is associated with sepsis-induced cardiac dysfunction [8, 29, 42]. Despite increased circulating catecholamine levels, the contractile response of cardiomyocytes to catecholamine stimulation is blunted in patients with sepsis [8, 43]. Downregulation of β-adrenergic receptor and disturbance of β-adrenergic signaling are the key mechanism in this autonomic dysregulation [8, 29]. Sepsis may cause an increased activity of inhibitory G protein and a decreased accumulation of intracellular cyclic adenosine monophosphate (cAMP). Stimulatory G protein activity may be depressed through overproduction of inflammatory cytokines, leading to attenuation of β-adrenergic response to catecholamines [44, 45]. In sepsis, catecholamine overstimulation and elevated levels of NO may contribute to decreased β-adrenergic receptor density on the myocardial cell surface [46–48].

Calcium trafficking   Sepsis causes alterations of calcium trafficking at various sites, resulting in reduced cardiomyocyte contraction [8, 28]. Under physiological conditions, opening of L-type voltage-gated calcium channels on the cardiomyocyte sarcolemma, due to depolarization of the cardiomyocyte sarcolemma, causes calcium influx into the cardiomyocytes, leading to the release of calcium from the sarcoplasmic reticulum, through ryanodine receptors. This increase in intracellular calcium concentration plays a very important role in cardiac contraction. Reports indicate that sepsis is associated with the suppression of calcium current through L-type voltage-gated calcium channels [49, 50], decreased density of L-type calcium channels [49] and ryanodine receptors [51, 52], and a decrease in calcium uptake into the sarcoplasmic reticulum during the diastolic phase. Furthermore, calcium trafficking may contribute to mitochondrial dysfunction. Further studies are warranted to elucidate how these alterations in calcium homeostasis affect the long-term prognosis of patients with sepsis.

Cardiomyocyte apoptosis   In an ex vivo experimental model, it was found that inhibition of caspase activity, a key enzyme in apoptosis, reduced the depression of cardiac function. Therefore, it was postulated that apoptotic cardiomyocyte cell death was one of the mechanisms of sepsis-induced cardiac dysfunction [53]. However, cardiomyocyte apoptosis is unlikely to cause myocardial dysfunction in sepsis as postmortem examination of patients with sepsis has revealed negligible myocardial apoptosis [36].

Protective effects of β-adrenergic blockers on sepsis-induced cardiac dysfunction

Although many studies have demonstrated that preventing cardiac injury is crucial to improving prognosis of septic patients [54, 55], effective treatment to attenuate cardiac dysfunction is not yet established. The mechanisms of sepsis-induced cardiac dysfunction have not been fully elucidated; nevertheless, some important factors contribute to the deterioration of cardiac dysfunction in the early stages of sepsis, as discussed above. Of these, catecholamine overstimulation plays a major role in sepsis-induced cardiac dysfunction [9, 56]. The elevated catecholamine level in sepsis can cause catecholamine-induced cardiomyopathy and cardiac damage by calcium overload, leading to cardiomyocyte necrosis. Furthermore, myocardial β-adrenergic receptor density is decreased and β-adrenergic stimulant signal transduction is impaired in sepsis [8, 29]. Therefore, prevention of further cardiomyocyte damage due to sympathetic nerve overstimulation could be a key component in the management of sepsis.

β-adrenergic blockers, first used for angina pectoris in the 1960s [57], have been widely prescribed for different diseases and conditions, such as ischemic heart disease and chronic heart failure [58], and perioperatively for patients with a high risk of cardiovascular events undergoing major surgery [59]. Berk et al. first reported the beneficial effects of β-adrenergic blockade therapy using an animal endotoxin shock model in the 1960s [60]; propranolol infusion reduced mortality from 78.2 to 19.4%. A further study, which included patients with refractory septic shock, reported a 27.3% mortality rate in patients treated with propranolol; this was low compared to the 30–40% mortality rate reported in recent studies. It is important to note that the management of patients with septic shock in these early studies was significantly different to the modern medical care available today [61]. Despite the beneficial effects in patients with septic shock, β-adrenergic blockade therapy in septic shock is not widely established, as results are conflicting. For example, a further study concluded that β-adrenergic blockade in an endotoxin dog model worsened cardiac function [62]. Following the publication of this animal study, which disputed the beneficial effects of β-adrenergic blockade therapy, this field of research received scarce attention.

Approximately 35 years after Berk et al. described the possibility of the beneficial effects of β-adrenergic modulation in septic shock, the authors showed that β-adrenergic blockade therapy for sepsis attenuated sepsis-induced cardiac dysfunction, in an ex vivo experiment using a septic rat model [48]. We examined whether the selective β1-adrenergic blocker esmolol, continuously administered immediately after CLP was performed, could restore cardiac function in an isolated anterograde perfused heart preparation 24 h after esmolol infusion was started. During esmolol infusion, heart rate and mean blood pressure were significantly reduced with no lactate elevation compared to saline infusion. Cardiac output, cardiac work, and cardiac efficiency, an indicator of how efficiently the heart can use oxygen, were well maintained in hearts harvested from esmolol-treated rats compared with those harvested from non-treated rats. Furthermore, esmolol infusion reduced plasma TNF-α concentration and limited the reduction of β-adrenergic receptor density on cardiomyocytes. Although this study has not considered the effect of esmolol infusion on mortality, it was the first to demonstrate the beneficial effect of β-adrenergic blockade therapy on cardiomyocytes in sepsis. Further experimental studies confirmed the beneficial effects of selective β1-adrenergic blockade therapy in sepsis [63, 64], following our study, published in 2005.

The most serious concern regarding the clinical use of β-adrenergic blockade therapy in sepsis is the risk of reducing cardiac output and blood pressure, resulting in a further decrease in blood flow to major organs and potentially compromising organ function. Despite the risk of reduced organ blood flow due to the usage of β-adrenergic blockers, one clinical study demonstrated that esmolol infusion in patients with sepsis maintained hepatic blood flow, despite a 20% decrease in cardiac output [65]. Another retrospective study, examining the effect of enteral metoprolol on the hemodynamic state of patients with septic shock, showed that stroke volume was increased and cardiac output remained stable despite increases in the administered dose of noradrenaline and milrinone in some patients [66]. These results indicate that β-adrenergic blockade in patients with sepsis may be safe if adequate volume resuscitation therapy is performed.

Morelli et al. evaluated the beneficial effect of esmolol on septic shock patients in a single-center randomized controlled study [67]. In this study, 154 patients with septic shock, requiring noradrenaline infusion to maintain blood pressure and presenting with persistent tachycardia [>95 beats per minute (bpm)] after adequate volume resuscitation, were assigned to an esmolol infusion therapy group to decrease the heart rate to 80–94 bpm or to a saline infusion group. All patients in the esmolol group achieved the target heart rate of 80–94 bpm, which was the primary outcome. Furthermore, esmolol infusion

increased the stroke volume index and reduced the fluid volume and norepinephrine dose to achieve a mean arterial pressure of 65–75 mmHg. Surprisingly, the 28-day mortality was significantly reduced from 80.5 to 49.4% in the esmolol group, without adverse events, compared with the control group. Despite the extremely high mortality in the control group and the widespread usage of levosimendan in both groups (49.4% in the esmolol group and 40.3% in the control group), this is the first clinical randomized controlled trial to show the beneficial effects of β-adrenergic blockade therapy in patients with septic shock.

Recently, an experimental study was conducted to identify the mechanisms underlying the beneficial effects of β-adrenergic blockade therapy in sepsis. Kimmoun et al. examined the effect of esmolol on cardiac and mesenteric vascular function in an ex vivo experiment, using a peritonitis-induced septic rat model [68]. Esmolol infusion counteracted the decreased cardiac contractility and the suppressed vasoreactivity to vasopressor treatment, induced by cecum ligation and puncture. Restored cardiac and vascular function through esmolol infusion was associated with decreased nuclear factor κB activation and reduced inducible nitrite oxide synthase expression, both at the cardiac and at the vessel level.

Further studies will be required to elucidate the effects of β-adrenergic blockade therapy in sepsis on cardiac function. The results of a multicenter controlled trial, evaluating the effect of β-adrenergic blockade therapy in a large number of patients with septic shock, are currently awaited.

Beneficial effects of β-adrenergic blockade other than cardioprotective effects in sepsis

A growing body of research is focusing on the effect of β-adrenergic blockade therapy in sepsis [9, 69], specifically examining the beneficial effects other than those on the cardiovascular system. These are discussed in the following section.

Metabolic alterations   Sepsis is associated with an overall catabolic state, leading to hyperglycemia, enhanced protein and fatty breakdown, increased resting energy expenditure, negative nitrogen balance, and loss of lean body mass [70, 71]. This hypermetabolic state is predominantly caused by catecholamine overstimulation, particularly by β2-adrenergic stimulation [72, 73]. Thus, non-selective β-adrenergic blockade may counteract this hypermetabolic state associated with sepsis, contributing to the maintenance of glucose homeostasis, improvement of net nitrogen balance, and reserved muscle protein. In children with severe burns, characterized by a pathophysiology similar to that of septic shock, propranolol treatment reduced muscle protein catabolism and suppressed resting energy expenditure, leading to increased lean body mass. In septic rat models, propranolol infusion improved the nitrogen balance, possibly through a reduction of muscle proteolysis [74]. Considering the benefits of esmolol infusion in patients with burns, non-selective β-adrenergic blockade in patients with sepsis may have the same beneficial effects.

Cytokine production and immune modulation In sepsis, the binding of lipopolysaccharides to toll-like receptor 4 promotes the translocation of the transcription factor NF-κB into nuclei, leading to a shower of cytokines. The increased levels of inflammatory cytokines further stimulate immunologically competent cells, contributing to a dysregulated hyper-inflammatory condition, with deleterious effects of activated neutrophils on different organs. Whether β-adrenergic blockade therapy in patients with sepsis has beneficial effects on the immune system requires further examination. However, it is well known that the β-adrenergic system is associated with immune system modulation [75]. Catecholamines have been shown to modulate the balance between pro-inflammatory and anti-inflammatory status through a β2-mediated pathway [76–78]. It has been reported that the pattern of cytokine production is strongly affected by the balance between CD4+ T-helper type 1 (Th1) and type 2 (Th2) cells. Th1 cell activation leads to activation of macrophages and natural killer T cells and production of pro-inflammatory cytokines, resulting in the promotion of cellular immunity. Conversely, Th2 cells inhibit macrophage activation, T cell proliferation, and pro-inflammatory cytokine production, through promotion of humoral immunity and production of anti-inflammatory cytokines [75]. Th1 cells, but not Th2 cells, have β2-adrenergic receptors on their surface. Stimulation of β2-adrenergic receptors suppresses Th1 cell activation, with a relative increase in Th2 cell response. Therefore, selective β1-adrenergic blockade could promote β2-adrenergic pathway activation, facilitating Th2 cell responses and contributing to the suppression of the pro-inflammatory status at the early stages of sepsis [9] and the activation of the anti-inflammatory pathway [79]. Conversely, β2-adrenergic blockade may enhance the inflammatory response, leading to pro-inflammatory cytokine production. The attenuation of the intense pro-inflammatory status at the early stages of sepsis, by selective β1-adrenergic blockade, may prevent the sequential immunosuppressive status.

In our study evaluating the effect of selective β1-adrenergic blockade on cardiac dysfunction in septic rat models, esmolol infusion significantly reduced plasma TNF-α concentration [48], and this may minimize cardiac dysfunction. A study by Hagiwara et al. demonstrated that a highly selective β1-adrenergic blocker, landiolol,

decreased the levels of circulating cytokines, such as TNF-α, IL-6, and high-mobility group box 1, in an experimental septic model [63]. While the precise mechanism of β1-adrenergic blockade-mediated suppression of cytokine production was not elucidated in these studies, relative β2-adrenergic pathway activation may contribute to a reduction of pro-inflammatory cytokine production, as described above. Further studies are required to identify the mechanism by which selective β1-adrenergic blockade affects cytokine release.

In sepsis, it has been shown that lymphocyte apoptosis may be induced by a high inflammatory status, contributing to a worse prognosis [80]. In an experimental septic model, Hotchkiss et al. found splenocyte apoptosis in postpartum patients with septic shock [81] and demonstrated that inhibition of caspase, a key enzyme causing lymphocyte apoptosis, improved the prognosis, by preventing lymphocyte apoptosis [80]. Therefore, modulation of lymphocyte apoptosis could be an attractive therapeutic option to improve the prognosis of sepsis. One of the key pro-inflammatory cytokines in sepsis, TNF-α, can cause T lymphocyte apoptosis [82], and β2-adrenergic blockade has been reported to induce splenocyte apoptosis [83]. Therefore, through attenuation of TNF-α production and relative β2-adrenergic pathway stimulation, selective β1-adrenergic blockade may prevent lymphocyte apoptosis causing secondary infection and increased mortality. In our laboratory, the effect of selective β1-adrenergic blockade on splenocyte apoptosis has been examined in a septic mouse model. Esmolol treatment restored the number of normal T lymphocytes in the spleen, which was severely reduced 24 h after CLP, compared with the control group receiving a saline infusion. This finding supports the hypothesis that attenuation of lymphocyte apoptosis is one of the major mechanisms through which β1-adrenergic blockade has a positive effect in sepsis.

Coagulation disorder Sepsis induces altered platelet function [84, 85], activation of the coagulation system, and suppression of fibrinolysis [9]. Increased levels of plasma tissue factor and von Willebrand factor amplify the coagulation cascade, leading to thrombin and fibrin formation [86]. Endothelial damage caused by thrombin formation further augments the coagulation cascade through more exposed tissue factor. Furthermore, impairment of the physiologic anticoagulation system occurs through downregulation of anticoagulant factors, such as tissue factor pathway inhibitor, antithrombin, and activated protein C, in sepsis [9]. Reports indicated that increased levels of TNF-α and IL-1β enhance the production of plasminogen activator inhibitor 1, leading to further impaired fibrinolysis [9]. A dysregulated coagulation system causes disseminated intravascular coagulation, leading to microcirculation disturbance and multiple organ injury.

Adrenergic pathways are associated with the coagulation system in different situations. Regarding platelet function, α2-adrenergic stimulation promotes platelet aggregation, while the β2-adrenergic pathway contributes to the suppression of platelet aggregation through cAMP stimulation [87]. β2-adrenergic stimulation promotes tissue plasminogen activator release, leading to enhanced fibrinolytic activity [88], while β1-adrenergic stimulation suppresses fibrinolysis through reduced prostacyclin synthesis [89].

Considering the association between the adrenergic pathway and the coagulation system described above, modulation of the β-adrenergic pathway could modify the hyper-coagulation status induced by sepsis. Regarding platelet function, β1-adrenergic blockade may reduce platelet activation through relative β2-adrenergic pathway activation. β1-adrenergic blockade could also enhance fibrinolysis through increased plasminogen activation and prostacyclin synthesis. Furthermore, reduction of pro-inflammatory cytokine production by β1-adrenergic blockade could reduce the increased plasminogen activator inhibitor 1 production, leading to improved fibrinolysis. There are few studies examining the beneficial effects of β1-adrenergic blockade on the disturbed coagulation system in sepsis, and this novel field should be examined in future studies.

β-adrenergic blockade therapy for sepsis in the clinical situation

Although many beneficial effects of β-adrenergic blockade therapy in sepsis have been recently described, few studies have evaluated the effects of β-adrenergic blockade therapy on sepsis in clinical situations. Table 1 shows the summary of four clinical trials that examined the effects of β-adrenergic blockers in patients with sepsis. Only one randomized controlled trial evaluated the effects of β-adrenergic blockade therapy in septic patients; therefore, it is difficult to determine when and how β-adrenergic blockade therapy should be used in clinical practice. One of the major concerns regarding the use of β-adrenergic blockers in sepsis is the reduction of blood pressure and cardiac output, resulting in decreased blood flow to major organs, which can cause organ injury. However, in a number of studies, cardiac output was maintained and stroke volume index was increased, despite the reduction in heart rate [66, 67]. A further study, investigating the effects of esmolol infusion on hepatic and peripheral blood flow in sepsis, found that hepatic and peripheral blood flow did not change, despite reduced cardiac output [65]. Therefore, it is likely that in patients with sepsis, administration of β-adrenergic blockers is relatively safe if patients have received adequate volume resuscitation. Sepsis-induced cardiac dysfunction develops in the early stages of sepsis; therefore, it seems reasonable to initiate β-adrenergic blockade therapy as early as possible after adequate volume resuscitation therapy, if persistent tachycardia does not improve. The duration of therapy and the target heart rate range are further important factors when administering β-adrenergic blockade therapy to septic patients. There are no studies investigating the optimum duration of β-adrenergic blockade therapy, which remains unknown. As the patient's condition improves, the heart rate may return to baseline levels, before the onset of sepsis, without β-adrenergic blocker therapy. In the four clinical trials [61, 65–67] presented in Table 1, β-adrenergic blocker administration was adjusted to achieve a heart rate <95 bpm, and the heart rate was

Table 1 Summary of four clinical trials evaluating the effects of β-adrenergic blockade therapy in patients with sepsis

Reference number	Generic name of β-blocker	Method of administration	Dose of drug	Duration of therapy	Effects on hemodynamics	Mortality
61	Propranolol	Continuous iv infusion	5 mg for 2–3 h, followed by 5 mg for 6–12 h	8–15 h	HR↓ Cardiac output↓ Blood pressure↑ Urinary output↑	27.3% No control
65	Esmolol	Continuous iv infusion	6–22 mg/min (dose to reduce HR by 20%)	3 h	HR↓ Cardiac output↓ SVR→ Hepatic blood flow→	No data
66	Metoprolol with milrinone	Enteral administration	25–47.5 mg/day (target range of 65–95 bpm)	48 h	HR↓ Cardiac output→ Catecholamine dose↓ SVI↑	28-day mortality: 33%
67	Esmolol	Continuous iv infusion	Median dose of 100 mg/h (dose to maintain HR from 80 to 94 bpm)	Until ICU discharge or death	HR↓ Cardiac index→ Mean blood pressure→ Norepinephrine dose↓ SVI↑	28-day mortality: Control 80.5% Esmolol 49.4%

bpm beats per minute, *HR* heart rate, *ICU* intensive care unit, *iv* intravenous, *SVI* stroke volume index

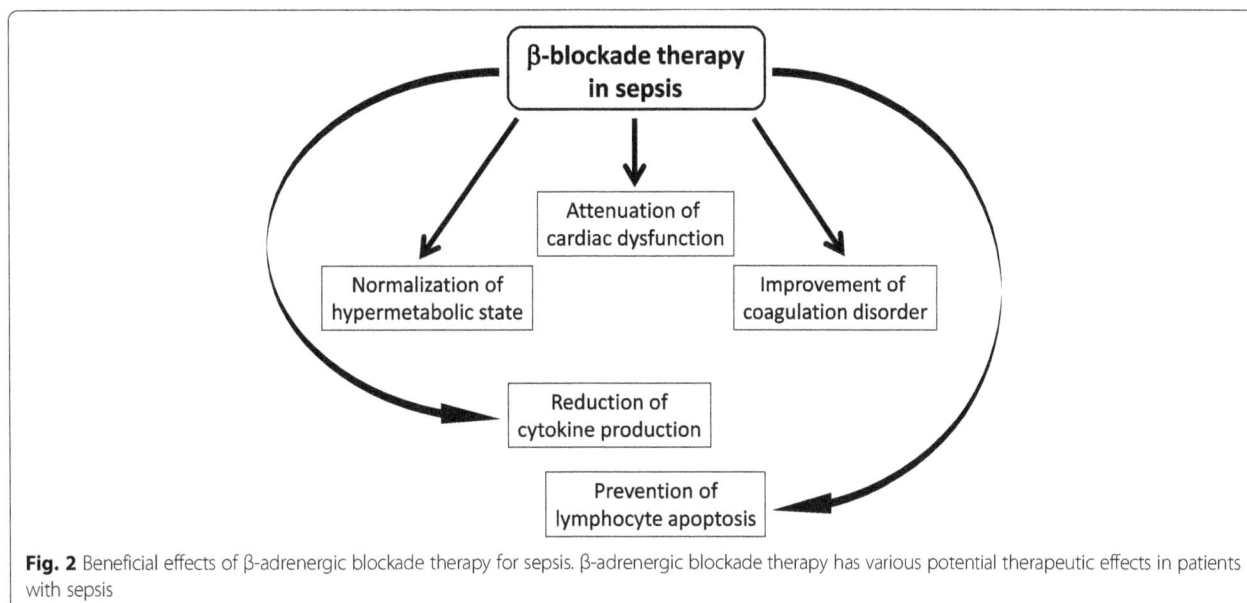

Fig. 2 Beneficial effects of β-adrenergic blockade therapy for sepsis. β-adrenergic blockade therapy has various potential therapeutic effects in patients with sepsis

maintained between 80 and 95 bpm. Therefore, the optimum heart rate may be between 80 and 95 bpm.

β-adrenergic blockade therapy for patients with sepsis remains controversial due to limited evidence in the clinical context. It is important to consider potential adverse effects and pitfalls of β-adrenergic blocker therapy before its use in patients with sepsis. As discussed above, the first adverse event to consider is the reduction of blood flow to major organs, due to decreased heart rate and cardiac output. Therefore, before administering β-blocker therapy, it is important to establish adequate volume resuscitation and the optimal dosage of norepinephrine, using the following parameters: diameter of the inferior vena cava evaluated by echocardiography, stroke volume variation, and systemic vascular resistance, which can be measured by arterial pressure-based cardiac output, and a central venous catheter. Interestingly, in the study by Morelli et al. evaluating the effect of β-blocker therapy following adequate volume resuscitation [67], mean arterial pressure was maintained, despite reduced norepinephrine and fluid requirements in the esmolol group. Furthermore, kidney function, evaluated by the estimated glomerular filtration rate, was maintained, and cardiac injury, assessed by troponin T and creatine kinase (CK)-MB, was reduced by esmolol administration. Taking into consideration that the heart rate was maintained between 80 and 94 bpm in the study by Morelli et al. [67], and mean heart rates were 78 and 90 bpm, respectively, in two recent clinical trials [65, 66], it could be unsafe to reduce the heart rate to <80 bpm. To achieve the beneficial effects of β-adrenergic blockade therapy in patients with sepsis, it appears that the heart rate should be maintained within a narrow range.

A further concern is the harmful effect of β2 receptor blockade on respiratory function. However, the effect on respiratory function may be negligible due to the high β1 receptor selectivity of esmolol and landiolol.

Conclusions

This review focuses on the mechanisms of sepsis-induced cardiac dysfunction and the beneficial effects of β-adrenergic blockade therapy, predominantly on the cardiovascular system and other organs (Fig. 2). Promising results are accruing and these show the beneficial effects of β-adrenergic blockade therapy in sepsis. β-adrenergic blocker therapy could be a promising novel therapeutic approach to modulate cardiovascular dysfunction, as well as metabolic and immune disorders and disorders of the coagulation system, as hyperactivation of the sympathetic nervous system could have deleterious effects on a wide range of organs. Experimental and clinical research is required to elucidate the β-adrenergic blocker therapy-mediated beneficial effects in sepsis, before β-adrenergic blocker therapy is widely used in clinical practice. It is our view that large multicenter randomized clinical trials could confirm the beneficial effects of β-adrenergic blockade therapy in patients with sepsis, improving the prognosis of sepsis which, to date, has a high mortality rate.

Abbreviations
ATP: Adenosine triphosphate; cAMP: Cyclic adenosine monophosphate; CK: Creatine kinase; CLP: Cecum ligation and puncture; EGDT: Early goal-directed therapy; ICU: Intensive care unit; IL-1β: Interleukin-1β; iNOS: Inducible nitric oxide synthase; MDF: Myocardial depressant factor; NO: Nitric oxide; ROS: Reactive oxygen species; ScVO$_2$: Oxygen saturation of central venous blood; Th1: CD4+ T-helper type 1; Th2: CD4+ T-helper type 2; TNF-α: Tumor necrosis factor-α

Acknowledgements
Not applicable.

Funding

Funding is derived from the departmental source.

Authors' contributions

TS, YS, JO, TK, TS, TU, HN, and HM participated in drafting and revising the manuscript. All authors have read and approved the final manuscript.

Competing interests

The authors declare that they have no competing interests.

References

1. Singer M, Deutschman CS, Seymour CW, Shankar-Hari M, Annane D, Bauer M, et al. The third international consensus definitions for sepsis and septic shock (Sepsis-3). JAMA. 2016;315:801–10.
2. Martin GS, Mannino DM, Eaton S, Moss M. The epidemiology of sepsis in the United States from 1979 through 2000. N Engl J Med. 2003;348:1546–54.
3. Annane D, Aegerter P, Jars-Guincestre MC, Guidet B. Current epidemiology of septic shock: the CUB-Rea Network. Am J Respir Crit Care Med. 2003;168:165–72.
4. Jawad I, Luksic I, Rafnsson SB. Assessing available information on the burden of sepsis: global estimates of incidence, prevalence and mortality. J Glob Health. 2012;2:010404.
5. Annane D, Bellissant E, Cavaillon JM. Septic shock. Lancet. 2005;365:63–78.
6. Parker MM, Shelhamer JH, Bacharach SL, Green MV, Natanson C, Frederick TM, et al. Profound but reversible myocardial depression in patients with septic shock. Ann Intern Med. 1984;100:483–90.
7. Price S, Anning PB, Mitchell JA, Evans TW. Myocardial dysfunction in sepsis: mechanisms and therapeutic implications. Eur Heart J. 1999;20:715–24.
8. Rudiger A, Singer M. Mechanisms of sepsis-induced cardiac dysfunction. Crit Care Med. 2007;35:1599–608.
9. de Montmolin E, Aboab J, Mansart A, Annane D. Bench-to-bedside review: β-adrenergic modulation in sepsis. Crit Care. 2009;13:1–8.
10. Fledman AM, Bristow MR. The beta-adrenergic pathway in the failing human heart: implications for inotropic therapy. Cardiology. 1990;77:s1–32.
11. Rudiger A. Beta-block the septic heart. Crit Care Med. 2010;38:s608–12.
12. Hotchkiss RS, Karl IE. The pathophysiology and treatment of sepsis. N Engl J Med. 2003;38:138–50.
13. Kakihara Y, Ito T, Nakahara M, Yamaguchi K, Yasuda T. Sepsis-induced myocardial dysfunction: pathophysiology and treatment. J Intensive Care. 2016;4:22.
14. Rivers E, Nguyen B, Havstad S, Ressler J, Muzzin A, Knoblich B, et al. Early goal-directed therapy in the treatment of severe sepsis and septic shock. N Engl J Med. 2001;345:1368–77.
15. Investigators PCESS, Yealy DM, Kellum JA, Huang DT, Barnato AE, Weissfeld LA, et al. A randomized trial of protocol-based care for early septic shock. N Engl J Med. 2014;370:1683–93.
16. Investigators ARISE, Clinical Trials Group ANZICS, Peake SL, Delaney A, Bailey M, Bellomo R, et al. Goal-directed resuscitation for patients with early septic shock. N Engl J Med. 2014;371:1496–506.
17. Mouncey PR, Osborn TM, Power GS, Harrison DA, Sadique MZ, Grieve RD, et al. Trial of early, goal-directed resuscitation for septic shock. N Engl J Med. 2015;372:1301–11.
18. Haas SA, Lange T, Saugel B, Petzoldt M, Fuhrmann V, Metschke M, et al. Severe hyperlactatemia, lactate clearance and mortality in unselected critically ill patients. Intensive Care Med. 2016;42:202–10.
19. Dellinger RP, Levy MM, Rhodes A, Annane D, Gerlach H, Opal SM, et al. Surviving sepsis campaign: international guideline for management of severe sepsis and septic shock: 2012. Crit Care Med. 2013;41:580–637.
20. Parillo JE, Packer MM, Natanson C, Suffredini AF, Danner RL, Cunnion RE, et al. Septic shock in humans. Advances in the understanding of pathogenesis, cardiovascular dysfunction, and therapy. Ann Intern Med. 1990;113:227–42.
21. Charpentier J, Luyt CE, Fulla Y, Vinsonneau C, Cariou A, Grabar S, et al. Brain natriuretic peptide: a marker of myocardial dysfunction and prognosis during severe sepsis. Crit Care Med. 2004;32:660–5.
22. Calvin JE, Driedger AA, Sibbald WJ. Assessment of myocardial function in human sepsis utilizing ECG gated cardiac scintigraphy. Chest. 1981;80:579–86.
23. Packer MM, Shelhamer JH, Natason C, Alling DW, Parillo JE. Serial cardiovascular variables in survivor and nonsurvivor of human septic shock heart rate as an early predictor of prognosis. Crit Care Med. 1987;15:923–9.
24. Morisaki H, Bloos F, Keys J, Martin C, Neal A, Sibbald WL. Compared with crystalloid, colloid therapy slow progression of extrapulmonary tissue injury in septic sheep. J Appl Physiol. 1994;77:1507–18.
25. Serita R, Morisaki H, Ai K, et al. Sevoflurane preconditions stunned myocardium in septic but not healthy isolated rat hearts. Br J Anaesth. 2002;89:896–903.
26. Kimchi A, Ellrodt AG, Berman DS, Riedinger MS, Swan HJ, Murata GH. Right ventricular performance in septic shock: a combined radionuclide and hemodynamic study. J Am Coll Cardiol. 1984;4:945–51.
27. Parker MM, McCarthy KE, Ognibene FP, Parillo JE. Right ventricular dysfunction and dilation, similar to left ventricular changes, characterize the cardiac depression of septic shock in humans. Chest. 1990;97:126–31.
28. Zaky A, Deem S, Bendjelid K, Treggiari MM. Characterization of cardiac dysfunction in sepsis: an ongoing challenge. Shock. 2014;41:12–24.
29. Hunter JD, Doddi M. Sepsis and the heart. Br J Anaesth. 2010;104:3–11.
30. Vieillard Baron A, Schmitt JM, Beauchet A, Augarde R, Prin S, Page B, Jardin F. Early preload adaptation in septic shock? A transesophageal echocardiographic study. Anesthesiology. 2001;94:400–6.
31. Merx MW, Weber C. Sepsis and the heart. Circulation. 2007;116:793–802.
32. Elkins RC, McCurdy JR, Brown PP, Greenfield LJ. Effects of coronary perfusion pressure on myocardial performance. Surg Gynecol Obstet. 1973;137:991–6.
33. Hinshaw LB, Archer LT, Spitzer JJ, Black MR, Peyton MD, Greenfield LJ. Effects of coronary hypotension and endotoxin on myocardial performance. Am J Physiol. 1974;227:1051–7.
34. Cunnion RE, Schaer GL, Paker MM, Natansos C, Parillo JE. The coronary circulation in human septic shock. Circulation. 1986;73:637–44.
35. Dhainaut JF, Huyghebaert MF, Monsallier JF, Lefevre G, Dall'Ava-Santucci J, Brunet F, et al. Coronary hemodynamics and myocardial metabolism of lactate, free acids, glucose, and ketones in patients with septic shock. Circulation. 1987;75:533–41.
36. Takasu O. Mechanisms of cardiac and renal dysfunction in patients dying of sepsis. Am J Respir Crit Care Med. 2013;187:509–17.
37. Parrillo JE, Burch C, Shelhamer JH, Parker MM, Natanson C, Schuette W. A circulating myocardial depressant substance in humans with septic shock. Septic patients with a reduced ejection fraction have a circulating factor that depresses in vitro myocardial cell performance. J Clin Invest. 1985;76:1539–53.
38. Cain BS, Meldrum DR, Dinarello CA, Meng X, Joo KS, Banerjee A, et al. Tumor necrosis factor-α and interleukin-1β synergistically depress human myocardial function. Crit Care Med. 1999;27:1309–18.
39. Khadour FH, Panas D, Ferdinandy P, Schulze C, Csont T, Lalu MM, et al. Enhanced NO and superoxide generation in dysfunctional hearts from endotoxemic rats. Am J Physiol Heart Circ Physiol. 2002;283:H1108–15.
40. Ferdinandy P, Daniel H, Ambrus I, Rothery RA, Schulz R. Peroxynitrite is a major contributor to cytokine-induced myocardial contractile failure. Circ Res. 2000;87:241–7.
41. Brealey D, Brand M, Hargreaves I. Association between mitochondrial dysfunction and severity and outcome of septic shock. Lancet. 2002;360:219–23.
42. Antonucci E, Friaccadori E, Donadello K, Taccone FS, Franchi F, Scolleta S. Myocardial depression in sepsis: from pathogenesis to clinical manifestations and treatment. J Crit Care. 2014;29:500–11.
43. Gulick TS, Chung MK, Pieper SJ, Lange LG, Schreiner GF. Interleukin 1 and tumor necrosis factor inhibit cardiac myocyte beta-adrenergic responsiveness. Proc Natl Acad Sci U S A. 1989;86:6753–7.
44. Bohm M, Kirchmayr R, Gierschik P, Erdmann E. Increased of myocardial inhibitory G-proteins in catecholamine-refractory septic shock or in septic multiorgan failure. Am J Med. 1995;98:183–6.
45. Matsuda N, Hattori Y, Akaishi Y, Suzuki Y, Kemmotsu O, Gando S. Impairment of cardiac β-adrenoceptor cellular signalling by decreased expression of $G^{s\alpha}$ in septic rabbits. Anesthesiology. 2000;93:1465–73.

46. Tang C, Liu MS. Initial externalization followed by internalization of β-adrenergic receptors in rat heart during sepsis. Am J Physiol. 1996;270:R254–63.

47. Shepherd RE, Lang CH, McDonough KH. Myocardial adrenergic responsiveness after lethal and nonlethal doses of endotoxin. Am J Physiol Heart Circ Physiol. 1987;252:410–6.

48. Suzuki T, Morisaki H, Serita R, Yamamoto M, Kotake Y, Ishizaka A, et al. Infusion of the β-adrenergic blocker esmolol attenuates myocardial dysfunction in septic rats. Crit Care Med. 2005;33:2294–301.

49. Zhong J, Hwang T-C, Adams HR, Rubin LJ. Reduced L-type calcium current in ventricular myocytes from endotoxemic guinea pigs. Am J Physiol Cell Physiol. 1997;273:2312–24.

50. Liu S, Schreur KD. G-protein-mediated suppression of L-type Ca2+ current by interleukin-1 beta in cultured rat ventricular myocytes. Am J Physiol Cell Physiol. 1995;268:339–49.

51. Wu LL, Liu MS. Altered ryanodine receptor of canine cardiac sarcoplasmic reticulum and its underlying mechanisms in endotoxin shock. J Surg Res. 1992;53:82–90.

52. Dong LW, Wu LL, Ji Y, Liu MS. Impairment of the ryanodine-sensitive calcium release channels in the cardiac sarcoplasmic reticulum and its underlying mechanisms during the hypodynamic phase of sepsis. Shock. 2001;16:33–9.

53. Lancel S, Joulin O, Favory R. Ventricular myocyte caspases are directly responsible for endotoxin-induced cardiac dysfunction. Circulation. 2005; 111:2596–604.

54. Sato R, Nasu M. A review of sepsis-induced cardiomyopathy. J Intensive Care. 2015;3:48.

55. Blamco J. incidence, organ dysfunction and mortality in severe sepsis: a Spanish multicentre study. Crit Care. 2008;12:R158.

56. Romanosky AJ, Giaimo ME, Shepherd RE, Burns AH. The effect of in vivo endotoxin on myocardial function in vitro. Circ Shock. 1986;19:1–12.

57. Prichard BN. Propranolol in the treatment of angina: review. Postgrad Med J. 1976;52:35–41.

58. Foody JM, Farrell M, Krumholz HM. β-blocker therapy in heart failure. JAMA. 2002;287:883–9.

59. Mangano DT, Layug EL, Wallance A, Tateo I. Effect of atenolol on mortality and cardiovascular morbidity after noncardiac surgery. N Engl J Med. 1996; 335:1713–20.

60. Berk JL, Hagen JF, Beyer WH, Gerber MJ, Dochat GR. The treatment of endotoxin shock by beta adrenergic blockade. Ann Surg. 1969;169:74–81.

61. Berk JL, Hagen JF, Maly G, Koo R. The treatment of shock with beta adrenergic blockade. Arch Surg. 1972;104:46–51.

62. Hinshaw L, Greenfield L, Archer L, Guenter C. Effects of endotoxin on myocardial hemodynamics, performance, and metabolism during beta adrenergic blockade. Proc Soc Exp Biol Med. 1971;137:1217–24.

63. Hagiwara S, Iwasaka H, Maeda H, Noguchi T. Landiolol, an ultrashort-acting beta1-adrenoceptor antagonist, has protective effects in an LPS-induced systemic inflammation model. Shock. 2009;31:515–20.

64. Ackland GL, Yao ST, Rudiger A, Dyson A, Stidwill R, Poputnikov D, et al. Cardioprotection, attenuated systemic inflammation, and survival benefit of beta1-adrenoceptor blockade in severe sepsis in rats. Crit Care Med. 2010;38:388–94.

65. Gore DC, Wolfe RR. Hemodynamic and metabolic effects of selective beta1 adrenergic blockade during sepsis. Surgery. 2006;139:686–94.

66. Schmittinger CA, Dunser MW, Haller M, Ulmer H, Luckner G, Torgersen C, et al. Combined milrinone and enteral metoprolol therapy in patients with septic myocardial depression. Crit Care. 2008;12:R99.

67. Morelli A, Ertmer C, Westphal M, Rehberg S, Kampmeier T, Ligges S, et al. Effect of heart rate control with esmolol on hemodynamic and clinical outcomes in patients with septic shock: a randomized clinical trial. JAMA. 2013;310:1683–91.

68. Kimmoun A, Louis H, Kattani NA, Delemazure J, Dessales N, Wei C, et al. b1-Adrenergic inhibition improves cardiac and vascular function in experimental septic shock. Crit Casre Med. 2015;43:e332–40.

69. Novotny NM, Lahm T, Markel TA, Crisostomo PR, Wang M, Wang Y, et al. β-Blockers in sepsis: re-examining the evidence. Shock. 2009;31:113–9.

70. Chiolero R, Revelly JP, Tappy L. Energy metabolism in sepsis and injury. Nutrition. 1997;13:45S–51S.

71. Trager K, DeBacker D, Radermacher P. Metabolic alteration in sepsis and vasoactive drug-related metabolic effects. Curr Opin Crit Care. 2003;9:271–8.

72. John GW, Doxey JC, Walter DS, Reid JL. The role of alpha-and beta-adrenoceptor subtypes in mediating the effects of catecholamines on

73. Haffner CA, Kendall MJ. Metabolic effects of beta 2-agonists. J Clin Pharm Ther. 1992;17:155–64.

74. Dickerson RN, Fried RC, Bailey PM, Stein TP, Mullen JL, Buzby GP. Effect of propranolol on nitrogen and energy metabolism in sepsis. J Surg Res. 1990;48:38–41.

75. Elenkov IJ, Wilder RL, Chrousos GP, Vizi ES. The sympathetic nerve—an integrative interface between two supersystems: the brain and the immune system. Pharmacol Rev. 2000;52:595–638.

76. Severn A, Rapsos NT, Hunter CA, Liew FY. Regulation of tumor necrosis factor production by adrenaline and beta-adrenergic agonists. J Immunol. 1992;148:3441–5.

77. Muthu K, Deng J, Gamelli R, Shankar R, Jones SB. Adrenergic modulation of cytokine release in bone marrow progenitor-derived macrophage following polymicrobial sepsis. J Neuroimmunol. 2005;158:50–7.

78. Deng J, Muthu K, Gamelli R, Shankar R, Jones SB. Adrenergic modulation of splenic macrophage cytokine release in polymicrobial sepsis. Am J Physiol Cell Physiol. 2004;287:C730–6.

79. Calzavacca P, Lankadeva YR, Bailey SR, Bailey M, Bellomo R, May CN. Effects of selective β1-adrenoceptor blockade on cardiovascular and renal function and circulating cytokines in ovine hyperdynamic sepsis. Crit Care. 2014;18:610.

80. Hotchkiss RS, Coopersmith CM, Karl IE. Prevention of lymphocyte apoptosis—a potential treatment of sepsis? Clin Infect Dis. 2005;41:S465–9.

81. Hotchkiss RS, Tinsley KW, Swanson PE, Schmieg Jr RE, Hui JJ, Chang KC, et al. Sepsis-induced apoptosis causes progressive profound depletion of B and CD4+ T lymphocytes in humans. J Immunol. 2001;166:6952–63.

82. Liu MW, Su MX, Zhang W, Zhang LM, Wang YH, Qian CY. Rhodiola rosea suppresses thymus T-lymphocyte apoptosis by downregulating tumor necrosis factor-α-induced protein 8-like-2 in septic rats. Int J Mol Med. 2015;36:386–98.

83. Oberbeck R. Catecholamines: physiological immunomodulators during health and illness. Curr Med Chem. 2006;13:1979–89.

84. Boldt J, Menges T, Wollbruck M, Sonneborn S, Hempelmann G. Platelet function in critically ill patients. Chest. 1994;106:899–903.

85. Gawaz M, Dickfeld T, Bogner C, Fateh-Moghadam S, Neumann FJ. Platelet function in septic multiple organ dysfunction syndrome. Intensive Care Med. 1997;23:379–85.

86. Amaral A, Opal SM, Vincent JL. Coagulation in sepsis. Intensive Care Med. 2004;30:1032–40.

87. Hjemdahl P, Larsson PT, Wallen NH. Effects of stress and beta-blockade on platelet function. Circulation. 1991;84:VI44–61.

88. Ogston D, Mc DG, Fullerton HW. The influence of anxiety in tests of blood coagulability and fibrinolytic activity. Lancet. 1962;2:521–3.

89. Adler B, Gimbrone Jr MA, Schafer AI, Handin RI. Prostacyclin and beta-adrenergic catecholamines inhibit arachidonate release and PGI2 synthesis by vascular endothelium. Blood. 1981;58:514–7.

fasting glucose and insulin concentrations in the rat. Br J Pharmacol. 1990; 100:699–704.

Light irradiation for treatment of acute carbon monoxide poisoning

Taku Tanaka[1*], Takeshi Kashimura[2], Marii Ise[2], Brandon D. Lohman[2] and Yasuhiko Taira[2]

Abstract

Background: Because treatment modalities for carbon monoxide (CO) poisoning, especially normobaric oxygen and hyperbaric oxygen therapies, have limited effects and hyperbaric oxygen is not available at the scene where treatment is most needed, we conducted a study to determine and compare rates of carboxyhemoglobin (COHb) dissociation achieved in human in vitro blood samples under light radiation emitted at three levels of illuminance. This was done with a view toward eventual on-site application.

Methods: We drew blood from 10 volunteers, prepared 10 red blood cell solutions, and subjected each solution to a CO bubbling procedure to increase the COHb saturation. Samples of each bubbled solution were then divided between 3 beakers (beakers A, B, and C) for a total of 30 beakers. The solution in each beaker was exposed to a continuous flow of oxygen at 50 mL/min, and simultaneously for a period of 15 min, the beaker A and B solutions were irradiated with light emitted at 500,000 and 100,000 lux, respectively, from a halogen light source. The beaker C solutions were exposed to room light. At 3, 6, 9, 12, and 15 min, a 50-μL sample was pipetted from each of the 30 beakers for determination of its light absorbance and the COHb dissociation rate.

Results: Under each of the experimental conditions, dissociation progressed but at different rates, and starting at 3 min, the differences in rates between conditions were significant ($P < 0.01$). The dissociation rate was greatest with light emitted at 500,000 lux.

Conclusions: Our results point toward the possibility of readily performed, acute photodissociation therapy for patients with CO poisoning.

Abbreviations: CO, Carbon monoxide; COHb, Carboxyhemoglobin; HBO, Hyperbaric oxygen; NBO, Normobaric oxygen; O_2Hb, Oxyhemoglobin

Background

Awareness of the deadly effects of carbon monoxide (CO) dates back to the time of the ancient Greeks and Romans, when the gas was used for executions [1]. To this day, CO poisoning remains one of the most common types of poisoning, accounting for more than 60 % of poisoning deaths in Japan, accidental or otherwise [2]. CO is a tasteless, odorless, and non-irritating but highly toxic gas that confers significant long-term morbidity and is often associated with severe delayed neuropathology [3].

Despite the aggressive treatment strategies available, morbidity and mortality rates attributable to CO poisoning remain high [4].

Because of the intrinsic properties of CO and lack of specific clinical features of CO poisoning, the condition is difficult to detect, and it can mimic other common disorders. Therefore, the true incidence of CO poisoning is unknown, and it is likely that many cases go unrecognized. CO is a by-product of the incomplete combustion of hydrocarbons, and it is commonly produced by domestic heating appliances and systems, charcoal burning, fires, and car exhaust. CO poisoning accounts for many deaths by suicide.

* Correspondence: taku040@gmail.com
[1]Medical Emergency and Disaster Center, Kawasaki Municipal Tama Hospital, 1-30-37 Shukugawara, Tama-ku, Kawasaki, Kanagawa 214-8525, Japan
Full list of author information is available at the end of the article

CO toxicity results from the formation of a carbon-hemoglobin complex, carboxyhemoglobin (COHb), which is over 200-fold more stable than oxyhemoglobin (O_2Hb) [5, 6]. An increased blood COHb concentration will compromise oxygen transport by hemoglobin and thus decrease oxygen delivery to vital organs and tissues. Furthermore, not only does COHb have a long half-life, but at a 20 % concentration, more than 8 h may be required for CO to fully dissociate from the complexed hemoglobin [7]. The importance of effectively eliminating the toxic effect of CO cannot be overemphasized. However, present treatment modalities, especially hyperbaric oxygen (HBO) and normobaric oxygen (NBO) therapies, have limited effects, and HBO therapy especially remains controversial and not readily available at the scene where treatment is most needed. Phototherapy, specifically photodissociation of COHb, appears to be a viable alternative because there are no known complications. With a view toward use in clinical cases of CO poisoning, we conducted a study to determine and compare rates of COHb dissociation achieved in human in vitro blood samples under light radiation emitted from two different light sources at three different levels of illuminance.

Methods
Blood samples
Under approval granted by the Ethics Committee of St. Marianna University School of Medicine, Japan, we drew blood from 10 adult volunteers (smokers $n – 2$, non-smokers $n = 8$) recruited from our staff. The volunteers ranged in age from 28 to 61 years, with a mean of 37.9 years. Thirty milliliters of blood was collected from each volunteer by direct venipuncture of the brachial vein, immediately anticoagulated with 0.1 mL heparin (Novoheparin, Mochida Seiyaku, Tokyo, Japan), and then washed. The specimen was then centrifuged at 3000 rpm for 10 min, the plasma supernatant was removed, the erythrocytes were re-suspended in a 9-g/L normal saline solution, and the suspension was centrifuged. This process was repeated three times before the tube was inverted two or three times until the contents were mixed to the point of turbidity. Next, 2 mL of the red blood cell solution was pipetted out of the tube and exposed continuously to 100 % pure oxygen at 60 mL/min to produce 100 % O_2-saturated hemoglobin (100 % O_2Hb) (Fig. 1).

CO bubbling
The remaining 28 mL of the red blood cell solution was prepared for CO bubbling, a procedure that is designed to increase the COHb saturation. The procedure consists of the following series of steps: (1) the red blood cell solution is placed at the bottom of a Ziploc freezer bag, and a flexible, plastic spray nozzle belonging to a CO canister (GL-Sciences, Ltd., Tokyo, Japan) is positioned at the mouth of the bag; (2) the air is squeezed out of the bag, which is then sealed by hand, and to avoid any tearing, the sealed bag is placed in a second Ziploc bag, which is also sealed; (3) the nozzle is attached to the CO canister, and CO is injected into the bag until it is fully inflated (Fig. 2a); and (4) the CO-inflated bag is then vigorously shaken for at least

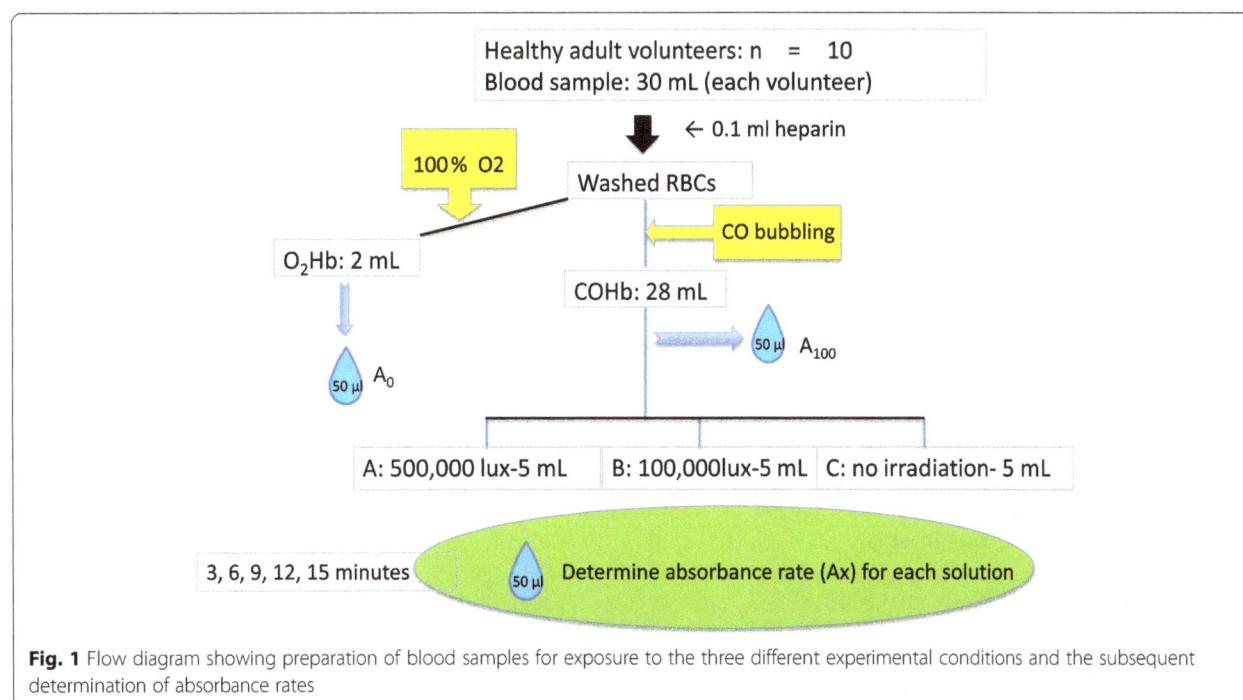

Fig. 1 Flow diagram showing preparation of blood samples for exposure to the three different experimental conditions and the subsequent determination of absorbance rates

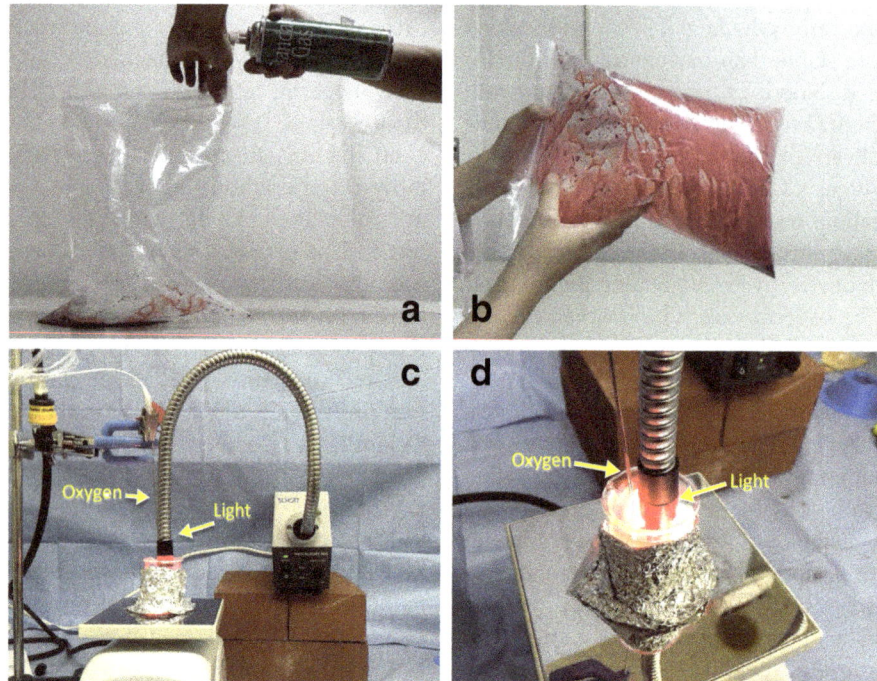

Fig. 2 CO bubbling. **a** CO is injected into a Ziploc bag containing the red blood cell solution until the bag is fully inflated. **b** The inflated bag is then vigorously shaken for at least 60 min, resulting in 90 % COHb production. **c**, **d** The sample solution, now in a beaker, is simultaneously exposed to light (500,000 lux, 300,000 lux, or simply room light) and to a continuous flow of oxygen at 50 mL/min. The oxygen is delivered via a copper nozzle connected to an oxygen gas cylinder

60 min, which we know will result in over 90 % COHb production (Fig. 2b).

After the CO bubbling procedure, three separate 5-mL samples of the solution were collected from the bag and placed into three separate 20-mL beakers: beaker A, beaker B, and beaker C. In all, 30 samples (3 samples × 10 volunteers) were obtained, and each was placed in its own beaker. A halogen light source (MegaLight 100, SHOTT-MORITEX, Tokyo, Japan) attached to a 25-cm-long flexible stainless steel gooseneck light guide was placed 10 mm above the surface of each sample. The light emitting end of the light guide was 6 mm in diameter. We administered a continuous flow of oxygen at 50 mL/min by plunging a copper nozzle (length 100 mm, diameter 4 mm) connected to an oxygen gas cylinder into the red blood cell solution, and at the same time, for a period of 15 min, we irradiated the beaker A blood sample with light at a total luminance of 500,000 lux and the beaker B sample with light at a total luminance of 100,000 lux. The beaker C sample was not irradiated but rather was left exposed to room light (Fig. 2c, d). At 3-min intervals (3, 6, 9, 12, and 15 min), a 50-μL sample was pipetted out of each beaker for determination of its light absorbance and its CO dissociation rate.

A distance of 10 mm between the light guide tip and the red blood cell surface is the optimal distance at which the flexible light guide can safely emit light without causing any blood splatter from the continuous oxygen administration. Under the optical illumination with 500,000 lux maintained for 15 min, the temperature of the blood in the beakers was below 32 °C, and therefore, hemoglobin protein denaturation was not a concern during the irradiation process. In addition, each beaker was firmly sealed with aluminum foil to prevent the escape of any irradiation light. The light reaches the bottom of the beaker and there measures 50–60 lux.

Measurement of the photodissociation rate

It is well established that O_2Hb and COHb each has its own specific light absorption spectra that are characterized by a bimodal curve, each with two maximal spectrophotometrically determined absorption peaks: 540 and 576 nm for O_2Hb and 538 and 568 nm for COHb. The absorption spectra may be altered by varying the ratio between the O_2Hb and COHb concentrations, and the morphology of the resulting waveforms will be by modified accordingly. It is also known that a small amount of sodium hydrosulfite can reduce O_2Hb, thereby altering its absorption curve from a bimodal to a monomodal wavelength with an absorption peak of 555 nm. (Fig. 3) [8, 9].

Because the aim of this study was to determine the rate of COHb dissociation resulting from exposure to

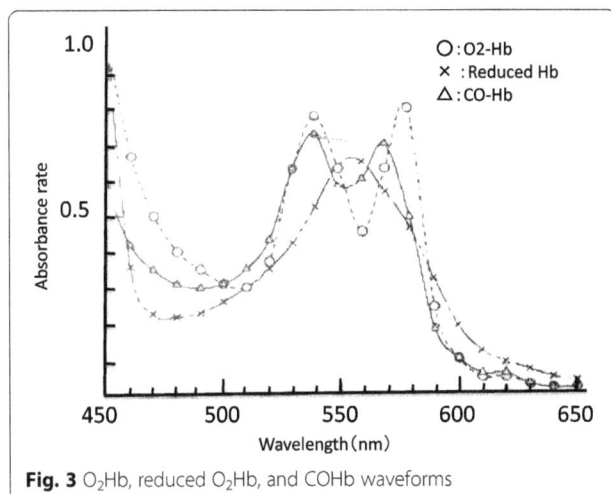

Fig. 3 O_2Hb, reduced O_2Hb, and COHb waveforms

light radiation, we selected a reduced O_2Hb monomodal curve absorption value of 555 nm and an absorption value of 538 nm from the COHb bimodal curve. To this end, we removed two samples of 50 µL each, one from the previously prepared sample containing 100 % O_2Hb, and one from the CO-bubbling bag, and we placed these samples in two separate test tubes before adding to each of them 10 mL 0.1 % sodium carbonate and then 0.0275 g (1 micro-spoon) sodium hydrosulfite, and we gently shook the samples for a few seconds. After allowing the solution to settle for 15 min, the samples were analyzed by spectrophotometry (BioSpectrometer Basic, Eppendorf, Hamburg, Germany) so that we could determine the parameters necessary to tabulate the O_2Hb (A_0) and COHb (A_{100}) constants that would be needed to calculate the COHb dissociation rate.

A 50-µL sample was then collected every 3 min over a period of 15 min (at 3, 6, 9, 12 and 15 min) from beaker A, beaker B, and beaker C, and these samples were subjected to the same buffering procedure described above. Subsequently, all collected samples were subjected to spectrophotometry in which the constant values were used to determine the light absorbance spectrum (A_x) of each sample.

Calculating CO saturation

For all samples, a bimodal curve was projected on a Cartesian coordinate system visible on the spectrophotometer screen. The abscissa and ordinate axes represent the wavelength and absorbance spectra, respectively. From the given E555 and E568 wavelengths on the x axis, we were able to identify the corresponding absorbance values on the y axis for O_2Hb and COHb in all samples tested.

Next, the respective constant values of A_0 and A_{100} for both O_2Hb and COHb and the A_x values for the three samples were calculated as follows: A_0 = E538/E555, A_{100} = E538/E555, and A_x = E538/E555, which were then

inserted and tabulated according to the following COHb concentration equation: COHb (%) = (A_x – A_0) / (A_{100} – A_0) * [9]. The value obtained is the dissociation rate, and the rate was calculated for each of the 30 samples obtained at each of the various time points.

Statistical analysis

For each of the 10 samples obtained at each time point, the mean ± SE COHb dissociation rate was calculated. The rates were then plotted per condition (i.e., per beaker A, B, or C), per time point. Differences in the mean ± SE dissociation rate between the three conditions were analyzed by repeated-measures ANOVA and Tukey's HSD test. Correlation between COHb saturation (shown as a percentage) and the rate of change was tested by Pearson's correlation coefficient. All statistical analyses were performed with Stat Flex ver. 6 (Artech Co., Ltd., Osaka, Japan), and $P < 0.05$ was considered significant.

Results

The study subjects, pertinent subject characteristics, and individual study data are shown in Table 1. We drew COHb dissociation curves (Fig. 4), and in comparing these curves, we found that the dissociation rate determined for the beaker B (100,000 lux) samples was higher than that for the beaker C (no irradiation) samples but lower than that for the beaker A (500,000 lux) samples. Under each of the experimental conditions, dissociation progressed at different rates, but starting at 3 min, the differences in rates between conditions were significant ($P < 0.01$). Under exposure to light at 500,000 lux, the dissociation rate decreased uniformly over time with no noticeable difference between the time periods (Fig. 5). Correlation between COHb saturation and the change in the dissociation rate was significant for the 0–3-min time period and the 12–15-min time period at $P = 0.020$ and $P = 0.023$, respectively (Fig. 6). Tukey's multiple comparisons analysis confirmed all statistical differences that we found ($P < 0.01$).

Two of the volunteers were chronic heavy smokers (subject 8: 2 packs/day for >30 years and subject 9: 1 pack/day for <10 years). Although the study group was too small for meaningful comparison between smokers and non-smokers, we noted that there was no significant difference in dissociation rates between them.

Discussion

An estimated 58,000 emergency cases of CO poisoning occur yearly in Japan, and the resulting estimated cost of over 1 trillion 75 billion yen (8,743,000,000 USD) per year [10] translates to a devastating socio-economic impact. The symptoms of CO poisoning are non-specific [11] and usually manifest when the CO concentration rises above 10 % [12]. However, the reported association

Table 1 Study subjects, pertinent subject characteristics, and individual study data

Subject	Age (years)	Sex	Smoking	500,000 lux		100,000 lux		No irradiation		Change rate
				3 min	15 min	3 min	15 min	3 min	15 min	0–3 min
1	44	M	No	83.9	54.3	87.9	62.0	95.1	91.5	−5.38
2	41	F	No	82.0	40.5	83.4	47.8	93.8	87.5	−6.02
3	28	F	No	83.1	47.7	97.9	70.9	97.8	90.3	−5.64
4	42	M	No	89.7	58.1	92.1	69.9	89.7	93.3	−3.43
5	40	F	No	83.3	49.2	92.4	71.6	98.6	91.1	−5.58
6	30	M	No	83.1	48.8	92.4	62.2	95.2	82.8	−5.64
7	32	M	No	84.5	54.3	89.4	69.6	91.4	84.7	−5.18
8	30	M	No	88.8	59.2	90.4	68.3	93.6	85.9	−3.72
9	61	M	Yes	90.0	51.7	89.9	64.9	94.4	90.4	−3.35
10	31	M	Yes	86.8	51.5	88.3	63.8	91.3	85.8	−4.41
Mean	37.9	–	–	85.5	51.5	90.4	65.1	94.5	88.3	−4.84

between a patient's blood level and that patient's clinical condition is poor [11, 12]. The general consensus is that levels below 60 % do not result in coma or death [5]. In non-smokers, the average CO concentration is 1 %, whereas in heavy smokers, the average concentration may reach 15 % [13]. CO causes hypoxia by combining with hemoglobin in the blood to form COHb and shifting the O_2Hb dissociation curve to the left [13]. Its affinity for hemoglobin is more than 200 times that of oxygen [14], and it easily displaces oxygen from hemoglobin, whereas COHb liberates CO very slowly, resulting in the formation of COHb with even negligible amounts of inhaled CO.

A small CO concentration can thus result in a toxic level of COHb in the blood and lead to a decrease in the amount of oxygen transported by hemoglobin to organs and tissues. Up to 46 % of CO poisoning victims develop

delayed neuropsychological sequelae, including cognitive deficits, motor disturbances, and vestibular abnormalities [15]. Recent reports have also highlighted the contribution of CO poisoning to the incidence of cardiac events [16, 17] because the affinity of CO for myoglobin is even greater than it is for Hb [1]. The binding of CO to cardiac myoglobin can cause myocardial depression, hypotension, arrhythmia, and even death [12].

To this day, one of the greatest challenges facing any emergency department in cases of CO poisoning is the need to promptly dissociate COHb to save patients' lives. However, the treatment options in the emergency physicians' arsenal remain limited and are often associated with severe side effects. Currently, the widely accepted methods of management, NBO therapy and HBO therapy, maximize the PaO_2 level, thereby increasing O_2Hb and indirectly dissociating CO from COHb. NBO treatment

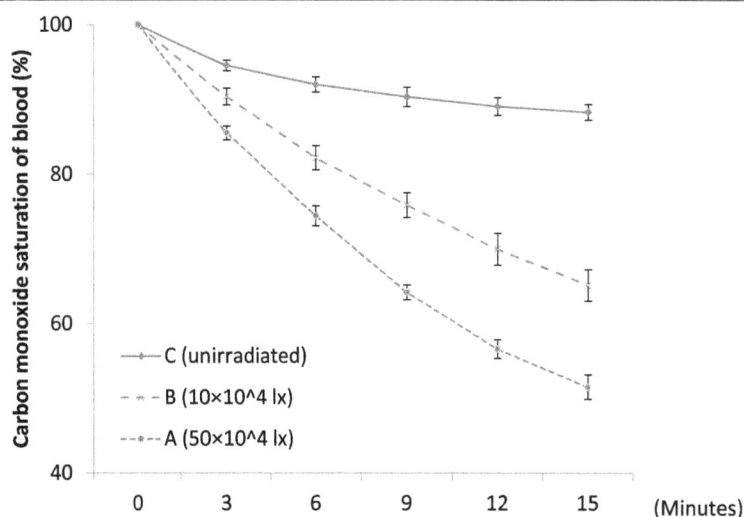

Fig. 4 COHb dissociation curves plotted from mean ± SE dissociation rates for the total solution samples under the three different light exposure conditions over a 15-min time period

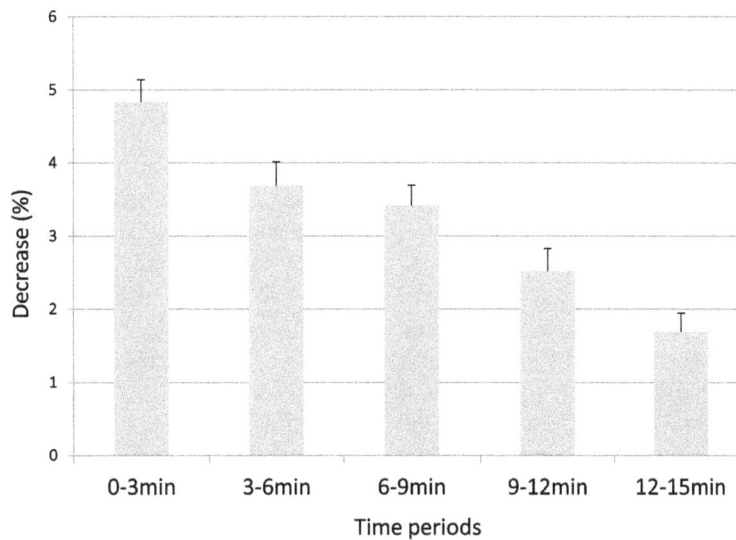

Fig. 5 Bar graph of the dissociation rate for each of the 3-minute time periods in samples exposed to light at 500,000 lux

involves removing the patient from the source of exposure and administering 100 % NBO for 4 to 6 h to remove over 90 % of the CO until the COHb concentration is less than 5 %. This regimen brings the half-life of COHb down to 74 min, as opposed to 320 min when breathing air [18]. The administration of oxygen speeds the elimination of CO from the body. Without oxygen therapy, the elimination half-life of CO is 4 to 5 h. Supplementation with 100 % oxygen via a tight-fitting mask at NBO pressure cuts the elimination half-life by approximately 50 %, whereas the use of HBO, i.e., the use of pure oxygen to speed and enhance the body's natural ability to heal, at 2.5 atm decreases the elimination half-life to 20 min [18, 19]. However, HBO should be administered within 6 h of exposure [7] for a duration of about 9 h [20],

and NBO should be administered when CO poisoning is suspected and before laboratory confirmation. For decades, HBO has been used for severe CO poisoning, but its indication remains controversial [21–25] because of the action of O_2, which can result in oxygen toxicity seizures and barotrauma, including pneumothorax and hemorrhage. Furthermore, there is no real evidence that HBO administration for CO poisoning reduces the incidence of adverse neurologic outcomes [26].

Additionally, because of the equipment required and its inconvenience, HBO therapy is often not a practical option. HBO therapy requires special equipment, and the institutions amenable to setting up a hyperbaric chamber are limited. Currently in Japan, according to the 2014 Japanese Society of Hyperbaric and Undersea

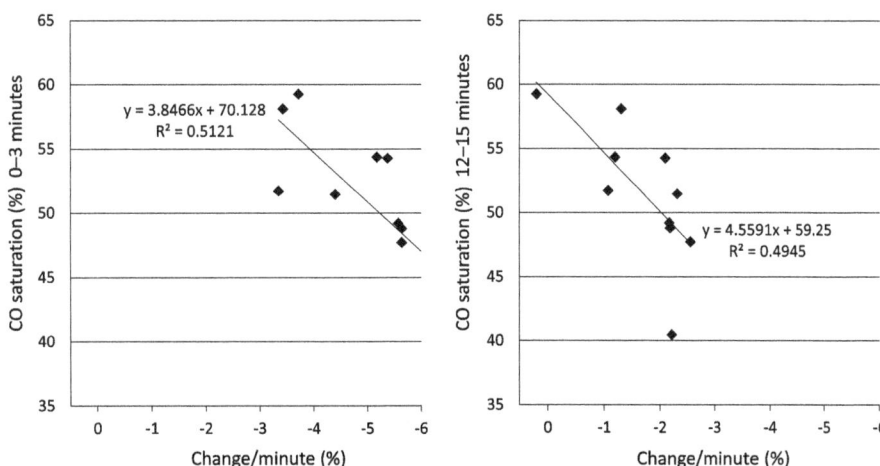

Fig. 6 Correlation between CO saturation and the change in the dissociation rate during the 0–3-min and 12–15-min time periods

Medicine registry, there are only 591 such facilities nationwide [27]. Phototherapy, i.e., the use of visible light to dissociate COHb, appears to be an appealing and viable alternative for addressing CO poisoning. Unlike NBO and HBO therapies, light irradiation therapy works directly to dissociate CO from COHb; it does not increase the PaO_2, is not known to result in any complications, and appears to be safe.

The phototherapy method was originally developed from an early hypothesis that light irradiation induces the photodissociation of O_2Hb. This hypothesis centers on the fact that O_2Hb absorbs the light radiation, and at a probability of approximately 10 %, the photodissociation will release the O_2 molecule and restore hemoglobin [28]. Extrapolating this finding to COHb, and despite the similarities in the absorption spectra of O_2Hb and COHb, with the significant difference (>10-fold) in the quantum yields of photodissociation (which is 98 % for COHb), it becomes possible to achieve selective decomposition of COHb in the bloodstream with a minimum effect on the O_2Hb. The typical absorption spectra of O_2Hb, COHb, and reduced O_2Hb, i.e., hemoglobin (Hb), in vitro are shown in Fig. 3. Light irradiation dissociates CO from the COHb complex and, with a constant O_2 supply, might re-establish the physiological O_2Hb bond. Irradiation of a COHb sample by light at various frequencies has been documented to split the CO-Hb bond and presumably restore O_2Hb binding. In a landmark study, Kashimura et al. [29] infused rats with synthetic artificial oxygen-carrying hemoglobin vesicles (HbV) and exposed the rats to light of 500,000 lux and showed that the COHb significantly dissociated (26.1 ± 2.4 %) after 90 min of exposure.

We further explored the theory and experimental success by examining the rate of dissociation achieved with light emitted at different illuminances (0, 100,000, and 500,000 lux) in human in vitro blood samples highly saturated with COHb. Results of the light irradiation were promising, with a relatively high dissociation rate achieved with exposure to 500,000 lux within a short (15-min) period.

In the in vitro study described herein, the Hb dissociated from the COHb complex presumably bound with O_2 and formed an O_2Hb molecule, and the remaining CO molecule most likely volatilized in air. In the human body, photodecomposition of COHb and CO removal will be most effective in the lungs and skin. However, the unbound CO has a strong propensity for attachment to Hb, and to prevent such de novo COHb complex formation, sufficient O_2 is required even in instances of low COHb dissociation.

Our application of light irradiation to in vitro human blood samples yielded encouraging data, and we consider this a first step toward clinical application of COHb dissociation for CO poisoning patients. The path to clinical application must include both tests in large animal models of CO poisoning and the conceptualization and design of devices, particularly devices that can be used at the scene.

The application of light irradiation to patients with a high COHb concentration will require application of the light as directly and closely as possible to the CO-contaminated blood. The optimal phototherapy effect will be achieved when the light is aimed as close to the oxygen source as possible, namely the lungs. The authors have envisioned a combination of options for the urgent care of CO poisoning patients. One is an extra-corporeal light radiation-emitting jacket that could ideally be used to provide COHb dissociation therapy at the scene of trauma, where the patient requires it most. Its easy handling would allow paramedics to place it on the patient during emergency transport to a hospital or trauma center. The second is a light-emitting catheter that, upon patient admission, could be introduced into the pulmonary artery or the right side of the heart to dissociate the COHb complex, thus allowing O2 to bind with Hb while CO is exhaled through the lungs. Development of a light radiation-emitting jacket would need to take into account the optical properties of the human skin for determination of the effective wavelength of the penetrating radiation. This could, however, be achieved by calculating the action spectra of HbCO within the cutaneous layers. Furthermore, the insertion and indwelling of the specifically designed light radiation-emitting catheter would probably require training.

Limitations

Our study had limitations. The first is the small sample size, and the second is the inherent disadvantage of an in vitro study, despite our use of human blood. Second, the refraction and barrier effect that the light would encounter in cutaneous and subcutaneous tissues of actual patients was not simulated. Third, medical histories, including any underlying chronic disorders, medications, or any prior hemoglobin studies, were not obtained from the volunteers who donated blood.

Conclusions

We attempted and achieved photodissociation of COHb in in vitro human blood samples by light irradiation. We anticipate performing a larger study to further confirm our results, which have convinced us of the real possibility of readily performed, acute photodissociation therapies for patients with CO poisoning, therapies that are imperative if we wish to meet the challenge of saving the lives of individuals exposed to CO.

Acknowledgements
We are indebted to Tina Tajima for her advice and editing of the English manuscript. We also thank Hirotsugu Komatsu of Interprotein Corporation for his assistance with our statistical analysis.

Funding
None.

Authors' contributions
All authors did research and assisted TT to write this paper. YT, on top of assisting the authors with research, provided guidance. All authors read and approved the final manuscript.

Competing interests
The authors declare that they have no competing interests.

Author details
[1]Medical Emergency and Disaster Center, Kawasaki Municipal Tama Hospital, 1-30-37 Shukugawara, Tama-ku, Kawasaki, Kanagawa 214-8525, Japan. [2]Emergency and Critical Care Medicine, St. Marianna University School of Medicine, 2-16-1 Sugao, Miyamae-ku, Kawasaki, Kanagawa 216-8511, Japan.

References
1. Barrett KE. Ganong's review of medical physiology 25th Edition. New York: McGraw-Hill; 2016.
2. Statistics and Information Department. Vital statistics. Tokyo: Ministry of Health, Labor and Welfare; 2011.
3. Varon J, Marik P. Carbon monoxide poisoning and gas powered equipment. J Emerg Med. 2001;21:283–4.
4. Omaye ST. Metabolic modulation of carbon monoxide toxicity. Toxicology. 2002;180:139–50. doi:10.1016/S0300-483X(02)00387-6.
5. Meredith T, Vale A. Carbon monoxide poisoning. BMJ. 1988;296:77–9.
6. Kao LW, Nañagas KA. Toxicity associated with carbon monoxide. Clin Lab Med. 2006;26:99–125. doi:10.1016/j.cll.2006.01.005.
7. Goulon M, Barois A, Rapin M. Carbon monoxide poisoning and acute anoxia due to breathing coal tar gas and hydrocarbons. J Hyperb Med. 1986;1:23–41.
8. Klendshoj NC, Feldstein M, Sprague AL. The spectrophotometric determination of carbon monoxide. J Biol Chem. 1950;183:297–303.
9. Kage S, Seto Y. Method of toxic gas measurement. In: Suzuki Y, editor. Method and annotation of measurement of chemical and toxic substances 2006. Tokyo: Tokyo Kagaku Dojin; 2006. p. 37–42.
10. Kohshi K, Ishitake T, Hoshiko M, Tamaki H, Kondo Y, Kukita I, et al. Social medical problems on carbon monoxide poisoning—estimating the social costs. Jpn J Occup Med Traumatol. 2012;60:18–22.
11. Hampson NB, Hauff NM. Carboxyhemoglobin levels in carbon monoxide poisoning: do they correlate with the clinical picture? Am J Emerg Med. 2008;26(6):665–9. doi:10.1016/j.ajem.2007.10.005.
12. Raub JA, Mathieu-Nolf M, Hampson NB, Thom SR. Carbon monoxide poisoning—a public health perspective. Toxicology. 2000;145:1–14. doi:10.1016/S0300-483X(99)00217-6.
13. Ernst A, Zibrak JD. Carbon monoxide poisoning. N Engl J Med. 1998;339:1603–8.
14. Hardy KR, Thom SR. Carbon monoxide pathophysiology and treatment of carbon monoxide poisoning. Clin Toxicol. 1994;32:613–29.
15. Weaver LK, Hopkins RO, Chan KJ, Churchill S, Elliott CG, Clemmer TP, et al. Hyperbaric oxygen for acute carbon monoxide poisoning. N Engl J Med. 2002;347:1057–67.
16. Henry CR, Satran D, Lindgren B, Adkinson C, Nicholson CI, Henry TD. Myocardial injury and long-term mortality following moderate to severe carbon monoxide poisoning. JAMA. 2006;295:398–402. doi:10.1001/jama.295.4.398.
17. Kalay N, Ozdogru I, Cetinkaya Y, Eryol NK, Dogan A, Gul I, et al. Cardiovascular effects of carbon monoxide poisoning. Am J Cardiol. 2007;99:322–4. doi:10.1016/j.amjcard.2006.08.030.
18. Weaver LK, Howe S, Hopkins R, Chan KJ. Carboxyhemoglobin half-life in carbon monoxide-poisoned patients treated with 100 % oxygen at atmospheric pressure. Chest. 2000;117:801–8.
19. Wolf SJ, Lavonas EJ, Sloan EP, Jagoda AS. Clinical policy: critical issues in the management of adult patients presenting to the emergency department with acute carbon monoxide poisoning. Ann Emerg Med. 2008;51:138–52. doi:10.1016/j.annemergmed.2007.10.012.
20. Hamilton-Farrell MR. British Hyperbaric Association carbon monoxide database, 1993-96. J Accid Emerg Med. 1999;16:98–103.
21. Buckley NA, Isbister GK, Stokes B, Juurlink DN. Hyperbaric oxygen for carbon monoxide poisoning: a systematic review and critical analysis of the evidence. Toxicol Rev. 2005;24:75–92.
22. Hampson NB, Little CE. Hyperbaric treatment of patients with carbon monoxide poisoning in the United States. Undersea Hyperb Med. 2005;32:21–6.
23. Raphael JC, Elkharrat D, Jars-Guincestre MC, Chastang C, Charles V, Vercken JB, et al. Trial of normobaric and hyperbaric oxygen for acute carbon monoxide intoxication. Lancet. 1989;2:414–9. doi:10.1016/S0140-6736(89)90592-8.
24. Scheinkestel CD, Bailey M, Myles PS, Jones K, Cooper DJ, Millar IL, et al. Hyperbaric or normobaric oxygen for acute carbon monoxide poisoning: a randomised controlled clinical trial. Med J Aust. 1999;170:203–10.
25. Annane D, Chadda K, Gajdos P, Jars-Guincestre M-C, Chevret S, Raphael J-C. Hyperbaric oxygen therapy for acute domestic carbon monoxide poisoning: two randomized controlled trials. Intensive Care Med. 2011;37:486–92. doi:10.1007/s00134-010-2093-0.
26. Buckley NA, Juurlink DN, Isbister G, Bennett MH, Lavonas EJ. Hyperbaric oxygen for carbon monoxide poisoning. Cochrane Database Syst Rev. 2011: CD002041. doi:10.1002/14651858.CD002041.pub3.
27. The Japanese Society of Hyperbaric and Undersea Medicine; n.d. http://www.jshm.net/shisetu.html. Accessed 12 Mar 2016.
28. Asimov MM, Asimov RM, Rubinov AN. Laser-induced photodissociation of carboxyhemoglobin: an optical method for eliminating the toxic effect of carbon monoxide. Opt Spectrosc. 2010;109:237–42. doi:10.1134/S0030400X1008014X.
29. Kashimura T, Hososan A, Furuya T, et al. New application of light irradiation to the treatment of acute CO poisoning. Jpn Kournal Hyperb Undersea Med. 2008;43:195–201.

Factors associated with increased pancreatic enzymes in septic patients

Anis Chaari[1*], Karim Abdel Hakim[1], Nevine Rashed[2], Kamel Bousselmi[1], Vipin Kauts[1], Mahmoud Etman[1] and William Francis Casey[1]

Abstract

Background: The perfusion of splanchnic organs is deeply altered in patients with septic shock. The aim of the study is to identify the predictive factors of septic shock-induced increase of serum lipase and amylase and to assess and evaluate its prognostic impact.

Methods: We conducted a prospective observational study. All adult patients admitted with septic shock were eligible for our study. Serum lipase and amylase were measured on admission. Patients with and those without increased pancreatic enzymes were compared. Predictive factors of pancreatic insult identified by the univariate analysis were integrated in a stepwise multivariate analysis. Odds ratios (OR) with the 95% confidence interval (CI) were calculated accordingly. Second, the sensitivity and the specificity of amylase and lipase to predict intensive care unit (ICU) mortality were identified through the Receiver Operator Curve.

Results: Fifty patients were included. Median [quartiles] age was 68.5 [58–81] years. The APACHE II score was 26 [20–31]. Twenty-three patients (46%) had increased serum amylase and/or serum lipase. Diabetes mellitus (OR = 16; 95% CI [1.7–153.5]; $p = 0.016$), increased blood urea nitrogen (OR = 1.12; 95% CI [1.02–1.20], $p = 0.016$), and decreased C-reactive protein (OR = 0.97; 95% CI [0.96–0.99]; $p = 0.027$) were identified as independent factors predicting increased pancreatic enzymes. Twenty patients (40%) died in the ICU. Neither serum amylase level nor serum lipase level was significantly different between survivors and non-survivors (respectively 49 [27.7–106] versus 85.1 [20.1–165] UI/L; $p = 0.7$ and 165 [88–316] versus 120 [65.5–592] UI/L; $p = 0.952$).

Conclusion: Increase of pancreatic enzymes is common in patients with septic shock. Diabetes and impaired renal function are predictive of increased pancreatic enzymes. Such finding does not carry any negative prognostic value.

Keywords: Amylase, Lipase, Septic shock, Prognosis

Background

Septic shock is a common cause of admission to the intensive care units (ICUs) [1, 2]. Despite subsequent improvement of management modalities and worldwide awareness of updated guidelines, it still carries a high mortality ranging from 30 to 60% [1, 2]. This high mortality is mainly related to the early onset of multiorgan failure due to increased demand and decreased supply of oxygen [3, 4]. Several studies have highlighted that renal, hepatic, and hematological dysfunctions in patients with septic shock are associated with poor outcome [4–6]. The aim of the study is to identify the predictive factors of septic shock-induced increase of serum lipase and amylase and to assess and evaluate its prognostic impact.

Methods

Study design

We conducted a prospective observational study in the intensive care unit of King Hamad University Hospital (KHUH) between 1 October 2015 and 31 May 2016. The study was approved by the ethics committee of KHUH.

* Correspondence: anischaari2004@yahoo.fr
[1]Critical Care Department, King Hamad University Hospital, Al Muharaq, Bahrain
Full list of author information is available at the end of the article

Patients

All the adult patients admitted with septic shock were eligible for inclusion in the study. We excluded patients with previous pancreatic disease, those with history of alcohol abuse, and those with biliary tract infections. Septic shock was defined according to the third international definition for sepsis and septic shock [7]. Therefore, serum lactate level was checked on admission and Sequential Organ Failure Assessment (SOFA) score was calculated [8]. The Increase of pancreatic enzymes was defined by a serum amylase level higher than 85 UI/L and/or serum lipase level higher than 286 UI/L. The diagnosis of acute pancreatitis was considered if two criteria among the following were met: (1) abdominal pain, (2) increased serum pancreatic enzymes (higher than threefold the upper limit of the normal range), (3) imaging findings suggesting acute pancreatitis [9].

Data collection and protocol of the study

For all the included patients, we recorded demographic characteristics (age, gender, comorbidities), cause of admission to the ICU, clinical findings on admission to the ICU (systolic and diastolic blood pressure, heart rate), laboratory results on admission to the ICU (arterial lactate, complete blood cell count, C-reactive protein, procalcitonin, renal function tests), and therapeutic interventions during the ICU stay (mechanical ventilation, vasopressors, antibiotics, nutritional support, and continuous renal replacement therapy). The source of sepsis and the identified microorganisms were also recorded. The severity on admission was assessed by calculating the Acute Physiology and Chronic Health Evaluation II (APACHE (II)) score [10].

Pancreatic enzymes (serum amylase and lipase) were checked on admission. Patients with increased pancreatic enzymes underwent either abdominal ultrasound or contrast-enhanced abdominal computed tomography.

We also recorded the duration of mechanical ventilation, the length of ICU stay, and the outcome (death/survival).

Statistics

Data were expressed as percentages for the qualitative variables and means ± standard deviation (SD) or median [quartiles] as appropriate for the quantitative variables. Two groups were compared: those with increased pancreatic enzymes (increased pancreatic enzymes (+)) and those with normal pancreatic enzymes levels (increased pancreatic enzymes (−)). The normal distribution of the quantitative variables was checked by Shapiro-Wilk test. The qualitative variables were compared by using the chi-square test or Fisher's exact test as appropriate. The quantitative variables were compared by using t test or Mann-Whitney test as appropriate. All the factors identified by the univariate analysis as statistically associated to the increase of pancreatic enzymes were integrated in a stepwise multivariate analysis. Odds ratios (OR) were therefore calculated with the corresponding 95% confidence interval (95% CI)

Second, the sensitivity and the specificity of pancreatic enzymes in predicting ICU mortality were assessed by constructing the Receiver Operator Curves (ROC). The area under curve was calculated for each parameter with the respective 95% confidence interval.

Results

Baseline characteristics

Fifty patients were included in the study. Median [quartiles] age was 68.5 [58–81] years. Sex ratio (M/F) was 1.2. The APACHE (II) score calculated within the first 24 h was 26 [20–31]. Median SOFA score on admission was 7 [6–10]. Thirty patients (60%) were diabetic, and 32 patients (64%) have previous history of hypertension. On admission to the intensive care unit (ICU), median systolic blood pressure was 88.5 [77–106] mmHg and median diastolic blood pressure was 50 [40–60] mmHg. Median heart rate was 102 [76–120] beats per minute. The source of sepsis was pneumonia in 20 patients (40%), urinary tract infection in 11 patients (22%), soft tissue infection in 9 patients (18%), and abdominal infection in 10 patients (20%). Cultures were positive in 24 patients (48%). The identified microorganisms were gram-positive cocci in 5 patients (10%) and gram-negative bacilli in 19 patients (38%).

Pancreatic function

Twenty-three patients (46%) had increased serum amylase and/or serum lipase. Median serum amylase level was 61 [24—139] UI/L. Nineteen patients (38%) had increased serum amylase, and 7 patients (14%) had a serum level higher than 3 times the upper limit. Median serum lipase level was 147 [77–316] UI/L. Thirteen patients (26%) had increased serum lipase level, and 5 patients (10%) had a level higher than 3 times the upper limit. All patients with increased pancreatic enzymes underwent imaging tests. Abdominal computed tomography was performed for 6 patients (12%) whereas abdominal ultrasound was performed for 17 patients (34%). Only one patient (2%) was diagnosed as acute pancreatitis Balthazar B whereas all the other patients had unremarkable imaging investigations.

Management

All our patients required vasopressor support on admission to the ICU. Median norepinephrine dose was 0.4

Table 1 Comparison of the baseline characteristics between patients with and those without increased pancreatic enzymes

Parameters	Increased pancreatic enzymes (+) (N = 23)	Increased pancreatic enzymes (−) (N = 27)	p
Age (years [quartiles])	71 [60–82]	67 [57–79]	0.190
Gender (M/F)	13/10	14/13	0.714
Hypertension (N/%)	17/73.9	15/55.6	0.178
Diabetes mellitus (N/%)	18/78.3	12/44.4	0.015
APACHE (II) ([quartiles])	28 [25–33]	24 [19–29]	0.032
SOFA score ([quartiles])	9 [6–12.3]	6 [5–9]	0.100

APACHE (II) Acute Physiology and Chronic Health Evaluation II, *SOFA* Sequential Organ Failure Assessment

[0.1–1.5] microgram/kg/min. Median duration of norepinephrine infusion was 3 [2–5] days. Mechanical ventilation was started on admission to the ICU in 32 patients (64%). Median duration of mechanical ventilation was 5 [2–14] days. All of our patients were started on enteral feeding within the first 24 h of admission and none of them received parenteral nutrition. Continuous renal replacement therapy was required for 24 patients (48%) and was started within 2 [1–3] days after admission.

Predictive factors of sepsis-induced increase of pancreatic enzymes

Univariate analysis showed that the incidence of diabetes mellitus as a morbidity was significantly higher in increased pancreatic enzymes (+) group (78.3 versus 44.4%; $p = 0.015$). The APACHE (II) score was also significantly higher in this group of patients (Table 1). The analysis of the biological findings on admission showed that patients with increased pancreatic enzymes had significant increase in renal function tests and lower serum C-reactive protein level (Table 2).

In multivariate analysis, independent factors predicting sepsis-induced increase of pancreatic enzymes were diabetes mellitus (OR = 16; 95% CI [1.7–153.5]; $p = 0.016$), increased blood urea nitrogen (OR = 1.12; 95% CI [1.02–1.20]; $p = 0.016$), and decreased C-reactive protein (OR = 0.97; 95% CI [0.96–0.99]; $p = 0.027$) (Table 3).

Outcome and prognostic factors

Twenty patients (40%) died in the ICU. Median ICU length of stay was 6 [3–12] days. There was no statistically significant difference between survivors and non-survivors regarding the baseline characteristics except for the APACHE (II) score which was significantly higher in non-survivors group (Table 4). Moreover, the rate of patients requiring mechanical ventilation support and/or renal replacement therapy was significantly higher in the non-survivors group (Table 5). Laboratory findings were comparable between the two studied groups. Neither serum amylase level nor serum lipase level was significantly different between survivors and non-survivors (respectively 49 [27.7–106] versus 85.1 [20.1–165] UI/L; $p = 0.7$ and 165 [88–316] versus 120 [65.5–592] UI/L; $p = 0.952$). Both pancreatic enzymes had poor value to predict ICU mortality (Fig. 1).

Discussion

Our study shows that the increase of pancreatic enzymes is common in patients with septic shock. In fact, 46% of the included patients had increased serum amylase and/or lipase. Previous studies have reported that the incidence of exocrine pancreatic dysfunction in critically ill patients ranges between 14 and 80% [6, 11, 12]. This wide range is due to the underlying diseases as the highest levels were

Table 2 Comparison of the laboratory findings on admission between patients with and those without increased pancreatic enzymes

Parameters	Increased pancreatic enzymes (+) (N = 23)	Increased pancreatic enzymes (−) (N = 27)	p
Amylase (UI [quartiles])	153 [97.2–445]	26 [16.6–44.7]	0.029
Lipase (UI [quartiles])	337 [146–744]	101 [68.5–166.3]	0.027
Lactate (mmol/L [quartiles])	3.9 [2.5–5.3]	3.4 [2–4.1]	0.228
CRP (mg/L [quartiles])	114.5 [55.5–196.8]	217 [120.5–281]	0.017
Procalcitonin (ng/mL [quartiles])	38.8 [2.2–97.6]	5.1 [1.8–46.6]	0.575
BUN (mmol/L [quartiles])	16.9 [9–33]	11.1 [5.4–17.4]	0.038
Creatinine (µmol/L [quartiles])	204 [131.3–331.8]	146 [84–209]	0.038

CRP C-reactive protein, *BUN* blood urea nitrogen

Table 3 Multivariate analysis of factors predicting sepsis-related increase of pancreatic enzymes

Factors	OR	p	95% CI	
			Min	Max
APACHE (II)	1.10	0.182	0.90	1.20
Diabetes mellitus	16	0.016	1.70	153.50
C-reactive protein	0.97	0.027	0.96	0.99
Blood urea nitrogen	1.12	0.016	1.02	1.20
Creatinine	1	0.929	0.99	1.10

APACHE (II) Acute Physiology and Chronic Health Evaluation II

recorded in surgical and trauma patients [13, 14]. However, epidemiological data regarding pancreatic dysfunction in patients with septic shock are lacking.

The increase of pancreatic enzymes in critically ill patients is mainly due to ischemic insults induced by prolonged hypotension [11, 15]. In fact, experimental studies have shown that the pancreas is extremely sensitive to hypoxia and that peripheral lobule necrosis can occur within 40 min of hypotension [16].

Other factors such as the activation of the coagulation cascade, cellular apoptosis, oxidative stress, and disturbed lipid profile have been reported as possible causes of sepsis-related increase of pancreatic enzymes [6]. Therefore, the involvement of these factors in the physiopathology of pancreatic insult may explain the occurrence of this complication in patients without significant hemodynamic compromise [6, 17]. Our study also showed that the impairment of renal function was significantly associated with sepsis-related increase of pancreatic enzymes. Previous studies have reported that acute kidney injury is a common complication of acute pancreatitis [18, 19]. Hypertriglyceridemia has been reported as a major factor responsible of acute kidney injury [18, 19].

Second, our study showed that independent factors predicting sepsis-related increase of pancreatic enzymes are diabetes mellitus and acute kidney injury. Previous studies have reported that patients with type 2 diabetes mellitus have two- to threefold higher risk of acute pancreatitis [20–23]. This higher risk has been confirmed even after adjusting for confounding factors such as alcohol abuse and obesity [21, 22]. The underlying mechanisms are still not fully elucidated but may involve disturbed lipid metabolism or drug toxicity [23]. Our study also showed that increased renal function tests were significantly associated with increased pancreatic enzymes. Previous studies showed that acute kidney injury is common in patients with acute pancreatitis [18, 19]. Hypertriglyceridemia has been reported as a major cause of renal dysfunction in this group of patients [18, 19].

The multivariate analysis also revealed that decreased C-reactive protein independently predicts increased pancreatic enzymes. Available data assessing the usefulness of this biomarker in predicting pancreatic necrosis are scarce. However, a systematic review showed that C-reactive protein, as well as procalcitonin and lactate deshydrogenase, is not reliable to predict pancreatic injury [24]. Further studies are required to confirm the correlation between decreased CRP and increased pancreatic enzymes and to investigate the underlying mechanisms that might explain this relationship.

Whether the increase of pancreatic enzymes carries per se a negative prognostic value or not is still a matter of debate. Manjuck et al. [12] reported that the level of pancreatic enzymes was not correlated to the mortality. However, the ICU length of stay and the duration of mechanical ventilation were significantly higher in patients with increased pancreatic enzymes. Similarly, Subramanian et al. [14]

Table 4 Comparison of baseline characteristics between survivors and non-survivors

Parameters	Survivors (N = 30)	Non-survivors (N = 20)	p
Age (years [quartiles])	66.5 [56.8–79.8]	70.5 [61.8–81]	0.220
Gender (M/F)	16/14	11/9	0.910
Diabetes mellitus (N/%)	17/56.7	13/65	0.556
Hypertension (N/%)	18/60	14/70	0.470
APACHE (II) ([quartiles])	21 [16.8–29]	29.5 [27–33.5]	<0.001
Leucocytes (mm³ [quartiles])	11,820 [8740–17,375]	19,380 [8805–26,125]	0.060
Hemoglobin (g/dL [quartiles])	10.6 [8.6–12.5]	10.4 [8.4–12.2]	0.400
Platelets count (g/L [quartiles])	233.5 [163.3–376.8]	279 [158.3–435]	0.318
CRP (mg/L [quartiles])	146 [79.9–271]	174 [129–226.5]	0.795
Lactate (mmol/L [quartiles])	3.7 [2.5–5.1]	3.2 [2.2–4.1]	0.707

APACHE (II) Acute Physiology and Chronic Health Evaluation II, *CRP* C-reactive protein

Table 5 Comparison of the therapeutic management between survivors and non-survivors

Parameters	Survivors (N = 30)	Non-survivors (N = 20)	p
MV (N/%)	12/40	20/100	<0.001
Duration of MV (days [quartiles])	6 [2.3–18.8]	3.5 [2–12.5]	0.344
CRRT (N/%)	10/33.3	14/70	0.011
NE (N/%)	30/100	20/100	1
NE dose (mcg/kg/min [quartiles])	0.2 [0.09–0.42]	2 [0.7–2]	<0.001

MV mechanical ventilation, *CRRT* continuous renal replacement therapy, *NE* norepinephrine

reported that the level of serum lipase was positively correlated with the incidence of organ failure in critically ill trauma patients. In patients with septic shock, Pizzelli et al. [15] reported that all the 21 included patients had increased pancreatic enzymes but none of them had clinical or radiological abnormalities suggesting acute pancreatitis. Our results corroborate these findings as only one of our patients had confirmed acute pancreatitis.

To the best of our knowledge, our study is the first to identify the predictive factor of sepsis-induced increase of pancreatic enzymes and to assess its prognostic value. However, several limitations should be mentioned. First, our study has a small sample size. Second, the involvement of the renal impairment in the rise of pancreatic enzymes needs to be investigated. In fact, the increase of amylase and lipase in patients with acute kidney injury might be related to a delayed clearance of these enzymes.

In this regard, Seno et al. [25] compared in an observational study the serum level of 6 pancreatic markers between 2 groups: 47 patients with impaired renal function and 24 healthy individuals. The authors reported that the serum levels of total amylase, pancreatic isoamylase (p-amylase), lipase, phospholipase A2, and elastase I were at least within 2.5-fold the upper limits of the normal ranges in patients with renal impairment The level was even higher (within 4.8-fold the upper limit) for trypsin(ogen). Finally, the diagnosis of acute pancreatitis was based on the levels of serum amylase and lipase. It has been shown that lipase is more specific than amylase for accurate diagnosis of acute pancreatitis [9]. Moreover, the alpha amylase fraction is more specific of pancreatic injury than total amylase. Yet only total amylase was measured in our study [9].

Conclusion

The increase of pancreatic enzymes is common in patients with septic shock. Diabetes mellitus, increased urea, and low C-reactive protein independently predict raise in pancreatic enzyme. Our results suggest that such finding is not associated with worse outcome and therefore should not trigger any specific therapeutic intervention. Further studies are required to confirm our conclusions.

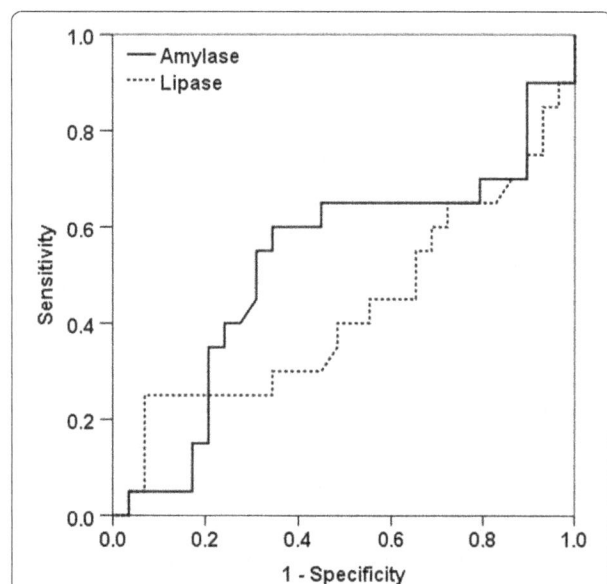

Fig. 1 ROC for sensitivity and specificity of serum amylase and serum lipase to predict ICU mortality. AUC for serum amylase 0.52 95% CI [0.35–0.7]. AUC for serum lipase 0.57 95% CI [0.40–0.74]. *ROC* Receiver Operator Curve, *AUC* area under curve, *CI* confidence interval

Abbreviations
APACHE (II): Acute Physiology and Chronic Health Evaluation II; BUN: Blood urea nitrogen; CI: Confidence interval; CRP: C-reactive protein; CRRT: Continuous renal replacement therapy; ICU: Intensive care unit; MV: Mechanical ventilation; NE: Norepinephrine; OR: Odds ratio; ROC: Receiver Operator Curve; SD: Standard deviation

Authors' contributions
All the authors equally contributed to the conception, data collection, statistical analysis, and drafting the manuscript. All the authors approved the final submitted version of the manuscript.

Acknowledgements
None.

Funding
None.

Competing interests
The authors declare that they have no competing interests.

Author details
[1]Critical Care Department, King Hamad University Hospital, Al Muharaq, Bahrain. [2]Gastroenterology Department, King Hamad University Hospital, Al Muharaq, Bahrain.

References
1. Angus DC, Linde-Zwirble WT, Lidicker J, Clermont G, Carcillo J, Pinsky MR. Epidemiology of severe sepsis in the United States: analysis of incidence, outcome, and associated costs of care. Crit Care Med. 2001;29(7):1303–10.
2. Annane D, Aegerter P, Jars-Guincestre MC, Guidet B. Current epidemiology of septic shock: the CUB-Rea Network. Am J Respir Crit Care Med. 2003; 168(2):165–72.
3. Angus DC, van der Poll T. Severe sepsis and septic shock. N Engl J Med. 2013;369(9):840–51.
4. Dellinger RP, Levy MM, Rhodes A, Annane D, Gerlach H, Opal SM, et al. Surviving sepsis campaign: international guidelines for management of severe sepsis and septic shock: 2012. Crit Care Med. 2013;41(2):580–637.
5. Honore PM, Jacobs R, Hendrickx I, Bagshaw SM, Joannes-Boyau O, Boer W, et al. Prevention and treatment of sepsis-induced acute kidney injury: an update. Ann Intensive Care. 2015;5(1):51.
6. Chaari A, Abdel Hakim K, Bousselmi K, Etman M, El Bahr M, El Saka A, et al. Pancreatic injury in patients with septic shock: a literature review. World J Gastrointest Oncol. 2016;8(7):526–31.
7. Singer M, Deutschman CS, Seymour CW, Shankar-Hari M, Annane D, Bauer M, et al. The Third International Consensus Definitions for Sepsis and Septic Shock (Sepsis-3). JAMA. 2016;315(8):801–10.
8. Vincent JL, Moreno R, Takala J, Willatts S, De Mendonça A, Bruining H, et al. The SOFA (Sepsis-related Organ Failure Assessment) score to describe organ dysfunction/failure. On behalf of the Working Group on Sepsis-Related Problems of the European Society of Intensive Care Medicine. Intensive Care Med. 1996;22(7):707–10.
9. Working Group IAPAPAAPG. IAP/APA evidence-based guidelines for the management of acute pancreatitis. Pancreatology. 2013;13(4 Suppl 2):e1–15.
10. Knaus WA, Draper EA, Wagner DP, Zimmerman JE. APACHE II: a severity of disease classification system. Crit Care Med. 1985;13(10):818–29.
11. Denz C, Siegel L, Lehmann KJ, Dagorn JC, Fiedler F. Is hyperlipasemia in critically ill patients of clinical importance? An observational CT study. Intensive Care Med. 2007;33(9):1633–6.
12. Manjuck J, Zein J, Carpati C, Astiz M. Clinical significance of increased lipase levels on admission to the ICU. Chest. 2005;127(1):246–50.
13. Takahashi M, Maemura K, Sawada Y, Yoshioka T, Sugimoto T. Hyperamylasemia in critically injured patients. J Trauma. 1980;20(11):951–5.
14. Subramanian A, Albert V, Mishra B, Sanoria S, Pandey RM. Association between the pancreatic enzyme level and organ failure in trauma patients. Trauma Mon. 2016;21(2), e20773.
15. Pezzilli R, Barassi A, Imbrogno A, Fabbri D, Pigna A, Morselli-Labate AM, Corinaldesi R, d'Eril GM. Is the pancreas affected in patients with septic shock?—a prospective study. Hepatobiliary Pancreat Dis Int. 2011;10(2):191–5.
16. Spormann H, Sokolowski A, Letko G. Effect of temporary ischemia upon development and histological patterns of acute pancreatitis in the rat. Pathol Res Pract. 1989;184(5):507–13.
17. Tribl B, Bateman RM, Milkovich S, Sibbald WJ, Ellis CG. Effect of nitric oxide on capillary hemodynamics and cell injury in the pancreas during Pseudomonas pneumonia-induced sepsis. Am J Physiol Heart Circ Physiol. 2004;286(1):H340–345.
18. Wu C, Ke L, Tong Z, Li B, Zou L, Li W, Li N, Li J. Hypertriglyceridemia is a risk factor for acute kidney injury in the early phase of acute pancreatitis. Pancreas. 2014;43(8):1312–6.
19. Nawaz H, Koutroumpakis E, Easler J, Slivka A, Whitcomb DC, Singh VP, et al. Elevated serum triglycerides are independently associated with persistent organ failure in acute pancreatitis. Am J Gastroenterol. 2015;110(10):1497–503.
20. Steinberg WM, Buse JB, Ghorbani MLM, Orsted DD, Nauck MA. Amylase, lipase, and acute pancreatitis in people with type 2 diabetes treated with liraglutide: results from the LEADER randomized trial. Diabetes care. 2017.
21. Girman CJ, Kou TD, Cai B, Alexander CM, O'Neill EA, Williams-Herman DE, Katz L. Patients with type 2 diabetes mellitus have higher risk for acute pancreatitis compared with those without diabetes. Diabetes Obes Metab. 2010;12(9):766–71.
22. Noel RA, Braun DK, Patterson RE, Bloomgren GL. Increased risk of acute pancreatitis and biliary disease observed in patients with type 2 diabetes: a retrospective cohort study. Diabetes care. 2009;32(5):834–8.
23. Urushihara H, Taketsuna M, Liu Y, Oda E, Nakamura M, Nishiuma S, et al. Increased risk of acute pancreatitis in patients with type 2 diabetes: an observational study using a Japanese hospital database. PloS one. 2012; 7(12), e53224.
24. Komolafe O, Pereira SP, Davidson BR, Gurusamy KS. Serum C-reactive protein, procalcitonin, and lactate dehydrogenase for the diagnosis of pancreatic necrosis. Cochrane Database Syst Rev. 2017;4, CD012645.
25. Seno T, Harada H, Ochi K, Tanaka J, Matsumoto S, Choudhury R, et al. Serum levels of six pancreatic enzymes as related to the degree of renal dysfunction. Am J Gastroenterol. 1995;90(11):2002–5.

Perspective on optimizing clinical trials in critical care: how to puzzle out recurrent failures

Bruno François[1,2]* , Marc Clavel[1], Philippe Vignon[1] and Pierre-François Laterre[3]

Abstract

Background: Critical care is a complex field of medicine, especially because of its diversity and unpredictability. Mortality rates of the diseases are usually high and patients are critically ill, admitted in emergency, and often have several overlapping diseases. This makes research in critical care also complex because of patients' conditions and because of the numerous ethical and regulatory requirements and increasing global competition. Many clinical trials in critical care have thus failed and almost no drug has yet been developed to treat intensive care unit (ICU) patients. Learning from the failures, clinical trials must now be optimized.

Main body: Several aspects can be improved, beginning with the design of studies that should take into account patients' diversity in the ICU. At the site level, selection should reflect more accurately the potential of recruitment. Management of all players that can be involved in the research at a site level should be a priority. Moreover, training should be offered to all staff members, including the youngest. National and international networks are also part of the future as they create a collective synergy potentially improving the efficacy of sites. Finally, computerization is another area that must be further developed with the appropriate tools.

Conclusion: Clinical research in the ICU is thus a discipline in its own right that still requires tailored approaches. Changes have to be initiated by the investigators themselves as they know all the specificities of the field.

Keywords: Clinical research, Intensive care unit, Trials, Ventilator-associated pneumonia, Investigation center, Performance

Background

Critical care is probably one of the most complex fields of medicine and has specific requirements. Severely ill patients who are hospitalized in the intensive care unit (ICU) require continuous monitoring and management and the presence of attending physicians 24/7, as opposed to most medical specialties with intermittent care [1]. Clinical research in the ICU setting is challenging because of an overall high mortality rate, the high number of healthcare workers including physicians with repeated rounds, the technological environment, and the unpredictable patients' course with potential sudden worsening of clinical status. In addition, ICU patients typically sustain life-threatening conditions with multiple organ failures and various underlying diseases. ICU admission is unpredictable and eligible patients present with various types of diseases, even in specialized ICUs (neurological, cardiovascular, trauma…).

Even if some ICU-specific diseases have been described such as sepsis, acute respiratory distress syndrome (ARDS) or ventilator-associated pneumonia (VAP), most of them remain identified as syndromes [2] with lack of specificity, as illustrated by regular updates of the definitions [3–5]. Accordingly, even when selected through strict inclusion/exclusion criteria within a trial, study population remains heterogeneous. Finally, ethical issues inherent to the severely ill patients include the discussion of care withdrawal in specific settings and the frequent inability of ICU patients to consent [6, 7].

Critical care is also a relatively recent field of medicine and even if a lot have been accomplished, as mentioned

---

* Correspondence: b.francois@unilim.fr
[1]Medical-surgical Intensive Care Unit, Dupuytren University Hospital, 2 avenue Martin Luther King, 87042 Limoges, France
[2]Inserm CIC 1435, Limoges University Hospital, Limoges, France
Full list of author information is available at the end of the article

by Takala, we are still in a learning phase for ICU-specific research development and especially for pharmaceutical-sponsored trials [8].

Accordingly, clinical trials have to be optimized both in terms of scientific approach and design. This perspective paper aims at understanding the current context of clinical trials in the ICU and its increasing difficulties and proposing solutions in terms of research organization and management.

Main text
Context
Increasing trial complexity
Within a decade, trial complexity has dramatically increased. In order to target the most appropriate study population, the inclusion/exclusion criteria have increased and become more precise (e.g., severity of sepsis and number and type of associated organ failures) [9]. This increased complexity associated with narrow time windows for patients' enrolment result in a time consuming and quite challenging screening process (Fig. 1). Pharmacokinetic explorations have also been added to most ICU randomized clinical trials (RCT). Finally, biomarkers are frequently used to better characterize the study population and increase the complexity of clinical research [10]. Some of them are commonly used, such as procalcitonin [11], but others such as HLA-DR result in a much more complex approach [12]. With the continuous progression of scientific knowledge, further complexity of future ICU clinical trials can be anticipated.

Increasing regulatory requirement
In order to address increasing safety concerns to protect the patients, strict regulations of clinical research have been developed. Between the last war when ethical rules have been proposed [13] and the early eighties, a few

regulatory texts have been written. The International Conference of Harmonization (ICH) [14] was the very first text to define a global regulatory approach (first presentation in April 1990 in Brussels). Good clinical practice (GCP) [15] is probably the best example of a universal regulatory requirement but remains the minimal standard to perform clinical research. In addition, legal requirements exist for each component of clinical research, especially in drug development trials, including data management, informed consent [16], biological sampling, case report form (CRF).... In some countries, national specificity still exists, such as the German *Bundesamt für Strahlenschutz* (Federal Office for Radiation Protection), a specific committee which evaluates the need of additional radiography or of CT scan prescription in clinical research projects to avoid useless detrimental radiation.

Thus, the regulatory work package has become central in clinical research and is often long to address, irrespective of the sponsor (academic or pharmaceutical). Because of its specificity, clinical research in critical care medicine has even more requirements since patients with life-threatening conditions are commonly unable to consent [17]. Emergency consent through legal representative or even waivers have been authorized to address this issue [18]. Agencies are currently paying particular attention to regulatory aspects with increasing control through audit or inspections [19], especially in high recruiting centers.

International competition
Clinical research has become an international competition and represents a strategic activity at a site level as well as at a country level [20]. Due to the financial investment required for the development of new drugs, there is a worldwide competition between pharmaceutical companies to obtain the leadership in specific medical fields. A similar

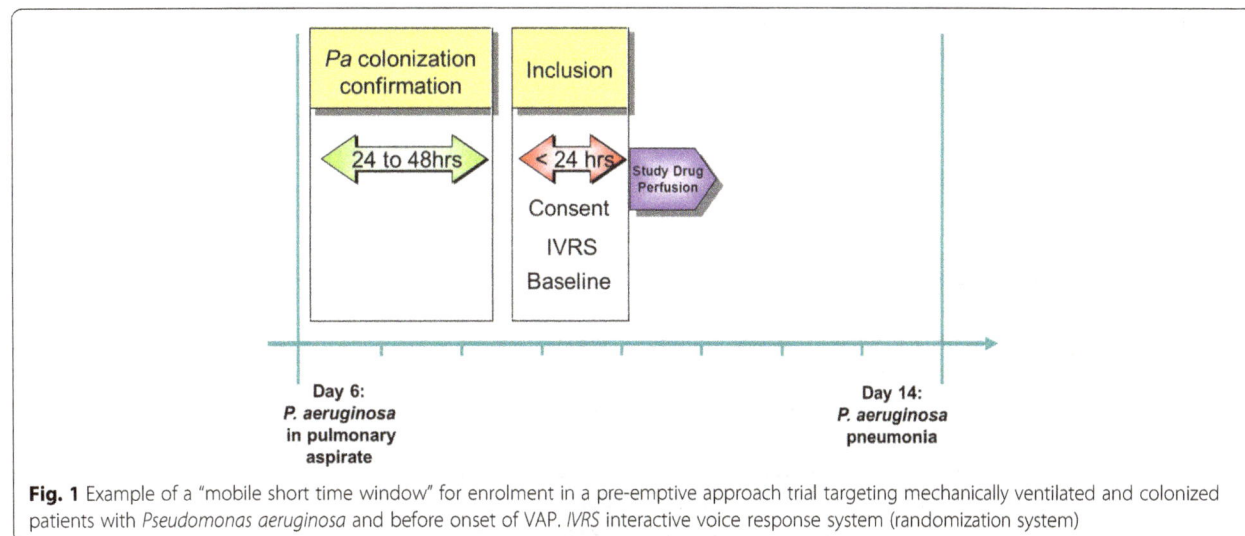

Fig. 1 Example of a "mobile short time window" for enrolment in a pre-emptive approach trial targeting mechanically ventilated and colonized patients with *Pseudomonas aeruginosa* and before onset of VAP. *IVRS* interactive voice response system (randomization system)

competition is observed in the academic area to become and remain a key player in clinical research and also because it constitutes a strong economic vector through allocated budgets, royalties, patents, grants.... While it was mostly a Northern American and Western European activity few decades ago, most of developed countries are now involved in clinical research. This increases the international competition to actively participate in RCTs, with some countries which are now offered to participate in research projects, or with a much lower number of sites. In pharmaceutical-sponsored trials, the competition is even initiated by the companies themselves or the clinical research organizations (CRO) to accelerate completion of the trial.

Inappropriate trial design resulting in absence of "ICU-specific" drug

Critical care remains one of the leading medical specialties in the conduction of pathophysiological and epidemiological studies and has validated several severity scoring systems [21, 22]. Nevertheless, and since Xigris® (Lilly, Indianapolis, IN) withdrawal, it is also one of the medical specialties in which most clinical trials have failed with nearly none or very few drugs specifically developed and validated for ICU patients [23] despite strong scientific rational and encouraging results on animal models. To date, the clinical phase of trials seems to be the main issue. Patients are included based on precise clinical criteria such as organ failure, but therapeutic criteria are not given enough attention. Moreover, monitoring of the drug activity and outcomes may not be sufficient to adequately evaluate the study drug. Diagnostic companions and biomarkers are thus needed to better assess new drugs as this weakness may have led to drop the development of appropriate molecules. In addition, the unmet medical need in critical care medicine is probably one of the most important when considering the high mortality rate of prevalent diseases leading to ICU admission even if a slight decrease have been recently evidenced in sepsis mortality [24]. Despite recurrent failure of RCTs testing the efficacy of new drugs, clinical trials are still designed to find the "golden success bullet," especially in the field of sepsis.

Proposed solutions
Scientific challenges to be addressed

How to learn from our failures Sepsis is a fascinating field in critical care medicine clinical research. After 25 years and >30,000 patients enrolled in successive clinical trials, not a single agent has yet been approved in this indication. The most recent RCTs were negative (e.g., TLR4 LPS antagonist) [25] or even early terminated (recombinant lactoferrin) despite strong scientific

rational and promising early phases. Similarly, ventilation strategies (e.g., low tidal volume, prone position) rather than specific drug development have been shown to be successful in ARDS [26, 27]. VAP might thus remain the most successful disease of critical care medicine in terms of drug development as several antibiotics have been validated in this indication [28, 29]. We need to understand the reasons for so many failures and how to puzzle them out. "Back to basics" remains a good approach since the understanding of pathophysiology has to be revisited before moving into clinical applications [30]. Results interpretation especially in early clinical phases should be less "emotional." Repeated phase II or II/III should also be encouraged in order to confirm results before implementing new drugs on clinical grounds [31].

When compared with oncology or even cardiology, most critical care diseases (VAP being one of the best examples) suffer from imprecise definition and lack of specific biomarkers. This results in heterogeneous study populations in which the demonstration of the efficacy and tolerance of a new drug or management strategy remains challenging. Accordingly, active research on specific biomarkers should be developed and once a biomarker is evidenced, it should be used as much as possible in the ICU setting to improve study population homogeneity [32]. Biomarkers can be considered as a diagnostic companion and part of the *theranostic* approach of a drug development.

Inclusion criteria must probably also be modified. As an example in sepsis trials, within a type of infection, different clinical phenotypes can exist depending on the pathogen (e.g., community-acquired pneumonia), and therefore, pathogen- or site-specific trials should be considered. Despite robust inclusion/exclusion criteria, large trials may also pool heterogeneous patients with limited discriminating data between subgroups with detrimental effects of studied drug. Accordingly, sample size could be redefined based on significance and on clinical relevance of endpoints.

It has also been demonstrated that the identification of eligible patients based on number of protocol violation improves in parallel with the number of patients enrolled in a trial. In some trials, violation of inclusion/exclusion criteria reached 20% in sites with low recruitment performance, whereas it fell to 5% in high recruiters. In fact, it seems that sites are following a research learning curve at every trial level [33].

Trial design (including personalized medicine) For a long time, placebo-controlled, double-blind, multicenter randomized trials have been considered as the gold standard of clinical research in the ICU with the dictatorship of the p value. ICU patients have numerous concomitant overlapping diseases, when compared to patients of other medical specialties [34]. Accordingly, proving the benefit of a unique drug or of a specific intervention becomes challenging and endpoints aside from mortality are always controversial as they remain less relevant. Nevertheless, the need for clinical trials in the ICU has never been so high since most of the standard of care remains based on bundles or low-grade recommendations with a high heterogeneity.

Therefore, time for innovative design is becoming a reality to be able to adapt our trials to critical care medicine. Adaptive design is an appealing approach. It enables to consider several interventions, pharmacological or not, at the same time and to eliminate the less relevant ones as patients are progressively enrolled [35]. In order to take into account inter-site variability, the cluster approach is also one methodological design to consider for the ICU setting. Even if critical care medicine remains far behind oncology for example, personalized medicine will probably be the most interesting paradigm shift in the coming years. Patients are not considered anymore as similar and homogenous within a specific disease. Accordingly, specific trial designs and approaches will have to be developed for critically ill patients. Some other interesting approaches might also be developed for rare diseases as those caused by multiresistant pathogen in the ICU. In this case, random trials comparing similar patients receiving drugs from different pharmaceutical companies could be the most innovative design.

Site selection

Even if the quality of the study protocol and of the tested intervention (drug, device, or other type of therapeutic approach) are probably the two most important factors to make a trial successful, research sites remain key players in patient recruitment. Therefore, particular attention should be paid to site selection. Even if it has improved over the past decade, it remains highly perfectible especially in the field of critical care medicine. The traditional 20/80 research rule in critical care medicine illustrates the weakness of research site selection. In most multicenter studies, some sites include many patients while other centers include only a few or even none. Thus, the majority of patients (around 80%) are recruited by the same sites (accounting for 20% of all the sites involved in the study). Site selection is frequently based on inaccurate investigators listing [36]. Some of these lists are issued by the sponsor for non-scientific reasons and include key opinion leaders not necessarily involved on clinical grounds. Most of the potential investigators are provided by the CROs based on previous collaborations but frequently these lists have not long been updated or are not even adapted to the

trial. Finally, some investigators can also be recommended by the principal investigator for personal reasons. Accordingly, optimization of trial delivery starts with a better site selection.

Feasibility process The feasibility process mainly based on declarative information is a key step in site selection [37]. Most of the feasibility questions remain focused on site resources, contracting, and GCP training and not on the actual recruitment capacity. In addition, items focused on the targeted population are usually vague asking the investigator for potential recruitment capacity. Investigators frequently overestimate their recruitment capacity in order to be selected, and CRO competition can also lead to further overestimation. Feasibility which is usually assessed far ahead in the selection process should specifically focus on: (1) actual recruitment capability and (2) prior performance of the site in the same topic of research. Actual recruitment capacity can be accurately estimated by recording retrospectively or prospectively over 1 or 2 months (or more in case of seasonality of the studied disease) the actual number of eligible patients based on inclusion and exclusion criteria. Each site should be able to record exhaustively all eligible patients for a trial project over a predefined period of time. This will improve the chance to successfully complete the trial but also guide the site in its decision to participate or not in the research project. Usually, investigators have a biased estimation of their patient flows when going through screening processes, since they commonly fail to take into account time window constraints or potential exclusion criteria. Prior performance is the second key factor for site selection. The ratio between the number of predicted enrollments and the number of patients finally included in a trial is a commonly used indicator to assess the recruitment performance of a research site. A site that was efficient in previous trials is probably well organized and has enough human resources to plug clinical research on routine patient flow. The last key factor is the absence of potential competing trials during the same period. However, if high recruitment capacity enables adequate conduction of competing trials, a local randomization table between trials is recommended to avoid any recruitment bias. Such an integrative approach will strengthen site selection and potentially allow reducing the number of sites needed to complete the trial.

Networking Networking may positively impact RCT delivery in critical care medicine. Since the development of multicenter RCTs, participating sites have developed informal networking. With the increasing requirements of clinical research, networking has become much more formal through charters in specific medical fields.

Networks have been progressively structured based on scientific collaborations and on synergy between research sites, sharing standard operating procedures and research tools to better reach common objectives. Among medical specialties, oncology is probably the most advanced in networking since most of RCTs are delivered through structured networks [38]. This approach makes trial process and delivery much more efficient and faster. Success is not only related to the active participation of all identified sites but also to the input of network coordinators and the collective synergy created by the network. Efficient networks have fully demonstrated their efficiency in the academic field of critical care medicine through the completion of numerous successful trials, including the ANZICS [39, 40] and ARDS networks [26]. In addition, well-structured network with a strong experience in pharmaceutical-sponsored trials may positively impact recruitment. As an example, CRICS, a French clinical research network, has contributed to 35% of the global recruitment of a very challenging sepsis phase II trial while representing only 15% of participating sites [41]. In addition to their recruitment capability, research networks may participate to the homogeneity of patient management through similar standard operating procedures. In addition, such network may facilitate the feasibility process when performing network-centralized feasibility. In the near future, networking will probably become a pillar of RCT optimization in critical care medicine. Accordingly, many countries are currently establishing clinical research network certifications.

Site management
Once site selection is performed, the optimization of trial recruitment also relies on site management. It has long been mainly based on principal investigators with little attention paid to their environment. Understanding that RCT must be considered as a team activity brings in light that local site management is another pillar of clinical research.

Study team management More than any other medical specialties, critical care medicine is based on a team activity for daily routine care. Regardless of the organization model, all staff members (physicians, fellows or residents, and nurses) are collectively in charge of patients, based on 24/7 shifts [1]. The same team approach has to be implemented in clinical research. Accordingly, all doctors and nurses should be involved in research activity, from patient enrollment to follow-up. Such as in oncology and hematology, all ICU care providers should incorporate clinical research as part of their daily routine care. Nevertheless, it is true that in many ICUs, physicians are overstrained with the routine

clinical practice and sometimes do not even have enough time to complete all essential tasks. Accordingly, different solutions can be proposed to address this challenge depending on local organization specificities. The easiest one is probably to have at least study nurses available 24/7 to help doctors with inclusions. A more global approach, such as a dedicated research physician on call, can be proposed at very experienced place with enough medical resources. A unique investigator cannot be fully efficient in the conduction of a research trial, even with the help of study coordinators. Every healthcare worker of the ICU has to be involved in the investigation activity to ensure research continuity. Therefore, before acceptance of any new protocol, a common agreement of all medical staff is needed. In order to ensure the motivation and commitment of all the staff, specific training must be developed at the site level. Communication is also a key factor within the team and research meetings should be encouraged on a regular basis. Study team management must result in a positive collaboration and encourage each staff member to be dedicated to the trial. Leadership is therefore needed since individual approaches may generate conflicting situations and negatively impact the study. The leader has to develop some strong management capability in order to achieve this goal.

Site interaction Regardless the type of ICU (surgical and/or medical, closed or open), they constitutively have transversal medical activities and receive patients from various clinical settings with a large panel of diseases. Accordingly, patient care requires interaction with numerous physicians and consultants but also easy and continuous access to technical platforms such as biology, microbiology, or radiology [42]. Thus, to ensure the appropriate participation of all these persons in clinical research, specific site interactions have to be developed through standard operating procedures. For example, close interactions with the microbiology department is crucial for sepsis or VAP trials. Indeed, most of the ICU trials on infectious diseases require microbiological availability at least 7/7, sometimes 24/7, using real-time techniques such as polymerase chain reaction. Involvement and valorization of these collaborators must be strengthened for a specific study but also more continuously with true interaction, routine common meeting, specific communications…. Pharmacy is another key actor of RCTs that has to work hand in hand with the ICU investigators and must not be considered as a simple "drug provider" [43]. At the ICU level, research is generally delivered by the study team including investigators, study nurses, and study coordinators. Nevertheless, interaction with the bedside nurses is key, these latter being patients' main interlocutors and so potentially considered as a relay at bedside to ensure good implementation of the study. Finally, collaboration with all other hospital departments involved in intra-hospital patient course is essential to ensure full commitment to the clinical research activity. It is important for the recruitment period but also for patient follow-up (including diagnosis of adverse events for example) when they are discharged from ICU. For research in critical care medicine, the emergency department from where many patients are referred to the ICU is probably one of the most important partners. It takes often years to develop strong hospital interaction but every players inside or outside the ICU should be considered as a potential study team member or at least part of the research activity. Conflicting situations can result in absence of such fruitful collaboration.

Recruitment strategy

Recruitment is a potential area of optimization of RCTs [44]. Despite robust pre-study calculation and estimation of study population size, under-recruitment remains an important issue in trials conducted in ICU setting. For decades, the recruitment rate of most participating centers to therapeutic trials in critical care medicine has remained fairly low without true learning from failures and efficient corrective actions. The fact that patient flow is fully unpredictable in the ICU even during closed hours may partially explain enrolment difficulties. Nevertheless, some sites are used to respect their commitment regardless their size while some other frequently overestimate their recruitment capacity, demonstrating that recruitment strategy is probably one piece of the puzzle of success [45]. This strategy must be general at the site level including involvement of every ICU physicians participating in patient care, systematic screening upon admission and during ICU stay, "helping resources" 24/7 making investigator life easier, screening binders for all trials...It has also to be study specific and recruitment capability should be carefully evaluated since the very beginning of the project (see feasibility paragraph). Thus, for every new trial, special attention should be paid to identify the key determinant of recruitment based on inclusion/exclusion criteria and where and when patients will be into the eligibility target, in order to set up specific study recruitment organization.

Quality of recruitment can also be improved and the use of a clinical coordinating center (CCC) can be one of the most efficient solutions. The function of a CCC is to facilitate testing of new interventions, develop high-quality protocols for the conduct of phase II and phase III clinical trials, generate consistent interpretation of enrolment criteria, and ultimately allow the strict respect of research protocols [46]. It is currently widely used in ICU trials.

While clinical research has greatly improved in the past decades in the ICU, recruitment may remain the most perfectible weak point and sites should work on specific strategies.

Tools development

Over the last 20 years, ICU took benefit of the technological revolution with a very large use of computerized and monitoring systems. Clinical research has incorporated these changes from generalization of eCRF to trial management system through centralized and computerized randomization systems. Nevertheless, very little has been made to "computerize" investigation and to develop tools facilitating investigators tasks. Optimization of RCT can start with the integration of all study specificities (e.g., drug traceability or specific biological sampling) in the computerized medical record and monitoring system. Nevertheless, some more practical instruments can be developed especially for patient screening, such as lab alerts plugged on the hospital biology results, automated notification systems for potential patients [47] or even screening tools (Fig. 2) that help the investigator at bedside but also confirm patient eligibility. After patient enrollment, schedule of event of ICU trials is usually cumbersome with very precise timing and follow-up 24/7. Accordingly, development of scheduling tools for bedside nurses can make acceptance of research easier but also avoid any omission or delay that could be harmful to both the patient and the trial (Fig. 3). For the long-term follow-up (sometimes 1 year) which is currently commonly required in trials, helping tracking tools with automatic reminder can also be developed in order not to miss any visit and avoid as much as possible loss of follow-up. This computerized approach will undoubtedly blow up in the coming years with pocket system or even with applications directly developed for smartphones [48].

Big data and bioinformatics

As stated previously, ICUs have now implemented many computerized and monitoring systems producing a huge quantity of data. To date, the data are mainly collected for patient routine care or for a specific purpose such as a trial and are not used "outside." This is progressively changing and big data is currently being implemented at patients' bedside and in clinical research. For example, "fused parametric measures" are routinely used to determine the level of severity [49]. In clinical trials, "pooled trial data" seems to be an inevitable evolution that might be very useful in the future. Datasets from existing clinical trials would be pooled to perform secondary analysis in order to acquire new knowledge or reveal trends that would have been missed in smaller datasets [50]. Pooled data could also be used to design the studies, for example to calculate more accurately the sample size or to identify the current problems that cause failure. Finally, big data

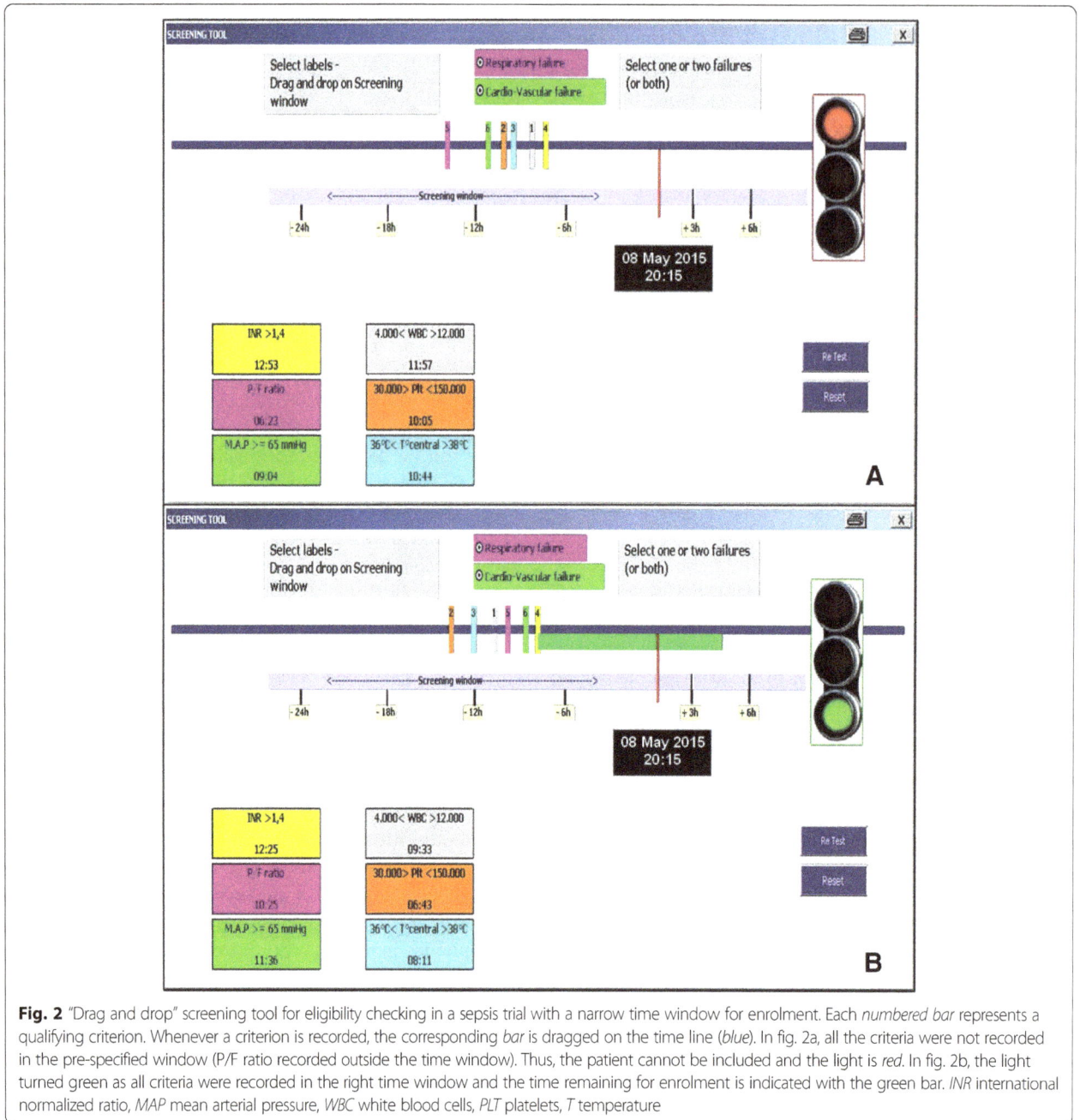

Fig. 2 "Drag and drop" screening tool for eligibility checking in a sepsis trial with a narrow time window for enrolment. Each *numbered bar* represents a qualifying criterion. Whenever a criterion is recorded, the corresponding *bar* is dragged on the time line (*blue*). In fig. 2a, all the criteria were not recorded in the pre-specified window (P/F ratio recorded outside the time window). Thus, the patient cannot be included and the light is *red*. In fig. 2b, the light turned green as all criteria were recorded in the right time window and the time remaining for enrolment is indicated with the green bar. *INR* international normalized ratio, *MAP* mean arterial pressure, *WBC* white blood cells, *PLT* platelets, *T* temperature

could also be implemented directly in the process of drug discovery. In oncology, this aspect is currently being investigated as physiologic information from national databases are compared to treatment information in order to connect specific phenotypes to molecular activity [51]. To date, the major limitation to big data implementation is the absence of ethical and legal context but some guidelines are already being published [50].

Training

In most of countries, physicians do not receive specific clinical research training during their medical training. Usually,

physicians start with basic science and sometimes move to clinical investigation mainly when they join a department participating in RCTs [52]. Most of the training is usually acquired through e-learning provided by pharmaceutical sponsors or CROs and mainly focused on GCP. Although GCPs are widely considered the standard background for participating in RCTs, it only covers a few aspects of clinical research. Thus, most of the investigators, especially in pharmaceutical-sponsored RCTs, are only involved in recruitment with little participation in the rest of the trial. In order to optimize the conduction and completion of clinical trials, physicians have to become more than "simple

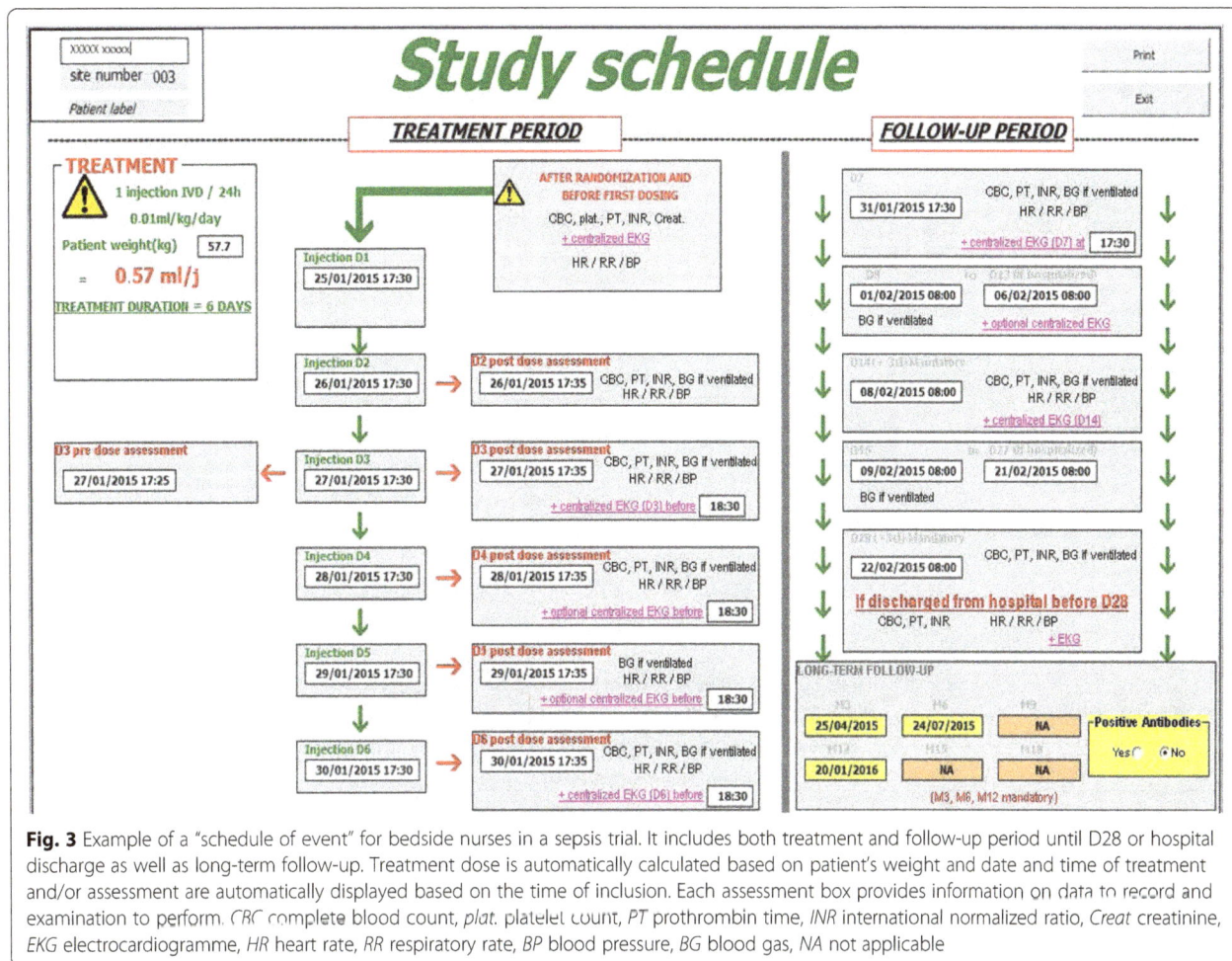

Fig. 3 Example of a "schedule of event" for bedside nurses in a sepsis trial. It includes both treatment and follow-up period until D28 or hospital discharge as well as long-term follow-up. Treatment dose is automatically calculated based on patient's weight and date and time of treatment and/or assessment are automatically displayed based on the time of inclusion. Each assessment box provides information on data to record and examination to perform. *CBC* complete blood count, *plat.* platelet count, *PT* prothrombin time, *INR* international normalized ratio, *Creat* creatinine, *EKG* electrocardiogramme, *HR* heart rate, *RR* respiratory rate, *BP* blood pressure, *BG* blood gas, *NA* not applicable

investigators" through specific training course, visiting all aspects of clinical research including methodology, trial management, pharmacovigilance, monitoring, audit, drug supplying, CRF... A perfect knowledge and understanding of clinical research will take part in the necessary professionalization of this activity. This training should become part of the medical studies but in the meantime, training of all the human resources of investigation sites is key, involving the physicians but also the nurses and other staff members that have usually less medical expertise.

Defining new collaborations with pharmaceutical companies

Since a long time, clinical investigation with pharmaceutical companies has been developed through site sub-contracting processes. Investigators are usually not involved in the trial design or management; most of these responsibilities being held by the steering committee and CROs are usually responsible for the overall trial management on behalf of the sponsor. This model should probably be revised, especially in the ICU setting

because of its huge specificity with a deeper participation of academic investigators in trial design, set-up of different committees, and trial management [53]. This would create a more collaborative research environment and increase site commitment. This paradigm shift is necessary in a period when lots of ICU professionals complain about trial realization. It could participate undoubtedly in a general improvement of RCT delivery. Some innovative experiences are currently developed in different countries and especially in Europe with the IMI collaboration [54] but also in the USA.

Comprehensive approach

From now on, clinical research in the ICU should not be any more considered as a stand-alone activity on top of routine patient care when people are available. The true change to perform to improve clinical research is to have a comprehensive approach, as it becomes part of patient care like in Oncology, and is not only an optional activity. While for years, treatment approaches have been very heterogeneous from site to site, standardization has started few

Table 1 Summary of issues identified and proposed solutions

Issues identified	Potential consequences for the study	Proposed solutions
Weakness of definitions of ICU diseases	Difficult to demonstrate trial and/or drug efficacy	Increase basic research, for example, on biomarkers
Current trial designs unadapted to ICU specificities	Lower impact of results and efficacy of trial	Adaptive design Personalized medicine
80 % of patients recruited by 20 % of sites	Possible bias, center effect	Improved site selection
Overestimation of recruitment capacity	Recruitment objectives not met, study closed	More precise calculation of recruitment capacity Evaluation of prior performance
Competing trials not considered during feasibility	Patients eligible for several studies	Tracking tables of all studies even potential
Caregivers not involved in research	Possible bias due to lack of information	Involvement of every member of the unit
Numerous players	Confusion, delay or lack of information	Standard operating procedures with different units Regular meetings
Under recruitment	Study closed for lack of patients	Research team available 24/7 Systematic screening procedures Clinical coordinating center
Complex and tight schedule of events	Missing data, delay	Computerized medical records Automatic alerts for results or treatment
Long-term follow-up of patients	Many patients lost to follow-up	Tracking tables with reminders
Lack of training for physicians	Physicians do not feel involved	Training included as soon as medical studies Specific training courses
Lack of involvement of investigators in pharmaceutical-sponsored trials	Design unadapted to ICU research Investigators do no feel involved	Involvement of physicians since the beginning of the process
Clinical research still considered as a stand-alone activity	Cares and treatments competing with routine	Clinical research implemented as part of routine care

years ago and nowadays, critical care medicine benefits from several international treatment recommendations, the most popular being the Surviving Sepsis Campaign [55]. In the meantime, a lot of universal definitions for the ICU-specific diseases have been validated, for care and research purposes. As an example, in 1992, the American College of Chest Physicians/Society of Critical Care Medicine Consensus Conference issued definitions regarding sepsis and the use of innovative therapies [3]; the Food and Drug Administration (FDA) has published recommendations and definition for VAP trials [56]. Accordingly, for sepsis and VAP, every patient wherever treated in the world should receive standard treatment and systematically be considered for eligibility in RCTs to potentially improve outcome and fill national and international database like for cancer [57] or cardiology patients. Continuous results from RCTs for these ICU topics with epidemiological prospective information will not only help understanding the diseases but also improve their management and thus outcome. Nevertheless, this requires a complete revolution at the site level in order to make clinical research part of routine care involving all staff members from the secretary to the physicians and the nurses. This is not an easy milestone in the ICU setting, its intrinsic specificities (emergency, life-threatening condition, ethical issues, number of players...) pushing back against it.

The problems identified and the potential solutions are summed up in Table 1.

Conclusions
Clinical research has become a true activity that not only provides new medical knowledge or brings validation of new drugs but also improves patient care through very high standard of quality and rigorous delivery. Because of its increasing requirements, it needs a global approach made of various competencies and professionalization. In this environment, ICU remains a very unique medical field with numerous specificities related to the type of admitted patients and to the 24/7 medical activity. This requires developing specific and optimized approach for clinical research in critical care medicine to create its own identity. The investigators have to make themselves the leaders of this transformation. Time for paradigm shift in clinical research in the ICU has come.

Abbreviations
ARDS: Acute respiratory distress syndrome; CCC: Clinical coordinating center; CRF: Case report form; CRO: Clinical research organization; FDA: Food and Drug Administration; GCP: Good clinical practice; ICH: International Harmonization Conference; ICU: Intensive care unit; RCT: Randomized clinical trial; VAP: Ventilator-associated pneumonia

Acknowledgements
The authors would like to thank Sarah Demai who provided medical writing services.

Funding
None.

Authors' contribution

BF drafted the manuscript. MC, PV, and PFL reviewed the manuscript. All authors read and approved the final manuscript.

Competing interests

The authors declare that they have no competing interests.

Author details

[1]Medical-surgical Intensive Care Unit, Dupuytren University Hospital, 2 avenue Martin Luther King, 87042 Limoges, France. [2]Inserm CIC 1435, Limoges University Hospital, Limoges, France. [3]Medical-surgical Intensive Care Unit, Cliniques Saint-Luc, Brussels, Belgium.

References

1. Ali NA, Hammersley J, Hoffmann SP, O'Brien Jr JM, Phillips GS, Rashkin M, et al. Continuity of care in intensive care units. A cluster-randomized trial of intensivist staffing. Am J Respir Crit Care Med. 2011;184(7):803–8.
2. Singh JM, Ferguson ND. Better infrastructure for critical care trials: nomenclature, etymology, and informatics. Crit Care Med. 2009;37 Suppl 1:S173–7.
3. Bone RC, Balk RA, Cerra FB, Dellinger RP, Fein AM, Knaus WA, et al. Definitions for sepsis and organ failure and guidelines for the use of innovative therapies in sepsis. The ACCP/SCCM Consensus Conference Committee. American College of Chest Physicians/Society of Critical Care Medicine. Chest. 1992;101(6):1644–55.
4. Levy MM, Fink MP, Marshall JC, Abraham E, Angus D, Cook D, Cohen J, Opal SM, Vincent JL, Ramsay G. SCCM/ESICM/ACCP/ATS/SIS. 2001 SCCM/ESICM/ ACCP/ATS/SIS International Sepsis Definitions Conference. Crit Care Med. 2003;31(4):1250–6.
5. Singer M, Deutschman CS, Seymour CW, Shankar-Hari M, Annane D, Bauer M, Bellomo R, Bernard GR, Chiche JD, Coopersmith CM, Hotchkiss RS, Levy MM, Marshall JC, Martin GS, Opal SM, Rubenfeld GD, van der Poll T, Vincent JL, Angus DC. The Third International Consensus Definitions for Sepsis and Septic Shock (Sepsis-3). JAMA. 2016;315(8):801–10.
6. Silverman HJ, Luce JM, Schwartz J. Protecting subjects with decisional impairment in research: the need for a multifaceted approach. Am J Respir Crit Care Med. 2004;169(1):10–4.
7. Luce JM, Cook DJ, Martin TR, Angus DC, Boushey HA, Curtis JR, et al. The ethical conduct of clinical research involving critically ill patients in the United States and Canada: principles and recommendations. Am J Respir Crit Care Med. 2004;170(12):1375–84.
8. Takala J. Better conduct of clinical trials: the control group in critical care trials. Crit Care Med. 2009;37 Suppl 1:S80–90.
9. Trzeciak S, Zanotti-Cavazzoni S, Parrillo JE, Dellinger RP. Inclusion criteria for clinical trials in sepsis. Did the American College of Chest Physicians/Society of Critical Care Medicine Consensus Conference definitions of sepsis have an impact? Chest. 2005;127:242–5.
10. Woodruff PG. Novel outcomes and endpoints. Biomarkers in chronic obstructive pulmonary disease clinical trials. Proc Am Thorac Soc. 2011;8:350–5.
11. Christ-Crain M, Jaccard-Stolz D, Bingisser R, Gencay MM, Huber PR, Tamm M, et al. Effect of procalcitonin-guided treatment on antibiotic use and outcome in lower respiratory tract infections: cluster-randomised, single-blinded intervention trial. Lancet. 2004;363(9409):600–7.
12. Meisel C, Schefold JC, Pschowski R, Baumann T, Hetzger K, Gregor J, et al. Granulocyte-macrophage colony-stimulating factor to reverse sepsis-associated immuno-suppression: a double-blind, randomized, placebo-controlled multicenter trial. Am J Respir Crit Care Med. 2009;180(7):640–8.
13. Rickham PP. Human experimentation. Code of ethics of the World Medical Association. Declaration of Helsinki. Br Med J. 1964;2(5402):177.
14. D'Arcy PF, Harron DWG. Proceedings of the First International Conference on Harmonisation. Belfast: Queen's University of Belfast; 1991.
15. ICH Expert Working Group. Guideline for good clinical practice E6(R1). In: International Conference on Harmonisation of technical requirements for registration of pharmaceuticals for human use. 1996
16. Grady C. Enduring and emerging challenges of informed consent. N Engl J Med. 2015;372(9):855–62.
17. Truog RD. Will ethical requirements bring critical care research to a halt? Intensive Care Med. 2005;31(3):338–44.
18. Asfar P, Meziani F, Hamel JF, Grelon F, Megarbane B, Anguel N, et al. High versus low blood-pressure target in patients with septic shock. N Engl J Med. 2014;370(17):1583–9.
19. European Medicines Agency. http://www.ema.europa.eu/ema/index. jsp?curl=pages/regulation/general/general_content_000161.jsp&mid= WC0b01ac0580024592. Accessed 19 Jul 2016.
20. Vincent JL. Logistics of large international trials: the good, the bad, and the ugly. Crit Care Med. 2009;37 Suppl 1:S75–9.
21. Le Gall JR, Lemeshow S, Saulnier F. A new Simplified Acute Physiology Score (SAPS II) based on a European/North American multicenter study. JAMA. 1993;270(24):2957–63.
22. Vincent JL, Moreno R, Takala J, Willatts S, De Mendonça A, Bruining H, et al. The SOFA (Sepsis-related Organ Failure Assessment) score to describe organ dysfunction/failure. On behalf of the Working Group on Sepsis-Related Problems of the European Society of Intensive Care Medicine. Intensive Care Med. 1996;22(7):707–10.
23. Opal SM, Patrozou E. Translational research in the development of novel sepsis therapeutics: logical deductive reasoning or mission impossible? Crit Care Med. 2009;37(1):S10–5.
24. Boucher HW, Talbot GH, Bradley JS, Edwards JE, Gilbert D, Rice LB, et al. Bad bugs, no drugs: no ESKAPE! An update from the Infectious Diseases Society of America. Clin Infect Dis. 2009;48(1):1–12.
25. Opal SM, Laterre PF, Francois B, LaRosa SP, Angus DC, Mira JP, et al. Effect of eritoran, an antagonist of MD2-TLR4, on mortality in patients with severe sepsis: the ACCESS randomized trial. JAMA. 2013;309(11):1154–62.
26. Network ARDS. Ventilation with lower tidal volumes as compared with traditional tidal volumes for acute lung injury and the acute respiratory distress syndrome. N Engl J Med. 2000;342(18):1301–8.
27. Guérin C, Reignier J, Richard JC, Beuret P, Gacouin A, Boulain T, et al. Prone positioning in severe acute respiratory distress syndrome. N Engl J Med. 2013;368(23):2159–68.
28. Corey GR, Kollef MH, Shorr AF, Rubinstein E, Stryjewski ME, Hopkins A, Barriere SL. Telavancin for hospital-acquired pneumonia: clinical response and 28-day survival. Antimicrob Agents Chemother. 2014;58(4):2030–7.
29. American Thoracic Society; Infectious Diseases Society of America. Guidelines for the management of adults with hospital-acquired, ventilator-associated, and healthcare-associated pneumonia. Am J Respir Crit Care Med. 2005;171(4):388–416.
30. Arnold DM, Burns KE, Adhikari NK, Kho ME, Meade MO, Cook DJ, et al. The design and interpretation of pilot trials in clinical research in critical care. Crit Care Med. 2009;37 Suppl 1:S69–74.
31. Reade MC, Angus DC. The clinical research enterprise in critical care: what's right, what's wrong, and what's ahead? Crit Care Med. 2009;37 Suppl 1:S1–9.
32. Kibe S, Adams K, Barlow G. Diagnostic and prognostic biomarkers of sepsis in critical care. J Antimicrob Chemother. 2011;66 Suppl 2:ii33–40.
33. Macias WL, Vallet B, Bernard GR, Vincent JL, Laterre PF, Nelson DR, et al. Sources of variability on the estimate of treatment effect in the PROWESS trial: implications for the design and conduct of future studies in severe sepsis. Crit Care Med. 2004;32(12):2385–91.
34. Silverman HJ, Miller FG. Control group selection in critical care randomized controlled trials evaluating interventional strategies: an ethical assessment. Crit Care Med. 2004;32(3):852–7.
35. Lewis RJ, Viele K, Broglio K, Berry SM, Jones AE. An adaptive, phase II, dose-finding clinical trial design to evaluate L-carnitine in the treatment of septic shock based on efficacy and predictive probability of subsequent phase III success. Crit Care Med. 2013;41(7):1674–8.
36. Gehring M, Taylor RS, Mellody M, Casteels B, Piazzi A, Gensini G, et al. Factors influencing clinical trial site selection in Europe: the Survey of Attitudes towards Trial sites in Europe (the SAT-EU Study). BMJ Open. 2013;3(11):e002957.
37. Wyse RKH. Feasibility studies. In: Ross C, editor. Accelerating patient recruitment in clinicals trials. Oxford: Network Pharma Ltd; 2006. p. 11.
38. Stahel R, Bogaerts J, Ciardiello F, de Ruysscher D. Dubsky P5 Ducreux M, et al. Optimising translational oncology in clinical practice: strategies to accelerate progress in drug development. Cancer Treat Rev. 2015;41(2):129–35.

39. Investigators ARISE, Clinical Trials Group ANZICS, Peake SL, Delaney A, Bailey M, Bellomo R, et al. Goal-directed resuscitation for patients with early septic shock. N Engl J Med. 2014;371(16):1496–506.

40. Doig GS, Simpson F, Sweetman EA, Finfer SR, Cooper DJ, Heighes PT, et al. Early parenteral nutrition in critically ill patients with short-term relative contraindications to early enteral nutrition: a randomized controlled trial. JAMA. 2013;309(20):2130–8.

41. Bernard GR, François B, Mira JP, Vincent JL, Dellinger RP, Russell JA, et al. Evaluating the efficacy and safety of two doses of AZD9773 in adult patients with severe sepsis and/or septic shock: randomized, double-blind, placebo-controlled Phase IIb study. Crit Care Med. 2014;42(3):504–11.

42. Deutschman CS, Ahrens T, Cairns CB, Sessler CN, Parsons PE. Critical Care Societies Collaborative/USCIITG Task Force on Critical Care Research. Multisociety task force for critical care research: key issues and recommendations. Chest. 2012;141(1):201–9.

43. Perreault MM, Thiboutot Z, Burry LD, Rose L, Kanji S, LeBlanc JM, et al. Canadian survey of critical care pharmacists' views and involvement in clinical research. Ann Pharmacother. 2012;46(9):1167–73.

44. Burns KE, Zubrinich C, Tan W, Raptis S, Xiong W, Smith O, et al. Research recruitment practices and critically ill patients. A multicenter, cross-sectional study (the Consent Study). Am J Respir Crit Care Med. 2013;187(11):1212–8.

45. Cook DJ, Blythe D, Rischbieth A, Hebert PC, Zytaruk N, Menon K, et al. Enrollment of intensive care unit patients into clinical studies: a trinational survey of researchers' experiences, beliefs, and practices. Crit Care Med. 2008;36(7):2100–5.

46. Sutton-Tyrrell K, Crow S, Hankin B, Trudel J, Faille C. Communication during the recruitment phase of a multicenter trial: the recruitment hotline. Control Clin Trials. 1996;17(5):415–22.

47. Weiner DL, Butte AJ, Hibberd PL, Fleisher GR. Computerized recruiting for clinical trials in real time. Ann Emerg Med. 2003;41(2):242–6.

48. Ozdalga E, Ozdalga A, Ahuja N. The smartphone in medicine: a review of current and potential use among physicians and students. J Med Internet Res. 2012;14(5):e128.

49. Pinsky MR, Dubrawski A. Gleaning knowledge from data in the intensive care unit. Am J Respir Crit Care Med. 2014;190(6):606–10.

50. Docherty AB, Lone NI. Exploiting big data for critical care research. Curr Opin Crit Care. 2015;21:467–72.

51. Taglang G, Jackson DB. Use of "big data" in drug discovery and clinical trials. Gyn Oncol. 2016;141:17–23.

52. Speicher LA, Fromell G, Avery S, Brassil D, Carlson L, Stevens E, et al. The critical need for academic health centers to assess the training, support, and career development requirements of clinical research coordinators: recommendations from the Clinical and Translational Science Award Research Coordinator Taskforce. Clin Transl Sci. 2012;5(6):470–5.

53. Cook D, Brower R, Cooper J, Brochard L, Vincent JL. Multicenter clinical research in adult critical care. Crit Care Med. 2002;30(7):1636–43.

54. Press Release Database. European Commission: a public-private research initiative to boost the competitiveness of Europe's pharmaceutical industry. 30 April 2008. http://europa.eu/rapid/press-release_IP-08-662_en.htm?locale=en. Accessed 15 May 2015.

55. Casserly B, Gerlach H, Phillips GS, Marshall JC, Lemeshow S, Levy MM. Evaluating the use of recombinant human activated protein C in adult severe sepsis: results of the Surviving Sepsis Campaign. Crit Care Med. 2012;40(5):1417–26.

56. U.S. Department of Health and Human Services, Food and Drug Administration, Center for Drug Evaluation and Research (CDER). Guidance for industry hospital-acquired bacterial pneumonia and ventilator-associated bacterial pneumonia: developing drugs for treatment. 2014.

57. Huang J, Ahmad U, Antonicelli A, Catlin AC, Fang W, Gomez D, et al. Development of the international thymic malignancy interest group international database: an unprecedented resource for the study of a rare group of tumors. J Thorac Oncol. 2014;9(10):1573–8.

Long-term recovery following critical illness in an Australian cohort

Kimberley J. Haines[1,2]* iD, Sue Berney[3], Stephen Warrillow[4] and Linda Denehy[2]

Abstract

Background: Almost all data on 5-year outcomes for critical care survivors come from North America and Europe. The aim of this study was to investigate long-term mortality, physical function, psychological outcomes and health-related quality of life in a mixed intensive care unit cohort in Australia.

Methods: This longitudinal study evaluated 4- to 5-year outcomes. Physical function (six-minute walk test) and health-related quality of life (Short Form 36 Version 2) were compared to 1-year outcomes and population norms. New psychological data (Center for Epidemiological Studies–Depression, Impact of Events Scale) was collected at follow-up.

Results: Of the 150 participants, 66 (44%) patients were deceased by follow-up. Fifty-six survivors were included with a mean (SD) age of 64 (14.2). Survivors' mean (SD) six-minute walk distance increased between 1 and 4 to 5 years (465.8 m (148.9) vs. 507.5 m (118.2)) (mean difference = − 24.5 m, CI − 58.3, 9.2, $p = 0.15$). Depressive symptoms were low: median (IQR) score of 7.0 (1.0–15.0). The mean level of post-traumatic stress symptoms was low—median (IQR) score of 1.0 (0–11.0)—with only 9 (16%) above the threshold for potentially disordered symptoms. Short-Form 36 Physical and Mental Component Scores did not change between 1 and 4 to 5 years (46.4 (7.9) vs. 46.7 (8.1) and 48.8 (13) vs. 48.8 (11.1)) and were within a standard deviation of normal.

Conclusions: Outcomes of critical illness are not uniform across nations. Mortality was increased in this cohort; however, survivors achieved a high level of recovery for physical function and health-related quality of life with low psychological morbidity at follow-up.

Keywords: Critical illness, Long-term outcomes

Background

Survivorship is the defining challenge of the twenty-first century in critical care [1] with increasing numbers of survivors experiencing new or worsened morbidity following critical illness [2, 3]. Attention has therefore focused on the quality of survivorship with adverse physical function, cognition and mental health outcomes, now recognised as post-intensive care syndrome (PICS) [1, 4, 5].

Existing long-term data suggests that ICU survivorship is associated with considerable long-term morbidity. Five-year data from North America indicate new and continued disability in physical function, cognition, and health-related quality of life (HRQoL) following adult respiratory distress syndrome (ARDS) [6, 7] and sepsis [2, 3, 6]. Five-year data from the United Kingdom (UK) and Europe indicate that in older, general ICU cohorts, survivors return to their pre-ICU HRQoL levels [8, 9], although often below population norms. Five-year data from other regions of the world are lacking. Previous findings may not be generalizable to other settings due to differences in models of care, patient cohorts, and differences in population HRQoL outcomes [10, 11].

* Correspondence: kimberley.haines@wh.org.au
[1]Physiotherapy Department, Western Health, Furlong Road, St. Albans, VIC 3021, Australia
[2]Department of Physiotherapy, Melbourne School of Health Sciences, The University of Melbourne, 200 Berkeley Street, Parkville, VIC 3010, Australia
Full list of author information is available at the end of the article

Given that ageing of the population is a global phenomenon, there are calls to define critical care survivorship in a way similar to cancer and stroke survivorship [2]. Current data on recovery from critical illness is incomplete and predominantly limited to the Northern Hemisphere. Intensive care unit (ICU) follow-up studies are typically clustered around the short and medium term of 6 [10, 12–15] to 12 months [14, 16–18] and typically describe HRQoL and physical function outcomes. Little is known about the overall experience for patients at 5 years, with a particular paucity of data relating to psychological outcomes beyond 1 to 2 years [13, 19–22].

Within Australia, no published long-term outcome data extends beyond 1 year [14, 17]. Comprehensive survivorship data from other healthcare contexts is important to contribute to the global understanding of critical care survivorship and improve generalizability across settings. Therefore, the primary aim of this study was to:

i) Investigate long-term mortality, physical function, psychological outcomes, and HRQoL in a mixed ICU cohort in Australia

The secondary aims of this study were to:

i) Compare the long-term physical function of Australian survivors with 1-year post-ICU physical function
ii) Investigate the long-term prevalence of symptoms of anxiety, depression, and post-traumatic stress disorder (PTSD) in Australian ICU survivors
iii) Compare the long-term HRQoL of Australian survivors with pre- and 1 year post-ICU
iv) Investigate long-term return to work and independent living status in Australian survivors

Methods

Study design, setting, and participants

This study was a prospective, observational follow-up study of a longer-stay (median ICU admission of 7 days) cohort. This randomised controlled trial (RCT) was conducted in a quaternary ICU in Melbourne, Australia, from 2007 to 2010 and detailed elsewhere [17]. RCT participants ($n = 150$) were screened and invited to participate, and informed consent sought for follow-up. Participants were included in the original RCT if they were > 18 years, ICU length of stay ≥ 5 days, understood English, resided within 50 km from the hospital and the intensive care specialist agreed to their participation. Patients were excluded if they had major disorders affecting the central nervous system or other conditions that would prevent participation in exercise, were approaching imminent death, length of stay > 5 days due to lack of general ward bed availability and unable to perform study physical outcome measures pre-morbidly.

The institutional ethics committee of Austin Health approved the study (H2012/04606), which is reported according to STROBE guidelines [23].

Procedure

From May 2012–December 2013, all patients enrolled in the RCT were screened for survival using hospital and general practitioner records. Patients not confirmed deceased were sent a letter describing the study and inviting participation, with an opt-out clause. Patients were contacted a week later via telephone to seek consent.

Outcome measures were performed at 4 to 5 years following ICU discharge in a standardised hospital environment and questionnaires completed in-person by a single assessor (KH). If participants were not within travelling distance (> 1 h via car journey) of the hospital, questionnaires were completed by phone interview. If participants were within travelling distance (< 1 h via car journey), but could not travel, the outcome assessor attended their home.

Outcome measurement

Demographic and 1-year follow-up data

Baseline demographic and 1-year follow-up data were drawn from the RCT [17] (Table 1). Additional demographic data was sought for the current study, including independent living status and employment status (devised questionnaire Additional file 1: Appendix E1), as well as the need for informal caregiver assistance following hospital discharge. ICU-acquired weakness (ICU-AW) was diagnosed when the Medical Research Council (MRC) score was less than 48/60 [24] and then dichotomized as either present or absent.

Mortality

Mortality data was sourced from hospital databases where available and all mortality data cross-referenced with the state-based Victorian Births and Deaths Registry (completed June 24, 2014).

Performance-based tests and patient-reported outcomes

Physical function was measured using the six-minute walk test (6MWT), a standardised walking test to measure functional exercise capacity, previously used in ICU cohorts [6, 14, 17, 25] and the Timed Up and Go Test (TUG) to assess functional mobility [26]. Bilateral handgrip strength was assessed using hand held dynamometry, modelled on a previously published protocol for ICU patients [27].

Psychological outcomes were assessed in the following domains: depression, anxiety, and post-traumatic stress disorder (PTSD). Depression and anxiety symptoms were screened using the Hospital Anxiety and Depression Scale (HADS) [28], one of the most commonly used measures in the critically ill [29]. Subscale scores of 0–7 are normal

Table 1 Demographics

	Whole cohort (n = 150)	Survivor cohort (n = 56)	Deceased (n = 66)
Age (years) at recruitment mean (SD)	61 (15.8)	59 (14.1) 64 (14.2) at 4–5 years	67 (14.6)
Male, n (%)	94 (62)	34 (61)	44 (66)
APACHE II mean (SD)	20 (7)	18 (6)	22 (7.9)
ICU diagnosis (%)			
Pneumonia	17	13	21
Cardiac[a]	39	43	33
Other surgery	15	16	14
Liver disease/transplant	10	13	9
Sepsis	8	5	12
Other	8	10	11
> 1 comorbidity, n (%)	53 (35%)	17 (30%)	30 (46%)
MV hours median (IQR)	92 (26–165)	96 (0–689.3)	84 (41–186)
ICU length of stay (days) median (IQR)	7 (6–11)	7 (5–11)	8 (6–11)
Hospital length of stay (days) median (IQR)	22 (15–36)	19 (11.3–29.5)	25 (18–45)

[a]Includes cardiogenic shock, cardiac arrest and complicated cardiac surgery

and > 8 indicates clinically significant symptoms [28]. The Centre for Epidemiological Studies-Depression Scale (CES-D) [30] was also included as it is the only measure of depression validated against clinician diagnoses in the post-ICU setting [29]. A cut-off score of 16 or more was used to define clinically significant depression [30]. PTSD was assessed using the Impact of Event Scale (IES) [31], a 15-item questionnaire, and a cut-off score of 19 was reported against, as originally described [32] and consistent with previous studies [33].

HRQoL was measured using the Short Form-36 Questionnaire, version 2 (SF-36v2) [34], and the Assessment of Quality of Life (AQoL) questionnaire [35]. The SF-36v2 has been widely used and validated in the critically ill [36, 37] and consists of eight subscales (including physical functioning, bodily pain, social functioning and mental health). Two summary scores (physical and mental, PCS and MCS respectively) based upon population norms [37] are produced and presented as standardised T-scores (mean = 50 and standard deviation = 10) [38]. The AQoL is a 15-item generic health, multi-attribute utility instrument [35] which has been previously used [17] and validated in the critically ill [39]. The AQoL utility instrument boundaries range from − 0.04 (state worse than death) to 1.00 (full HRQoL).

Statistical analysis

Descriptive data are presented as median [interquartile range (IQR)] and mean [standard deviation (SD)] as appropriate. Imputation of missing data for survivors was not undertaken as there was little missing data between baseline, 1-year, and 4–5-year time points for the outcomes of interest.

Multiple variable logistic regression was conducted as a post hoc analysis to investigate the factors associated with mortality at follow-up. A priori selected baseline variables were compared between survivors and non-survivors, using univariate analyses with $p \leq 0.1$ used to determine which variables were entered into the final model. Six independent variables (baseline age, APACHE II scores, acute hospital length of stay, pre-ICU HRQoL (AQoL utility score), Physical Component Summary Score of the SF36v2, ability to perform the Physical Function in Intensive Care Test by day 10 of ICU admission [40]) were included in the final model. The Hosmer-Lemeshow test was used to assess goodness of fit, and pseudo R^2 statistics were calculated with Nagelkerke R-square. The Wald test was used to assess the significance of the association of the individual variables with mortality. Odds ratios (95% CIs) and sensitivity and specificity of the model are reported. A Kaplan-Meier analysis was conducted to investigate differences in survival between those without comorbidities and those with one or more.

For repeated measures at one with either 4 or 5 years (e.g. 6MWT, TUG), the paired t test was used for normally distributed data and Wilcoxon signed-rank test for non-normally distributed data. One-way repeated measures ANOVA was used to compare HRQoL (AQoL utility score, SF36v2 PCS, MCS and PF) across the three time points. Where appropriate, analyses are reported as mean change in scores with 95% CI and compared with reported minimal clinically important differences as a secondary analysis, where available.

Data analysis was performed using SPSS™ (Mac SPSS™ Statistical Version 20, IBM, New York, NY) and $p < 0.05$ was taken to indicate statistical significance.

Results

Of the 150 patients in the original RCT, 84 were assessed for eligibility with 16 lost to follow-up. Of the 68 still alive at follow-up and able to be contacted, 56 (82% of 68) agreed to participate. At follow-up, the survivor cohorts had a mean (SD) age of 64 (14.2), were mostly male, were previously a moderately unwell cohort with mean (SD) APACHE II scores of 18 (6), and had been mechanically ventilated for a median of 4 days (Table 1). The flow of participants through the study is provided in Fig. 1.

Mortality

In the entire group of 150, 66 (44%) patients were deceased (cause of death listed in Additional file 1: Appendix E2). Date of death was only available for 43

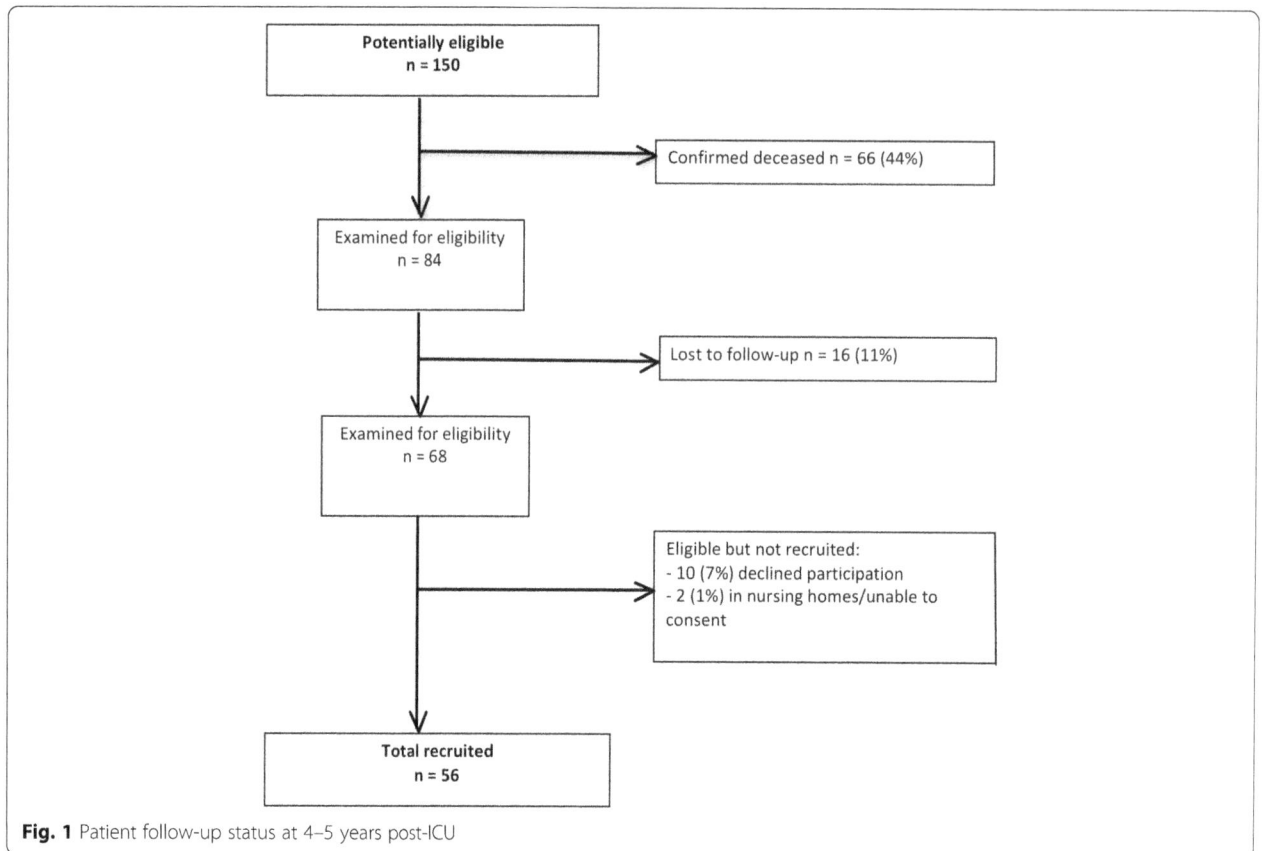

Fig. 1 Patient follow-up status at 4–5 years post-ICU

(65%) patients, and mortality was highest (*n* = 19, 44%) during the first year following ICU discharge. In the multivariable regression, those who were deceased by follow-up were older (*p* = 0.05), with higher APACHE II scores (*p* = 0.001) and comorbidities (46% with one or more) compared to survivors (Table 2). Survival rates were significantly improved in the group who had no comorbidities compared to those who had one or more (Fig. 2, log rank *p* = 0.03).

Physical function

At longer-term follow-up, 48 of the 56 survivors (86%) completed the 6MWT with data unable to be collected on 8 survivors due to the travel distance outside defined inclusion criteria. Whilst there was an improvement in the survivors' 6MWT distance between 1 year (mean 465.8 m, SD 148.9) and 4–5 years (mean 507.5 m, SD 118.2), this difference was not statistically significant *p* = 0.15 (mean difference = – 24.5 m, CI – 58.3, 9.2). Survivors' 6MWT distance at 4–5 years was 70% of the predicted distance for Australian age and gender-matched norms [41]. In comparison, survivors' scores were 89% of predicted North American normative values [42], derived from a sample size more than double that of the Australian reference equation.

More than a third of survivors had an improvement in their walk distance greater than the reported minimal clinically important difference (MCID) of 20 m as reported for ICU survivors [43] and similarly for the previously reported MCID of 30 m for patients with chronic respiratory disease [44, 45]. The frequency distribution of distances for the 6MWT is displayed in Fig. 3.

The survivors had an improvement in their TUG time from a median (IQR) of 7.5 s (6.0–9.0) at 1 year to 6.5 s (6.0–9.0) at 4–5 years. This improvement was statistically significant (*p* = 0.001) and survivors outperformed normative values for their age range (mean (CI) 8.1 (7.1–9.0) [46] although did not improve by one of the few available reports of MCID for the TUG in acutely hospitalised older medical patients of 9.5 s [47].

Baseline outcome measures for strength included Medical Research Council (MRC) scores and diagnosis of ICU-AW. Survivors' mean (SD) MRC score was 51/ 60 (8.0), and 73% did not have ICU-AW as measured during their ICU admission. At longer-term follow-up, grip strength in males was 76% of age-matched normative values [48] at mean (SD) 34 (12.5) kg. Females had a mean (SD) grip strength of 20 (9.9) kg, which was 77% of age-matched normative values [48].

Table 2 Logistic regression predicting the likelihood of death by longer-term follow-up

	B	SE	Wald	df	P	OR	95% CI
Baseline MRC score	− 0.76	0.05	2.16	1	0.14	0.93	0.84 to 1.03
Baseline age	0.05	0.02	4.23	1	0.04*	1.05	1.00 to 1.10
APACHE II	0.17	0.07	6.46	1	0.01*	1.18	1.04 to 1.34
Acute hospital length of stay	0.12	0.01	1.59	1	0.21	1.01	0.99 to 1.03
Baseline AQoL utility score	− 2.16	1.28	2.85	1	0.09	0.12	0.01 to 1.41
Baseline SF36v2 PCS	− 0.04	0.03	1.58	1	0.21	0.96	0.91 to 1.02
Constant	0.41	3.47	0.01	1	0.91	1.51	

B beta coefficient, *SE* standard error, *Wald* Wald test, *df* degrees of freedom, *OR* odds ratio, *CI* confidence interval *MRC score* Medical Research Council score, *APACHE II* Acute Physiological and Chronic Health Evaluation II, *AQoL* Assessment of Quality of Life, *SF36v2 PCS* Short Form 36 Health Survey Version 2 Physical Component Score
*Statistically significant $p \leq 0.05$

Psychological outcomes

As measured by the CES-D, depressive symptoms were low with a median (IQR) CES-D score of 7.0 (1.0–15.0). Forty (71%) survivors had no depression, 10 (18%) had mild depression and 6 (11%) had major depression. As measured by the HADS, survivors' symptoms of anxiety and depression were within normal ranges with respective median (IQR) scores of 3.0 (1.0–6.0) and 1.0 (0–4). Forty-five (80%) survivors had no symptoms of anxiety, whilst 11 (20%) had clinically significant symptoms. Forty-eight (86%) survivors reported no symptoms of depression whilst 8 (14%) had clinically significant symptoms. The incidence of PTSD was also sub-clinical with a median (IQR) score of 1.0 (0–11.0) as measured by the IES. Nine (16%) survivors had 'clinically significant' symptoms for PTSD.

Health-related quality of life

At follow-up, survivors' mean SF36v2 PCS scores were normal for age-matched Australian values (Table 3), whilst the MCS were below population normative values but within one SD [38]. For survivors with available data at both time points, there was no significant difference in PCS ($p = 0.32$, $n = 37$) over time although there was a significant improvement for the MCS ($p = 0.01$, $n = 37$). Only the differences in MCS between pre-ICU and 1 year follow-up exceeded the reported MCID of 5-point difference [37].

At longer-term follow-up survivors' mean (SD), AQoL utility score was 0.74 (0.23), below age-matched normative values of 0.79 (0.19) [49]. There were no differences in AQoL scores over time ($p = 0.14$, $n = 38$). Between pre-ICU and 1-year follow-up, the change in the

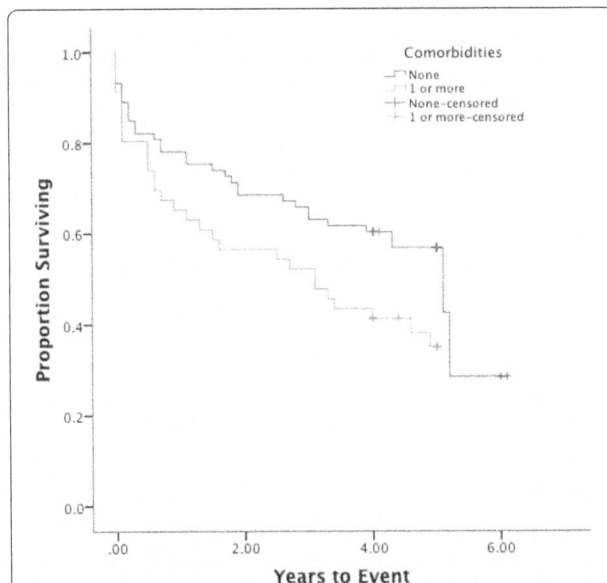

Fig. 2 Kaplan-Meier curve for survival from 0 to 5 years for different numbers of premorbid comorbidities

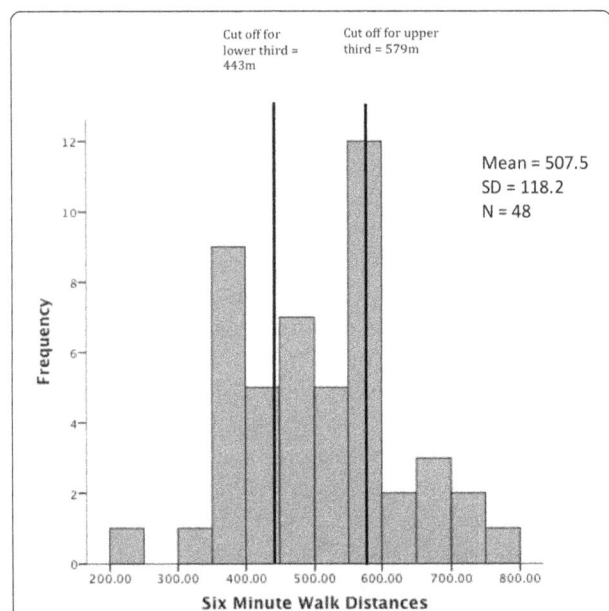

Fig. 3 Histogram of frequency distribution for Six Minute Walk Distances

Table 3 Descriptive statistics for health-related quality of life scores over time for survivors and age-matched normative values

Outcome measure	Baseline		1 year		4–5 years		Age-matched Australian normative values[a]
	n	Mean (SD)	n	Mean (SD)	n	Mean (SD)	Mean (SD)
AQoL utility	43	0.70 (0.25)	49	0.77 (0.24)	56	0.74 (0.23)	0.79 (0.19)
SF36v2 PCS	43	43.4 (12.1)	44	46.4 (7.9)	56	46.7 (8.1)	46.8 (11.6)
SF36v2 MCS	43	42.9 (12.8)	44	48.8 (13)	56	48.8 (11.1)	50.1 (10.8)
Physical functioning	43	45.3 (12.3)	44	44.7 (10)	56	43.6 (11.5)	47.4 (10.7)
Role physical	43	40.4 (14.1)	44	46.0 (10.1)	56	46.3 (11.6)	47.5 (12.0)
Bodily pain	43	47.2 (15.7)	44	53.4 (11.0)	56	50.7 (10.7)	47.3 (10.4)
General health	43	41.6 (10.5)	44	44.2 (9.9)	56	45.6 (9.9)	47.4 (11.9)
Vitality	43	39.7 (13.3)	44	46.6 (11.9)	56	50.7 (8.4)	49.0 (10.9)
Social functioning	43	42.3 (15.1)	44	48.4 (12.9)	56	50.0 (8.8)	49.3 (11.1)
Role emotional	43	45.4 (15.3)	44	48.5 (11.5)	56	44.2 (14.3)	49.2 (11.5)
Mental health	43	42.2 (13.5)	44	48.5 (14.2)	56	49.2 (12.0)	49.4 (11.2)

AQoL utility Assessment of Quality of Life Utility score range − 0.04 (state worse than death) to 1.00 (perfect health), *SF36v2* Short Form 36 Health Survey version 2 in which higher scores indicate greater performance and data is presented as *T* scores where the population mean is 50 and the SD is 10, *PCS* Physical Component Score, *MCS* Mental Component Score, *PF* Physical Function Subscale
[a]Age-matched Australian population for mean (SD) age 64 (14.2) of survivors at 4–5-year follow-up

survivors' mean difference in AQoL scores exceeded the reported MCID of 0.06 [49]. Between 1 year and 4–5 years, there was a smaller clinically insignificant improvement. Between 1 and 4 or 5-year follow-up, 11 (23%) survivors improved more than the AQoL MCID [49], 22 (45%) deteriorated and 16 (32%) did not differ compared to the MCID.

Return to work

Twenty (69%) survivors who had been working prior to ICU (*n* = 29, 52% of original cohort) had returned to work. Five (17%) survivors had not, reporting poor health as the reason. Twenty-seven (48%) survivors were not working prior to ICU, with 21 (81%) being retired whilst only 4 (15%) survivors were not working due to ill health.

Discussion

This first longitudinal Australian study provides a contrasting perspective to other international reports of critical care survivorship [2, 3, 6–8, 50]. Survivors were characterised by a low burden of impairments in their physical, HRQoL and psychological outcomes. This study comprehensively evaluated multiple outcomes including physical function and HRQoL in a long-stay, heterogeneous cohort representative of Australian ICUs [51]. It is also one of the first reports to provide empirical psychological data at 4 to 5 years. A particular strength is the combined use of performance-based and patient-reported measurement, an important consideration in ICU follow-up studies [52].

Mortality

The long-term mortality rate of 44% was unexpectedly high compared to previous reports of 19% [6] and 30% [8] in landmark studies at 5-year follow-up. Differences observed in our study may be attributable to increased baseline age and higher APACHE II scores comparative to these previous reports [6, 8]. The Kaplan-Meier curve highlights the contribution of comorbidity to mortality although these analyses were not adjusted for age and APACHE II scores. Overall, the original cohort had a high prevalence of comorbid illness [53]. Almost half of the non-survivors had one or more comorbidities compared to a third of survivors. Pre-existing comorbid illness may be an important consideration for post-ICU trajectories of recovery [53] with worse outcomes attributed to pre-existing illness, particularly for HRQoL [54, 55]. We hypothesise our observed mortality rate could be influenced by local healthcare system factors including physician decision-making regarding ICU admission and rationing and socioeconomic factors. For example, the Australian healthcare model may be relatively well resourced compared to other regions, with a greater ratio of ICU beds to ward beds, a 'closed' ICU model and 1:1 nurse to patient ratios [11]. As a result, the threshold for ICU admission may be lower in Australian units than more resource-limited regions.

Physical function

The majority of survivors had minimal decrements in their physical function as evidenced by their 6MWD and TUG values relative to population normative data. Most recovery appears to be gained by 1 year although this was a heterogeneous group, with some survivors still experiencing physical impairment at follow-up. This demonstrates the variability in trajectories of recovery [56] that may influence response to targeted intervention [57, 58] and the importance of stratification according to disability [59]. The greatest deficits were seen in the survivors' grip strength compared to normative data although this is difficult to interpret as the majority did not have an earlier diagnosis of ICU-AW and grip strength was not measured during the original RCT. Reasons for observed differences in our physical function outcomes could be related to a high proportion of patients admitted for cardiac causes. These patients have a relatively unimpeded recovery following surgery and critical care with resolution of some premorbid co-morbidities [10, 60]. The majority of our cohort did not have a diagnosis of ICU-AW during their ICU admission, and this may explain the overall level of high performance in the physical function tests. Comparatively, Herridge and colleagues hypothesised that in their younger cohort with a lower prevalence of comorbid illness, the adverse physical outcomes observed in their cohort likely stemmed from persistent weakness although the incidence of ICU-AW was not specifically reported [6].

HRQoL

The HRQoL findings of our study were comparable to the patterns demonstrated in the study by Cuthbertson and colleagues [8]. In both of these studies, by 5 year follow-up, survivors' HRQoL scores were comparable if not better than their premorbid scores. However, in the study by Cuthberston and colleagues, the survivors' HRQoL remained lower than population norms at 5 years whereas in our study, scores were comparable to Australian population norms at this time point which is consistent with the findings of more recent research [9, 61]. The similarity in trends in the SF36 scores over time between these two studies is likely attributable to similarities in demographics (both were conducted in mixed older age cohorts with comparable APACHE II scores) and consistency in the administration of the SF36 to capture premorbid HRQoL.

Psychological outcomes

We provide one of the first reports at 4 to 5 years of directly measured, comprehensive psychological outcome data. Consistent with the other outcomes we have described for this cohort, the incidence and prevalence of psychological morbidity was low. Although not evaluated, these survivors may have possessed higher levels of attributes such as resiliency and self-efficacy as well as access to greater familial and social support. This may have assisted their overall high level of recovery. This concept has been demonstrated in other ICU survivors

where resilience has an inverse correlation with neuropsychological impairment and other outcomes such as pain and self-care [62].

Our data are influenced by survivor bias and loss to follow-up inherent in longitudinal studies. The findings suggest most recovery occurs within the first year, and this may be important to consider in the design of future interventional studies. Patients and their families may be at greatest risk of adverse outcomes during this time, and promising interventions such as peer support may assist their recovery transition [63]. A limitation of this study is the lack of follow-up from 1 to 4 and 5 years. This may have assisted in improved follow-up rates through repeated contact with participants although overall attrition was comparable if not better than previous studies. We approached the measurement of psychological outcomes using screening tools rather than diagnostic tools although this was consistent with other reports [21, 22, 29, 33, 64]. Further, the IES was selected as the best measure to screen for PTSD at the time of study design, although more recent reports support the use of the IES-Revised [65] which may limit comparability of our findings.

This study highlights the need for a co-ordinated and collaborative international approach to describe the spectrum of critical care survivorship, particularly as we are starting to see better outcomes reported in other regions such as Europe [9]. In order to improve the outcomes for critical care survivors, consensus is required between clinicians, researchers and policymakers regarding time points for follow-up and which outcome measures to use. Further, there may be other important factors to evaluate that mediate recovery such resilience [62] and post-traumatic growth and the role of caregivers and their ability to provide support following exposure to critical illness [66, 67]. By establishing large international datasets for a range of patient and family outcomes, we may be able to better understand survivorship from critical illness and develop interventions that will be sensitive to these specific domains.

Conclusions

In conclusion, this Australian cohort had an increased mortality rate compared to existing studies that may be attributable to differences in healthcare models and delivery of care. However, survivors achieved recovery in their physical function and HRQoL comparable with population norms and had low psychological morbidity. Further exploration through large datasets is warranted to understand regional differences in outcomes to truly define critical care survivorship from an international perspective.

Additional file

Additional file 1: Appendix E1. Independent living status and employment status questions. Appendix E2. Cause of death information provided by the Victorian Births and Deaths Registry. (DOC 44 kb)

Abbreviations

6MWT: Six-minute walk test; AQoL: Assessment of Quality of Life; ARDS: Adult respiratory distress syndrome; CES-D: Centre for Epidemiological Studies–Depression Scale; HADS: Hospital Anxiety and Depression Scale; HR-QoL: Health-related Quality of Life; ICU: Intensive care unit; ICU-AW: Intensive care unit-acquired weakness; IES : Impact of events scale; MCID: Minimal clinically important difference; MCS: Mental Component Summary Scale (of SF-36); MRC: Medical Research Council; PCS: Physical Component Summary Scale (of SF-36); PICS: Post-intensive care syndrome; PTSD: Post-traumatic stress disorder; RCT: Randomised controlled trial; SF-36: Short Form-36; STROBE: STrengthening the Reporting of OBservational Studies in Epidemiology; TUG: Timed Up and Go Test; UK: United Kingdom

Acknowledgements
The authors would like to thank Dr. Elizabeth Skinner and Associate Professor Theodore 'Jack' Iwashyna for their critical review of the manuscript.

Funding
Dr. Haines was supported by an Australian National Health and Medical Research Council Dora Lush Scholarship, and this work was supported by the Austin Medical Research Foundation.

Authors' contributions
KH, SB, and LD conceived and designed the study. KH collected the data of the study. All authors contributed to the analysis and interpretation of the study and revised and drafted the manuscript. All authors read and approved the final manuscript.

Competing interests
The authors declare that they have no competing interests.

Author details
[1]Physiotherapy Department, Western Health, Furlong Road, St. Albans, VIC 3021, Australia. [2]Department of Physiotherapy, Melbourne School of Health Sciences, The University of Melbourne, 200 Berkeley Street, Parkville, VIC 3010, Australia. [3]Department of Physiotherapy, Austin Hospital, 145 Studley Road, Heidelberg, VIC 3084, Australia. [4]Department of Intensive Care, Austin Hospital, 145 Studley Road, Heidelberg, VIC 3084, Australia.

References
1. Iwashyna TJ. Survivorship will be the defining challenge of critical care in the 21st century. Ann Intern Med. 2010;153:204–5. doi: https://doi.org/10.7326/0003-4819-153-3-201008030-00013.

2. Iwashyna TJ, Cooke CR, Wunsch H, Kahn JM. Population burden of long-term survivorship after severe sepsis in older Americans. J Am Geriatr Soc. 2012;60:1070–7. doi: https://doi.org/10.1111/j.1532-5415.2012.03989.x.

3. Iwashyna TJ, Ely EW, Smith DM, Langa KM. Long-term cognitive impairment and functional disability among survivors of severe sepsis. JAMA. 2010;304: 1787–94. doi: https://doi.org/10.1001/jama.2010.1553.

4. Elliott D, Davidson JE, Harvey MA, Bemis-Dougherty A, Hopkins RO, Iwashyna TJ, Wagner J, Weinert C, Wunsch H, Bienvenu OJ, Black G, Brady S, Brodsky MB, Deutschman C, Doepp D, Flatley C, Fosnight S, Gittler M, Gomez BT, Hyzy R, Louis D, Mandel R, Maxwell C, Muldoon SR, Perme CS, Reilly C, Robinson MR, Rubin E, Schmidt DM, Schuller J, Scruth E, Siegal E, Spill GR, Sprenger S, Straumanis JP, Sutton P, Swoboda SM, Twaddle ML, Needham DM. Exploring the scope of post-intensive care syndrome therapy and care: engagement of non-critical care providers and survivors in a second stakeholders meeting. Crit Care Med. 2014;42:2518–26. doi: https://doi.org/10.1097/CCM.0000000000000525.

5. Needham DM, Davidson J, Cohen H, Hopkins RO, Weinert C, Wunsch H, Zawistowski C, Bemis-Dougherty A, Berney SC, Bienvenu OJ, Brady SL, Brodsky MB, Denehy L, Elliott D, Flatley C, Harabin AL, Jones C, Louis D, Meltzer W, Muldoon SR, Palmer JB, Perme C, Robinson M, Schmidt DM, Scruth E, Spill GR, Storey CP, Render M, Votto J, Harvey MA. Improving long-term outcomes after discharge from intensive care unit: report from a stakeholders' conference. Crit Care Med. 2012;40:502–9. doi: https://doi.org/10.1097/CCM.0b013e318232da75.

6. Herridge MS, Tansey CM, Matte A, Tomlinson G, Diaz-Granados N, Cooper A, Guest CB, Mazer CD, Mehta S, Stewart TE, Kudlow P, Cook D, Slutsky AS, Cheung AM, Canadian Critical Care Trials G. Functional disability 5 years after acute respiratory distress syndrome. N Engl J Med. 2011;364:1293–304. doi: https://doi.org/10.1056/NEJMoa1011802.

7. Pfoh ER, Wozniak AW, Colantuoni E, Dinglas VD, Mendez-Tellez PA, Shanholtz C, Ciesla ND, Pronovost PJ, Needham DM. Physical declines occurring after hospital discharge in ARDS survivors: a 5-year longitudinal study. Intensive Care Med. 2016;42:1557–66. doi: https://doi.org/10.1007/s00134-016-4530-1.

8. Cuthbertson BH, Roughton S, Jenkinson D, Maclennan G, Vale L. Quality of life in the five years after intensive care: a cohort study. Crit Care. 2010;14: R6. doi: https://doi.org/10.1186/cc8848.

9. Hofhuis JG, van Stel HF, Schrijvers AJ, Rommes JH, Spronk PE. ICU survivors show no decline in health-related quality of life after 5 years. Intensive Care Med. 2015;41:495–504. doi: https://doi.org/10.1007/s00134-015-3669-5.

10. Skinner EH, Warrillow S, Denehy L. Health-related quality of life in Australian survivors of critical illness. Crit Care Med. 2011;39:1896–905. doi: https://doi.org/10.1097/CCM.0b013e31821b8421.

11. Bellomo R, Stow PJ, Hart GK. Why is there such a difference in outcome between Australian intensive care units and others? Curr Opin Anaesthesiol. 2007;20:100–5. doi: https://doi.org/10.1097/ACO.0b013e32802c7cd5.

12. Garland A, Dawson NV, Altmann I, Thomas CL, Phillips RS, Tsevat J, Desbiens NA, Bellamy PE, Knaus WA, Connors AF Jr, Investigators S. Outcomes up to 5 years after severe, acute respiratory failure. Chest. 2004;126:1897–904. doi: https://doi.org/10.1378/chest.126.6.1897.

13. Jackson JC, Pandharipande PP, Girard TD, Brummel NE, Thompson JL, Hughes CG, Pun BT, Vasilevskis EE, Morandi A, Shintani AK, Hopkins RO, Bernard GR, Dittus RS, Ely EW, Bringing to light the Risk F, Incidence of Neuropsychological dysfunction in ICUssi (2014). Depression, post-traumatic stress disorder, and functional disability in survivors of critical illness in the BRAIN-ICU study: a longitudinal cohort study. Lancet Respir Med 2:369–79 doi: https://doi.org/10.1016/S2213-2600(14)70051-7.

14. Elliott D, McKinley S, Alison J, Aitken LM, King M, Leslie GD, Kenny P, Taylor P, Foley R, Burmeister E. Health-related quality of life and physical recovery after a critical illness: a multi-centre randomised controlled trial of a home-based physical rehabilitation program. Crit Care. 2011;15:R142. doi: https://doi.org/10.1186/cc10265.

15. Investigators TS, Hodgson C, Bellomo R, Berney S, Bailey M, Buhr H, Denehy L, Harrold M, Higgins A, Presneill J, Saxena M, Skinner E, Young P, Webb S. Early mobilization and recovery in mechanically ventilated patients in the ICU: a bi-national, multi-centre, prospective cohort study. Crit Care. 2015;19: 81. doi: https://doi.org/10.1186/s13054-015-0765-4.

16. Cuthbertson BH, Scott J, Strachan M, Kilonzo M, Vale L. Quality of life before and after intensive care. Anaesthesia. 2005;60:332–9. doi: https://doi.org/10.1111/j.1365-2044.2004.04109.x.

17. Denehy L, Skinner EH, Edbrooke L, Haines K, Warrillow S, Hawthorne G, Gough K, Hoorn SV, Morris ME, Berney S. Exercise rehabilitation for patients

with critical illness: a randomized controlled trial with 12 months of follow-up. Crit Care. 2013;17:R156. doi: https://doi.org/10.1186/cc12835.

18. Herridge MS, Cheung AM, Tansey CM, Matte-Martyn A, Diaz-Granados N, Al-Saidi F, Cooper AB, Guest CB, Mazer CD, Mehta S, Stewart TE, Barr A, Cook D, Slutsky AS, Canadian Critical Care Trials G. One-year outcomes in survivors of the acute respiratory distress syndrome. N Engl J Med. 2003;348:683–93. doi: https://doi.org/10.1056/NEJMoa022450.

19. Duggan MC, Wang L, Wilson JE, Dittus RS, Ely EW, Jackson JC. The relationship between executive dysfunction, depression, and mental health-related quality of life in survivors of critical illness: results from the BRAIN-ICU investigation. J Crit Care. 2017;37:72–9. doi: https://doi.org/10.1016/j.jcrc.2016.08.023.

20. Jackson JC, Girard TD, Gordon SM, Thompson JL, Shintani AK, Thomason JW, Pun BT, Canonico AE, Dunn JG, Bernard GR, Dittus RS, Ely EW. Long-term cognitive and psychological outcomes in the awakening and breathing controlled trial. Am J Respir Crit Care Med. 2010;182:183–91. doi: https://doi.org/10.1164/rccm.200903-0442OC.

21. Needham DM, Dinglas VD, Bienvenu OJ, Colantuoni E, Wozniak AW, Rice TW, Hopkins RO, Network NNA. One year outcomes in patients with acute lung injury randomised to initial trophic or full enteral feeding: prospective follow-up of EDEN randomised trial. BMJ. 2013;346:f1532. doi: https://doi.org/10.1136/bmj.f1532.

22. Nikayin S, Rabiee A, Hashem MD, Huang M, Bienvenu OJ, Turnbull AE, Needham DM. Anxiety symptoms in survivors of critical illness: a systematic review and meta-analysis. Gen Hosp Psychiatry. 2016;43:23–9. doi: https://doi.org/10.1016/j.genhosppsych.2016.08.005.

23. von Elm E, Altman DG, Egger M, Pocock SJ, Gotzsche PC, Vandenbroucke JP, Initiative S. The Strengthening the Reporting of Observational Studies in Epidemiology (STROBE) statement: guidelines for reporting observational studies. J Clin Epidemiol. 2008;61:344–9. doi: https://doi.org/10.1016/j.jclinepi.2007.11.008.

24. De Jonghe B, Sharshar T, Lefaucheur JP, Authier FJ, Durand-Zaleski I, Boussarsar M, Cerf C, Renaud E, Mesrati F, Carlet J, Raphael JC, Outin H, Bastuji-Garin S, Groupe de Reflexion et d'Etude des Neuromyopathies en R. Paresis acquired in the intensive care unit: a prospective multicenter study. JAMA. 2002;288:2859–67.

25. Holland AE, Spruit MA, Troosters T, Puhan MA, Pepin V, Saey D, McCormack MC, Carlin BW, Sciurba FC, Pitta F, Wanger J, MacIntyre N, Kaminsky DA, Culver BH, Revill SM, Hernandes NA, Andrianopoulos V, Camillo CA, Mitchell KE, Lee AL, Hill CJ, Singh SJ. An official European Respiratory Society/American Thoracic Society technical standard: field walking tests in chronic respiratory disease. Eur Respir J. 2014;44:1428–46. doi: https://doi.org/10.1183/09031936.00150314.

26. Podsiadlo D, Richardson S. The timed "up & go": a test of basic functional mobility for frail elderly persons. J Am Geriatr Soc. 1991;39:142–8.

27. Baldwin CE, Paratz JD, Bersten AD. Muscle strength assessment in critically ill patients with handheld dynamometry: an investigation of reliability, minimal detectable change, and time to peak force generation. J Crit Care. 2013;28:77–86. doi: https://doi.org/10.1016/j.jcrc.2012.03.001.

28. Zigmond AS, Snaith RP. The hospital anxiety and depression scale. Acta Psychiatr Scand. 1983;67:361–70.

29. Davydow DS, Gifford JM, Desai SV, Bienvenu OJ, Needham DM. Depression in general intensive care unit survivors: a systematic review. Intensive Care Med. 2009;35:796–809. doi: https://doi.org/10.1007/s00134-009-1396-5.

30. Radloff LS. The CES-D scale: a self-report depression scale for research in the general population. Appl Psychol Meas. 1977;1:385–401.

31. Griffiths J, Fortune G, Barber V, Young JD. The prevalence of post traumatic stress disorder in survivors of ICU treatment: a systematic review. Intensive Care Med. 2007;33:1506–18. doi: https://doi.org/10.1007/s00134-007-0730-z.

32. Horowitz M, Wilner N, Alvarez W. Impact of event scale: a measure of subjective stress. Psychosom Med. 1979;41:209–18.

33. Davydow DS, Gifford JM, Desai SV, Needham DM, Bienvenu OJ. Posttraumatic stress disorder in general intensive care unit survivors: a systematic review. Gen Hosp Psychiatry. 2008;30:421–34. doi: https://doi.org/10.1016/j.genhosppsych.2008.05.006.

34. Ware JEK MA, Dewey JE. How to score version 2 of the SF-36 health survey. Lincoln: Quality Metric Inc; 2000.

35. Hawthorne G, Richardson J, Osborne R. The assessment of quality of life (AQoL) instrument: a psychometric measure of health-related quality of life. Qual Life Res. 1999;8:209–24.

36. Chrispin PS, Scotton H, Rogers J, Lloyd D, Ridley SA. Short form 36 in the intensive care unit: assessment of acceptability, reliability and validity of the questionnaire. Anaesthesia. 1997;52:15–23.

37. Ware JE, Snow KK, Kosinski M, Gandek B. SF-36 health survey: manual and interpretation guide. The Health Institute, New England Medical Centre: Boston, MA; 1993.

38. Hawthorne G, Osborne RH, Taylor A, Sansoni J. The SF36 version 2: critical analyses of population weights, scoring algorithms and population norms. Qual Life Res. 2007;16:661–73. doi: https://doi.org/10.1007/s11136-006-9154-4.

39. Skinner EH, Denehy L, Warrillow S, Hawthorne G. Comparison of the measurement properties of the AQoL and SF-6D in critical illness. Crit Care Resusc. 2013;15:205–12.

40. Skinner EH, Berney S, Warrillow S, Denehy L. Development of a physical function outcome measure (PFIT) and a pilot exercise training protocol for use in intensive care. Crit Care Resusc. 2009;11:110–5.

41. Jenkins S, Cecins N, Camarri B, Williams C, Thompson P, Eastwood P. Regression equations to predict 6-minute walk distance in middle-aged and elderly adults. Physiother Theory Pract. 2009;25:516–22. doi: https://doi.org/10.3109/09593980802664711.

42. Enright PL, Sherrill DL. Reference equations for the six-minute walk in healthy adults. Am J Respir Crit Care Med. 1998;158:1384–7. doi: https://doi.org/10.1164/ajrccm.158.5.9710086.

43. Chan KS, Pfoh ER, Denehy L, Elliott D, Holland AE, Dinglas VD, Needham DM. Construct validity and minimal important difference of 6-minute walk distance in survivors of acute respiratory failure. Chest. 2015;147:1316–26. doi: https://doi.org/10.1378/chest.14-1808.

44. Puhan MA, Gimeno-Santos E, Scharplatz M, Troosters T, Walters EH, Steurer J. Pulmonary rehabilitation following exacerbations of chronic obstructive pulmonary disease. Cochrane Database Syst Rev:CD005305. 2011; doi: https://doi.org/10.1002/14651858.CD005305.pub3.

45. Holland AE, Nici L. The return of the minimum clinically important difference for 6-minute-walk distance in chronic obstructive pulmonary disease. Am J Respir Crit Care Med. 2013;187:335–6. doi: https://doi.org/10.1164/rccm.201212-2191ED.

46. Bohannon RW. Reference values for the timed up and go test: a descriptive meta-analysis. J Geriatr Phys Ther. 2006;29:64–8.

47. de Morton NA, Keating JL, Jeffs K (2007) Exercise for acutely hospitalised older medical patients. Cochrane Database Syst Rev:CD005955 doi: https://doi.org/10.1002/14651858.CD005955.pub2.

48. Gunther CM, Burger A, Rickert M, Crispin A, Schulz CU. Grip strength in healthy Caucasian adults: reference values. J Hand Surg Am. 2008;33:558–65. doi: https://doi.org/10.1016/j.jhsa.2008.01.008.

49. Hawthorne G, Osborne R. Population norms and meaningful differences for the assessment of quality of life (AQoL) measure. Aust N Z J Public Health. 2005;29:136–42.

50. Cuthbertson BH, Elders A, Hall S, Taylor J, Maclennan G, Mackirdy F, Mackenzie SJ, the Scottish Critical Care Trials G, the Scottish Intensive Care Society Audit G. Mortality and quality of life in the five years after severe sepsis. Crit Care. 2013;17:R70. doi: https://doi.org/10.1186/cc12616.

51. Berney SC, Harrold M, Webb SA, Seppelt I, Patman S, Thomas PJ, Denehy L. Intensive care unit mobility practices in Australia and New Zealand: a point prevalence study. Crit Care Resusc. 2013;15:260–5.

52. Denehy L, Nordon-Craft A, Edbrooke L, Malone D, Berney S, Schenkman M, Moss M. Outcome measures report different aspects of patient function three months following critical care. Intensive Care Med. 2014;40:1862–9. doi: https://doi.org/10.1007/s00134-014-3513-3.

53. Puthucheary ZA, Denehy L. Exercise interventions in critical illness survivors: understanding inclusion and stratification criteria. Am J Respir Crit Care Med. 2015;191:1464–7. doi: https://doi.org/10.1164/rccm.201410-1907LE.

54. Orwelius L, Nordlund A, Edell-Gustafsson U, Simonsson E, Nordlund P, Kristenson M, Bendtsen P, Sjoberg F. Role of preexisting disease in patients' perceptions of health-related quality of life after intensive care. Crit Care Med. 2005;33:1557–64.

55. Orwelius L, Nordlund A, Nordlund P, Simonsson E, Backman C, Samuelsson A, Sjoberg F. Pre-existing disease: the most important factor for health related quality of life long-term after critical illness: a prospective, longitudinal, multicentre trial. Crit Care. 2010;14:R67. doi: https://doi.org/10.1186/cc8967.

56. Iwashyna TJ. Trajectories of recovery and dysfunction after acute illness, with implications for clinical trial design. Am J Respir Crit Care Med. 2012; 186(4):302. doi: https://doi.org/10.1164/rccm.201206-1138ED.

57. Cuthbertson BH, Wunsch H. Long-term outcomes after critical illness. The best predictor of the future is the past. Am J Respir Crit Care Med. 2016;194: 132–4. doi: https://doi.org/10.1164/rccm.201602-0257ED.

58. Herridge MS, Batt J, Santos CD. ICU-acquired weakness, morbidity, and death. Am J Respir Crit Care Med. 2014;190:360–2. doi: https://doi.org/10.1164/rccm.201407-1263ED.

59. Herridge MS, Chu LM, Matte A, Tomlinson G, Chan L, Thomas C, Friedrich JO, Mehta S, Lamontagne F, Levasseur M, Ferguson ND, Adhikari NK, Rudkowski JC, Meggison H, Skrobik Y, Flannery J, Bayley M, Batt J, Santos CD, Abbey SE, Tan A, Lo V, Mathur S, Parotto M, Morris D, Flockhart L, Fan E, Lee CM, Wilcox ME, Ayas N, Choong K, Fowler R, Scales DC, Sinuff T, Cuthbertson BH, Rose L, Robles P, Burns S, Cypel M, Singer L, Chaparro C, Chow CW, Keshavjee S, Brochard L, Hebert P, Slutsky AS, Marshall JC, Cook D, Cameron JI, Investigators RP, Canadian Critical Care Trials G. THE RECOVER program: disability risk groups and 1-year outcome after 7 or more days of mechanical ventilation. Am J Respir Crit Care Med. 2016;194:831–44. doi: https://doi.org/10.1164/rccm.201512-2343OC.

60. Soliman IW, de Lange DW, Peelen LM, Cremer OL, Slooter AJ, Pasma W, Kesecioglu J, van Dijk D. Single-center large-cohort study into quality of life in Dutch intensive care unit subgroups, 1 year after admission, using EuroQoL EQ-6D-3L. J Crit Care. 2015;30:181–6. doi: https://doi.org/10.1016/j.jcrc.2014.09.009.

61. Orwelius L, Fredrikson M, Kristenson M, Walther S, Sjoberg F. Health-related quality of life scores after intensive care are almost equal to those of the normal population: a multicenter observational study. Crit Care. 2013;17: R236. doi: https://doi.org/10.1186/cc13059.

62. Maley J, Brewster I, Mayoral I, Siruckova R, Adams S, McGraw K, Piech A, Detsky M, Mikkelsen M. Resilience in survivors of critical illness in the context of the survivors' experience and recovery. Ann Am Thorac Soc. 2016;13:1351–60.

63. Mikkelsen ME, Jackson JC, Hopkins RO, Thompson C, Andrews A, Netzer G, Bates DM, Bunnell AE, Christie LM, Greenberg SB, Lamas DJ, Sevin CM, Weinhouse G, Iwashyna TJ. Peer support as a novel strategy to mitigate post-intensive care syndrome. AACN Adv Crit Care. 2016;27:221–9. doi: https://doi.org/10.4037/aacnacc2016667.

64. Mikkelsen ME, Christie JD, Lanken PN, Biester RC, Thompson BT, Bellamy SL, Localio AR, Demissie E, Hopkins RO, Angus DC. The adult respiratory distress syndrome cognitive outcomes study: long-term neuropsychological function in survivors of acute lung injury. Am J Respir Crit Care Med. 2012; 185:1307–15. doi: https://doi.org/10.1164/rccm.201111-2025OC.

65. Bienvenu OJ, Williams JB, Yang A, Hopkins RO, Needham DM. Posttraumatic stress disorder in survivors of acute lung injury: evaluating the impact of event scale-revised. Chest. 2013;144:24–31. doi: https://doi.org/10.1378/chest.12-0908.

66. Cameron JI, Chu LM, Matte A, Tomlinson G, Chan L, Thomas C, Friedrich JO, Mehta S, Lamontagne F, Levasseur M, Ferguson ND, Adhikari NK, Rudkowski JC, Meggison H, Skrobik Y, Flannery J, Bayley M, Batt J, dos Santos C, Abbey SE, Tan A, Lo V, Mathur S, Parotto M, Morris D, Flockhart L, Fan E, Lee CM, Wilcox ME, Ayas N, Choong K, Fowler R, Scales DC, Sinuff T, Cuthbertson BH, Rose L, Robles P, Burns S, Cypel M, Singer L, Chaparro C, Chow CW, Keshavjee S, Brochard L, Hebert P, Slutsky AS, Marshall JC, Cook D, Herridge MS, Investigators RP, Canadian Critical Care Trials G. One-year outcomes in caregivers of critically ill patients. N Engl J Med. 2016;374:1831–41. doi: https://doi.org/10.1056/NEJMoa1511160.

67. Haines KJ, Denehy L, Skinner EH, Warrillow S, Berney S. Psychosocial outcomes in informal caregivers of the critically ill: a systematic review. Crit Care Med. 2015;43:1112–20. doi: https://doi.org/10.1097/CCM.00000000000008.

Extrasystoles for fluid responsiveness prediction in critically ill patients

Simon Tilma Vistisen[1,2,3]* (ID), Martin Buhl Krog[2], Thomas Elkmann[2], Mikael Fink Vallentin[1], Thomas W. L. Scheeren[3] and Christoffer Sølling[2,4]

Abstract

Background: Fluid responsiveness prediction with continuously available monitoring is an unsettled matter for the vast majority of critically ill patients, and development of new and reliable methods is desired. We hypothesized that the post-ectopic beat, which is associated with increased preload, could be analyzed in relation to preceding sinus beats and that the change in cardiac performance (e.g., systolic blood pressure) at the post-ectopic beat could predict fluid responsiveness.

Methods: Critically ill patients were observed when scheduled for a 500-ml volume expansion. The 30-min ECG prior to volume expansion was analyzed for the occurrence of extrasystoles. Classification variables were defined as the change in a variable (e.g., systolic blood pressure or pre-ejection period) from the median of ten preceding sinus beats to extrasystolic post-ectopic beat. A stroke volume increase > 10% following volume expansion defined fluid responsiveness.

Results: Twenty-six patients were included. The change in systolic blood pressure predicted fluid responsiveness with receiver operating characteristic (ROC) area 0.79 (CI [0.52:1.00]), specificity 100%, sensitivity 67%, positive predictive value 100%, and negative predictive value 91% (threshold: 5%). The change in pre-ejection period predicted fluid responsiveness with ROC area 0.74 (CI [0.53:0.94]), specificity 78%, sensitivity 67%, positive predictive value 50%, and negative predictive value 88% (threshold 7.5 ms).

Conclusions: Based on standard critical care monitoring, analysis of the extrasystolic post-ectopic beat predicts fluid responsiveness in critical care patients with good accuracy. The presented results are considered preliminary proof-of-concept results, and further validation is needed to confirm these preliminary findings.

Keywords: Hemodynamic monitoring, Fluid responsiveness, Extrasystole, Ectopic beat, Stroke volume, Cardiac output

Background

Fluid responsiveness prediction remains an unresolved issue for most ICU patients. Ventilator-induced dynamic variables, such as pulse pressure variation (PPV) or stroke volume variation (SVV), are only optimally reliable in 2–3% of admitted ICU patients [1], and passive leg raising (PLR) is time-consuming to perform and requires cardiac output monitoring to give optimal prediction [2]. Still, when used within their limitations, these two monitoring concepts are by far the best validated methods for fluid responsiveness prediction across various patient populations in the ICU setting [3–6]. However, sparsely reported data from the largest PLR study to date [7] indicate that PLR may have a slightly reduced predictive power [8] compared with the estimates from a meta-analysis [4]. The two techniques are at the core of fluid responsiveness research, and both concepts rely on the assumption that a standardized preload fluctuation will induce large fluctuations in, e.g., stroke volume (SV) or pulse pressure (PP) in fluid responders compared with non-responders. So, in the search for equally reliable but easier and more applicable fluid responsiveness methods for ICU patients, the preload fluctuation concept is likely the way forward.

* Correspondence: vistisen@clin.au.dk
[1]Research Centre for Emergency Medicine, Institute of Clinical Medicine, Aarhus University, Palle Juul-Jensens Boulevard 99, 8200 Aarhus N, Denmark
[2]Department of Anesthesiology and Intensive Care, Aarhus University Hospitals, Aarhus, Denmark
Full list of author information is available at the end of the article

Recently, we suggested that an extrasystole could be considered as a preload varying mechanism [9, 10]. While the ectopic beat itself is a poor heartbeat due to its premature nature, the post-ectopic beat is associated with an increased preload due to the compensatory pause and probably also due to a poor ejection at the ectopic beat [11, 12]. The post-ectopic beat is otherwise a sinus beat, and therefore, the post-ectopic beat is likely to elucidate the effect of increased preload and can be seen as a one-heartbeat reversible fluid challenge to the heart.

In a recent study, we showed that the post-ectopic change in the systolic blood pressure (SBP) and pre-ejection period (PEP) predicted fluid responsiveness with good accuracy in postoperative cardiac surgery patients [10] (both had an area under the receiver operating characteristic (ROC) curve of 0.81). However, post-cardiac surgery patients in their recovery phase are clinically very different from critically ill patients in the ICU. In the present study, we investigated the post-ectopic beat characteristics' ability to predict fluid responsiveness in critically ill patients admitted to a more general ICU and scheduled for a volume expansion.

Methods

The Regional Ethics Committee, Central Region, Denmark, and the Danish Health and Medicines Authority considered the study design observational. The study was approved by the Danish Data Agency (1-16-02-83-15), and it was registered at ClinicalTrials.gov (NCT02520037). Data was collected from June 2015 to September 2016.

Patients and inclusion/exclusion criteria

Critically ill patients aged 18 years or more admitted to our intensive care unit were observed if a volume expansion of 500 ml crystalloid was scheduled to be infused within 30 min or less on clinical reasons. Patients had been assessed with ultrasonography (Focus Assessed Transthoracic Echocardiography) as part of the clinical decision-making of prescribing a volume expansion (including crude assessment of left ventricular function by eyeballing). Patients with arrhythmia precluding the use of the extrasystoles method (i.e., atrial fibrillation, trigemini, or obscure pacing rhythm) were not observed. The study time frame was up to 30 min prior to volume expansion until 5 min after volume expansion. Any changes made in hemodynamically relevant treatments during this period excluded the observation, i.e., any changes in vasopressor, inotropic, analgesic or anesthetic infusion rates, changes in positive end-expiratory pressure (PEEP), and body position in the bed.

Sepsis was defined according to the previous criteria [13] because the study was initiated prior to the publication of the new sepsis criteria [14].

Data acquisition

The 30-min ECG and arterial pressure waveforms prior to volume expansion were extracted using Philips Research Data Export software. These waveforms were sampled at 125 Hz and subsequently upsampled to 1000 Hz as previously described [15]. Stroke volume (SV) before and after fluid infusion was measured with a non-invasive bioreactance-based cardiac output monitor (NICOM®, Cheetah Medical, Newton Center, MA, USA). The 5-min average of ten consecutive SV measurements before fluid infusion defined the baseline SV, and the 5-min SV average immediately following the fluid infusion defined the SV after fluid infusion. No hemodynamic changes were made during SV measurements. Other hemodynamic variables, ventilator settings, and blood gases were manually registered.

Detection and eligibility of extrasystoles

Detection of extrasystoles was done semi-automatically by custom-made R spike detection algorithms in Matlab (Version 2014a, Mathworks Inc., MA, USA). Potential extrasystoles were visually checked for eligibility defined by being preceded by ten sinus beats (representing baseline heartbeats) and the coupling interval being 80% or less than the preceding sinus beat (resulting in a relevant preload change [9]). For each eligible extrasystole, the fluctuation in SBP, PEP, PP, and maximal slope of systolic upstroke (dP/dt) was derived from the arterial blood pressure curve. The fluctuation was defined as the difference from the post-ectopic beat and the median value for the ten preceding sinus beats as previously described (supplemental material in [10]). Differences were calculated as both relative and absolute changes for SBP, PEP, PP, and dP/dt and referred to as, for example, SBP_{rel} and PEP_{abs}.

In case of more than one eligible extrasystole in the 30-min period before volume expansion, the derived variables for all extrasystoles were averaged (median) to represent a single number for an extrasystolic change in that variable per patient. The ten most recent extrasystoles prior to the volume expansion were used if there were more than ten extrasystoles in the 30-min period prior to the volume expansion.

Classification, data analysis, and statistics

Fluid responsiveness was initially defined as a 15% or more increase in SV, and results for this threshold is reported, but the limit was reduced to 10% upon data collection for statistical purposes due to only a few cases of fluid responsiveness to classify at the initial fluid response threshold of 15%.

Paired t test was used to compare hemodynamic variables prior to and after volume expansion. PPV was calculated for patients meeting the ventilator setting criteria for PPV. Central venous pressure is not standard monitoring in our ICU but was collected when available. We did not investigate additional variables for fluid responsiveness prediction since these were not readily available. All waveform data signal processing were done with Matlab. ROC area statistics are reported as "estimate [confidence interval]" along with optimal sensitivity and specificity measures according to the Youden index. The combined classification results from this and our previous clinical study in post-cardiac surgery patients are also reported. All statistical tests were performed with R (R studio, version 3.2.3 using package "pROC" for ROC statistics with the DeLong method used for ROC area confidence intervals). Spearman correlation is reported. Paired t test was used to compare the hemodynamic variables before and after fluid infusion. Student's t test was used to compare the hemodynamic variables between responders and non-responders. Based on previous data, we calculated the sample size. Using a significance level of 0.05 and power of 0.8 and assuming equal numbers of fluid responders and non-responders, we needed 23 patients with extrasystoles to provide a ROC area significantly different from 0.5. Assuming that half of the patients had one or more extrasystoles in the observation window, we aimed at 46 patients.

Results

Patient inclusion is shown in Fig. 1. Demographic and clinical data are presented in Table 1 for the included patients with extrasystoles. Twenty-six out of 41 (63%) patients eligible for ECG analysis had at least one eligible extrasystole prior to the scheduled fluid challenge, and they were included in the fluid responsiveness prediction analysis. Sixteen of the included patients were intubated but only three patients were ventilated in controlled mode and fully adapted to the ventilator, and tidal volumes for these patients were 6.4, 6.7, and 8.8 ml/kg

predicted body weight. CVP was monitored in two patients. Therefore, the classification performance of PPV and CVP is not reported.

In two cases, the post-ectopic change in PEP and PP could not be calculated for technical reasons (waveform "cut" near the diastolic pressure level), leaving 24 datasets for these variables.

Six (23%) patients responded to fluids with an increase in SV of at least 10%.

Classification characteristics of the four variables investigated during post-ectopic beats are shown in Table 2 and Fig. 2. SBP_{rel} predicted fluid responsiveness with ROC area of 0.79, with sensitivity of 67%, specificity of 100%, negative predictive value of 91%, and positive predictive value of 100%. PEP_{abs} predicted fluid responsiveness with ROC area of 0.74, with sensitivity of 67%, specificity of 78%, negative predictive value of 88%, and positive predictive value of 50%. Table 3 presents the baseline values and absolute post-ectopic changes of SBP, PEP, PP, and dP/dt for fluid responders and fluid non-responders. The correlation between variables presented in Fig. 2 did not reach a statistical significance (rho = 0.19, $p = 0.36$, for SBP_{rel} and rho = 0.14, $p = 0.50$, for PEP_{abs}). The present study's data combined with previously reported clinical data (SBP_{rel} and PEP_{abs}) is shown in Additional file 1: Figure S1, where AUC point estimates ranged from 0.72 to 0.81.

Discussion

In the present study, we investigated the post-ectopic beat characteristics' ability to predict fluid responsiveness in critically ill patients. Four out of six fluid responders (increasing SV by 10% or more) had a post-ectopic SBP_{rel} change exceeding 5%, whereas none of the 20 non-responders had post-ectopic SBP changes exceeding that level, resulting in estimated sensitivity and specificity of 67% and 100%,

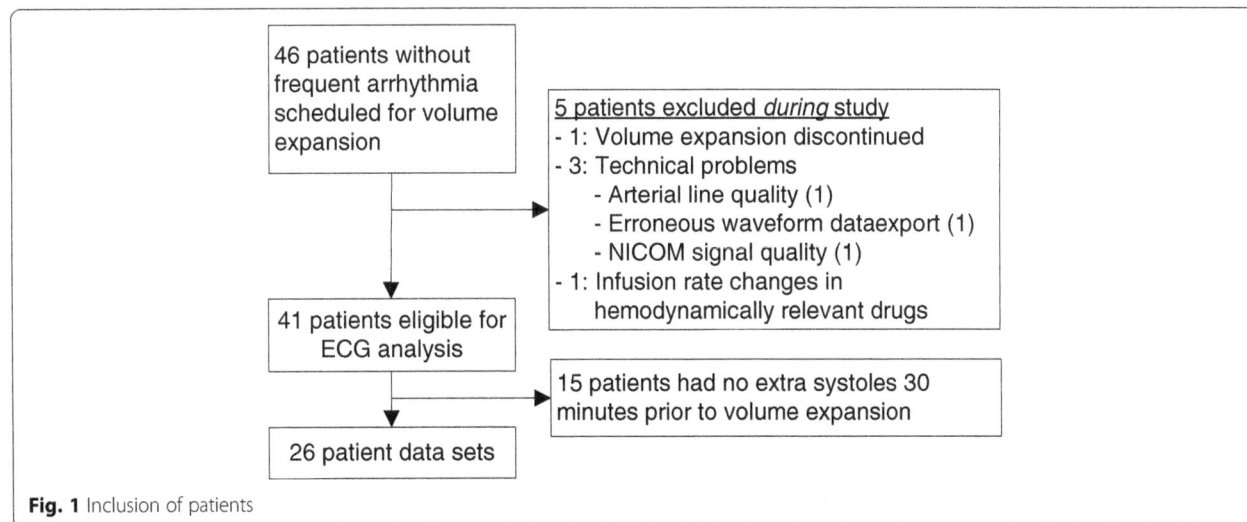

Fig. 1 Inclusion of patients

Table 1 Demographic and clinical characteristics of patients

n = 26	
Age, years	70.1 (11.2)
Gender, male/female	9/17
Height, cm	168 (7.9)
Weight, kg	65.7 (16.7)
SOFA score	7.2 (3.2)
Lactate	2.1 (1.5)
Primary diagnosis	
-Severe sepsis	4
-GI origin	2
-Origin not confirmed	2
-Septic shock	14
-GI origin	5
-Pneumonia	5
-Origin not confirmed	4
-Severe hypotension after major orthopedic surgery	2
-Cerebral event	2
-GI bleeding	1
-Chronic pancreatitis	1
-Rhabdomyolysis	1
-Acute liver failure	1
Vasoactive/inotropic drugs	
-Norepinephrine	17
-Dobutamine	1

Hemodynamics	Before fluids	After fluids
HR, min^{-1}	90 (18)	88 (19)
MAP, mmHg	73 (15)	82 (14)*
SV, ml	72 (23)	71 (22)

GI gastro-intestinal, *HR* heart rate, *MAP* mean arterial pressure, *SV* stroke volume
*$p < 0.00001$

respectively. As such, our study confirms our previous clinical findings that a post-ectopic SBP change of more than 5% appears a safe threshold for predicting a significant increase in SV after fluid loading, which, however, is on the expense of a sensitivity level of around 70% [10].

Extrasystoles were available in 63% of the observed non-atrial fibrillation patients in this study. In our previous clinical study in post-cardiac surgery patients, we found a similar incidence (61%). Still, both of these studies' samples are considered convenience samples, but these figures are in alignment with a more detailed extrasystolic occurrence analysis (paper under review). The detection of extrasystoles was done semi-automatically in this study because the monitor's automatic annotation of hearts beat was not available. Eventually, detection of extrasystoles should be automated by existing monitor software as well as the interbeat calculation of SPB, PP, etc. These detections are already done in existing monitoring, but not combined. The steady-state period of 30 min observation for extrasystoles is obviously not suggested as a waiting time for clinicians, rather the idea is that clinicians facing hemodynamically unstable patients could look back in time and supplement their intervention decision with the arterial waveform characteristics of recent extrasystoles (< 30 min). This is (as estimated) possible in more than half of non-atrial fibrillation patients. While not directly comparable, this stands in contrast to 2–3% of patients where PPV is reliable in the ICU. Still, there is a large group of patients (here, estimated 37%), where extrasystoles had not spontaneously occurred prior to volume expansion. In these cases, the extrasystole method is not applicable. It is up to the clinicians to decide whether the glass is half full or half empty with this extrasystolic occurrence. We think of it as half full because the information held in extrasystoles is, in principle, freely and readily available in half of the ICU patients monitored with ECG and invasive arterial pressure. Obviously, however, post-ectopic beat characteristics need to be calculated by monitors since eyeballing small changes in SBP is difficult and

Table 2 Classification characteristics of post-ectopic changes in variables

Variable	Prediction at 10% SV change threshold				Prediction at 15% SV change threshold			
	ROC curve area	Spec (%)	Sens (%)	Threshold	ROC curve area	Spec (%)	Sens (%)	Threshold
SBP$_{abs}$	0.78 [0.54; 1]	90	67	5.5 mmHg	0.66 [0.33; 0.99]	82	50	5.5 mmHg
PEP$_{abs}$	0.74 [0.53; 0.95]	78	67	7.5 ms	0.73 [0.47; 1]	75	75	7.5 ms
PP$_{abs}$	0.77 [0.52; 1]	78	83	8.46 mmHg	0.73 [0.36; 1]	75	75	8.46 mmHg
dP/dt$_{abs}$	0.76 [0.53; 0.99]	85	67	0.195 mmHg/s^2	0.64 [0.33; 0.94]	32	100	0.030 mmHg/s^2
SBP$_{rel}$	0.79 [0.52; 1]	100	67	5%	0.66 [0.27; 1]	95	50	5.5%
PEP$_{rel}$	0.70 [0.50; 0.90]	65	83	2.5%	0.69 [0.44; 0.95]	68	75	3%
PP$_{rel}$	0.70 [0.48; 0.93]	67	83	15%	0.71 [0.41; 1]	80	75	15%
dP/dt$_{rel}$	0.68 [0.39; 98]	70	83	14%	0.68 [0.39; 0.98]	64	75	14%

SBP systolic blood pressure, *PEP* pre-ejection period, *PP* pulse pressure, *dP/dt* maximal systolic upstroke, *SV* stroke volume, *ROC* receiver operating characteristic, *Spec* specificity, *Sens* sensitivity, *rel* post-ectopic change calculated on relative scale, *abs* post-ectopic change calculated on absolute scale

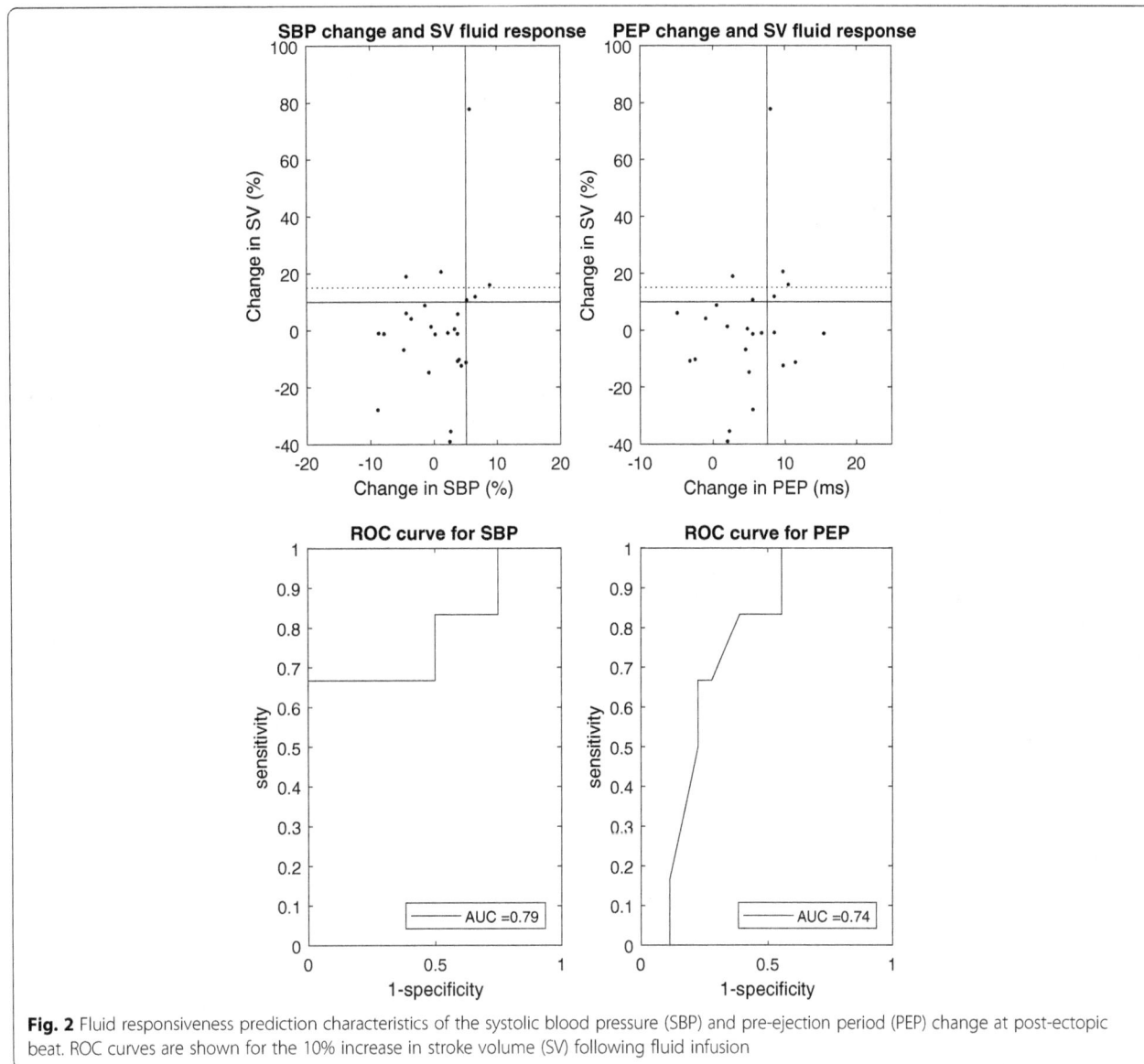

Fig. 2 Fluid responsiveness prediction characteristics of the systolic blood pressure (SBP) and pre-ejection period (PEP) change at post-ectopic beat. ROC curves are shown for the 10% increase in stroke volume (SV) following fluid infusion

Table 3 Hemodynamic characteristics of sinus beats prior to ectopy and the post-ectopic beat for fluid non-responders and fluid responders

	Non-responders	Responders	p value
Baseline SBP (mmHg)	116 (21)	125 (35)	0.46
Post-ectopic SBP change (mmHg)	− 0.1 (5.6)	5.9 (6.6)	0.04
Baseline PEP (ms)	212 (39)	212 (34)	0.99
Post-ectopic PEP change (ms)	4.0 (5.3)	7.5 (2.9)	0.14
Baseline PP (mmHg)	58 (21)	65 (22)	0.51
Post-ectopic PP change (mmHg)	4.0 (6.7)	10.6 (7.0)	0.05
Baseline dP/dt (ms)	0.88 (0.47)	0.94 (0.39)	0.77
Post-ectopic dP/dt change (mmHg/ms)	0.08 (0.11)	0.16 (0.08)	0.10

SBP systolic blood pressure, *PEP* pre-ejection period, *PP* pulse pressure

even impossible for PEP changes. For the method to work, these calculations have to be automated by monitors.

Our study is associated with some limitations that should be taken into account when interpreting the data. In this observational study, we included a heterogenic patient population. The study was small (*n* = 26), and we encountered few responders to classify with our method. Therefore, we have to pay discrete and meticulous caution for the data interpretation. The low number of responders leads to the choice of reducing the otherwise prospectively defined SV response threshold from 15 to 10%, which is a suboptimal modification to the registered study design. Still, combining the study results with previously reported clinical data (Additional file 1: Figure S1) is supporting the conclusion that the extrasystolic method is predicting fluid responsiveness in ICU patients with good accuracy. However, while Additional file 1: Figure S1 is summarizing the classification accuracy of the existing data for the extrasystoles method, it has to be kept in mind that the combined data originates from two different ICU patient populations, namely postoperative cardiac surgery patients [10] and in this study more regular ICU patients not including any post-cardiac surgery patients.

While not anticipating the low number of responders, we speculate that it could be related to the fact that most of the patients could be described as being in their "optimization/stabilization" phase, where a massive increase in stroke volume upon fluid loading is less likely as opposed to, for example, the early "rescue" hours in sepsis [16], where a future study preferentially could be conducted. Infusion time (30 min) might also be considered long, but patients increased their mean arterial pressure (MAP) significantly to the fluid challenge as opposed to their SV (Table 1), so from some clinical viewpoints, more than six patients responded to fluids. In addition, our SV monitoring technique, NICOM®, may also be an explanation for the few fluid responders. CO measurements fluctuate as a consequence of both interventions (e.g., fluids), physiologic variation over time and measurement error. NICOM® bias was reported to be + 4.1% ± 11.3%, and sensitivity and specificity for significant directional changes were both 93% [17]. In another study, the measured SV response on fluid loading as measured by NICOM® was also modest (4 out of 48 patients increased NICOM®-derived SV by 15% or more upon volume expansion) [18]. The validity of NICOM® to detect these changes has therefore been debated [17, 18], and the use of bioreactance techniques for measuring CO and/or SV in the everyday *clinical setting* may not be ready for expert panel endorsement [19], because absolute values are of importance. Still, NICOM®-derived SV is a reasonable outcome measure for fluid responsiveness *research* [17, 20]. Finally, we did

not compare the extrasystolic method with other fluid responsiveness predictors such as PLR and CVP. PLR, despite the need for intervention and reliable, fast responding SV measurements, is currently the most applicable method in ICUs. Additionally, PLR has reportedly a very high accuracy of predicting fluid responsiveness as estimated by systematic reviews [3–5]. However, the largest and probably best-conducted PLR study to date [7] is revealing somewhat lower prediction accuracy (sensitivity and specificity *estimated* at 84% and 62%, respectively [8]). Surprisingly, the authors of that study did not wish to provide exact classification statistics in their study [7] despite data for it was undoubtedly available and despite the authors were encouraged to [8]. Consequently, and since we did not directly compare with PLR in this study, it becomes difficult to discuss what classification accuracy should be considered acceptable for competing methods like the one presented. It is up to the readers to judge, but we think that the available clinical data shows that post-ectopic beat characteristics could supplement the decision of whether or not to give a fluid infusion in ICU patients since the method does not rely on an intervention. However, the extrasystolic morphologic configuration in ABP should not be the sole reason for administering or not administering fluids since the classification accuracy is not excellent and since a lot of other clinical factors should be taken into account in the decision of administering fluids, including risk of side effects to fluids, which fluid responsiveness methods generally cannot assess.

There are fundamental differences between supraventricular and ventricular extrasystoles. Particularly, the compensatory pause is different (longer) for ventricular extrasystoles compared with supraventricular extrasystoles. However, in the clinical studies conducted so far, the post-ectopic changes encountered in, for example, SBP and PEP are not different when comparing the supraventricular and ventricular extrasystoles and they appear equally predictive of fluid responsiveness. This was the reason why we included both types of extrasystoles in the study. It has been hypothesized that both preload and contractility of the heart are altered during the ectopic activity, contributing to the compensatory mechanism of reduced stroke volume at the ectopic beat [11]. While left ventricular end-diastolic pressure is always increased at the post-ectopic beat compared with the preceding sinus beats [11], contractility may also contribute to the observed changes in cardiac performance at the post-ectopic beat [11], and it has been hypothesized that calcium derangements occur at the post-ectopic beat. A contractility altering mechanism could explain why the simple post-ectopic evaluation of blood pressure characteristics does not excellently predict fluid responsiveness with a ROC AUC exceeding 0.90. Still, in vivo studies testing the contractility derangements have so far not investigated this mechanism under various preload conditions in the intact heart, so it remains unclear how much a contractility altering effect contributes to the contraction at the post-ectopic beat compared with the preload altering the effect.

Respiration, particularly mechanical ventilation, influences the beat-to-beat level of hemodynamic variables such as SBP. In our data analyses, we averaged out this effect as we calculated a median value from ten preceding heartbeats. However, the exact occurrence of an extrasystole within a respiratory cycle may influence the value of SBP at the post-ectopic beat.

In our study, we did not evaluate the exclusion of frequent arrhythmia (predominantly atrial fibrillation), but the overall occurrence of atrial fibrillation in medical and non-cardiac surgical adult intensive care unit patients is estimated at 10.5% [21].

The magnitude of the post-ectopic PEP_{abs} change was markedly different between this and our previous study as reflected in the optimal classification thresholds (7.5 ms in this study and 19 ms in our previous study [10]). We do not have any reason to believe that the difference could be related to the monitoring technology, since pressure transducers, monitors, the data extraction, and the algorithms to derive PEP were the same across studies. It must be related to the patient category and/or how patients were treated. Looking detailed into this and the previous study's data, indeed, there appears to be an explanation: baseline PEP (at sinus beats and according to our definition) was 253 ms (SD: 33 ms) for cardiac surgery patients in their first postoperative hours, whereas PEP was 212 ms (SD 37 ms) in the present study's patients. The vascular transit time (time from pressure upstroke in the aorta to pressure upstroke in the radial artery) is around 80–100 ms and probably does not vary much across our populations. Since the post-ectopic PEP change is defined by us as an absolute value (in ms and not percent), this physiologic difference between the two patient populations may—in combination with patient characteristics and the low number of fluid responders in the present study—explain the observed difference in the magnitude of absolute post-ectopic PEP changes. No matter the underlying explanation for the differences in post-ectopic PEP changes, which we speculate to be related to cardiac function and/or cardiac medication differences, it should be noted that this variable has to be investigated more thoroughly in various patient categories before it can be suggested to be used for fluid responsiveness prediction.

Conclusion

This study's data further supports the notion that extrasystoles may be useful for fluid responsiveness prediction, but we have not encountered excellent prediction with the extrasystoles method. Due to the limitations of our study

along with the amount of available clinical data on extrasystoles' ability to predict fluid responsiveness, we still consider the data at hand preliminary proof-of-concept results and we would be cautious and not yet recommend the method for clinical use before more validation studies point in the same direction as the currently available data, preferably carried out by other research groups. So far, however, a 5% post-ectopic increase in systolic blood pressure appears a consistent indicator of a positive fluid response, and this observation may be useful in situations where other reliable fluid responsiveness monitoring is not available.

Additional file

Additional file 1: Figure S1. Data combining previous clinical data with the present study's data. Dot markers constitute data from this study. Star markers constitute data from the previous study. Middle panels are ROC curves for predicting fluid responsiveness at the 15% stroke volume (SV) increase threshold (dashed horizontal lines in upper panels), whereas the lower panels are ROC curves for the 10% SV increase threshold (full horizontal lines in upper panels). (PDF 8 kb)

Funding
STV is financially supported by the Danish Medical Research Council (DFF – 4183-00540).

Authors' contributions
STV contributed to the conception of the study, study design, data collection, data analysis, interpretation of data, and writing of the first draft of the paper and revising it critically for important intellectual content and gave final approval of the version to be published. MBK and TE contributed to the study design and data collection, revised the first draft critically for important intellectual content, and gave final approval of the version to be published. MFV contributed to the conception of study and study design, revised the first draft critically for important intellectual content, and gave final approval of the version to be published. TWLS contributed to the interpretation of data, revised the first draft critically for important intellectual content, and gave final approval of the version to be published. CS contributed to the study design and data collection, revised the first draft critically for important intellectual content, and gave final approval of the version to be published.

Competing interest
The extrasystoles method was previously protected by a patent application owned by Aarhus University (PCT/DK2014/050094; STV as sole inventor). The application did, however, not lead to the granting of a patent at priority expiry date.
TWLS is an associate editor of the Journal of Clinical Monitoring and Computing. TWLS received honoraria for consulting from Edwards Lifesciences and Masimo Corp. TWLS is currently the Chair of the Section Cardiovascular Dynamics of the European Society of Intensive Care Medicine as well as the Chair of the Scientific Subcommittee 14 (Monitoring, Ultrasound, and Equipment) of the European Society of Anaesthesiology. Apart from this, all other authors declare that they have no competing interests.

Author details
[1]Research Centre for Emergency Medicine, Institute of Clinical Medicine, Aarhus University, Palle Juul-Jensens Boulevard 99, 8200 Aarhus N, Denmark. [2]Department of Anesthesiology and Intensive Care, Aarhus University Hospitals, Aarhus, Denmark. [3]University Medical Center Groningen, Department of Anesthesiology, University of Groningen, Groningen, the Netherlands. [4]Department of Anesthesiology and Intensive Care, Viborg Regional Hospital, Viborg, Denmark.

References
1. Mahjoub Y, Lejeune V, Muller L, Perbet S, Zieleskiewicz L, Bart F, Veber B, Paugam-Burtz C, Jaber S, Ayham A, Zogheib E, Lasocki S, Vieillard-Baron A, Quintard H, Joannes-Boyau O, Plantefeve G, Montravers P, Duperret S, Lakhdari M, Ammenouche N, Lorne E, Slama M, Dupont H. Evaluation of pulse pressure variation validity criteria in critically ill patients: a prospective observational multicentre point-prevalence study. Br J Anaesth. 2014 Apr; 112(4):681–5.
2. Marik PE, Monnet X, Teboul JL. Hemodynamic parameters to guide fluid therapy. Ann Intensive Care. 2011 Mar 21;1(1):1,5820-1-1.
3. Cherpanath TG, Hirsch A, Geerts BF, Lagrand WK, Leeflang MM, Schultz MJ, Groeneveld AB. Predicting fluid responsiveness by passive leg raising: a systematic review and meta-analysis of 23 clinical trials. Crit Care Med. 2016 May;44(5):981–91.
4. Cavallaro F, Sandroni C, Marano C, La Torre G, Mannocci A, De Waure C, Bello G, Maviglia R, Antonelli M. Diagnostic accuracy of passive leg raising for prediction of fluid responsiveness in adults: systematic review and meta-analysis of clinical studies. Intensive Care Med. 2010 Sep;36(9):1475–83.
5. Monnet X, Marik P, Teboul JL. Passive leg raising for predicting fluid responsiveness: a systematic review and meta-analysis. Intensive Care Med. 2016 Dec;42(12):1935–47.
6. Marik PE, Cavallazzi R, Vasu T, Hirani A. Dynamic changes in arterial waveform derived variables and fluid responsiveness in mechanically ventilated patients: a systematic review of the literature. Crit Care Med. 2009 Sep;37(9):2642–7.
7. Vignon P, Repesse X, Begot E, Leger J, Jacob C, Bouferrache K, Slama M, Prat G, Vieillard-Baron A. Comparison of echocardiographic indices used to predict fluid responsiveness in ventilated patients. Am J Respir Crit Care Med. 2017 Apr 15;195(8):1022–32.
8. Vistisen ST, Enevoldsen J, Scheeren TW. Can passive leg raising be considered the gold standard in predicting fluid responsiveness? Am J Respir Crit Care Med. 2017 Apr 15;195(8):1075–6.
9. Vistisen ST, Andersen KK, Frederiksen CA, Kirkegaard H. Variations in the pre-ejection period induced by ventricular extra systoles may be feasible to predict fluid responsiveness. J Clin Monit Comput. 2014 Aug;28(4):341–9.
10. Vistisen ST. Using extra systoles to predict fluid responsiveness in cardiothoracic critical care patients. J Clin Monit Comput. 2017 Aug; 31(4):693–9.
11. Takada H, Takeuchi S, Ando K, Kaito A, Yoshida S. Experimental studies on myocardial contractility and hemodynamics in extrasystoles. Jpn Circ J. 1970 May;34(5):419–30.
12. Yellin EL, Kennish A, Yoran C, Laniado S, Buckley NM, Frater RW. The influence of left ventricular filling on postextrasystolic potentiation in the dog heart. Circ Res. 1979 May;44(5):712–22.
13. Dellinger RP, Levy MM, Rhodes A, Annane D, Gerlach H, Opal SM, Sevransky JE, Sprung CL, Douglas IS, Jaeschke R, Osborn TM, Nunnally ME, Townsend SR, Reinhart K, Kleinpell RM, Angus DC, Deutschman CS, Machado FR, Rubenfeld GD, Webb S, Beale RJ, Vincent JL, Moreno R, Surviving Sepsis Campaign Guidelines Committee including The Pediatric Subgroup. Surviving Sepsis Campaign: International Guidelines For Management Of Severe Sepsis And Septic Shock, 2012. Intensive Care Med. 2013 Feb;39(2):165–228.
14. Singer M, Deutschman CS, Seymour CW, Shankar-Hari M, Annane D, Bauer M, Bellomo R, Bernard GR, Chiche JD, Coopersmith CM, Hotchkiss RS, Levy MM, Marshall JC, Martin GS, Opal SM, Rubenfeld GD, van der Poll T, Vincent JL, Angus DC. The Third International Consensus Definitions for Sepsis and Septic Shock (Sepsis-3). Jama. 2016 Feb 23;315(8):801–10.
15. Vistisen ST, Koefoed-Nielsen J, Larsson A. Automated pre-ejection period variation predicts fluid responsiveness in low tidal volume ventilated pigs. Acta Anaesthesiol Scand. 2010 Feb;54(2):199–205.
16. Hoste EA, Maitland K, Brudney CS, Mehta R, Vincent JL, Yates D, Kellum JA, Mythen MG, Shaw AD, ADQI XII Investigators Group. Four phases of intravenous fluid therapy: a conceptual model. Br J Anaesth. 2014 Nov; 113(5):740–7.
17. Squara P. Bioreactance for estimating cardiac output and the effects of passive leg raising in critically ill patients. Br J Anaesth. 2014 May;112(5):942.
18. Kupersztych-Hagege E, Teboul JL, Artigas A, Talbot A, Sabatier C, Richard C, Monnet X. Bioreactance is not reliable for estimating cardiac output and the effects of passive leg raising in critically ill patients. Br J Anaesth. 2013 Dec; 111(6):961–6.
19. Teboul JL, Saugel B, Cecconi M, De Backer D, Hofer CK, Monnet X, Perel A, Pinsky MR, Reuter DA, Rhodes A, Squara P, Vincent JL, Scheeren TW. Less invasive hemodynamic monitoring in critically ill patients. Intensive Care Med. 2016 Sep;42(9):1350–9.
20. Jakovljevic DG, Trenell MI, MacGowan GA. Bioimpedance and bioreactance methods for monitoring cardiac output. Best Pract Res Clin Anaesthesiol. 2014 Dec;28(4):381–94.
21. Kanji S, Williamson DR, Yaghchi BM, Albert M, McIntyre L. Canadian Critical Care Trials Group. Epidemiology and management of atrial fibrillation in medical and noncardiac surgical adult intensive care unit patients. J Crit Care. 2012 Jun;27(3):326.e1,326.e8.

Seizure prophylaxis in the neuroscience intensive care unit

Sushma Yerram[1], Nakul Katyal[1]* [iD], Keerthivaas Premkumar[2], Premkumar Nattanmai[1] and Christopher R. Newey[1,3]

Abstract

Background: Seizures are a considerable complication in critically ill patients. Their incidence is significantly high in neurosciences intensive care unit patients. Seizure prophylaxis with anti-epileptic drugs is a common practice in neurosciences intensive care unit. However, its utility in patients without clinical seizure, with an underlying neurological injury, is somewhat controversial.

Body: In this article, we have reviewed the evidence for seizure prophylaxis in commonly encountered neurological conditions in neurosciences intensive care unit and discussed the possible prognostic role of continuous electroencephalography monitoring in detecting early seizures in critically ill patients.

Conclusion: Based on the current evidence and guidelines, we have proposed a presumptive protocol for seizure prophylaxis in neurosciences intensive care unit. Patients with severe traumatic brain injury and possible subarachnoid hemorrhage seem to benefit with a short course of anti-epileptic drug. In patients with other neurological illnesses, the use of continuous electroencephalography would make sense rather than indiscriminately administering anti-epileptic drug.

Keywords: Seizure prophylaxis, Critically ill patients, Anti-epileptic drugs, Continuous electroencephalography

Background

Seizures are a considerable complication in critically ill patients. Their incidence is higher in neurosciences intensive care unit (NSICU) patients [1]. Seizure prophylaxis with anti-epileptic drugs (AED) is a common practice in NSICU. However, its utility in patients without clinical seizure, with an underlying neurological injury is somewhat controversial. AEDs for seizure prophylaxis are used in various acute neurological insults including traumatic brain injury (TBI), epidural hemorrhage (EDH), subdural hemorrhage (SDH), aneurysmal subarachnoid hemorrhage (SAH), intracerebral hemorrhage (ICH), brain neoplasms, ischemic stroke, cavernoma and arteriovenous malformation (AVM), cerebral venous sinus thrombosis (CVST), posterior reversible encephalopathy syndrome (PRES), and meningitis. The underlying risk for seizure varies significantly in all these disease states. In this article, we have reviewed the evidence for seizure prophylaxis in commonly encountered neurological conditions in NSICU and discussed the possible prognostic role of continuous electroencephalography (CEEG) monitoring in detecting early seizures in critically ill patients.

Traumatic brain injury

Post traumatic seizures (PTS) in TBI patients are classified as early PTS, with seizure occurring within 7 days of injury and late PTS, with seizure occurring after 7 days of injury [1, 2]. According to a civilian study [1], the incidence rate for early PTS ranges between 4 and 25%, whereas the incidence rate for late PTS ranges between 9 and 42% [1]. Studies have identified multiple risk factors increasing the likelihood of PTS in TBI patients [3]. Penetrating injuries are associated with highest incidence of PTS with more than 50% of patients developing seizures over 15 years [1] (Table 1).

The risk factors for early and late PTS include [3]:

Seizure prophylaxis in traumatic brain injury

Given the high incidence of seizures in TBI patients, AEDs are frequently used as prophylactic therapy. Temkin et al. [4] conducted a randomized, double-blinded,

* Correspondence: Katyal.nakul@gmail.com
[1]Department of Neurology, University of Missouri, 5 Hospital Drive, CE 540, Columbia, MO 65211, USA
Full list of author information is available at the end of the article

Table 1 Risk factors for seizure in patients with traumatic brain injury

Risk factors for early PTS [3]	Risk factors for late PTS [3]
• Glasgow coma scale < 10	• Early PTS
• Penetrating brain injuries	• Acute intracerebral hematoma
• Acute intracerebral hematoma	• Brain contusion
• Acute subdural hematoma	• Loss of consciousness
• Younger age	• Post traumatic amnesia lasting
• Loss of consciousness	> 24 h
• Post traumatic amnesia	• Age > 65 at the time of injury
lasting > 30 min	
• Chronic alcoholism	

placebo-controlled trial to evaluate the effects of phenytoin (20 mg/kg load) on early and late PTS. A significant reduction was observed in the incidence of early PTS in phenytoin group from 14.2 to 3.6% ($p < 0.001$) whereas, no significant reduction was noted in the incidence of late PTS with phenytoin use. Unfortunately, patients with seizures were included in the prophylaxis group making the data difficult to interpret. No significant side effects or mortality differences were observed between phenytoin and placebo groups [5]. Significant impairment was noted on neuropsychological testing in phenytoin group patients at 1 month time after starting therapy, which later was not apparent after 1 year of injury [6].

In another RCT, the effects of valproate on early and late PTS were studied. The trial later compared valproate (20 mg/kg load) to phenytoin (20 mg/kg load) for prevention of early PTS valproate to placebo for prevention of late PTS [7]. It was reported that the rate of early PTS was low and similar in both valproate (4.5%) and phenytoin (1.5%) groups [7]. The rate of late PTS was also similar, being high in both groups (valproate 16%, phenytoin 15%). However, a significantly higher mortality rate was observed in valproate group (13.4%) as compared to phenytoin (7.2%) [7]. No potential added benefits and higher mortality rates suggest that valproate should not be used for seizure prophylaxis. A meta-analysis study conducted in 2001 showed that out of all AED, only phenytoin and carbamazepine were effective in reducing early PTS. No AED was found to be effective in reducing late PTS [8].

Levetiracetam has been studied for seizure prophylaxis [9]. Levetiracetam has no known drug interactions, excellent bioavailability and relatively safer pharmacological profile; these make it somewhat ideal for prophylactic use [9]. In a study to compare effectiveness of levetiracetam (500 mg BD) to that of phenytoin (historical controls) for preventing seizures in patients with TBI, no differences were observed in seizure activity between the two (levetiracetam 6.7 and phenytoin 0%, $p = 0.556$) [10]. Strikingly, an increased incidence of EEG abnormalities (seizure tendency with epileptiform activity) was noted in levetiracetam group ($p = 0.003$). No difference in EEG findings of seizures

($p = 0.556$) was seen in the two groups [10]. In another study comparing seizure prophylaxis with levetiracetam (1500 mg BD) versus phenytoin (20 mg/kg load followed by 5 mg/kg/d maintenance), no significant differences were seen in early seizure rates (phenytoin 3 of 18 vs levetiracetam 5 of 34; $p = 1.0$) [11]. However, levetiracetam group reportedly had lower disability rating scale scores at 3 and 6 months ($p = 0.006$ and $p = 0.037$, respectively) and higher extended Glasgow outcome scale scores at 6 months [11] (Table 2).

Current recommendations
Aneurysmal subarachnoid hemorrhage

Abnormal seizure like moments is common in patients with aneurysmal subarachnoid hemorrhage (aSAH) [12, 13]. Their incidence can be as high as 26% [12, 13]. They may be associated more with the posturing event during rupture of aneurysm than actual seizures [12, 13]. Clinical seizures occur in about 1 to 7% of patients with aSAH and typically are manifestations of rerupture of an unsecured aneurysm [14, 15]. The incidence rate for nonconvulsive seizures in patients with aSAH is reportedly 8 to 18% [16–18]. Risk factors increasing the likelihood of seizures in aSAH patients are [12, 13] (Table 3).

Seizure prophylaxis in aneurysmal subarachnoid hemorrhage

AED prophylaxis for aSAH is somewhat controversial [19]. Limited randomized controlled trials (RCT) justifying the prophylactic use and serious adverse effects of AED make the decision even more challenging [19, 20]. Seizures in acutely ill patients with aSAH can lead to additional injury or rebleeding from an unsecured aneurysm, which make AED prophylaxis critical in some cases.

In a study to assess the utility of phenytoin (900–1100 mg load followed by 300 mg/d) for seizure prophylaxis in patients with aSAH, investigators observed a low seizure incidence of about 5.4% after 2.4 years of follow-up [21]. In a retrospective study, undertaken to compare different duration of phenytoin (1 g load followed by 300 mg/d) prophylaxis (3 days prophylaxis versus 14 days prophylaxis), no significant differences were observed in seizure incidences during hospitalization (1.9 vs 1.3%, $p = 0.6$) and after a follow-up period of 3 to 12 months (4.6 vs 5.7%,

Table 2 Brain trauma guidelines for management of TBI patients

According to latest brain trauma foundation guidelines (2016) [75]

• Phenytoin is recommended for prevention of early PTS and it should be used for first 7 days after TBI [75].

• Phenytoin or valproate use is not recommended for prevention against late PTS [75].

• Given its safety profile levetiracetam could be a potential alternative to phenytoin for prophylaxis against early PTS. Presently there is not enough corroborative evidence to support its use over phenytoin [75].

Table 3 Risk factors for seizures in aSAH patients

Risk factors for seizures in aSAH patients [12, 13]
• Prior seizures
• History of HTN
• Intraparenchymal hemorrhage
• Infarction
• Middle cerebral artery aneurysm
• Thickness of aSAH clot
• Rebleeding
• Poor neurological grade
• Intervention: endovascular coiling associated with a lower risk of seizure compared to open craniotomy for clipping

Table 4 Neurocritical Care Society guidelines and 2012 American Heart Association/American stroke Association guidelines for management of patients with aSAH

As per the 2011 Neurocritical Care Society guidelines [71] and 2012 American Heart Association/American stroke Association guidelines [76]
• Phenytoin is not recommended routinely for seizure prophylaxis after SAH [71].
• Other AED may be considered for seizure prophylaxis [71].
• A short course is preferable (3–7 days) in case prophylaxis is needed [71].
• CEEG monitoring should be used in patients who failed to improve or have poor grade SAH [71].
• Prophylactic use of AED can be considered in immediate post hemorrhagic period [76].
• Long-term use of AED can be considered for patients with known risk factors for delayed seizure disorder, such as prior seizure, intracerebral hematoma, intractable hypertension, infarction, or aneurysm at the middle cerebral artery [76].

$p = 0.6$) [22]. A significant reduction was noticed in incidence of adverse drug reactions with 3 days prophylaxis (0.5 vs 8.8%, $p = 0.002$), which indicates that a 3-day regimen is a superior treatment protocol [22]. This study was further scrutinized to assess the relationship between phenytoin exposure and harm by quantifying phenytoin burden and estimating its impact on outcomes [20]. Phenytoin burden was identified as an independent predictor for poor functional outcome at 14 days (OR per quartile 1.5%, 95% CI 1.2–1.9) and for poor cognitive outcome at 3 months ($p = 0.003$) [20]. A study estimating the impact of AED on outcomes by analyzing data from four RCTs reported that the use of AED in patients with aSAH was associated with poor a 3-month outcomes with worse Glasgow outcome scale (OR 1.56, $p = 0.003$), vasospasm (OR 1.87, $p < 0.001$), neurological deterioration (OR 1.61, $p < 0.001$), cerebral infarction (OR 1.33, $p = 0.04$), and fever (OR 1.36, $p = 0.03$) [19].

A possible risk for drug-drug interaction exist in patients taking phenytoin and nimodipine, a calcium channel blocker commonly used to counter vasospasm in patients with aSAH [23]. A single-dose pharmacokinetic study of nimodipine in patients on chronic enzyme inducing AED showed a mean decrease of 70% ($p < 0.01$) in plasma nimodipine concentration in patients taking enzyme inducing AED and an increase of 50% in plasma nimodipine concentration in patients taking valproate [23].

Given its relatively safer profile, there is a growing interest in support of using levetiracetam for seizure prophylaxis [9]. A retrospective study comparing phenytoin (15–20 mg/kg load; 13.7 days) to levetiracetam (500 mg BD; 3.6 days) in aSAH patients reported a higher seizure incidence in levetiracetam group (8.3 vs 3.4%) [24]. A lower incidence of poor outcome (death or nursing home discharge) was noticed in levetiracetam group (16 vs 24%, $p = 0.06$) [24]. Nonetheless, the concerns like lack of loading dose of levetiracetam, a shorter course of therapy renders the study statistically insignificant (Table 4).

Current recommendations
Brain neoplasm
Seizures are commonly reported in patients with brain neoplasms [25, 26]. The incidence rate of seizures at or before the time diagnosis of brain tumor diagnosis ranges from 14 to 51%, whereas after the diagnosis, it varies between 10 and 45% [25].

Risk factors for seizures in patients with brain neoplasm vary according to [26]:

• Type of tumor: primary tumor > metastatic
• Grade of tumor: low-grade glioma > high-grade glioma
• Specific tumor types: dysembryoplastic neuroepithelial tumors > meningiomas

Seizure prophylaxis in brain neoplasms
A meta-analysis study of five trials from 1999 through 2004 evaluated the efficacy of AED phenobarbital, phenytoin, and valproic acid versus placebo or no treatment for seizure prophylaxis in patients with brain neoplasm [27]. Four of the trials showed no significant benefits of seizure prophylaxis at 1 week (OR 0.91, CI 0.45–1.83) or at 6 months (OR 1.01, CI 0.51–1.98) in patients with brain neoplasm [27]. AED prophylaxis showed no preventive benefits for specific tumor pathologies, including primary glial tumors (OR 3.46, 95% CI 0.32–37.47), cerebral metastasis (OR 2.50, 95% CI 0.25–24.72), and meningiomas (OR 0.62, 95% CI 0.10–3.85) [27]. The cochrane review in 2008 came to similar conclusions but did find higher incidence of adverse effects in patients on AEDs (NNH 3; RR 6.1, CI 1.1–34.63; $p = 0.046$) [28]. The American Academy of Neurology (AAN) introduced practice parameters for seizure prophylaxis in patients with brain neoplasms [25]. Based on results from 12 studies evaluating efficacy of AED phenobarbital, phenytoin and valproic acid over a

median follow-up time of 5.4 to 19 months, it was concluded that AED prophylaxis had no significant preventive effect on either seizure incidence (OR 1.09, CI 0.63–1.89; $p = 0.08$) or seizure free survival (OR 1.03, CI 0.74–1.44; $p = 0.9$) [25]. Significant side effects were reported in the trials including rash (14%), nausea/vomiting (5%), encephalopathy (5%), myelosuppression (3%), ataxia, increased liver enzymes, and gum pain (5%) [25].

Guidelines for prophylactic use of AED in patients with metastatic brain neoplasms were derived from analysis of a RCT, evaluating the efficacy of AED phenobarbital, phenytoin versus no treatment [29, 30]. No significant differences were observed in seizure incidence between two groups in the trial [29]. It was concluded that seizure prophylaxis was not beneficial in patients with metastatic brain tumors [29]. Another RCT comparing the efficacy of short course AED prophylaxis with phenytoin for 7 days versus no prophylaxis in patients with intraparenchymal tumors showed no significant difference in seizure incidence between two groups (24 vs 18%; $p = 0.51$) [31]. However, significant adverse effects were reported in phenytoin group (18 vs 0%; $p < 0.01$) [31]. The most commonly reported side effects were thrombocytopenia, confusion, aphasia, decreased level of consciousness, nausea, vomiting, dry itchy skin, ataxia, and photophobia [31].

A meta-analysis review of 19 studies from 1979 through 2010 evaluated the efficacy of AED including phenytoin, valproic acid, carbamazepine, lamotrigine, and levetiracetam versus that of no treatment in patients undergoing resection of supratentorial meningioma [32]. No significant differences were observed in incidence of both early (1.4 vs 1.4%, $p > 0.05$) and late seizures (8.8 vs 9.0%, $p > 0.05$) in two groups. It was concluded that seizure prophylaxis with AED is not beneficial in patients undergoing supratentorial meningioma resection [32].

A retrospective study was conducted to evaluate the efficacy of levetiracetam (1000 to 3000 mg) for seizure prophylaxis in patients undergoing surgery for brain tumors [33]. A seizure incidence of 2.6% was reported in levetiracetam group 1 week following surgery, which was significantly lower than the previously known seizure incidence in patients who did not receive prophylactic AED (15–20%) [33]. 6.4% of patients receiving levetiracetam reportedly had progressive somnolence and reactive psychosis [33]. Another retrospective study was conducted to compare the efficacy of a 750-mg load dose of phenytoin to that of a 1000-mg load dose of levetiracetam, both followed by taper over 5 days for seizure prophylaxis in patients undergoing surgery for brain tumors [34]. No significant differences were observed in rate of postoperative seizures between the two groups (levetiracetam 2.5 vs phenytoin 4.5%, $p = 0.66$) [34].

Current recommendations

- AED are not recommended for routine prophylactic use in patients with newly diagnosed brain neoplasm, as they are not effective in preventing first seizure and have potential side effects [32].

- In patients with brain neoplasm, who never had seizure, discontinuation or taper of AED after first postoperative week is recommended. This is particularly beneficial in medically stable patient or in those experiencing side effects [32].

- Seizure prophylaxis is not considered beneficial in patients with metastatic brain tumors [29].

- Seizure prophylaxis with AED is not beneficial in patients undergoing supratentorial meningioma resection [32].

Intracerebral hemorrhage

The risk of seizure is highest within first few days after ictus in patients with intracerebral hemorrhage. More than 50% of seizures occurs in the first 24 h [35–43]. The incidence of early seizures in patients with ICH is reported to be 28 to 31% on CEEG monitoring [38, 43]. Clinical seizures are seen from 5.5 to 24% of the patients with ICH [38, 43]. The underlying cause of early seizures is believed to be immediate metabolic and physical disturbances in brain following ICH [39, 40, 44]. Late seizures are seen less frequently in patients with ICH and are believed to be due underlying gliotic scarring [37, 39, 44]. Risk factors increasing the likelihood of seizures in patients with ICH are not well known because of limited clinical studies [37, 40, 41].

Seizure prophylaxis in intracerebral hemorrhage

A prospective study conducted on 761 patients with nontraumatic, nonaneurysmal ICH, without seizure in first 24 h, grouped on the basis of ICH location showed significant decrease in incidence of early seizures in patients with lobar ICH receiving phenobarbital prophylaxis as compared to patients with no treatment (5.9 vs 13.6%) [41]. It was reported that early prophylaxis could be beneficial in patients with lobar ICH [41].

A placebo-controlled RCT evaluated the association between the use of AED and poor outcomes (severe disability or death) by using modified Rankin scale. AED was started in 23 patients (8%) without documented seizure. The use of AED was associated with poorer outcomes after adjustment for other known predictors of outcome after ICH (OR 6.83; CI 2.2–21.23; $p = 0.001$). It was concluded that prophylactic use of AED especially phenytoin was associated with poor outcomes in patients with acute ICH [45].

Another study reported poor outcomes with prophylactic AED therapy in patients with ICH. This study evaluated data from 98 patients with ICH taking phenytoin, levetiracetam, or both [46]. It was reported that phenytoin use was associated with more fever ($p = 0.03$), worse scores on National Institutes of Health Stroke Scale at 14 days (23 [9 to 42] versus 11 [4 to 23], $P = 0.003$), and worse scores on modified Rankin scale at 14 and 28 days and 3 months as compared to levetiracetam [46]. It was speculated that poor outcomes could be related to reportedly larger ICH volume in patients on phenytoin prophylaxis [46] (Table 5).

Current recommendations
Ischemic stroke
Ischemic stroke is the most common cause of seizure in elderly patients [47]. Incidence rate of seizure in ischemic stroke patients ranges from 4 to 23% [48]. Post stroke seizures can be classified into early seizures, occurring within 7 days of stroke and late seizure, occurring after 7 days of stroke [49, 50]. Early seizure occurs from 2 to 6% of stroke patients and is believed to be related to edema and cytotoxicity associated with ischemic insult [49, 51]. Late seizure occurs in 3–5% of stroke patients and is related to underlying gliosis and meningo cerebral scarring [49, 51].

A higher risk for seizure development exists in certain patients:

- Patients with hemorrhagic stroke or with hemorrhagic transformation are at higher risk of developing seizures (12.5%) as compared to ischemic stroke without hemorrhagic transformation (4.2%, $p < 0.0001$) [49, 51].
- Cortical involvement in stroke patients predisposes them to higher seizure risk (9.8%) as compared to those with subcortical involvement (3.8%, $p < 0.005$) [49, 51].
- Patients with involvement of more than one lobe are at higher risk (21.2%) as compared to those with single lobe involvement (5.2%) [49, 51].

Seizure prophylaxis in ischemic stroke
Currently, there is limited corroborative data available to support the use of AED for seizure prophylaxis in post stroke patients.

Table 5 AHA/ASA guidelines for management of patients with ICH

As per the AHA/ASA guidelines for management of ICH [72]

- Prophylactic use of AED is not recommended in patients with ICH [72].
- Clinical seizures should be treated with anti-epileptic drugs [72].
- Continuous EEG monitoring is probably indicated in ICH patients with depressed mental status out of proportion to the degree of brain injury [72].
- Patients with a change in mental status who are found to have electrographic seizures on EEG should be treated with anti-epileptic drugs [72].

Current recommendations

As per the AHA guidelines for management of patients with acute ischemic stroke (2013) [52] and malignant cerebral edema (2014) [53]:

- Prophylactic use of AED is not recommended in patients with ischemic stroke [52].
- Seizure prophylaxis in patients without seizures at presentation is not recommended [53].

Postoperative craniotomy
Incidence of seizure in patients with craniotomy varies greatly and depends upon the type of procedure performed and underlying pathology [54]. Incidence rate of seizures in patients with post supratentorial craniotomy is estimated to be 15 to 20% [54]. Risk of seizure varies between 3 and 92% over a 5-year period post craniotomy [54].

Seizure prophylaxis in postoperative patients
A retrospective study compared prophylactic use of phenytoin ($n = 210$; most common dosage 300 mg/d, range 200–800 mg/d) to that of levetiracetam ($n = 105$; most common dosage 1000 mg/d, range 500–3000 mg/d) in 315 patients, who underwent supratentorial neurosurgery for wide range of disease pathologies [55]. An early seizure incidence (within 7 days) of 1% was reported in levetiracetam group as compared to 4.3% ($p = 0.17$) in phenytoin group [55]. Incidence of late seizure (within 30 days) was 1.9% in levetiracetam group as compared to 5.2% in phenytoin group ($p = 0.23$) [55]. No significant difference was observed in incidence of postoperative seizures between the levetiracetam and phenytoin groups (0 vs 1.8%, $p = 0.56$) in patients with a history of preoperative seizures [55]. Patients on levetiracetam prophylaxis had significantly lower incidence of adverse effects as compared to those on phenytoin prophylaxis (1 vs 18%, $p < 0.001$) [55]. Both the AEDs were associated with low risk of early as well as late seizures. The safety profile of levetiracetam (fewer adverse effects) makes it somewhat ideal for prophylactic use in post neurosurgery patients.

Current recommendations

As per the cochrane review 2013 [54]:

- There is a limited evidence to support the prophylactic use of AED in post neurosurgery patients.

Vascular lesions
Cavernous and arteriovenous malformations
A recent prospective study evaluated a 5-year seizure risk in 368 patients with either cavernous malformation

(CM) ($n = 139$) or arteriovenous malformation (AVM) ($n = 229$) [56]. Five-year seizure risk was reportedly higher in patients with AVM presenting with intracranial hemorrhage or focal neurologic deficit (ICH/FND) 23% ($n = 119$; 95% confidence interval (CI) 9–37%) compared to incidental AVM 8% ($n = 40$; 95% CI 0–20%) [56]. Risk of developing epilepsy in incidental AVM was reportedly 2% per person-year, annualized over 5 years [56].

Five-year risk of seizure in patients with CM presenting with focal neurological deficit or ICH was 6% ($n = 38$; 95% CI 0–14%) compared to incidentally found cavernoma 4% ($n = 57$; 95% CI 0–10%) [56]. Risk of developing epilepsy in incidental cavernoma was reportedly 0.9% per person-year, annualized over 5 years [56].

Current recommendations

As per the current ASA guidelines for management of patients with either cavernous or arteriovenous malformations [57]:

• Surgical or radiosurgical obliteration of AVM is generally considered effective in reducing seizure activity [57].

• Currently there are not enough studies available to formulate recommendations regarding type and duration of AED prophylaxis after treatment [57].

Other conditions
Cerebral venous thrombosis (CVT)
Seizures occur in about 40% of patients with CVT [58].

Risk factors increasing likelihood of seizure in patients with CVT are [58]:

• Motor deficit (OR 5.8, CI 2.98–11.42, $p < 0.001$) [58]
• ICH (OR 2.8, CI 1.46–5.56, $p = 0.002$) [58]
• Cortical vein thrombosis (OR 2.9, CI 1.43–5.96, $p = 0.003$) [58]

Prophylactic use of AED in patients with CVT is somewhat controversial. As per the cochrane review (2014) [59], there is no evidence to support or refute the use of anti-epileptic drugs for the primary or secondary prevention of seizures related to intracranial venous thrombosis [59].

Current recommendations

As per the AHA guidelines for management of patients with acute CVT [58]:

• In absence of seizure, routine use of AED in patients with CVT is not recommended [58].

Posterior reversible leukoencephalopathy syndrome (PRES)
Seizures occur in up to 68.8% patients with PRES [60]. However, there is not enough literature evidence to support prophylactic use of AED in patients with PRES.

Meningitis
Seizures occur in up to 27% of patients with meningitis [61]. There is not enough literature evidence to support prophylactic use of AED in patients with meningitis.

Guidelines for prophylactic use of AED in various neurological conditions encountered in the neurocritical ICU are generally derived from corroborative evidence provided by various RCT. For the majority of conditions, currently, there are not enough studies available to formulate recommendations regarding type and duration of AED prophylaxis [57]. In conditions without definite recommendations, the decision regarding prophylactic use of AED is usually derived from physician's personal belief and local practice trends. However, under such circumstances, an ideal approach should be diagnosing seizure or epileptiform abnormalities rather than prophylaxis.

Recognizing seizures in neurocritical ICU
Seizures can be difficult to recognize in critically ill patients. Prompt recognition of nonconvulsive seizures (NCSz) or nonconvulsive status epilepticus (NCSE) is crucial. Certain clinical presentations can indicate the ongoing NCS [62], these are as follows:

• An apparently prolonged "postictal state" following generalized convulsive seizures or with prolonged reduction of alertness from an operative procedure or neurologic insult [62]
• Acute onset of impaired consciousness or fluctuating picture with episodes of normal mentation [62]
• Impaired mentation or consciousness with myoclonus of facial muscles or nystagmoid eye movements [62]
• Episodic blank staring, aphasia, automatisms (lip smacking, fumbling with fingers), perseverative activity [62]
• Aphasia without an acute structural lesion
• Other acutely altered behavior without other obvious etiology [62]

A high degree of clinical suspicion is required to recognize these clinical presentations [62]. Prompt recognition is critical as NCS are associated with high mortality rate of 33% [63]. However, clinical presentations are not always reliable in accurately predicting the ongoing NCS. In a retrospective review of 208 patients admitted to neurocritical ICU from emergency department (ED) with either acute transient neurological deficits, loss of consciousness (LOC), or unclear motor phenomena, 13.9% of the patients were incorrectly diagnosed with epileptic seizures, whereas in 15.6% of patients who were eventually admitted to neurocritical ICU, diagnosis of epilepsy was missed in the ED [64]. The most common factors associated with missing seizure diagnosis were no prior history of epilepsy, older age (mean 76.4 years), multimorbidities, CT showing cerebrovascular lesion, seizure description given by nonprofessionals, negative seizure phenomenon (e.g., aphasia, LOC, paresis), and lack of tongue biting [64].

A retrospective review study evaluated 52 video EEGs over 18-month period in a neurocritical ICU [65]. These EEGs were from patients with possible seizures due to motor phenomenon [65]. Fourteen patients (27%) were found to have epileptic seizures [65]. That included four focal motor status epilepticus, three focal clonic, three myoclonus, two generalized status epilepticus, one focal tonic, and one generalized tonic clonic [65]. Thirty-eight patients (73%) had nonepileptic events, out of which 12 patients (23%) had tremor like events, 7 (13.5%) had multifocal jerks, 7 (13.5%) had slow semi purposeful movements, and the rest 12 (23%) had "other movements" [65]. These studies indicate that diagnosing seizures based on clinical presentation alone can be misleading. CEEG monitoring can be helpful in such circumstances. In a study of 236 patients with coma and no overt seizure activity, 8% of the patients were found to have NCSE on CEEG monitoring [66].

Role of CEEG monitoring in neuro ICU

Continuous electroencephalography (CEEG) monitoring is commonly used in critically ill patients. CEEG is tightly linked to cerebral metabolism and, thus, sensitive to changes in cerebral blood flow [67]. Several patterns on CEEG are of diagnostic and prognostic significance in patients with cerebral edema that lie on the ictal-interictal continuum [68]. EEG patterns that correlate with increased intracranial pressure (ICP) include focal slowing of underlying rhythms or global EEG suppression progressing to burst suppression or flat EEG [67]. CEEG monitoring provides real-time dynamic information about brain functioning and allows for detection of any early change in neurological status of a patient that may not be evident on neurological examination alone [67]. CEEG is also tightly linked to cerebral metabolism and thus sensitive to changes in cerebral blood flow [67]. CEEG monitoring can identify NCS and NCSE in critically ill patients. Evaluation for suspected NCS is the most common indication for CEEG [69]. Studies have reported that the use of CEEG monitoring in ICU patients at risk for NCS can change the treatment protocol

in the majority of patients [70]. In a retrospective study, Kilbride et al. showed that CEEG monitoring leads to AED modifications in 52% of patients, which included therapy initiation in 14%, modification in 33%, and discontinuation in 5% [70]. The NCS 2011 guidelines advocated use of CEEG monitoring in patients who failed to improve or have poor grade SAH (low-quality evidence-strong recommendation) [71]. The AHA/ASA guidelines also supported use of CEEG monitoring in patients with depressed mental status out of proportion to the degree of brain injury (Class IIa; Level of Evidence:B) [72]. According to AHA/ASA guidelines for management of ICH, only patients with "Clinical seizures should be treated with anti-epileptic drugs (Class I; Level of Evidence:A)" [72]. AED may be initiated for these events, but as they carry a significant risk for serious adverse effects including rash (Stevens Johnson syndrome), hematological abnormalities, behavioral changes, drug-drug interactions [1], it is ideal to diagnose the seizure before initiating prophylactic therapy in such circumstances [1].

The duration of CEEG monitoring is also an important aspect in diagnosing seizures in neurocritical ICU. In a retrospective review, Claassen et al. [73] reviewed CEEG data of 100 patients and reported time to seizure duration [73]. Sixty percent of noncomatose patients had seizure during the first hour of monitoring, whereas 95% of noncomatose patients had seizure in first 24 h [73]. In comparison to noncomatose patients, 50% of comatose patients had seizure in the first hour and only 80% had seizure in the first 24 h [73]. Eighty-seven percent of comatose patients reportedly had seizure within 48 h of monitoring [73]. This study concluded that comatose patients may require monitoring longer than the usual 24 h for detection of their first electrographic seizure [73].

Regarding the management of patients on CEEG monitoring, generally, if NCS or NCSE are detected, most physicians recommend initiating treatment, although the management approach can be highly variable [74]. Physicians tend to treat NCSE more aggressively than NCS, with a trend toward lesser use of anti-convulsants like levetiracetam and more willingness to induce coma and intubation if necessary [74]. Given the limited literature evidence regarding treatment of NCS and NCSE for adult or pediatric patients, management is pretty much similar across age groups.

CEEG monitoring can be helpful in conditions lacking sufficient evidence to support the use of AED for prophylactic use. Until there is more data available to provide supporting evidence, a potential seizure prophylaxis protocol can be summarized as follows (Table 6):

Table 6 Seizure prophylaxis protocol in neuro-ICU

Seizure prophylaxis	Conditions
Definitive prophylaxis	• Severe TBI (7 days)
Probable prophylaxis	• Unsecured aneurysm in SAH • Elevated intracranial pressure (ICP) and concern for poor compliance
Possible/no prophylaxis	• ICH • AVM • Cavernoma • Brain neoplasm • Malignant ischemic stroke • Postoperative craniotomy • Meningitis • Cerebral venous sinus thrombosis (CVST) • PRES

Conclusion

The data for prophylactic use of AEDS in neuro critically ill patients lacks robustness. Patients with severe TBI and possible SAH seem to benefit with a short course of AED. In patients with injury to their brain, the use of CEEG would make sense rather than indiscriminately administering AED. Only observed seizures should be treated in such patients.

Abbreviations

AED: Anti-epileptic drugs; AVM: Arteriovenous malformation; CEEG: Continuous electroencephalography; CVST: Cerebral venous sinus thrombosis; ED: Emergency department; EDH: Epidural hemorrhage; ICH: Intracerebral hemorrhage; LOC: Loss of consciousness; NCSE: Nonconvulsive status epilepticus; NCSz: Nonconvulsive seizures; NSICU: Neurosciences intensive care unit; PRES: Posterior reversible encephalopathy syndrome; PTS: Post traumatic seizures; SAH: Aneurysmal subarachnoid hemorrhage; SDH: Subdural hemorrhage; TBI: Traumatic brain injury

Acknowledgements

No other acknowledgements to report.

Funding

There is no funding information to report.

Authors' contributions

SY, NK, KP, PN, and CN worked equally on writing and editing the manuscript. All authors read and approved the final manuscript.

Authors' information

Christopher R. Newey has served on speaker's bureau for BARD medical. Dr. Nattanmai has served on speaker bureau of Chiesi.

Competing interests

The authors declare that they have no competing interests.

Author details

[1]Department of Neurology, University of Missouri, 5 Hospital Drive, CE 540, Columbia, MO 65211, USA. [2]Department of Biological Sciences, University of Missouri, Columbia, MO 65211, USA. [3]Cleveland Clinic, Cerebrovascular Center, 9500 Euclid Avenue, Cleveland, OH 44195, USA.

References

1. Temkin NR, Dikmen SS, Winn HR. Posttraumatic seizures. In: Eisenberg HM, Aldrich EF, editors. Management of head injury. Philadelphia: W.B. Saunders; 1991. p. 425–35.
2. Yablon SA. Posttraumatic seizures. Arch Phys Med Rehabil. 1993;74:983–1001.
3. Frey LC. Epidemiology of posttraumatic epilepsy: a critical review. Epilepsia. 2003;44:11–7.
4. Temkin NR, Dikmen SS, Wilensky AJ, et al. A randomized, double-blind study of phenytoin for the prevention of post-traumatic seizures. N Engl J Med. 1990;323:497–502.
5. Haltiner AM, Newell DW, Temkin NR, et al. Side effects and mortality associated with use of phenytoin for early posttraumatic seizure prophylaxis. J Neurosurg. 1999;91:588–92.
6. Dikmen SS, Temkin NR, Miller B, et al. Neurobehavioral effects of phenytoin prophylaxis of posttraumatic seizures. JAMA. 1991;265:1271–7.
7. Temkin NR, Dikmen SS, Anderson GD, et al. Valproate therapy for prevention of posttraumatic seizures: a randomized trial. J Neurosurg. 1999; 91:593–600.
8. Temkin NR. Antiepileptogenesis and seizure prevention trials with antiepileptic drugs: meta-analysis of controlled trials. Epilepsia. 2001;4:515–24.
9. Kruer RM, Harris LH, Goodwin H, et al. Changing trends in the use of seizure prophylaxis after traumatic brain injury: a shift from phenytoin to levetiracetam. J Crit Care. 2013;28:9–13.
10. Jones KE, Puccio AM, Harshman KJ, et al. Levetiracetam versus phenytoin for seizure prophylaxis in severe traumatic brain injury. Neurosurg Focus. 2008;4:E3.
11. Szaflarski JP, Sangha KS, Lindsell CJ, Shutter LA. Prospective, randomized, single-blinded comparative trial of intravenous levetiracetam versus phenytoin for seizure prophylaxis. Neurocrit Care. 2010;2:165–72.
12. Choi KS, Chun HJ, Yi HJ, Ko Y, Kim YS, Kim JM. Seizures and epilepsy following aneurysmal subarachnoid hemorrhage: incidence and risk factors. J Korean Neurosurg Soc. 2009;46:93–8.
13. Rhoney DH, Tipps LB, Murry KR, Basham MC, Michael DB, Coplin WM. Anticonvulsant prophylaxis and timing of seizures after aneurysmal subarachnoid hemorrhage. Neurology. 2000;55:258–65.
14. Molyneux AJ, Kerr RS, Yu LM, et al. International subarachnoid aneurysm trial (ISAT) of neurosurgical clipping versus endovascular coiling in 2143 patients with ruptured intracranial aneurysms: a randomised comparison of effects on survival, dependency, seizures, rebleeding, subgroups, and aneurysm occlusion. Lancet. 2005;366:809–17.
15. Claassen J, Peery S, Kreiter KT, et al. Predictors and clinical impact of epilepsy after subarachnoid hemorrhage. Neurology. 2003;60:208–14.
16. Little AS, Kerrigan JF, McDougall CG, et al. Nonconvulsive status epilepticus in patients suffering spontaneous subarachnoid hemorrhage. J Neurosurg. 2007;106:805–11.
17. Claassen J, Hirsch LJ, Frontera JA, et al. Prognostic significance of continuous EEG monitoring in patients with poor-grade subarachnoid hemorrhage. Neurocrit Care. 2006;4:103–12.
18. Dennis LJ, Claassen J, Hirsch LJ, Emerson RG, Connolly ES, Mayer SA. Nonconvulsive status epilepticus after subarachnoid hemorrhage. Neurosurgery. 2002;51:1136–43.
19. Rosengart AJ, Huo JD, Tolentino J, et al. Outcome in patients with subarachnoid hemorrhage treated with antiepileptic drugs. J Neurosurg. 2007;2:253–60.
20. Naidech AM, Kreiter KT, Janjua N, et al. Phenytoin exposure is associated with functional and cognitive disability after subarachnoid hemorrhage. Stroke. 2005;3:583–7.
21. Baker CJ, Prestigiacomo CJ, Solomon RA. Short-term perioperative anticonvulsant prophylaxis for the surgical treatment of low-risk patients with intracranial aneurysms. Neurosurgery. 1995;5:863–70.
22. Chumnanvej S, Dunn IF, Kim DH. Three-day phenytoin prophylaxis is adequate after subarachnoid hemorrhage. Neurosurgery. 2007;1:99–102.

23. Tartara A, Galimberti CA, Manni R, et al. Differential effects of valproic acid and enzyme-inducing anticonvulsants on nimodipine pharmacokinetics in epileptic patients. Br J Clin Pharmacol. 1991;3:335–40.

24. Murphy-Human T, Welch E, Zipfel G, Diringer MN, Dhar R. Comparison of short-duration levetiracetam with extended course phenytoin for seizure prophylaxis after subarachnoid hemorrhage. World Neurosurg. 2011;2:269–74.

25. Glantz MJ, Cole BF, Forsyth PA, et al. Practice parameter: anticonvulsant prophylaxis in patients with newly diagnosed brain tumors. Report of the Quality Standards Subcommittee of the American Academy of Neurology. Neurology. 2000;10:1886–93.

26. van Breemen MS, Wilms EB, Vecht CJ. Epilepsy in patients with brain tumours: epidemiology, mechanisms, and management. Lancet Neurol. 2007;5:421–30.

27. Sirven JI, Wingerchuk DM, Drazkowski JF, Lyons MK, Zimmerman RS. Seizure prophylaxis in patients with brain tumors: a meta-analysis. Mayo Clin Proc. 2004;12:1489–94.

28. Tremont-Lukats IW, Ratilal BO, Armstrong T, Gilbert MR. Antiepileptic drugs for preventing seizures in people with brain tumors. Cochrane Database Syst Rev. 2008;2:CD004424.

29. Mikkelsen T, Paleologos NA, Robinson PD, et al. The role of prophylactic anticonvulsants in the management of brain metastases: a systematic review and evidence-based clinical practice guideline. J Neuro-Oncol. 2010;1:97–102.

30. Forsyth PA, Weaver S, Fulton D, et al. Prophylactic anticonvulsants in patients with brain tumour. Can J Neurol Sci. 2003;2:106–10.

31. Wu AS, Trinh VT, Suki D, et al. A prospective randomized trial of perioperative seizure prophylaxis in patients with intraparenchymal brain tumors. J Neurosurg. 2013;4:873–83.

32. Komotar RJ, Raper DM, Starke RM, Iorgulescu JB, Gutin PH. Prophylactic antiepileptic drug therapy in patients undergoing supratentorial meningioma resection: a systematic analysis of efficacy. J Neurosurg. 2011;3:483–90.

33. Zachenhofer I, Donat M, Oberndorfer S, Roessler K. Perioperative levetiracetam for prevention of seizures in supratentorial brain tumor surgery. J Neuro-Oncol. 2011;1:101–6.

34. Kern K, Schebesch KM, Schlaier J, et al. Levetiracetam compared to phenytoin for the prevention of postoperative seizures after craniotomy for intracranial tumours in patients without epilepsy. J Clin Neurosci. 2012;1:99–100.

35. Beghi E, D'Alessandro R, Beretta S, et al. Incidence and predictors of acute symptomatic seizures after stroke. Neurology. 2011;20:1785–93.

36. Berger AR, Lipton RB, Lesser ML, Lantos G, Portenoy RK. Early seizures following intracerebral hemorrhage: implications for therapy. Neurology. 1988;9:1363–5.

37. Bladin CF, Alexandrov AV, Bellavance A, et al. Seizures after stroke: a prospective multicenter study. Arch Neurol. 2000;11:1617–22.

38. Claassen J, Jette N, Chum F, et al. Electrographic seizures and periodic discharges after intracerebral hemorrhage. Neurology. 2007;13:1356–65.

39. De Herdt V, Dumont F, Henon H, et al. Early seizures in intracerebral hemorrhage: incidence, associated factors, and outcome. Neurology. 2011;20:1794–800.

40. Lamy C, Domigo V, Semah F, et al. Early and late seizures after cryptogenic ischemic stroke in young adults. Neurology. 2003;3:400–4.

41. Passero S, Rocchi R, Rossi S, Ulivelli M, Vatti G. Seizures after spontaneous supratentorial intracerebral hemorrhage. Epilepsia. 2002;10:1175–80.

42. Szaflarski JP, Rackley AY, Kleindorfer DO, et al. Incidence of seizures in the acute phase of stroke: a population-based study. Epilepsia. 2008;6:974–81.

43. Vespa PM, O'Phelan K, Shah M, et al. Acute seizures after intracerebral hemorrhage: a factor in progressive midline shift and outcome. Neurology. 2003;9:1441–6.

44. Gilmore E, Choi HA, Hirsch LJ, Claassen J. Seizures and CNS hemorrhage: spontaneous intracerebral and aneurysmal subarachnoid hemorrhage. Neurologist. 2010;3:165–75.

45. Messe SR, Sansing LH, Cucchiara BL, Herman ST, Lyden PD, Kasner SE. Prophylactic antiepileptic drug use is associated with poor outcome following ICH. Neurocrit Care. 2009;1:38–44.

46. Naidech AM, Garg RK, Liebling S, et al. Anticonvulsant use and outcomes after intracerebral hemorrhage. Stroke. 2009;12:3810–5.

47. Forsgren L, Bucht G, Eriksson S, Bergmark L. Incidence and clinical characterization of unprovoked seizures in adults: a prospective population-based study. Epilepsia. 1996;3:224–9.

48. Burn J, Dennis M, Bamford J, Sandercock P, Wade D, Warlow C. Epileptic seizures after a first stroke: the Oxfordshire Community Stroke Project. BMJ. 1997;7122:1582–7.

49. Gupta SR, Naheedy MH, Elias D, Rubino FA. Postinfarction seizures. A clinical study. Stroke. 1988;12:1477–81.

50. Horner S, Ni XS, Duft M, Niederkorn K, Lechner H. EEG, CT and neurosonographic findings in patients with postischemic seizures. J Neurol Sci. 1995;1:57–60.

51. Lancman ME, Golimstok A, Norscini J, Granillo R. Risk factors for developing seizures after a stroke. Epilepsia. 1993;1:141–3.

52. Jauch EC, Saver JL, Adams HP Jr, Bruno A, Connors JJ, Demaerschalk BM, Khatri P, PW MM Jr, Qureshi AI, Rosenfield K, Scott PA, Summers DR, Wang DZ, Wintermark M, Yonas H, American Heart Association Stroke Council; Council on Cardiovascular Nursing; Council on Peripheral Vascular Disease; Council on Clinical Cardiology. Guidelines for the early management of patients with acute ischemic stroke: a guideline for healthcare professionals from the American Heart Association/American Stroke Association. Stroke. 2013;44(3):870–947.

53. Wijdicks EF, Sheth KN, Carter BS, Greer DM, Kasner SE, Kimberly WT, Schwab S, Smith EE, Tamargo RJ, Wintermark M, American Heart Association Stroke Council. Recommendations for the management of cerebral and cerebellar infarction with swelling: a statement for healthcare professionals from the American Heart Association/American Stroke Association. Stroke. 2014;45:1222–38.

54. Pulman J, Greenhalgh J, Marson AG. Antiepileptic drugs as prophylaxis for post-craniotomy seizures. Cochrane Database Syst Rev. 2013;2:CD007286.

55. Milligan TA, Hurwitz S, Bromfield EB. Efficacy and tolerability of levetiracetam versus phenytoin after supratentorial neurosurgery. Neurology. 2008;9:665–9.

56. Josephson CB, Leach JP, Duncan R, Roberts RC, Counsell CE, Al-Shahi SR. Seizure risk from cavernous or arteriovenous malformations: prospective population-based study. Neurology. 2011;18:1548–54.

57. Ogilvy CS, Stieg PE, Awad I, et al. AHA Scientific Statement: recommendations for the management of intracranial arteriovenous malformations: a statement for healthcare professionals from a special writing group of the Stroke Council, American Stroke Association. Stroke. 2001;6:1458–71.

58. Ferro JM, Canhão P, Bousser MG, Stam J, Barinagarrementeria F, ISCVT Investigators. Early seizures in cerebral vein and dural sinus thrombosis: risk factors and role of antiepileptics. Stroke. 2008;39:1152–8.

59. Price M, Günther A, Kwan JS. Antiepileptic drugs for the primary and secondary prevention of seizures after intracranial venous thrombosis. Cochrane Database Syst Rev. 2014;8:CD005501.

60. Kastrup O, Gerwig M, Frings M, Diener HC. Posterior reversible encephalopathy syndrome (PRES): electroencephalographic findings and seizure patterns. J Neurol. 2012;259:1383–9.

61. Rosman NP, Peterson DB, Kaye EM, Colton T. Seizures in bacterial meningitis: prevalence, patterns, pathogenesis, and prognosis. Pediatr Neurol. 1985;1:278–85.

62. Drislane FW. Presentation, evaluation, and treatment of nonconvulsive status epilepticus. Epilepsy Behav. 2000;1:301–14.

63. Young GB, Jordan KG, Doig GS. An assessment of nonconvulsive seizures in the intensive care unit using continuous EEG monitoring: an investigation of variables associated with mortality. Neurology. 1996;47:83–9.

64. Boesebeck F, Freermann S, Kellinghaus C, Evers S. Misdiagnosis of epileptic and non-epileptic seizures in a neurological intensive care unit. Acta Neurol Scand. 2010;122:189–95.

65. Benbadis SR, Chen S, Melo M. What's shaking in the ICU? The differential diagnosis of seizures in the intensive care setting. Epilepsia. 2010;51:2338–40.

66. Towne AR, Waterhouse EJ, Boggs JG, Garnett LK, Brown AJ, Smith JR Jr, DeLorenzo RJ. Prevalence of nonconvulsive status epilepticus in comatose patients. Neurology. 2000;54:340–5.

67. Newey CR, Sarwal A, Hantus S. Continuous electroencephalography (cEEG) changes precede clinical changes in a case of progressive cerebral edema. J Neurocrit Care. 2013;18:261–5.

68. Katyal N, Sarwal A, George P, Banik B, Newey CR. The relationship of triphasic waves with intracranial pressure as a possible prognostic marker in traumatic brain injury. Case Rep Neurol Med. 2017;2017:4742026. 4 pages

69. Abend NS, Dlugos DJ, Hahn CD, Hirsch LJ, Herman ST. Use of EEG monitoring and management of nonconvulsive seizures in critically ill patients: a survey of neurologists. Neurocrit Care. 2010;12:382–9.

70. Kilbride RD, Costello DJ, Chiappa KH. How seizure detection by continuous electroencephalographic monitoring affects the prescribing of antiepileptic medications. Arch Neurol. 2009;66:723–8.

71. Diringer MN, Bleck TP, Claude Hemphill J 3rd, Menon D, Shutter L, Vespa P, Bruder N, Connolly ES Jr, Citerio G, Gress D, Hänggi D, Hoh BL, Lanzino G, Le Roux P, Rabinstein A, Schmutzhard E, Stocchetti N, Suarez JI, Treggiari M, Tseng MY, Vergouwen MD, Wolf S, Zipfel G, Neurocritical Care Society. Critical care management of patients following aneurysmal subarachnoid hemorrhage: recommendations from the Neurocritical Care Society's Multidisciplinary Consensus Conference. Neurocrit Care. 2011;15:211–40.

72. Morgenstern LB, Hemphill JC III, Anderson C, et al. Guidelines for the management of spontaneous intracerebral hemorrhage: a guideline for healthcare professionals from the American Heart Association/American Stroke Association. Stroke. 2010;9:2108–29.

73. Claassen J, Mayer SA, Kowalski RG, Emerson RG, Hirsch LJ. Detection of electrographic seizures with continuous EEG monitoring in critically ill patients. Neurology. 2004;62:1743–8.

74. Abend NS, Dlugos DJ, Hahn CD, Hirsch LJ, Herman ST. Use of EEG monitoring and management of non-convulsive seizures in critically ill patients: a survey of neurologists. Neurocrit Care. 2010;12(3):382–9.

75. Carney N, Totten AM, O'Reilly C, Ullman JS, Hawryluk GWJ, Bell MJ, Bratton SL, Chesnut R, Harris OA, Kissoon N, Rubiano AM, Shutter L, Tasker RC, Vavilala MS, Wilberger J, Wright DW, Ghajar J. Guidelines for the management of severe traumatic brain injury, fourth edition. Neurosurgery. 2017;80:6–15.

76. Connolly ES Jr, Rabinstein AA, Carhuapoma JR, Derdeyn CP, Dion J, Higashida RT, Hoh BL, Kirkness CJ, Naidech AM, Ogilvy CS, Patel AB, Thompson BG, Vespa P, American Heart Association Stroke Council; Council on Cardiovascular Radiology and Intervention; Council on Cardiovascular Nursing; Council on Cardiovascular Surgery and Anesthesia; Council on Clinical Cardiology. Guidelines for the management of aneurysmal subarachnoid hemorrhage: a guideline for healthcare professionals from the American Heart Association/american Stroke Association. Stroke. 2012;43:1711–137.

Interleukin-6 is a key factor for immunoglobulin-like transcript-4-mediated immune injury in sepsis

De Wen Zhang[*] and Jian He

Abstract

Background: ILT4+ monocytes seem to be associated with poor prognosis of sepsis in humans, but the exact mechanisms are unknown. This study aimed to examine the biological behaviors and effects of immunoglobulin-like transcript-4 (ILT4) levels on monocytes during sepsis and on the prognosis of sepsis.

Methods: ILT4$^{+/+}$ (WT) and ILT4-knockout (ILT4$^{-/-}$) male BALB/c mice were used for sepsis modeling using cecal ligation puncture (CLP). Flow cytometry was used to measure the levels of ILT4 and major histocompatibility complex class II (MHC-II) on peripheral blood monocytes 24 h after CLP. ELISA was used to measure the serum levels of tumor necrosis factor-alpha (TNF-α), interleukin (IL)-1β, IL-6, and IL-12 at 0, 6, 12, and 24 h after CLP. Survival and prognosis were monitored over the course of 168 h.

Results: ILT4 was highly expressed in peripheral blood monocytes of septic mice 24 h after CLP (1292.00 ± 143.70 vs. 193.50 ± 52.54, $p < 0.05$). MHC-II levels on peripheral blood monocytes in ILT4$^{-/-}$ mice were significantly higher than those in WT mice (49.38 ± 5.66% vs. 24.25 ± 6.76%, $p < 0.05$). Serum IL-6 was significantly elevated 24 h after CLP (470.75 ± 88.03 vs. 54.25 ± 20.04, $p < 0.05$). The serum IL-6 levels were significantly lower in ILT4$^{-/-}$ mice compared with those in WT mice after CLP (241.25 ± 45.10 vs. 470.75 ± 88.03, $p < 0.05$), but TNF-α, IL-1β, and IL-12 were not changed. The survival of ILT4$^{-/-}$ mice was significantly better after CLP compared with that of WT mice.

Conclusions: High levels of ILT4 on monocytes were observed in peripheral blood during sepsis and found to be associated with high serum IL-6 levels and low MHC-II levels on monocytes, possibly associated with higher mortality. ILT-4-IL-6-MHC-II could be a potential signaling pathway involved in sepsis.

Keywords: Sepsis, Monocytes, Immunoglobulin-like transcript-4 (ILT4), Major histocompatibility complex class II molecules (MHC-II), Interleukin (IL)-6

Background

Sepsis is a life-threatening condition caused by dysregulated host response to infection [1]. Ever since the concept of sepsis was proposed in 1991, the understanding of its pathogenesis and clinical patterns has made great progress. Mortality from sepsis remains high, and the management of severe sepsis is still a clinical challenge [2]. A previous study in China reported an incidence of sepsis in surgical intensive care units (ICU) of 8.68% and a mortality rate of 48.7% [3].

The pathogenesis of sepsis is very complex, involving derangements in infection, inflammation, immunity, and coagulation [4]. Studies have shown that the poor prognosis of sepsis is not entirely and directly caused by the pathogens or their toxins. Indeed, the immune responses of the host also play important roles in the progression of sepsis. The innate immune response is activated through pattern-recognition receptors (PRRs) and pathogen-pathogen interaction. These PRRs also react with some danger-associated molecular patterns (DMAPs), leading to excessive inflammatory response and immune system imbalance [5, 6]. Sepsis is a biphasic process showing first a hyper-inflammatory phase, followed by a hypo-inflammatory phase characterized by monocyte deactivation [7]. Sepsis

* Correspondence: zhangdewen120@hotmail.com
Department of Emergency and Critical Care Medicine, Eastern Hepatobiliary Surgery Hospital, Second Military Medical University, No. 700 North Moyu Road, Shanghai 201805, China

after major surgery has been associated with defects in the production of monocyte cytokines [8]. The exact mechanisms of this deactivation are still poorly understood.

Immunoglobulin-like transcripts (ILTs), also known as leukocyte immunoglobulin-like receptors (LiLRs), monocyte/macrophage Ig-like receptor (MIRs), and CD85, are a family of genes encoded on the human chromosome 19q13.4 [9]. ILT4 is mainly expressed on monocytes/macrophages in the peripheral blood. It is a transmembrane protein with a long cytoplasmic tail containing two to four immunoreceptor tyrosine-based inhibitory motifs (ITIMs) to deliver inhibitory signals through protein tyrosine phosphatase (SHP) [10]. Upregulation of ILT4 in the serum of septic patients is directly correlated with the degree of organ dysfunction [11]. ILT4$^+$ monocytes from septic patients display an alteration in the cytokine response to endotoxin stimulation [11]. Furthermore, ILT4 participates in the regulation of neutrophils in inflammatory disorders [12].

Therefore, we hypothesized that ILT4 is involved in the deregulation of the monocytes during sepsis. The aim of the present study was to determine the biological behaviors and effects of ILT4 levels on peripheral blood monocytes of septic mice.

Methods
Animals
Male 8-week-old wild type (WT) and ILT4-knockout (ILT4$^{-/-}$) mice of the BALB/c background (weight, 25–30 g) were used in this study. The mouse homology of ILT4 is PIR-B [13]. To be discussed conveniently in this paper, the mice will be referred to as ILT4. WT BALB/c mice were purchased from Shanghai Laboratory Animal Center of Chinese Academy of Science (Shanghai, China). The ILT4$^{-/-}$ mice were generated and bred by MultiSciences/Lianke Biotech Co., Ltd. (Zhejiang Province, China). The genotype of each mouse used in this study had been confirmed by PCR genotyping of tail DNA before the study.

Sepsis modeling with CLP
Based on a previous study [14], sepsis modeling was conducted using cecal ligation puncture (CLP) in BALB/c mice. Animals were fasted for 12 h, followed by anesthesia with 10% chloral hydrate intraperitoneal injection (0.5 ml/100 g bodyweight) and abdominal midline incision (1.5 cm length) to ligate the cecum at the three-fourth point from its free end using no. 4 suture thread. A 21 gauge needle was used to perforate the midpoint of the ligated area along the longitudinal axis of the mesentery to extrude a small drop of intestinal content from each of the two puncture holes. The bowel was then put back in the abdominal cavity, which was sutured layer by layer. Animals received subcutaneous injection of 37 °C normal saline (5 mL/100 g

bodyweight) after surgery and were housed in the animal facility with 12 h/12 h circadian rhythm and free access to water and food.

Specimen collection
Blood samples were collected by heart puncture at 0, 6, 12, and 24 h after CLP and centrifuged at 2500 rpm for 20 min after sitting at room temperature for 20 min for serum collection. Serum samples were stored at – 20 °C. Whole blood samples collected at 24 h after CLP were stored in tubes containing EDTA anticoagulant for immediate flow cytometry.

Flow cytometry analysis of ILT4 and MHC-II on monocytes
Red blood cells from 50 μL of EDTA-anticoagulated blood were lysed to prepare a cell suspension (1×10^8 cells/ml) after washing, followed by fluorescent labeling for CD14 (1 μL of APC-CD14 monoclonal antibody, eBioscience, San Diego, CA, USA), ILT4 (2 μL of PE-ILT4 monoclonal antibody, eBioscience), and MHC-II (2 μL of FITC-MHC-II monoclonal antibody, eBioscience) separately and incubated at room temperate according to the manufacturer's instructions. Then, levels of ILT4 and MHC-II in monocytes were quantified using a MACSQuant flow cytometry system (Miltenyi Biotec GmbH, Bergisch Gladbach, Germany).

ELISA detection of serum tumor necrosis factor-alpha (TNF-α), interleukin (IL)-1β, IL-6, and IL-12
Fifty microliters of each serum sample was added into wells of ELISA plates. Buffer, biotinylated anti-mouse TNF-α, IL-1β, IL-6, and IL-12, horseradish peroxidase (HRP)-labeled streptavidin, and 3,3',5,5'-tetramethyl-benzidine (TMB) substrate were added according to the instructions included with the kit (Bender, MedSystems GmbH, Vienna, Austria). The plates were shaken and incubated at room temperature. After color development was complete, the stopping solution was added to terminate the reaction and optical density (OD) was immediately measured at 450 nm (using 650 nm as reference wavelength) using a Multiskan Ascent microplate reader (LabSystems Diagnostic Ltd., Helsinki, Finland) to calculate the concentrations using the standard curve (prepared using different dilutions of standard sample provided in the kit).

Survival and prognosis
Twenty animals from each of the BALB/c WT and ILT4$^{-/-}$ groups were evaluated. The number of surviving mice was recorded every 12 h after sepsis modeling by CLP, for a total of 168 h.

Statistical analyses
SPSS 18.0 (IBM, Armonk, NY, USA) was used for statistical analysis. Continuous data were presented as mean

± standard deviation and analyzed using the Student t test and two-way ANOVA. Cox-Mantel log-rank and Breslow tests were used for statistical analysis of mouse survival. $p < 0.05$ was considered indicative of significant differences.

Results

Monocytes highly expressed ILT4 during sepsis

ILT4 was highly expressed on peripheral blood monocytes of septic mice 24 h after CLP (1292.00 ± 143.70 vs. 193.50 ± 52.54, + 566%, $p < 0.05$, Fig. 1).

ILT4 inhibited MHC-II levels on monocytes during sepsis

MHC-II levels on peripheral blood monocytes in ILT4$^{-/-}$ mice were significantly higher than those in WT mice ($49.38 \pm 5.66\%$ vs. $24.25 \pm 6.76\%$, + 103%, $p < 0.05$, Fig. 2).

ILT4 regulated IL-6 but not TNF-α, IL-1β, or IL-12 levels during sepsis

Serum TNF-α showed a one-way trend peaking at 6 h after CLP (53.13 ± 5.49 vs. 24.50 ± 4.57, + 117%, $p < 0.05$) that reverted to preoperative levels 12 h after CLP in WT mice. ILT4 knockout showed no significant impact of CLP on TNF-α levels (50.88 ± 6.38 vs. 53.13 ± 5.49, − 4%, $p > 0.05$, Fig. 3a). Twenty-four hours after CLP, serum IL-1β was significantly elevated in the WT mice (3639.13 ± 627.20 vs. 581.75 ± 152.89, + 525%, $p < 0.05$) while serum IL-1β was not affected in ILT4$^{-/-}$ mice (3144.63 ± 549.74 vs. 3639.13 ± 627.20, − 14%, $p > 0.05$, Fig. 3b). IL-6 was significantly elevated 24 h after CLP in the WT mice (470.75 ± 88.03 vs. 54.25 ± 20.04, + 772%, $p < 0.05$). The IL-6 levels were significantly lower in ILT4$^{-/-}$ mice compared with those in WT mice after CLP (241.25 ± 45.10 vs. 470.75 ± 88.03, − 49%, $p < 0.05$, Fig. 3c). Serum IL-12 levels were significantly high 12 h after CLP in WT mice compared with controls (3508.99 ± 326.77 vs. 1641.57 ± 314.13, + 114%, $p < 0.05$) but was not significantly affected by ILT4

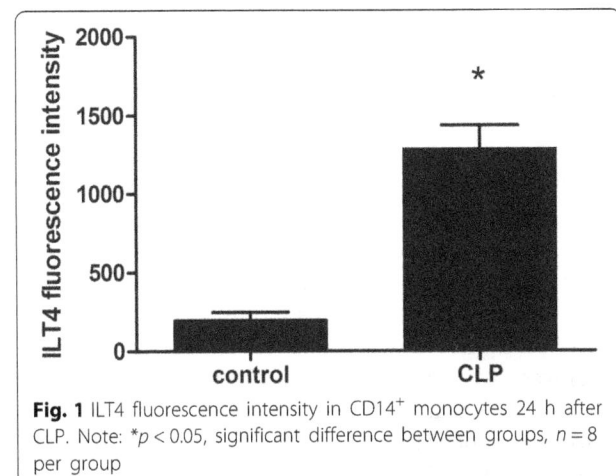

Fig. 1 ILT4 fluorescence intensity in CD14$^+$ monocytes 24 h after CLP. Note: *$p < 0.05$, significant difference between groups, $n = 8$ per group

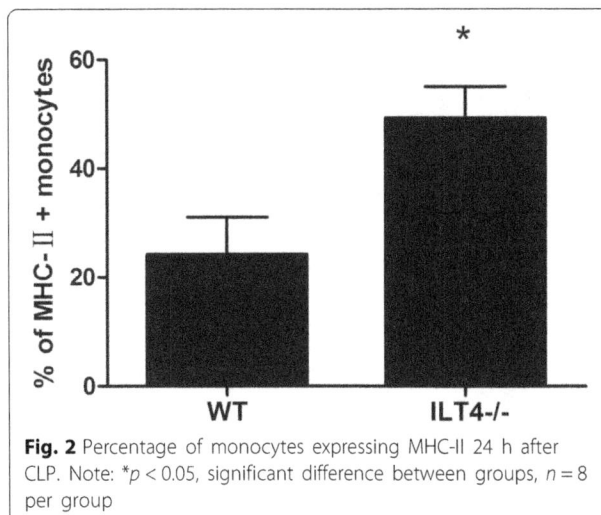

Fig. 2 Percentage of monocytes expressing MHC-II 24 h after CLP. Note: *$p < 0.05$, significant difference between groups, $n = 8$ per group

knockout (3198.74 ± 221.12 vs. 3508.99 ± 326.77, − 9%, $p > 0.05$, Fig. 3d).

High levels of ILT4 increased the mortality of sepsis

The survival of ILT4$^{-/-}$ mice after CLP was significantly higher than that of WT mice ($p < 0.05$, Fig. 4).

Discussion

Sepsis is a complex pathophysiological process caused by the interaction between the host and pathogens. Monocytes are the main effector cells in innate immunity and antigen presentation and show diverse manifestations in infectious diseases according to their subtype and stimulation by lipopolysaccharide (LPS). In the past, immunophenotypes and biological behaviors of monocytes were roughly divided into two groups [15]. CD14^{++}CD16$^-$ "classical monocytes" are the dominant subgroup under normal circumstances, accounting for 90–95% of the total monocytes in healthy humans. LPS stimulation leads to more active phagocytosis and causes the synthesis and secretion of IL-10 [16], which is anti-inflammatory. CD14$^+$ CD16$^+$ "non-classical monocytes" account for 5–10% of the total monocytes in healthy humans. LPS can induce the massive secretion of TNF-α by non-classical monocytes [16, 17]. The populations of these cell subgroups increases during infection and sepsis and are positively correlated with the poor prognosis of sepsis [18]. In the present study, the specific high ILT4 levels on peripheral blood monocytes during sepsis was associated with high serum IL-6 concentrations and low MHC-II levels on monocytes, leading to poor prognosis. Nevertheless, the specific properties of these cell populations have not been clarified yet, but Baffari et al. [11] showed that ILT4 is crucial to the tolerogenic function of monocytes. Indeed, high levels of ILT4 appear to be induced by soluble factors present in the serum of

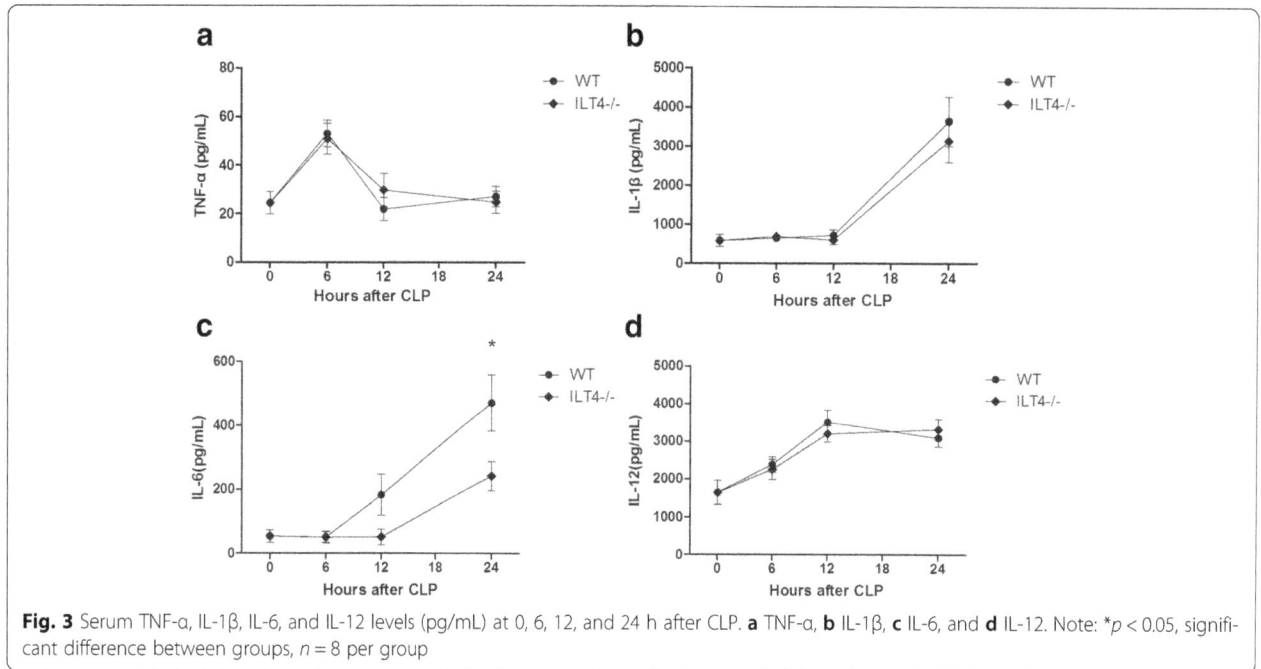

Fig. 3 Serum TNF-α, IL-1β, IL-6, and IL-12 levels (pg/mL) at 0, 6, 12, and 24 h after CLP. **a** TNF-α, **b** IL-1β, **c** IL-6, and **d** IL-12. Note: *$p < 0.05$, significant difference between groups, $n = 8$ per group

septic patients and directly correlates with the degree of organ dysfunction in human subjects [11]. ILT4+ monocytes from septic patients also display an alteration in the cytokine response to endotoxin stimulation characterized by reduced IL-12 production and increased IL-10 production [11]. Therefore, ILT4 probably plays important roles in sepsis.

In this study, ILT4 was highly expressed by peripheral blood monocytes of septic mice 24 h after CLP, while mortality of ILT4-knockout sepsis mice was significantly reduced. In view of this phenomenon, this study detected the relevant inflammatory mediators and antigen-presenting cells in order to identify the potential pathogenic mechanisms of ILT4. The results showed that serum IL-6 was significantly increased 24 h after CLP,

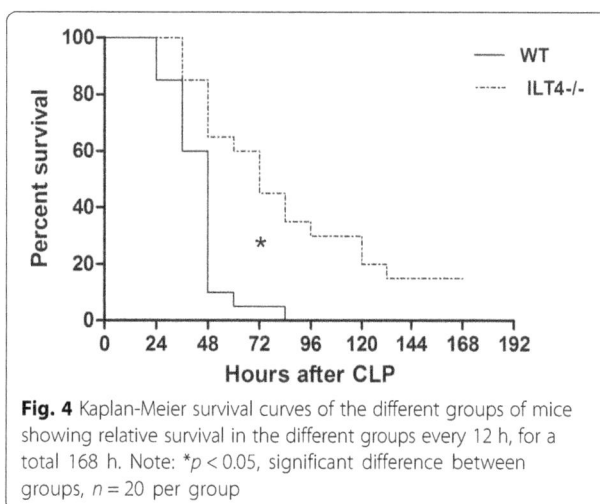

Fig. 4 Kaplan-Meier survival curves of the different groups of mice showing relative survival in the different groups every 12 h, for a total 168 h. Note: *$p < 0.05$, significant difference between groups, $n = 20$ per group

and ILT4 knockout significantly suppressed this phenomenon, which was negatively correlated with survival. These findings were consistent with the clinical study by Gomez et al. [19]. An earlier study suggested that septic patients with serum IL-6 > 1000 pg/mL had 56% mortality, while patients with < 1000 pg/mL serum IL-6 had a mortality of only 40% [20].

Nevertheless, ILT4 had no significant impact on other inflammatory mediators, including TNF-α, IL-1β, and IL-12. ILT4 gene knockout demonstrated significant protective effects on septic mice at high serum levels of TNF-α, IL-1β, and IL-12, which was surprisingly different from our expectations. High levels of TNF-α [21] and IL-1β [22] in sepsis are generally considered to be correlated with high mortality, while IL-12, the primary effector of monocytes, can synergize IFN-γ to promote the inflammatory response, leading to poor prognosis of sepsis [23]. This could be explained by the existence of a numerous inflammatory mediators during sepsis, each playing multiple roles in a complex network and it is still unclear which are the ultimate key factors. This study showed that the effects of IL-6 were independent from the effects of TNF-α, IL-1β, and IL-12, but IL-6 was regulated by ILT4, which was associated with poor prognosis of sepsis. Further investigation of the regulation of IL-6 levels by ILT4 and its correlation with poor prognosis should be conducted in the future.

This study also showed that MHC-II levels on monocytes were significantly higher in the peripheral blood of ILT4$^{-/-}$ mice than in WT mice. MHC-II mediates the transmission of extracellular signals. Following bacterial infection, macrophages phagocytose the bacteria and use

MHC-II to supply T helper cells with bacterial fragments to initiate the immune response. In this way, MCH-II plays an essential role in the response to infection. Indeed, patients with < 30% HLA-DR (a member of the MHC-II family) in monocytes had 100% mortality, while patients with < 40% HLA-DR in monocytes had 80% mortality [24, 25]. High MHC-II levels on monocytes rather than the reduction of serum IL-6 was here found to be key to the survival of the ILT4$^{-/-}$ mice. Nevertheless, the correlation between IL-6 and MHC-II has been reported [26].

The present study is not without limitations. The experiments were performed in the CLP animal model of sepsis, which is of course not perfect and could not completely mimic what is observed in humans.

Conclusions

In conclusion, this study showed that high levels of ILT4 in monocytes during sepsis were associated with high serum IL-6 levels and low MHC-II levels on monocytes, resulting in higher mortality of sepsis. This study provides a new focus and further understanding of the pathology of sepsis. Nevertheless, further in-depth studies of the interplay among cytokines and molecular pathways are necessary.

Abbreviations

CLP: Cecal ligation puncture; DMAPs: Danger-associated molecular patterns; IL: Interleukin; ILT4: Immunoglobulin-like transcript-4; ITIMs: Immunoreceptor tyrosine-based inhibitory motifs; LPS: Lipopolysaccharide; MHC-II: Major histocompatibility complex class II molecules; PRRs: Pattern-recognition receptors; TNF-α: Tumor necrosis factor-alpha

Acknowledgements

Not applicable

Funding

Not applicable

Authors' contributions

DWZ designed the subject and performed the biological experiment and was a major contributor in writing the manuscript. JH analyzed and interpreted the study data. Both authors read and approved the final manuscript.

Competing interests

The authors declare that they have no competing interests.

References

1. Singer M, Deutschman CS, Seymour CW, Shankar-Hari M, Annane D, et al. The third international consensus definitions for sepsis and septic shock (sepsis-3). JAMA. 2016;315:801–10.
2. Finfer S, Bellomo R, Lipman J, French C, Dobb G, et al. Adult-population incidence of severe sepsis in Australian and New Zealand intensive care units. Intensive Care Med. 2004;30:589–96.
3. Cheng B, Xie G, Yao S, Wu X, Guo Q, et al. Epidemiology of severe sepsis in critically ill surgical patients in ten university hospitals in China. Crit Care Med. 2007;35:2538–46.
4. Cohen J. The immunopathogenesis of sepsis. Nature. 2002;420:885–91.
5. van der Poll T, Opal SM. Host-pathogen interactions in sepsis. Lancet Infect Dis. 2008;8:32–43.
6. Anas AA, Wiersinga WJ, de Vos AF, van der Poll T. Recent insights into the pathogenesis of bacterial sepsis. Neth J Med. 2010;68:147–52.
7. Volk HD, Reinke P, Krausch D, Zuckermann H, Asadullah K, et al. Monocyte deactivation—rationale for a new therapeutic strategy in sepsis. Intensive Care Med. 1996;22(Suppl 4):S474–81.
8. Weighardt H, Heidecke CD, Emmanuilidis K, Maier S, Bartels H, et al. Sepsis after major visceral surgery is associated with sustained and interferon-gamma-resistant defects of monocyte cytokine production. Surgery. 2000;127:309–15.
9. Barrow AD, Trowsdale J. The extended human leukocyte receptor complex: diverse ways of modulating immune responses. Immunol Rev. 2008;224:98–123.
10. Borges L, Cosman D. LIRs/ILTs/MIRs, inhibitory and stimulatory Ig-superfamily receptors expressed in myeloid and lymphoid cells. Cytokine Growth Factor Rev. 2000;11:209–17.
11. Baffari E, Fiume D, Caiazzo G, Sinistro A, Natoli S, et al. Upregulation of the inhibitory receptor ILT4 in monocytes from septic patients. Hum Immunol. 2013;74:1244–50.
12. Baudhuin J, Migraine J, Faivre V, Loumagne L, Lukaszewicz AC, et al. Exocytosis acts as a modulator of the ILT4-mediated inhibition of neutrophil functions. Proc Natl Acad Sci U S A. 2013;110:17957–62.
13. Takai T. Paired immunoglobulin-like receptors and their MHC class I recognition. Immunology. 2005;115:433–40.
14. Rittirsch D, Huber-Lang MS, Flierl MA, Ward PA. Immunodesign of experimental sepsis by cecal ligation and puncture. Nat Protoc. 2009;4:31–6.
15. Ziegler-Heitbrock L, Ancuta P, Crowe S, Dalod M, Grau V, et al. Nomenclature of monocytes and dendritic cells in blood. Blood. 2010;116:e74–80.
16. Auffray C, Sieweke MH, Geissmann F. Blood monocytes: development, heterogeneity, and relationship with dendritic cells. Annu Rev Immunol. 2009;27:669–92.
17. Geissmann F, Jung S, Littman DR. Blood monocytes consist of two principal subsets with distinct migratory properties. Immunity. 2003;19:71–82.
18. Pinheiro da Silva F, Aloulou M, Skurnik D, Benhamou M, Andremont A, et al. CD16 promotes Escherichia coli sepsis through an FcR gamma inhibitory pathway that prevents phagocytosis and facilitates inflammation. Nat Med. 2007;13:1368–74.
19. Gomez HG, Gonzalez SM, Londono JM, Hoyos NA, Nino CD, et al. Immunological characterization of compensatory anti-inflammatory response syndrome in patients with severe sepsis: a longitudinal study*. Crit Care Med. 2014;42:771–80.
20. Oberhoffer M, Karzai W, Meier-Hellmann A, Bogel D, Fassbinder J, et al. Sensitivity and specificity of various markers of inflammation for the prediction of tumor necrosis factor-alpha and interleukin-6 in patients with sepsis. Crit Care Med. 1999;27:1814–8.
21. Waage A, Halstensen A, Espevik T. Association between tumour necrosis factor in serum and fatal outcome in patients with meningococcal disease. Lancet. 1987;1:355–7.
22. Goldie AS, Fearon KC, Ross JA, Barclay GR, Jackson RE, et al. Natural cytokine antagonists and endogenous antiendotoxin core antibodies in sepsis syndrome. The Sepsis Intervention Group. JAMA. 1995;274:172–7.
23. Nakahira M, Ahn HJ, Park WR, Gao P, Tomura M, et al. Synergy of IL-12 and IL-18 for IFN-gamma gene expression: IL-12-induced STAT4 contributes to IFN-gamma promoter activation by up-regulating the binding activity of IL-18-induced activator protein 1. J Immunol. 2002;168:1146–53.

24. Su L, Zhou DY, Tang YQ, Wen Q, Bai T, et al. Clinical value of monitoring
     CD14+ monocyte human leukocyte antigen (locus) DR levels in the early
     stage of sepsis. Zhongguo Wei Zhong Bing Ji Jiu Yi Xue. 2006;18:677–9.
25. Lekkou A, Karakantza M, Mouzaki A, Kalfarentzos F, Gogos CA. Cytokine
     production and monocyte HLA-DR expression as predictors of outcome for
     patients with community-acquired severe infections. Clin Diagn Lab
     Immunol. 2004;11:161–7.
26. Kitamura H, Kamon H, Sawa S, Park SJ, Katunuma N, et al. IL-6-STAT3
     controls intracellular MHC class II alphabeta dimer level through cathepsin S
     activity in dendritic cells. Immunity. 2005;23:491–502.

21

The impact of smoking on patient outcomes in severe sepsis and septic shock

Fahad Alroumi[1,2]* (iD), Ahmed Abdul Azim[1,2], Rachel Kergo[1], Yuxiu Lei[1,2] and James Dargin[1,2]

Abstract

Background: To assess, in the setting of severe sepsis and septic shock, whether current smokers have worse outcomes compared to non-smokers.

Methods: This is a retrospective analysis of immunocompetent adult patients with severe sepsis and septic shock at a tertiary medical center. The primary outcome was the effect of active smoking on hospital mortality. Chi-square test and logistic regression were used to assess categorical outcomes. Wilcoxon rank-sum was utilized to test the differences in continuous outcomes among the varied smoking histories. Multivariable logistic regression was used to evaluate the association of smoking and mortality, need for vasopressors, mechanical ventilation, and ICU admission.

Results: Of the 1437 charts reviewed, 562 patients were included. Current smokers accounted for 19% (107/562) of patients, while 81% (455/562) were non-smokers. The median hospital length of stay in survivors was significantly longer in current smokers versus non-smokers (8 vs 7 days, $p = 0.03$). There was a trend towards a higher mortality among current smokers, but this failed to meet statistical significance (OR 1.81, 95% CI 0.92–3.54, $p = 0.08$). On multivariable analysis, current smoking was associated with the need for mechanical ventilation (OR 2.38, 95% CI 1.06–5.34, $p = 0.04$), but that association was not observed with the need for vasopressors (OR 2.10, 95% CI 1.01–4.36, $p = 0.58$) nor ICU admission (OR 0.93, 95% CI 0.41–2.13, $p = 0.86$).

Conclusions: In patients with severe sepsis or septic shock, current smoking was associated with a longer hospital stay, the need for mechanical ventilation, and trended towards a higher mortality. Larger multicenter prospective case-control studies are needed to confirm these findings.

Keywords: Sepsis, Smoking, Septic shock, Mortality, Cigarettes, Tobacco

Background

Tobacco smoking remains the leading cause of preventable illness and death worldwide, accounting for approximately six million deaths annually [1]. Smoking imposes a heavy economic toll, costing countries billions of dollars in productivity and medical care [1]. In addition, it negatively impacts patient outcomes from acute illnesses, including influenza, pneumococcal pneumonia, and acute respiratory distress syndrome [2–4]. Although tobacco smoking is a risk factor for pulmonary and extra-pulmonary infections alike, its role in sepsis remains unclear [4–7].

Sepsis affects over one million individuals annually in the USA, and the mortality can be as high as 30% [8]. The costs incurred by sepsis have been estimated at $20 billion annually, making it one of the most expensive conditions treated in hospitals [8]. Smoking predisposes to infection through both structural and immunologic mechanisms [2]. Tobacco smoke causes peribronchiolar inflammation and fibrosis, which results in an alteration in mucosal permeability and deterioration in the function of the mucociliary escalator therefore increasing susceptibility to infection [2, 9]. Cigarette smoking also affects cell-mediated and humoral immune responses to infection, resulting in a number of seemingly contradictory influences on immune function, including both pro-inflammatory and immunosuppressive effects [10–13]. Such immunosuppressive effects may be expected to increase the severity and duration of infection

* Correspondence: fahad.alroumiMD@baystatehealth.org
[1]Department of Pulmonary and Critical Care Medicine, Lahey Hospital and Medical Center, Burlington, MA, USA
[2]Tufts University School of Medicine, Boston, MA, USA

[14–16]. Contrarily, there is some evidence that current smoking is associated with a decreased risk of mortality in pneumococcal pneumonia with bacteremia [17]. Given the complex nature of the effect of smoking on immune function, it is difficult to predict the overall impact of tobacco smoking on clinical outcomes in sepsis [5]. Furthermore, there is a paucity of published data and the results are conflicting with regard to the effects of smoking on sepsis-related morbidity and mortality [8, 18, 19]. Here, we describe the association between smoking status and patient outcomes in severe sepsis and septic shock.

Methods
Study population
The study was conducted at Lahey Hospital & Medical Center, a 317-bed tertiary care, academic hospital with approximately 40,000 emergency department visits annually. The institutional review board approved this study and waived the need for informed consent. Consecutive adults (≥ 18 years) discharged with a sepsis-related diagnosis between February 1, 2013, and January 30, 2014, were identified using ICD-9 codes (038, 0380, 0389, 77181, 78552, 99802, 99591, and 99592). The medical records were then manually reviewed to confirm that the patients met the criteria for either severe sepsis or septic shock. The sepsis-2 consensus definitions were utilized because data collection commenced prior to the publication of the sepsis-3 definition [20]. We included only patients meeting criteria for either severe sepsis or septic shock. In patients who had multiple episodes of severe sepsis or septic shock during a single hospitalization, only the first episode was included. Likewise, for patients with multiple admissions for severe sepsis or septic shock during the study period, solely their first admission was included.

Patients were excluded if they met the criteria for sepsis alone (without organ dysfunction), had systemic inflammatory response syndrome (SIRS) without a suspected infection, they had a history of immunosuppression (solid organ transplantation, stem cell transplantation; cytotoxic chemotherapy in the past 3 months; HIV infection; chronic corticosteroid therapy with ≥ 10 mg of prednisone or equivalent; neutropenia with an absolute neutrophil count < 1000/mm^3; congenital immunodeficiency; or immunosuppressive therapy in the past 3 months, including azathioprine, methotrexate, TNF-alpha antagonists, or other biologic immunosuppressants), they were pregnant, smoking history was unavailable, were transitioned to comfort care only within 24 h of admission, and if treatment for sepsis was commenced at an outside hospital.

We retrospectively collected, from the medical record, demographics including age, gender, co-morbid conditions, sequential organ failure assessment (SOFA) score at the time of diagnosis with sepsis, and smoking status, as well as other predictors of outcomes related to sepsis.

In order to characterize smoking status, the Center for Disease Control and Prevention's (CDC) definitions of current, former, and never smoker were adapted [21]. A current smoker was defined as an individual who smoked ≥ 100 cigarettes and still smoked daily on admission or quit within 1 year of admission. A former smoker smoked ≥ 100 cigarettes and quit more than 1 year of admission. A never smoker never smoked a cigarette or smoked less than 100 cigarettes during her/his lifetime. A non-smoker was defined as the combination of all former and never smokers. In addition, data on sepsis-related outcomes, including intensive care unit (ICU) and hospital mortality, ICU and hospital length of stay, the need for and duration of treatment with vasopressors, the need for and duration of renal replacement therapy, and the need for and duration of mechanical ventilation were collected.

Statistics
The primary outcome was inpatient mortality, and secondary outcomes were hospital length of stay, ICU length of stay, and the need for vasopressors, dialysis, and mechanical ventilation. The continuous variables were tested for normality. Nonparametric continuous variables were compared between current smokers, never smokers, and former smokers using Wilcoxon rank-sum test. Categorical variables were compared using chi-square test. The impact of smoking and other covariates on mortality was explored. Variables showing a significant difference ($p \leq 0.10$) in univariate analysis were included in the multivariable logistic regression analysis. Chronic obstructive pulmonary disease (COPD) was also included in the multivariable analysis as the authors felt that clinically, it was an important mediator in the association. The statistical analysis for this study was generated using Statistical Analysis Software (SAS), version 9.4 for Windows.

Results
Patient characteristics
There were 1437 patients identified with a sepsis-related discharge diagnosis based on ICD-9 codes. After manually reviewing the medical records, 562 individuals met criteria for inclusion in this study (Fig. 1). Current smokers accounted for 19% (107/562) of patients, and 81% (455/562) were non-smokers. As a reference, the prevalence of smoking reported in the state of Massachusetts was 17% (95% CI, 16–18) for the year this study was conducted [22]. Of the non-smokers in our study, 55% (249/455) were former smokers and the rest (45%, 206/455) never smoked. Details on smoking history were available for 86/107(80%) of current smokers. The mean number of cigarettes smoked per day in this group was 23.3 ± 13.4, and the mean number of pack years smoked was 45.7 ± 30.5. In former smokers, a detailed smoking history was available in 176/

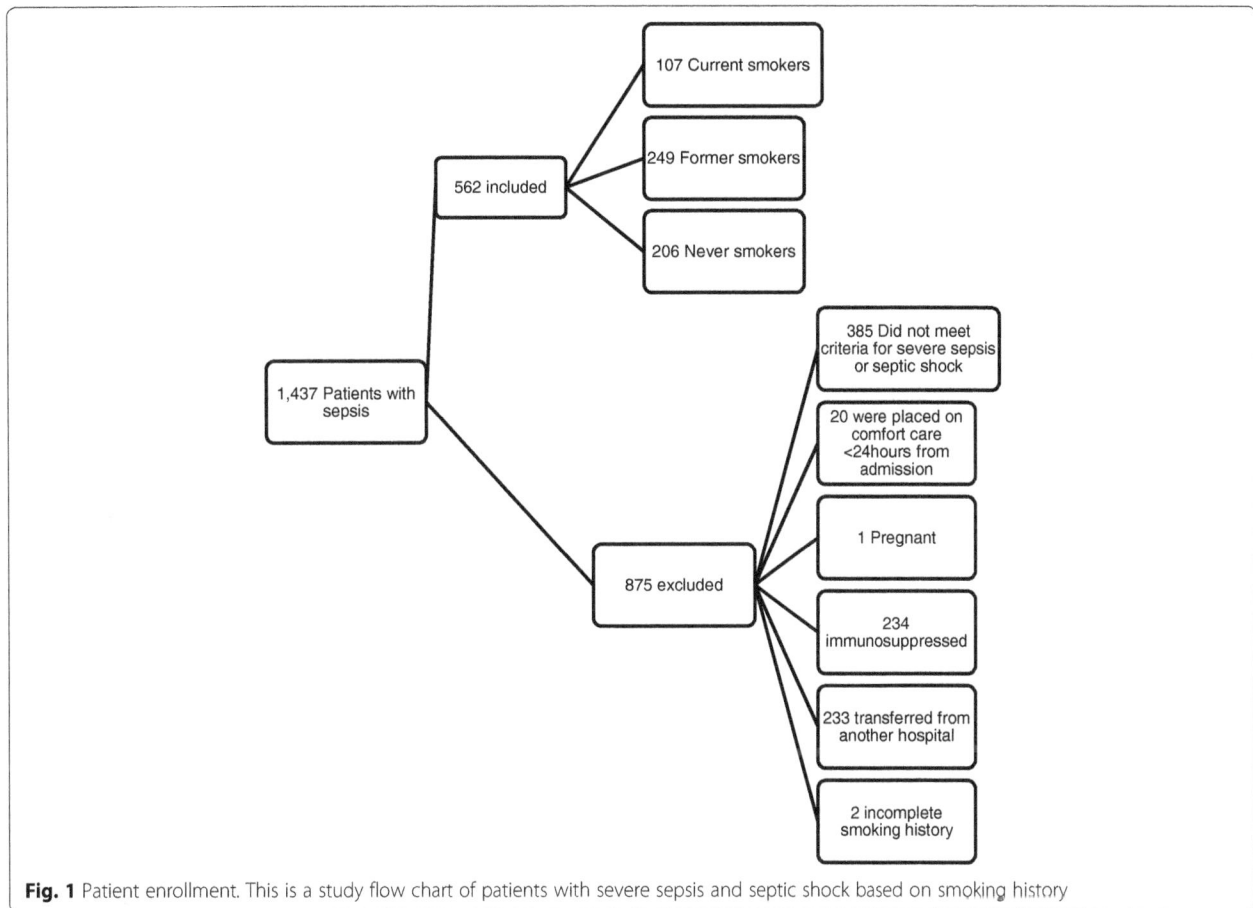

Fig. 1 Patient enrollment. This is a study flow chart of patients with severe sepsis and septic shock based on smoking history

249 (71%) of patients. In this group, the mean number of cigarettes smoked per day was 22.9 ± 13.5 and the mean number of pack-years smoked was 37.1 ± 25.6. The majority of patients were male (62%, 347/562), and there was no difference in gender distribution among the groups (Table 1). Current smokers were significantly younger than non-smokers (age 58, IQR 50–69 vs 78, IQR 66–85, $p < 0.01$). The median Charlson Comorbidity Index (CCI) was significantly lower in current smokers compared to non-smokers (4, IQR 2–5 vs 5, IQR 4–7, $p < 0.01$). Current smokers had fewer cardiac, neuro-logic, and renal co-morbidities but had more cirrhosis, COPD, and alcohol abuse than non-smokers (Table 1).

The overall percentage of patients with severe sepsis was 57% (319/562) and 43% (243/562) had septic shock. The proportion of patients with septic shock was signifi-cantly higher among current smokers (56%, 60/107 vs 40%, 183/455; $p < 0.01$), and pneumonia was the com-monest source of sepsis among all groups. Abdominal sepsis was commoner in current smokers, whereas soft tissue and genitourinary infections were more frequently seen in non-smokers (Table 1). Current smokers had a significantly higher SOFA score than non-smokers at the time of diagnosis of severe sepsis or septic shock (7, IQR 4–12 vs 5, IQR 3–9; $p < 0.01$). Specifically, the respira-tory component of the SOFA score was higher in the current smokers versus non-smokers (2, IQR 0–3 vs 1, IQR 0–2; $p < 0.001$).

Clinical outcomes

The proportion of patients who died during their hos-pital stay was higher in current smokers (32%, 34/107) when compared to non-smokers (22%, 101/455, $p = 0.04$) (Table 2). In the multivariable analysis, when current smokers were compared to non-smokers, there was a trend towards higher mortality among current smokers but this failed to meet statistical significance (OR 1.81, 95% CI 0.92–3.54, $p = 0.08$) (Table 3). In comparison with former smokers, mortality was higher among current smokers (OR 2.18, 95% CI 1.002–4.743, $p < 0.05$) (Table 4). This association was not observed when mortality was compared between current smokers and never smokers (OR 1.47, 95% CI 0.612–3.516, $p = 0.39$) (Table 5). The percentage of patients who required ICU admission was higher in current smokers versus non-smokers (70% 75/107 vs 53% 243/455, $p < 0.01$). There was a trend towards a longer ICU length of stay in survivors in that same cohort (6, IQR 3–11 vs 4, IQR 2–10 days, $p = 0.06$). The

Table 1 Baseline characteristics stratified by smoking history

Demographics	All (N = 562)	Current smokers (N = 107)	Non-smokers (N = 455)	P value* (current vs. non)	Former smokers (N = 249)	P value** (current vs. former)	Never smokers (N = 206)	P value§ (current vs. never)
Age—median years (IQR)	74 (61–84)	58 (50–69)	78 (66–85)	<0.0001	78 (69–85)	<0.0001	76.5 (61–85)	<0.0001
Male—n (%)	347 (62%)	69 (65)	278 (61)	0.52	166 (67)	0.69	112 (54)	0.09
BMI, median (IQR)	26 (23–31)	26 (23–32)	26 (23–31)	0.87	26 (23–31)	0.66	26 (22–31)	0.86
FEV1 mean (std)^f	1.76 (0.78)	2.11 (1.05)	1.65 (0.64)	0.048	1.64 (0.64)	0.049	1.67 (0.65)	0.09
FEV1 % pred mean (std)^f	68.4 (24.5)	66.6 (23.3)	68.9 (24.9)	0.69	69.3 (24.2)	0.65	67.9 (27.5)	0.87
FVC mean (std)^f	2.54 (0.97)	3.07 (1.13)	2.37 (0.85)	<0.01	2.39 (0.83)	0.004	2.32 (0.93)	0.03
FVC % pred mean (std)^f	73.2 (20.9)	75.9 (20.5)	72.3 (21.0)	0.46	73.0 (19.0)	0.54	70.2 (26.6)	0.44
FEV1/FVC mean (std)^f	68.6 (15.9)	67.3 (16.0)	69.0 (15.9)	0.65	69.1 (14.6)	0.64	68.7 (19.8)	0.79
Hospital acquired sepsis#	52 (9.3%)	15 (14%)	37 (8.1%)	0.06	21 (8.4%)	0.11	16 (7.8%)	0.08
Charlson Score, median (IQR)	5 (4–7)	4 (2–5)	5 (4–7)	<0.0001	6 (4–7)	<0.0001	5 (3–7)	0.0005
MI, n (%)	151 (27)	19 (18)	132 (29)	0.002	93 (37)	0.0003	39 (19)	0.80
CHF, n (%)	137 (24)	14 (13)	123 (27)	0.003	75 (30)	0.0007	48 (23)	0.03
CVA, n (%)	75 (13)	6 (6)	69 (15)	<0.01	38 (15)	0.01	31 (15)	0.01
Dementia, n (%)	64 (11)	3 (3)	61 (13)	<0.01	34 (14)	0.002	27 (13)	0.003
COPD, n (%)	110 (20)	35 (33)	75 (17)	<0.01	68 (27)	0.30	7 (3)	<0.0001
DM, n (%)	161 (29)	27 (25)	134 (30)	0.39	72 (29)	0.48	62 (30)	0.37
Cirrhosis, n (%)	56 (10)	24 (22)	32 (7)	<0.01	15 (6)	<0.0001	17 (8)	0.0004
CKD, n (%)	55 (10)	5 (5)	50 (11)	0.05	33 (13)		17 (8)	
Source of infection								
Pneumonia, n (%)	241 (43)	53 (50)	188 (41)	0.12	116 (47)	0.61	72 (35)	0.01
Genitourinary	154 (27)	21 (20)	133 (29)	0.05	66 (27)	0.17	67 (32)	0.02
Abdominal	108 (19)	31 (29)	77 (17)	<0.01	42 (17)	0.01	35 (17)	0.01
Soft tissue	39 (7)	2 (2)	37 (8)	0.02	23 (9)	0.01	14 (7)	0.06
CNS	3 (1)	1 (1)	2 (0.4)	0.53	0 (0)	0.13	2 (1)	0.98
Cardiovascular	9 (2)	2 (2)	7 (2)	0.81	2 (1)	0.38	5 (2)	0.75
Blood stream	73 (13)	12 (11)	61 (13)	0.54	28 (11)	0.99	33 (16)	0.25
CVC	10 (2)	0 (0)	10 (2)	0.12	4 (2)	0.19	6 (3)	0.07
Other	0	0	0	–	0	–	0	–
Unknown	16 (3)	2 (2)	14 (3)	0.50	6 (2)	0.75	8 (4)	0.34
Medical, n (%)	481 (86)	84 (79)	397 (87)	0.02	218 (88)	0.03	179 (87)	0.05
Surgical	81 (13)	23 (22)	58 (13)		31 (13)		27 (13)	

Table 1 Baseline characteristics stratified by smoking history (Continued)

Demographics	All (N = 562)	Current smokers (N = 107)	Non-smokers (N = 455)	P value* (current vs. non)	Former smokers (N = 249)	P value** (current vs. former)	Never smokers (N = 206)	P value§ (current vs. never)
Alcohol abuse, n (%)	64 (11)	37 (35)	27 (6)	<0.01	19 (8)	<0.0001	8 (4)	<0.0001
Severe sepsis, n (%)	319 (57)	47 (44)	272 (60)	<0.01	144 (58)	0.02	128 (62)	0.002
Septic shock, n (%)	243 (43)	60 (56)	183 (40)		105 (42)		78 (38)	
Lactate—median (IQR)	2.1 (1.3–3.4)	2.1 (1.5–3.1)	2.05 (1.2–3.5)	0.53	2.0 (1.2–3.2)	0.53	2.1 (1.2–3.7)	0.61
SOFA score median (IQR)	6 (3–9)	7 (4–12)	5 (3–9)	<0.01	5 (3–9)	0.001	5 (3–8)	<0.0001
Respiratory‡ median (IQR)	1 (0–2)	2 (0–3)	1 (0–2)	<0.001	1 (0–3)	0.015	0 (0–2)	<0.0001
72 h fluid balance—median L (IQR)	2.1 (0.2–4.35)	2.3 (0.01–5.9)	2.1 (0.26–4.1)	0.32	2.1 (0.01–4.1)	0.18	2.2 (0.5–4.1)	0.67
Stress steroids given—n (%)	38 (7)	9 (8)	29 (6)	0.45	17 (7)	0.60	12 (6)	0.38
Time to appropriate antibiotics after hypotension—minutes, median (IQR)	60 (−60–159)	35 (−117–120)	61 (−60–165)	0.23	60 (−76–165)	0.44	68.5 (−22–170)	0.14
Appropriate empiric antibiotics given based on culture data								
Yes, n (%)	248 (44)	53(50)	195/454 (43)	0.17	107 (43)	0.17	88/205 (43)	0.26
No, n (%)	50 (9)	5(5)	45/454 (10)		26 (10)		19/205 (9)	
Unknown, n (%)	263 (47)	49(46)	214/454 (47)		116 (47)		98/205 (48)	

Abbreviations: *IQR* interquartile range, *BMI* body mass index, *std.* standard deviation, *FEV1* forced expiratory volume in 1 s, *FVC* forced vital capacity, *MI* myocardial infarction, *CHF* congestive heart failure, *CVA* cerebrovascular accident, *COPD* chronic obstructive pulmonary disease, *DM* diabetes mellitus, *CKD* chronic kidney disease, *CNS* central nervous system, *CVC* central venous catheter, *SOFA* sequential organ failure assessment

*P value refers to comparison between current smokers and non-smokers

**P value refers to comparison between current smokers and former smokers

§P value refers to comparison between current smokers and never smokers

†There were only 98/562 (17.4%) patients that had available pulmonary function testing recorded prior to data collection. Therefore, the N in this section is unique: current smokers N = 24, former smoker N = 55, never smoker N = 19. Additionally, the reported spirometry is pre-bronchodilator

#Individuals who acquired sepsis more than 48 h following hospital admission

‡Independent evaluation of respiration as part of SOFA score. 0 = PaO₂/FiO₂ ratio > 400, 1 = PaO₂/FiO₂ 301–400 or SaO2/FiO₂ > 400, 1 = PaO₂/FiO₂ 301–400 or SaO2/FiO₂ 221–301, 2 = PaO₂/FiO₂ 201–300 or SaO2/FiO₂ 142–220, 3 = PaO₂/FiO₂ 101–200 or SaO2/FiO₂ 67–141, 4 = PaO₂/FiO₂ < 100 or SaO2/FiO₂ 67

Table 2 Outcomes in smokers, former smokers, and never smokers with severe sepsis or septic shock

Outcomes	Current smokers (N = 107)	Non-smokers (N = 455)	P value*	Former smokers (N = 249)	P value**	Never smokers (N = 206)	P value§
Mortality‡—n (%)	34 (32)	101 (22)	0.04	60 (24)	0.13	41 (20)	0.02
Hospital LOS—median days (IQR)	7 (4–17)	7 (4–12)	0.19	7 (4–12)	0.26	7 (4–12)	0.20
Hospital LOS in survivors	8 (4–18) (N = 73)	7 (4–12) (N = 354)	0.03	7 (4–12) (N = 189)	0.05	7 (4–11) (N = 165)	0.05
ICU LOS	5 (3–10) (N = 75)	4 (2–11) (N = 243)	0.36	5 (2–11) (N = 135)	0.67	4 (2–10) (N = 108)	0.20
ICU LOS survivors	6 (3–11) (N = 47)	4 (2–10) (N = 162)	0.06	4 (2–10) (N = 84)	0.10	4 (2–10) (N = 78)	0.07
Required ICU admission—n (%)	75 (70)	243 (53)	<0.01	135 (54)	<0.01	108 (52)	<0.01
Required vasopressors—n (%)	57 (53)	175 (39)	<0.01	104 (42)	0.05	71 (34)	<0.01
Vasopressor days—median (IQR)	3 (2–4) (N = 57)	3 (2–5) (N = 175)	0.97	3 (2–5.5) (N = 104)	0.72	3 (2–5) (N = 71)	0.68
Required mechanical ventilation—n (%)	62 (58)	133 (29)	<0.01	77 (31)	<0.01	56 (27)	<0.01
Ventilator days	5 (2–9) (N = 62)	5 (2–9) (N = 133)	0.99	6 (2–11) (N = 77)	0.42	4 (2–8) (N = 56)	0.32
Required dialysis—n (%)	10 (9)	42 (9)	0.97	27 (11)	0.67	15 (7)	0.52
Dialysis days	4 (2–6) (N = 10)	4 (2–9) (N = 42)	0.58	6 (3–13) (N = 27)	0.30	3 (2–6) (N = 15)	0.74

LOS length of stay, ICU intensive care unit
*P value refers to comparison between current smokers and non-smokers
**P value refers to comparison between current smokers and former smokers
§P value refers to comparison between current smokers and never smokers
‡Includes death or discharge to hospice

Table 3 Multivariable logistic regression analysis of active smoking and mortality in severe sepsis and septic shock (current smokers vs. non-smokers)

Risk factor	Odds ratio (95% CI)	P value
Current smoking	1.81 (0.92–3.54)	0.08
Alcohol abuse	1.17 (0.54–2.49)	0.69
72 h fluid balance	1.06 (0.99–1.13)	0.08
Age	1.02 (0.99–1.05)	0.06
Charlson score	1.16 (1.02–1.31)	0.02
SOFA	1.15 (1.068–1.238)	< 0.01
COPD	0.98 (0.539–1.794)	0.96
Hospital acquired sepsis	1.51 (0.711–3.201)	0.28
Severe sepsis	0.54 (0.288–1.011)	0.05
Genitourinary infect	0.52 (0.282–0.970)	0.04
Abdominal	0.93 (0.487–1.757)	0.81
Soft tissue	1.03 (0.394–2.713)	0.95
Medical ICU admission	1.62 (0.765–3.411)	0.21

All survival predictors (except for "respiratory") that were noted to be significant ($p < 0.1$) on univariate analysis were included in this multivariate model
SOFA sequential organ failure assessment, *COPD* chronic obstructive pulmonary disease

overall hospital length of stay in survivors was significantly longer when comparing current smokers versus non-smokers (8, IQR 4–18 vs 7 IQR 4–12 days, $p = 0.03$). There was a greater need for mechanical ventilation (58 vs 29%, $p < 0.01$) and vasopressors (53 vs 39%, $p < 0.01$) in current smokers vs non-smokers, respectively, though the ventilator days, vasopressor days, the need for dialysis, and dialysis days did not significantly differ between the compared groups (Table 2). After controlling for other confounders, current smoking predicted the need for

Table 4 Multivariable logistic regression analysis of active smoking and mortality in severe sepsis and septic shock (current smokers vs. former smokers)

Risk factor	Odds ratio (95% CI)	P value
Current smoking	2.18 (1.00–4.74)	0.049
Alcohol abuse	1.61 (0.67–3.85)	0.29
72 h fluid balance	1.03 (0.95–1.12)	0.42
Age	1.02 (0.99–1.05)	0.17
Charlson score	1.18 (1.00–1.38)	0.05
SOFA	1.15 (1.05–1.25)	< 0.01
COPD	0.98 (0.49–1.93)	0.94
Hospital acquired sepsis	1.77 (0.704–0.4.442)	0.23
Severe sepsis	0.40 (0.176–0.895)	0.03
Genitourinary infect	0.29 (0.12–0.71)	< 0.01
Abdominal	0.95 (0.43–2.10)	0.90
Soft tissue	1.99 (0.61–6.51)	0.25
Medical ICU admission	1.65 (0.66–4.15)	0.29

mechanical ventilation (OR 2.38, 95% CI 1.06–5.34, $p = 0.04$) but did not predict the need for vasopressors or ICU admission (Tables 6, 7, and 8).

Clinical outcomes in patients with pneumonia

There was no statistically significant difference in the proportion of patients with pneumonia who died during their hospital stay when current smokers (34%, 18/53) were compared to non-smokers (24%, 45/188, $p = 0.14$) and former smokers (28%, 33/116, $p = 0.47$) (Table 9). However, the percentage of deaths was significantly less in never smokers (12%, 12/72) when compared to current smokers ($p = 0.03$).

The percentage of patients who required ICU admission was higher in current smokers versus non-smokers (77% 41/53 vs 55% 104/188, $p < 0.01$). There was a longer overall hospital length of stay in survivors in that same cohort (10, IQR 5–21 vs 7, IQR 4–12 days, $p = 0.02$), but ICU length of stay did not differ. There was a greater need for mechanical ventilation (74 vs 35%, $p < 0.01$) and vasopressors (62 vs 38%, $p < 0.01$) in current smokers vs non-smokers, respectively. Ventilator days, vasopressor days, need for dialysis, and dialysis days did not significantly differ among the compared groups (Table 9).

Discussion

Sepsis is one of the most expensive conditions treated in US hospitals, and its impact on the morbidity and mortality of those afflicted is substantial [23]. Tobacco smoking has well-documented effects on immune function, but the overall impact of smoking on clinical outcomes in sepsis has been poorly defined. Our results suggest that smoking is a potentially modifiable risk factor that can impact the course of those who have severe sepsis or septic shock. Despite being a younger group with fewer comorbidities, there was a trend towards a higher mortality in current smokers especially when compared to former smokers. Previous studies have primarily focused on the effect of smoking on outcomes in patients with respiratory infection, with conflicting results reported. For example, there is evidence that active smoking is associated with a higher mortality in patients with respiratory infections, particularly pneumonia and influenza [19, 24]. Contrarily, a large South African retrospective study noted that with the exception of tuberculosis, there was no significant risk of tobacco-attributable mortality from lung infections in smokers compared to non-smokers [25]. In other studies, bacteremic patients with pneumococcal pneumonia who were current smokers had decreased mortality or no difference in mortality when compared to non-smokers with the same infection [17, 26]. However, none of these studies looked at the effect of smoking on a broad population with sepsis [7, 18, 19]. To our knowledge, this is the first study to specifically examine

Table 5 Multivariable logistic regression analysis of active smoking and mortality in severe sepsis and septic shock (current smokers vs. never smokers)

Risk factor	Odds ratio (95% CI)	P value
Current smoking	1.47 (0.61–3.52)	0.39
Alcohol abuse	0.73 (0.29–1.86)	0.51
72 h fluid balance	1.04 (0.95–1.13)	0.45
Age	1.03 (0.99–1.06)	0.10
Charlson score	1.21 (1.02–1.43)	0.03
SOFA	1.12 (1.02–1.24)	0.02
COPD	1.62 (0.59–4.41)	0.35
Hospital acquired sepsis	1.13 (0.40–3.17)	0.28
Severe sepsis	0.65 (0.29–1.01)	0.82
Genitourinary infect	0.86 (0.39–1.90)	0.71
Abdominal	0.98 (0.42–2.33)	0.97
Soft tissue	0.557 (0.10–3.08)	0.50
Medical ICU admission	1.06 (0.39–2.84)	0.91

Table 7 Multivariable analysis of active smoking and requiring vasopressors in severe sepsis and septic shock (current smokers vs. non-smokers)

Risk factor	Odds ratio (95% CI)	P value
Current smoking	2.10 (1.01–4.36)	0.58
Alcohol abuse	1.25 (0.50–3.10)	0.99
72 h fluid balance	1.05 (0.98–1.13)	< 0.01
Age	1.02 (0.98–1.07)	0.34
Charlson score	0.89 (0.67–1.176)	0.40
SOFA	1.59 (1.34–1.88)	< 0.01
COPD	1.62 (0.39–6.68)	0.51
Hospital acquired sepsis	3.94 (0.61–25.4)	0.15
Severe sepsis	0.004 (0.001–0.01)	< 0.01
Genitourinary infect	1.01 (0.33–3.03)	0.99
Abdominal	0.61 (0.17–2.19)	0.45
Soft tissue	1.03 (0.14–7.37)	0.98
Medical ICU admission	1.23 (0.28–5.43)	0.79

the effect of active smoking on a general population of patients with severe sepsis and septic shock.

Our data also suggest that smokers have a higher proportion of sepsis-related organ dysfunction. We observed a greater percentage of septic shock and an increased need for vasopressors and mechanical ventilation in current smokers despite this population being younger and having fewer comorbidities. Furthermore, current smokers had a higher SOFA score at the time of diagnosis and were more likely to require ICU admission, suggesting a higher severity of illness on presentation and a more fulminant sepsis course. There is convincing biological plausibility for these findings considering the reported effects of smoking on several pro-inflammatory mediators, including TNFα, interleukin 6 and 8 NF-κB [27–30]. Furthermore, smoking increases levels of pro-inflammatory cytokines, including tumor necrosis factor (TNF) alpha and interleukin (IL)-6 [13]. Such an exaggerated pro-inflammatory response to microorganisms could potentially result in worse outcomes from sepsis. We also observed a longer hospital length of stay and a trend towards a longer ICU length of stay, suggesting a longer recovery from sepsis. This may be related to the immunosuppressive effects of smoking, which renders the host less able to combat infection. The increased rates of mechanical ventilation and worse hypoxia in current smokers can partially be explained by the higher rates of COPD in that group.

Table 6 Multivariable analysis of active smoking and requiring ICU admission in severe sepsis and septic shock (current smokers vs. non-smokers)

Risk factor	Odds ratio (95% CI)	P value
Current smoking	0.93 (0.41–2.13)	0.86
Alcohol abuse	0.83 (0.31–2.23)	0.71
72 h fluid balance	1.04 (0.94–1.16)	0.42
Age	0.987 (0.96–1.01)	0.31
Charlson score	1.03 (0.89–1.19)	0.70
SOFA	1.42 (1.27–1.60)	< 0.01
COPD	1.35 (0.67–2.76)	0.40
Hospital acquired sepsis	3.87 (1.11–13.5)	0.03
Severe sepsis	0.08 (0.04–0.16)	< 0.01
Genitourinary infect	0.55 (0.29–1.04)	0.07
Abdominal	1.02 (0.44–2.35)	0.97
Soft tissue	0.95 (0.27–3.26)	0.93
Medical ICU admission	0.71 (0.27–1.91)	0.50

Table 8 Multivariable analysis of active smoking and requiring mechanical ventilation in severe sepsis and septic shock (current smokers vs. non-smokers)

Risk factor	Odds ratio (95% CI)	P value
Current smoking	2.38 (1.06–5.34)	0.04
Alcohol abuse	0.99 (0.37–2.66)	0.99
72 h fluid balance	1.05 (0.97–1.11)	0.21
Age	0.98 (0.96–1.01)	0.21
Charlson score	0.92 (0.78–1.09)	0.33
SOFA	1.53 (1.37–1.70)	< 0.01
COPD	1.13 (0.52–2.43)	0.76
Hospital acquired sepsis	1.25 (0.45–3.45)	0.66
Severe sepsis	0.45 (0.23–0.88)	0.02
Genitourinary infect	0.26 (0.12–0.55)	< 0.01
Abdominal	0.40 (0.18–0.88)	0.02
Soft tissue	0.31 (0.10–0.96)	0.04
Medical ICU admission	0.13 (0.05–0.33)	< 0.01

Table 9 Outcomes in smokers, former smokers, and never smokers with severe sepsis or septic shock due to pneumonia (N = 241)

Outcomes	Current smokers (N = 53)	Non-smokers (N = 188)	P value*	Former smokers (N = 116)	P value**	Never smokers (N = 72)	P value§
Mortality‡—n (%)	18 (34)	45 (24)	0.14	33 (28)	0.47	12 (17)	0.03
Hospital LOS—median days (IQR)	8 (5–20)	7 (4–12)	0.13	7.5 (4–13)	0.16	7 (5–12)	0.20
Hospital LOS in survivors	10 (5–21)	7 (4–12)	0.02	7 (4–13)	0.03	7 (5–12)	0.05
ICU LOS	7 (3–13)	6 (3–12)	0.70	6 (3–11)	0.77	6 (2–12)	0.68
ICU LOS survivors	8 (4–13)	5 (2–12)	0.14	4 (2–11)	0.14	6 (3–12)	0.28
Required ICU admission—n (%)	41 (77)	104 (55)	< 0.01	66 (57)	0.01	38 (53)	< 0.01
Required vasopressors—n (%)	33 (62)	72 (38)	< 0.01	48 (41)	0.01	24 (33)	< 0.01
Vasopressor days—median (IQR)	3 (2–5)	3 (2–6)	0.73	3 (2–6)	0.62	3 (2–5)	0.97
Required mechanical ventilation—n (%)	39 (74)	66 (35)	< 0.01	42 (36)	< 0.01	24 (33)	< 0.01
Ventilator days	5 (3–12)	6 (3–10)	0.78	6 (3–11)	0.60	4 (3–8)	0.85
Required dialysis—n (%)	6 (11)	15 (8)	0.45	10 (9)	0.58	5 (7)	0.39
Dialysis days	4.5 (3–10)	6 (2–14)	0.70	10 (4–14)	0.32	2 (2–2)	0.52

LOS length of stay, *ICU* intensive care unit

*P value refers to comparison between current smokers and non-smokers

**P value refers to comparison between current smokers and former smokers

§P value refers to comparison between current smokers and never smokers

‡Includes death or discharge to hospice

Smokers also have an increased susceptibility to respiratory tract infections and acute respiratory distress syndrome (ARDS), which puts them at risk for respiratory failure and the need for mechanical ventilation [2–4].

Another possible explanation for the trend towards higher mortality in smokers is its association with worse health habits. In concordance with other studies, our data illustrate that smoking is accompanied by alcohol abuse [4, 31]. However, alcohol abuse was not an independent predictor of mortality in our multivariable analysis. In other studies, smoking was associated with less vaccination uptake [4, 32]. As a behavior pattern, smokers may potentially delay seeking medical attention and that is reflected in a higher severity of illness on presentation. This association has been observed in lung cancer patients, where smokers often avoided medical advice for lung cancer symptoms [33].

Because pneumonia was observed to be the most common source of infection and due to its association with smoking, we performed a subgroup analysis of patients with respiratory infections. Overall, the outcome trends were similar in patients with sepsis due to pneumonia as compared to outcomes observed in other sources of sepsis. However, as one would expect, the contrast between current smokers and non-smokers' need for mechanical ventilation was more pronounced in patients with pneumonia.

Our study is subject to a number of limitations. This was a single-center study, thus limiting the generalizability of our findings. Furthermore, the retrospective study design and small sample size potentially introduce bias into the results. Because the data were collected retrospectively, the smoking history and spirometry were limited to what was documented in the medical record a priori. However, the proportion of smokers observed in our study (19%, CI 95% 16–22) is similar to the prevalence of smoking reported in the state of Massachusetts (17%, CI 95% 16–18) for the year this study was conducted [22]. A larger sample size detailing patients' smoking history including pack years would have shed light on any potential dose-dependent effect on sepsis. Additionally, a prospective study design with the use of a validated biomarker to quantify tobacco exposure such as NNAL would have provided an objective measure to corroborate the smoking history. Finally, we did not determine whether the study patients received nicotine supplementation during their hospitalization and did not assess for second-hand smoke exposure in the non-smokers.

Conclusions

This study identified that current smokers trended towards a higher mortality in severe sepsis and septic shock despite being younger and with fewer comorbid illnesses. In addition, current smoking was associated with more than a twofold increase in the need for mechanical ventilation. Thus, tobacco smoking may represent a modifiable risk factor for worse outcomes in severe sepsis and septic shock. This was an exploratory study to evaluate the effects of smoking on severe sepsis and septic shock. Ultimately, large-scale multicenter prospective case-control studies are needed to confirm our findings.

Abbreviations
ARDS: Acute respiratory distress syndrome; BMI: Body mass index; CCI: Charlson Comorbidity Index; CDC: Center for Disease Control and Prevention; CHF: Congestive heart failure; CKD: Chronic kidney disease; CNS: Central nervous system; COPD: Chronic obstructive pulmonary disease; CVA: Cerebrovascular accident; CVC: Central venous catheter; DM: Diabetes mellitus; ICU: Intensive care unit; IL: Interleukin; IQR: Interquartile range; LOS: Length of stay; MI: Myocardial infarction; SIRS: Systemic inflammatory response syndrome; SOFA: Sequential organ failure assessment; TNF: Tumor necrosis factor

Authors' contributions
All authors had full access to the data. FA takes responsibility for the integrity of the data and accuracy of the data analysis. He contributed to the conception, design, and drafting of the manuscript. AAA and RK contributed to data acquisition and drafting of parts of the manuscript. YL contributed to analysis and interpretation. JD contributed to the final design, creation, and authorship of this manuscript. All authors read and approved the final manuscript.

Competing interests
The authors declare that they have no competing interests.

References
1. World Health Organization. Report on the global tobacco epidemic, 2013. http://www.who.int/tobacco/global_report/2013/en/. Accessed 14 June 2018.
2. Arcavi L, Benowitz NL. Cigarette smoking and infection. Arch Intern Med. 2004;164(20):2206–16.
3. Calfee CS, Matthay MA, Kangelaris KN, Siew ED, Janz DR, Bernard GR, May AK, Jacob P, Havel C, Benowitz NL, Ware LB. Cigarette smoke exposure and the acute respiratory distress syndrome. Crit Care Med. 2015;43(9):1790–7.
4. Bello S, Menéndez R, Antoni T, et al. Tobacco smoking increases the risk for death from pneumococcal pneumonia. Chest. 2014;146(4):1029–37.
5. Huttunen R, Heikkinen T, Syrjänen J. Smoking and the outcome of infection. J Intern Med. 2011;269(3):258–69.
6. Carter BD, Abnet CC, Feskanich D, et al. Smoking and mortality—beyond established causes. N Engl J Med. 2015;372(7):631–40.
7. Leithead JA, Ferguson JW, Hayes PC. Smoking-related morbidity and mortality following liver transplantation. Liver Transpl. 2008;14(8):1159–64.
8. Centers for Disease Control and Prevention. Inpatient care for septicemia or sepsis: a challenge for patients and hospitals. National Center for Health Statistics Data Brief No. 62, 2011. https://www.cdc.gov/nchs/data/databriefs/db62.pdf. Accessed 14 June 2018.
9. Dye JA, Adler KB. Effects of cigarette smoke on epithelial cells of the respiratory tract. Thorax. 1994;49(8):825–34.
10. Reinherz EL, Rubinstein A, Geha RS, et al. Abnormalities of immunoregulatory T cells in disorders of immune function. N Engl J Med. 1979;301(19):1018–22.
11. Gulsvik A, Fagerhoi MK. Smoking and immunoglobulin levels. Lancet. 1979; 1(8113):449.
12. Gerrard JW, Heiner DC, Ko CG, et al. Immunoglobulin levels in smokers and nonsmokers. Ann Allergy. 1980;44:261–2.

13. Arnson Y, Shoenfeld Y, Amital H. Effects of tobacco smoke on immunity, inflammation and autoimmunity. J Autoimmun. 2010;34(3):258–65.

14. Gualano RC, Hansen MJ, Vlahos R, et al. Cigarette smoke worsens lung inflammation and impairs resolution of influenza infection in mice. Respir Res. 2008;9:53.

15. Robbins CS, Bauer CM, Vujicic N, Gaschler GJ, Lichty BD, Brown EG, Stämpfli MR. Cigarette smoke impacts immune inflammatory responses to influenza in mice. Am J Respir Crit Care Med. 2006;174(12):1342–51.

16. Drannik AG, Pouladi MA, Robbins CS, Goncharova SI, Kianpour S, Stämpfli MR. Impact of cigarette smoke on clearance and inflammation after Pseudomonas aeruginosa infection. Am J Respir Crit Care Med. 2004; 170(11):1164–71.

17. Beatty JA, Majumdar SR, Tyrrell GJ, Marrie TJ, Eurich DT. Current smoking and reduced mortality in bacteremic pneumococcal pneumonia: a population-based cohort study. Chest. 2016;150(3):652–60.

18. Pittet D, Thiévent B, Wenzel RP, et al. Importance of pre-existing co-morbidities for prognosis of septicemia in critically ill patients. Intensive Care Med. 1993;19(5):265–72.

19. Huttunen R, Laine J, Lumio J, et al. Obesity and smoking are factors associated with poor prognosis in patients with bacteraemia. BMC Infect Dis. 2007;7:13.

20. Levy MM, Fink MP, Marshall JC, et al; SCCM/ESICM/ACCP/ATS/SIS. 2001 SCCM/ESICM/ACCP/ATS/SIS International Sepsis Definitions Conference. Crit Care Med. 2003;31:1250–1256.

21. Centers for Disease Control and Prevention. Adult tobacco use information: glossary, Last reviewed 2015. https://www.cdc.gov/nchs/nhis/tobacco/tobacco_glossary.htm. Accessed 14 June 2018.

22. Centers for Disease Control and Prevention. State Tobacco Activities Tracking and Evaluation (STATE) System: Massachusetts State Report, 2013. https://nccd.cdc.gov/STATESystem/rdPage.aspx?rdReport=OSH_STATE.Highlights&rdRequestForwarding=Form. Accessed 14 June 2018.

23. Torio CM, Moore BJ. National inpatient hospital costs: the most expensive conditions by payer, 2013. HCUP statistical brief no. 204. Rockville: Agency for Healthcare Research and Quality; 2016. https://www.hcup-us.ahrq.gov/reports/statbriefs/sb204-Most-Expensive-Hospital-Conditions.pdf. Accessed 14 June 2018

24. Pirie K, Peto R, Reeves GK, et al. The 21st century hazards of smoking and benefits of stopping: a prospective study of one million women in the UK. Lancet. 2013;381:133–41.

25. Sitas F, Urban M, Bradshaw D, et al. Tobacco attributable deaths in South Africa. Tob Control. 2004;13:396–9.

26. Kalin M, Ortqvist A, Almela M, et al. Prospective study of prognostic factors in community-acquired bacteremic pneumococcal disease in 5 countries. J Infect Dis. 2000;182(3):840–7.

27. Liu SF, Malik AB. NF-kappa B activation as a pathological mechanism of septic shock and inflammation. Am J Physiol Lung Cell Mol Physiol. 2006; 290(4):622–45.

28. Zappacosta B, Persichilli S, Minucci A, et al. Effects of aqueous cigarette smoke extract on the chemiluminescence kinetics of polymorphonuclear leukocytes and on their glycolytic and phagocytic activity. Luminescence. 2001;16:315–9.

29. Goncalves RB, Coletta RD, Silvério KG, et al. Impact of smoking on inflammation: overview of molecular mechanisms. Inflamm Res. 2011;60(5):409–24.

30. Rom O, Avezov K, Aizenbud D, et al. Cigarette smoking and inflammation revisited. Respir Physiol Neurobiol. 2013;187(1):5–10.

31. Bobo JK, Husten C. Sociocultural influences on smoking and drinking. Alcohol Res Health. 2000;24(4):225–32.

32. Pearson WS, Dube SR, Ford ES, Mokdad AH. Influenza and pneumococcal vaccination rates among smokers: data from the 2006 Behavioral Risk Factor Surveillance System. Prev Med. 2009;48(2):180–3.

33. Friedemann Smith C, Whitaker KL, Winstanley K, Wardle J. Smokers are less likely than non-smokers to seek help for a lung cancer 'alarm' symptom. Thorax. 2016;71(7):659–61.

22

Management of patients with high-risk pulmonary embolism

Takeshi Yamamoto (iD)

Abstract

High-risk pulmonary embolism (PE) is a life-threatening disorder associated with high mortality and morbidity. Most deaths in patients with shock occur within the first few hours after presentation, and rapid diagnosis and treatment is therefore essential to save patients' lives. The main manifestations of major PE are acute right ventricular (RV) failure and hypoxia. RV pressure overload is predominantly related to the interaction between the mechanical pulmonary vascular obstruction and the underlying cardiopulmonary status. Computed tomography angiography allows not only adequate visualization of the pulmonary thromboemboli down to at least the segmental level but also RV enlargement as an indicator of RV dysfunction. Bedside echocardiography is an acceptable alternative under such circumstances. Although it does not usually provide a definitive diagnosis or exclude pulmonary embolism, echocardiography can confirm or exclude severe RV pressure overload and dysfunction. Extracorporeal membrane oxygenation support can be an effective procedure in patients with PE-induced circulatory collapse. Thrombolysis is generally accepted in unstable patients with high-risk PE; however, thrombolytic agents cannot be fully administered to patients with a high risk of bleeding. Conversely, catheter-directed treatment is an optimal treatment strategy for patients with high-risk PE who have contraindications for thrombolysis and is a minimally invasive alternative to surgical embolectomy. It can be performed with a minimum dose of thrombolytic agents or without, and it can be combined with various procedures including catheter fragmentation or embolectomy in accordance with the extent of the thrombus on a pulmonary angiogram. Hybrid catheter-directed treatment can reduce a rapid heart rate and high pulmonary artery pressure and can improve the gas exchange indices and outcomes. Surgical embolectomy is also performed in patients with contraindications for or an inadequate response to thrombolysis. Large hospitals having an intensive care unit should preemptively establish diagnostic and therapeutic protocols and rehearse multidisciplinary management for patients with high-risk PE. Coordination with a skilled team comprising intensivists, cardiologists, cardiac surgeons, radiologists, and other specialists is crucial to maximize success.

Keywords: Pulmonary embolism, Multidisciplinary management, Thrombolytic therapy, Catheter-directed treatment, Surgical embolectomy

Background

High-risk pulmonary embolism (PE), which presents as shock or persistent hypotension, is a life-threatening disorder associated with high mortality and morbidity [1–3]. The 30-day mortality rate of patients with PE who develop shock ranges from 16 to 25% and that of patients with cardiac arrest ranges from 52 to 65% [4, 5]. Most deaths in patients presenting with shock occur within the first hour after presentation [6]; therefore, rapid therapeutic action is essential to save patients' lives. PE is caused by abrupt obstruction of pulmonary arteries by thrombi that have mostly formed in the deep veins of the lower limbs or pelvis in more than 90% of affected patients. It is estimated that nearly half of PEs occur in a hospital or health care-related institution [4, 7, 8]. Hospitalized critically ill patients are at high risk for PE [9, 10]. The management of PE in a critically ill patient admitted to the intensive care unit can be exceedingly complex [11]. Intensivists should know how to appropriately care for patients with high-risk PE of both in-hospital onset and out-of-hospital onset [12, 13]. The present review critically assesses data that have contributed to substantial improvement in the management strategies for high-risk PE in recent years.

Correspondence: yamamoto56@nms.ac.jp
Division of Cardiovascular Intensive Care, Nippon Medical School Hospital, 1-1-5 Sendagi, Bunkyo-ku, Tokyo 113-8603, Japan

Pathophysiology

Circulatory failure

The main manifestations of major PE are acute right ventricular (RV) failure and hypoxia. RV pressure overload is predominantly related to the interaction between the mechanical pulmonary vascular obstruction and the underlying cardiopulmonary status. Additional factors of pulmonary vasoconstriction include neural reflexes, the release of humoral factors from platelets (i.e., serotonin and platelet-activating factor), plasma (i.e., thrombin and vasoactive peptides C3a, C5a), tissue (i.e., histamine), and systemic arterial hypoxia, all of which are associated with increased RV afterload [14]. Heart failure induced by major PE results from a combination of increased wall stress and cardiac ischemia, which compromise RV function and impair left ventricular (LV) output in multiple interactions (Fig. 1) [2]. With increasing RV load and wall stress, RV systolic function becomes depressed and cardiac output begins to decrease. The LV preload consequently decreases because the ventricles are aligned in series. LV preload is additionally impaired by decreased LV distensibility as a consequence of a leftward shift of the interventricular septum and of pericardial restraint, both of which are related to the degree of RV dilatation [15, 16]. A further decrease in LV flow results in systemic hypotension. Decreases in the mean arterial pressure associated with increases in the RV end-diastolic pressure impair the subendocardial perfusion and oxygen supply [17]. Increased oxygen demands associated with elevated wall stress coupled with the decreased oxygen supply have been shown to precipitate RV ischemia, which is thought to be the cause of RV failure. Clinical evidence of RV infarction as a consequence of the preceding condition has been demonstrated in patients with and without obstructive coronary disease.

The mean pulmonary arterial pressure that can be generated by the right ventricle is 40 mmHg in individuals without cardiopulmonary disease [18]. Therefore, when the pulmonary arterial pressure exceeds 40 mmHg

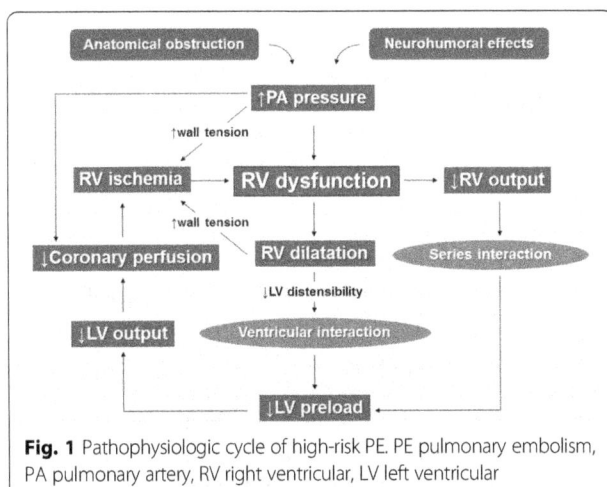

Fig. 1 Pathophysiologic cycle of high-risk PE. PE pulmonary embolism, PA pulmonary artery, RV right ventricular, LV left ventricular

during the acute phase of PE, physicians should suspect recurrent PE or chronic thromboembolic pulmonary hypertension.

Respiratory failure

Gas exchange abnormalities in patients with PE are complex and related to the size and characteristics of the embolic material, the extent of the occlusion, the underlying cardiopulmonary status, and the length of time since embolization [2]. Hypoxia has been attributed to an increase in alveolar dead space, right-to-left shunting, ventilation–perfusion mismatch, and a low mixed venous oxygen level [2, 19, 20]. The two latter mechanisms are proposed to account for most cases of observed hypoxia and hypocapnia before and after treatment. Zones of reduced flow in obstructed vessels combined with zones of overflow in the capillary bed served by unobstructed vessels result in ventilation–perfusion mismatch, which contributes to hypoxia. In addition, low cardiac output results in a low mixed venous oxygen level [20].

Diagnosis

The diagnostic strategy [12, 13, 19, 21, 22] for patients with suspected high-risk PE is shown in Fig. 2. Computed tomography (CT) angiography allows not only adequate visualization of the pulmonary thromboemboli down to at least the segmental level but also RV enlargement as an indicator of RV dysfunction. CT venography has been advocated as a simple way to diagnose deep vein thrombosis (DVT) in stable patients with suspected PE because it can be combined with chest CT angiography as a single procedure using only one intravenous injection of contrast dye [23]. If CT angiography is not immediately available or cannot be performed because of hemodynamic instability, bedside transthoracic echocardiography, which will yield evidence of acute pulmonary hypertension and RV dysfunction, is the most useful initial test. In highly unstable patients, the presence of echocardiographic RV dysfunction is sufficient to prompt immediate definitive treatment without further testing. Ancillary bedside imaging tests include transesophageal echocardiography, which may allow direct visualization of thrombi in the pulmonary artery and its main branches, and bilateral compression venous ultrasonography, which may confirm proximal DVT; these techniques may be helpful in emergency management decisions [19].

Treatment

Hemodynamic and respiratory support

Acute RV failure with resulting low systemic output is the leading cause of death in patients with high-risk PE.

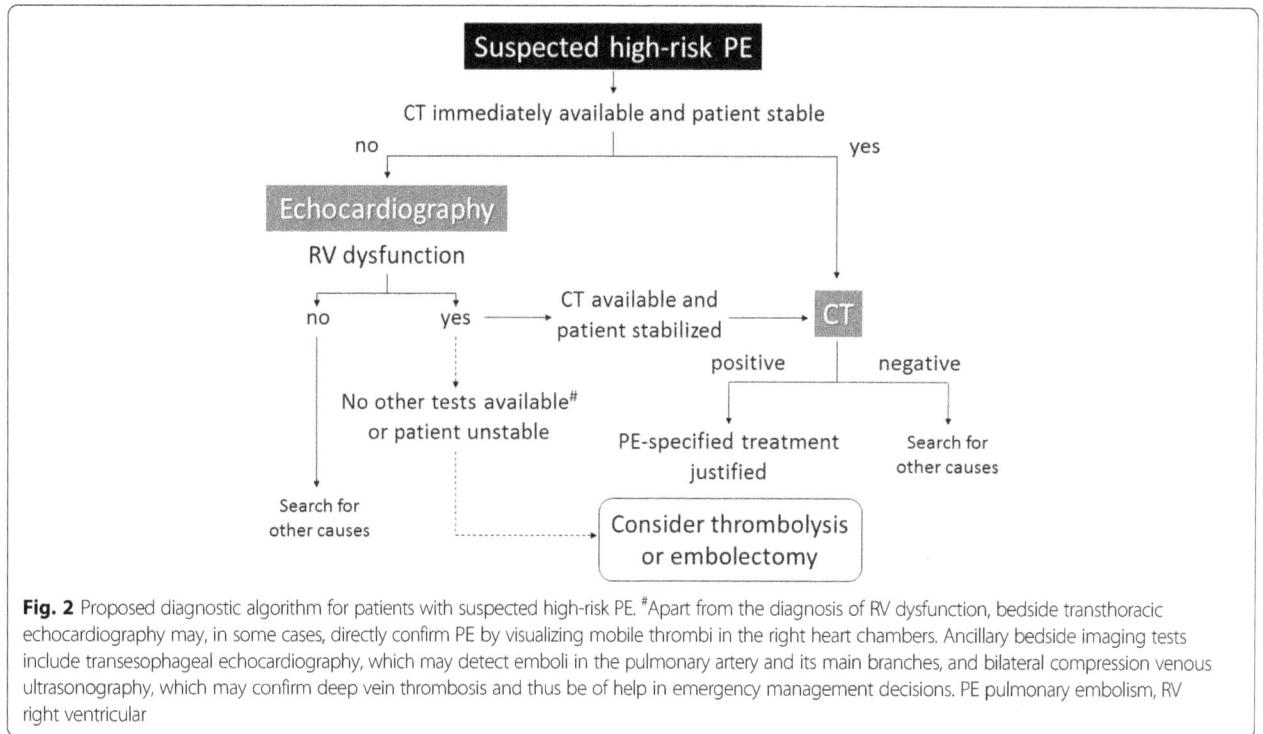

Fig. 2 Proposed diagnostic algorithm for patients with suspected high-risk PE. #Apart from the diagnosis of RV dysfunction, bedside transthoracic echocardiography may, in some cases, directly confirm PE by visualizing mobile thrombi in the right heart chambers. Ancillary bedside imaging tests include transesophageal echocardiography, which may detect emboli in the pulmonary artery and its main branches, and bilateral compression venous ultrasonography, which may confirm deep vein thrombosis and thus be of help in emergency management decisions. PE pulmonary embolism, RV right ventricular

Therefore, supportive treatment is of vital importance in patients with PE who develop shock.

Administration of oxygen

Hypoxia is usually reversed with administration of oxygen. When mechanical ventilation is required, care should be taken to limit its adverse hemodynamic effects. In particular, the positive intrathoracic pressure induced by mechanical ventilation may reduce venous return and worsen RV failure in patients with shock; therefore, positive end-expiratory pressure should be applied with caution. Low tidal volumes (approximately 6 ml/kg lean body weight) should be used in an attempt to keep the end-expiratory plateau pressure at < 30 cmH$_2$O [19].

Modest fluid loading

Experimental studies have shown that aggressive volume loading may worsen RV function by causing mechanical overstretch and/or inducing reflex mechanisms that depress contractility. However, a small clinical study revealed an increase in the cardiac index from 1.7 to 2.1 l/min/m^2 after infusion of 500 ml of dextran during a 15-min period in normotensive patients with acute PE and a low cardiac index [24]. This finding suggests that a modest fluid challenge may help to increase the cardiac index in patients with PE, a low cardiac index, and normal blood pressure. However, excessive volume loading is not recommended because of the possibility of an increased leftward shift of the interventricular septum

[1, 19]. Therefore, the permitted fluid loading volume ranges from 500 to 1000 ml[1].

Vasopressors

Use of vasopressors is often necessary in parallel with (or while waiting for) definitive treatment. Norepinephrine appears to improve RV function via a direct positive inotropic effect while also improving RV coronary perfusion by peripheral vascular alpha receptor stimulation and an increase in systemic blood pressure. No clinical data are available on the effects of norepinephrine in patients with PE, and its use should probably be limited to patients with hypotension [19].

In a small series of patients requiring admission to an intensive care unit for PE, dobutamine increased cardiac output and improved oxygen transport and tissue oxygenation at a constant arterial partial pressure of oxygen. In another study [25] of 10 patients with PE, a low cardiac index, and normal blood pressure, a 35% increase in the cardiac index was observed under intravenous dobutamine infusion at a moderate dosage without significant changes in the heart rate, systemic arterial pressure, or mean pulmonary arterial pressure. Accordingly, the use of dobutamine can be considered for patients with PE, a low cardiac index, and normal blood pressure [19, 21]. However, an increased cardiac index above physiological values may aggravate ventilation–perfusion mismatch by further redistributing flow from partly obstructed to unobstructed vessels. Epinephrine combines the beneficial properties of norepinephrine and dobutamine without the systemic vasodilatory effects of the latter drug. Epinephrine may exert beneficial effects in patients with PE and shock.

Inhalation of nitric oxide
Inhalation of nitric oxide improves ventilation–perfusion mismatch in association with selective dilation of the pulmonary artery without systemic vasodilation. It is considered one therapeutic option in patients whose condition is unresponsive to standard treatment [26].

Extracorporeal membrane oxygenation
Experimental evidence suggests that extracorporeal membrane oxygenation (ECMO) support can be an effective procedure in patients with PE-induced circulatory collapse. This notion is supported by the results of a series of 10 patients with massive PE requiring ECMO with catheter-based treatment [27]. The mean duration of ECMO was 48 ± 44 h, and the 30-day mortality rate was 30% [27].

Pharmacological treatment
Anticoagulation
Anticoagulant treatment plays a pivotal role in the management of patients with PE. The need for immediate anticoagulation in patients with PE is based on a landmark study [28] that was performed in the 1960s and demonstrated the benefits of unfractionated heparin (UFH) in comparison with no treatment. The efficacy of UFH is attributed to impairment of clot propagation and prevention of recurrent PE. The risk of recurrent PE is highest in the early stages, during which time it is crucial to rapidly achieve a therapeutic level of anticoagulation. An inability to establish a therapeutic activated partial thromboplastin time (aPTT) early in the disease course is associated with a higher rate of recurrence [29].

Because of the high mortality rate in untreated patients, anticoagulant treatment should be considered in patients with suspected PE while awaiting definitive diagnostic confirmation. When high- or intermediate-risk PE is first suspected, patients should receive a bolus of UFH provided that no contraindications to anticoagulation are present.

If intravenous UFH is given, a weight-adjusted regimen of 80 U/kg as a bolus injection followed by infusion at the rate of 18 U/kg/h is preferred to fixed doses of UFH [19, 21, 22]. Subsequent doses of UFH should be adjusted using an aPTT-based nomogram to rapidly reach and maintain aPTT prolongation (1.5–2.5 times control) corresponding to therapeutic heparin levels [19, 21, 22]. The aPTT should be measured 4 to 6 h after the bolus injection and then 3 h after each dose adjustment or once daily when the target therapeutic dose has been reached. Oral anticoagulants can be initiated after hemodynamic stabilization has been achieved. When

using warfarin, UFH infusion should be continued until the international normalized ratio has been maintained at therapeutic levels for 2 consecutive days. The UFH infusion can be switched to direct oral anticoagulants; however, direct oral anticoagulants have not been assessed in patients with high-risk PE who have been initially treated with thrombotic therapy. According to an expert comment [30], the introduction of any anticoagulant should be postponed until after the patient has been stabilized with hemodynamic support and after the period of increased bleeding risk related to thrombolytic therapy has passed, which usually lasts 48 to 72 h.

Thrombolytic treatment
Thrombolytic treatment of acute PE restores pulmonary perfusion more rapidly than anticoagulation with UFH alone [31, 32]. The early resolution of pulmonary obstruction leads to a prompt reduction in pulmonary artery pressure and resistance, with a concomitant improvement in RV function [32]. In one study, the pulmonary diffusing capacity after 1 year was higher in patients treated with thrombolytic treatment than in those treated with only anticoagulation [33].

The hemodynamic benefits of thrombolysis are confined to the first few days; in survivors, differences are no longer apparent at 1 week after treatment [31]. Accelerated regimens involving administration of tissue plasminogen activator (t-PA) during a 2-h period are preferable to prolonged infusions of first-generation thrombolytic agents during a 12- to 24-h period [34]. Compared with the properties of native t-PA, third-generation bioengineered thrombolytic agents (tenecteplase and monteplase) have a longer half-life, greater clot sensitivity, and more rapid lytic capacity [19, 35, 36]. Monteplase has been approved for acute PE with hemodynamic instability in Japan [35, 36]. Overall, more than 90% of patients appear to respond favorably to thrombolysis as judged by clinical and echocardiographic improvement within 36 h [37]. The greatest benefit is observed when treatment is initiated within 48 h of symptom onset, but thrombolysis can still be useful in patients who have had symptoms for 6 to 14 days [38].

However appealing the rapid resolution of embolic obstruction may be, only one trial has demonstrated a benefit in terms of mortality [39]. However, the results of this small trial of only eight patients should be viewed with caution. All four patients randomized to thrombolytic therapy were treated within 4 h of presentation, whereas those patients randomized to heparin therapy had previously failed to respond to it and developed recurrent PE with severe respiratory failure. A review of randomized trials performed before 2004 indicated that thrombolysis was associated with a significant reduction in mortality or recurrent PE in high-risk patients presenting with hemodynamic instability as compared with anticoagulation (9.4 vs. 19.0%, respectively; odds ratio, 0.45; number needed to treat = 10) [40].

Thrombolytic treatment carries a risk of major bleeding, including intracranial hemorrhage. A meta-analysis of pooled data from trials using various thrombolytic agents and regimens showed an intracranial bleeding rate of 1.46% [41]. In a meta-analysis comparing thrombolysis vs. anticoagulation with UFH alone [42], major bleeding including intracranial or retroperitoneal bleeding, bleeding requiring blood transfusion, or bleeding requiring surgical hemostasis was observed significantly more often in patients undergoing thrombolysis than anticoagulation (13.7 vs. 7.7%, respectively). In the subgroup analysis of that study [42], major bleeding was not significantly increased in patients aged ≤ 65 years (odds ratio, 1.25; 95% confidence interval, 0.50–3.14). However, there was an association with a greater risk of major bleeding in those aged > 65 years (odds ratio, 3.10; 95% confidence interval, 2.10–4.56). Increasing age and the presence of comorbidities including cancer, diabetes, a high prothrombin time–international normalized ratio, or concomitant use of catecholamines have been associated with a higher risk of bleeding complications [43]. In a recent study, a strategy using reduced-dose recombinant t-PA appeared to be safe in patients with hemodynamic instability or massive pulmonary obstruction [44]. In patients with mobile right heart thrombi, the therapeutic benefits of thrombolysis remain controversial [45–47].

Some researchers have proposed that anticoagulation therapy with heparin will prevent the accretion of new fibrin on the thrombus, thereby facilitating lysis by thrombolytic agents and reducing the risk of re-extension after thrombolysis [48]. Unfractionated heparin infusion can be continued during recombinant t-PA infusion.

Absolute contraindications for thrombolysis are active bleeding, ischemic stroke within 2 months, and a history of hemorrhagic stroke. Relative contraindications include a major operation within 10 days, multiple trauma within 2 weeks, neurosurgery or ophthalmologic operations within 1 month, and similar conditions [12]. However, these relative contraindications are also associated with inducible risks for PE. Therefore, thrombolytic therapy may still be appropriate for patients with severe PE complicated by relative contraindications. In patients with confirmed PE as the precipitant of cardiac arrest, thrombolysis is a reasonable emergency treatment option. Thrombolysis may be considered when cardiac arrest is suspected to be caused by PE [49].

Catheter-directed treatment
Catheter-directed treatment (CDT) can be performed as an alternative to thrombolysis when a patient has

absolute contraindications to thrombolysis, as adjunctive therapy when thrombolysis has failed to improve hemodynamics, or as an alternative to surgery if immediate access to cardiopulmonary bypass is unavailable [19]. The objective of CDT is the removal of obstructing thrombi from the main pulmonary arteries to facilitate RV recovery and improve symptoms and survival [50]. For patients with absolute contraindications to thrombolysis, interventional options include thrombus fragmentation with a pigtail or balloon catheter, rheolytic thrombectomy with hydrodynamic catheter devices, and suction thrombectomy with aspiration catheters. Conversely, for patients without absolute contraindications to thrombolysis, catheter-directed thrombolysis or pharmacomechanical thrombolysis are preferred approaches. With respect to thrombus fragmentation, the fact that the cross-sectional area of the distal arterioles is more than four times that of the central circulation and that the volume of the peripheral circulatory bed is about twice that of the pulmonary arteries suggests that the redistribution of large central clots into smaller clots in the peripheral pulmonary arteries may acutely improve cardiopulmonary hemodynamics, with significant increases in the total pulmonary blood flow and RV function [51]. The action of these thrombectomy devices can sometimes be facilitated by softening the thrombotic mass using thrombolytic therapy, which helps to speed up the debulking and fragmentation of the occlusive clots. Fragmentation can also be used as a complement to thrombolytic therapy because fragmentation of a large clot exposes fresh surfaces on which endogenous urokinase and infused thrombolytic drugs can work to further break down the resulting emboli [51]. One review on CDT included 35 nonrandomized studies involving 594 patients [52]. The rate of clinical success, defined as stabilization of hemodynamic parameters, resolution of hypoxia, and survival to discharge, was 87%. The contribution of the mechanical catheter intervention per se to clinical success is unclear because 67% of patients also received adjunctive local thrombolysis. Publication bias probably resulted in underreporting of major complications (reportedly affecting 2% of interventions), which may include death from worsening RV failure, distal embolization, pulmonary artery perforation with lung hemorrhage, systemic bleeding complications, pericardial tamponade, heart block or bradycardia, hemolysis, contrast-induced nephropathy, and puncture-related complications [50]. While anticoagulation with heparin alone has little effect on improvement of RV size and performance within the first 24 to 48 h, the extent of early RV recovery after low-dose catheter-directed thrombolysis appears comparable with that after standard-dose systemic thrombolysis. In a randomized controlled clinical trial of 59 patients with intermediate-risk PE, when compared with treatment by heparin alone, catheter-directed ultrasound-accelerated thrombolysis (administration of 10 mg t-PA per treated lung over 15 h) significantly reduced the subannular RV/LV dimension ratio between baseline and the 24-h follow-up without an increase in bleeding complications [53].

According to a recent guideline [19], CDT should be considered as an alternative to surgical pulmonary embolectomy for patients in whom full-dose systemic thrombolysis is contraindicated or has failed.

Surgical embolectomy

Traditionally, surgical embolectomy has been reserved for patients with PE who may need cardiopulmonary resuscitation. It is also performed in patients with contraindications or inadequate responses to thrombolysis and in those with patent foramen ovale and intracardiac thrombi [19]. Pulmonary embolectomy is technically a relatively simple operation. ECMO can be helpful in critical situations, ensuring circulation and oxygenation until a definitive diagnosis is obtained [54]. After rapid transfer to the operating room and induction of anesthesia and median sternotomy, normothermic cardiopulmonary bypass should be instituted. Aortic cross-clamping and cardioplegic cardiac arrest should be avoided [55]. With bilateral pulmonary artery incisions, clots can be removed from both pulmonary arteries down to the segmental level under direct vision. Prolonged periods of postoperative cardiopulmonary bypass and weaning may be necessary for recovery of RV function. With a rapid multidisciplinary approach and individualized indications for embolectomy before hemodynamic collapse, perioperative mortality rates of ≤ 6% have been reported [55, 56]. Preoperative thrombolysis increases the risk of bleeding, but it is not an absolute contraindication to surgical embolectomy [57]. The long-term postoperative survival rate, World Health Organization functional class, and quality of life were favorable in published series [54, 58]. Patients presenting with an episode of acute PE superimposed on a history of chronic dyspnea and pulmonary hypertension are likely to develop chronic thromboembolic pulmonary hypertension. These patients should be transferred to an expert center for pulmonary endarterectomy.

Inferior vena cava filters

In general, inferior vena cava (IVC) filters are indicated in patients with acute PE who have absolute contraindications to anticoagulant drugs and in patients with objectively confirmed recurrent PE despite adequate anticoagulation treatment. Observational studies have suggested that insertion of a venous filter might reduce PE-related mortality rates in the acute phase [59, 60], this benefit possibly coming at the cost of an increased risk of recurrence of venous thromboembolism (VTE) [60]. Although complications associated with permanent

IVC filters are common, they are rarely fatal [61]. Overall, early complications, which include insertion-site thrombosis, occur in approximately 10% of patients. Late complications are more frequent and include recurrent DVT in approximately 20% of patients and post-thrombotic syndrome in up to 40% of patients. Occlusion of the IVC affects approximately 22% of patients at 5 years and 33% at 9 years, regardless of the use and duration of anticoagulation [62]. Impermanent IVC filters are classified as temporary or retrievable devices. Temporary filters must be removed within a few days, while retrievable filters can be left in place for longer periods. Impermanent filters should be removed as soon as it is safe to use anticoagulants. The Prévention du Risque d'Embolie Pulmonaire par Interruption Cave II trial enrolled patients with acute symptomatic PE with concomitant DVT and at least one independent risk factor for fatal PE (age of > 75 years, RV dysfunction and/or elevated troponin and/or hypotension, bilateral DVT and/or iliocaval DVT, active cancer, or chronic cardiac or respiratory failure) [63]. The primary end point was fatal and nonfatal PE recurrence at 3 months. The investigators found no significant reduction in the primary end point for patients who received an IVC filter (relative risk with filter, 2.00; 95% confidence interval, 0.51–7.89) [63].

Although some observational data suggest that IVC filter placement in addition to anticoagulation might improve survival in patients with unstable PE or after thrombolytic therapy, controlled data do not support its routine use in patients at high risk of death unless there is a contraindication to anticoagulant therapy [60]. There are no data to support the routine use of venous filters in patients with high-risk PE.

Treatment algorithm for high-risk PE

An institutional protocol for high-risk PE should be adopted. Figure 3 shows a treatment algorithm for high-risk PE.

VTE prevention

VTE is a well-recognized life-threatening complication in patients admitted to the intensive care unit (ICU). Patients in the ICU often have multiple thrombotic and bleeding risk factors and should undergo prevention of VTE based on individual assessment of the level of risk. An institution-wide protocol for the prevention of VTE is recommended [64, 65]. The routine use of ultrasonographic screening for DVT is not recommended when thromboprophylactic measures are in place because the detection of asymptomatic DVT may prompt therapeutic anticoagulation that may increase the bleeding risk and has not been proven to reduce significant VTE events. Pharmacological prophylaxis for critically ill patients is effective and is advocated by recent guidelines. Mechanical devices such as intermittent pneumatic

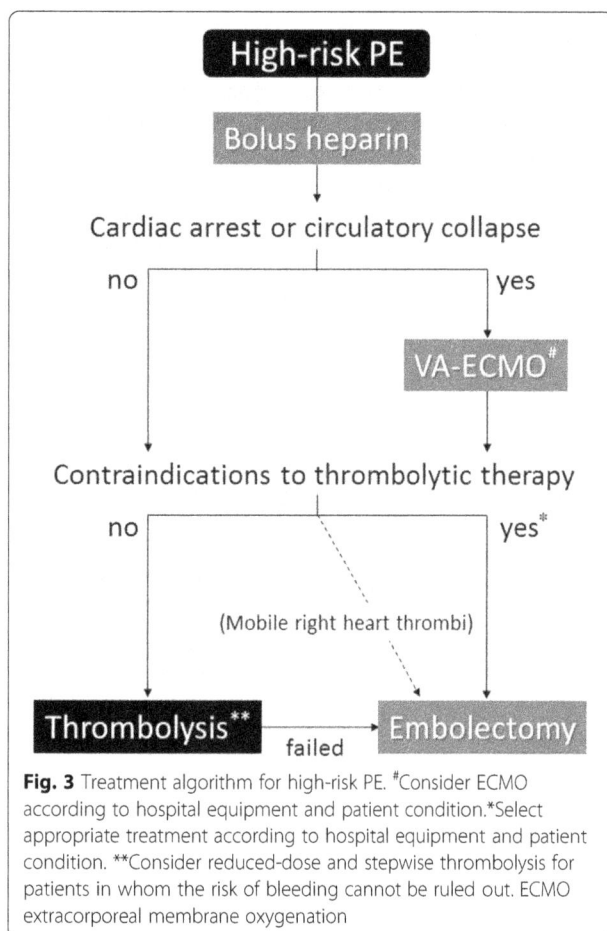

Fig. 3 Treatment algorithm for high-risk PE. #Consider ECMO according to hospital equipment and patient condition.*Select appropriate treatment according to hospital equipment and patient condition. **Consider reduced-dose and stepwise thrombolysis for patients in whom the risk of bleeding cannot be ruled out. ECMO extracorporeal membrane oxygenation

compression devices are recommended for patients with contraindications to pharmacological prophylaxis. Generally, pharmacological prophylaxis with low-molecular-weight heparin (LMWH) is recommended over low-dose UFH [64]. Prophylaxis using LMWH and indirect factor Xa inhibitors has stable effects without significant individual differences, and these drugs can be administered subcutaneously once or twice a day without close monitoring. The incidence of adverse drug reactions such as thrombocytopenia and osteopenia is low. In Japan, enoxaparin, a type of LMWH, and fondaparinux, an indirect factor Xa inhibitor, are officially indicated only for patients following orthopedic surgery of a lower limb or abdominal surgery associated with a high risk of development of VTE [21]. Therefore, ICU patients in Japan are prevented by adjusted-dose UFH, which is administered to maintain the aPTT at the upper limit of the normal range. For ICU patients with severe renal insufficiency, the use of low-dose UFH, dalteparin, or reduced-dose enoxaparin is recommended. No study has prospectively evaluated the efficacy and safety of DVT prophylaxis in ICU patients with severe liver dysfunction. Thus, the use of pharmacological prophylaxis in these patients should be carefully balanced against the

risk of bleeding. For ICU patients, the routine use of inferior vena cava filters is not recommended for the primary prevention of VTE [64]. When the diagnosis of heparin-induced thrombocytopenia is suspected or confirmed, all forms of heparin must be discontinued and immediate anticoagulation with non-heparin anticoagulants such as argatroban is recommended [64].

Future perspective
Patients with high-risk PE have a potential for circulatory collapse, and thrombolysis is therefore often contraindicated. Physicians should rapidly and properly evaluate patients with PE, formulate a treatment plan, and mobilize the necessary resources to provide the highest level of care. Some centers have recently introduced a formalized system involving a multidisciplinary pulmonary embolism response team to streamline the care of these patients [1, 66]. The team comprises specialists in cardiology, emergency medicine, radiology, cardiovascular surgery, and critical care with an interest in PE. However, how widespread these models have become and whether a multidisciplinary approach to patients with life-threatening PE will be accompanied by improvements in clinical outcomes remain unclear.

Conclusions
High-risk PE is a life-threatening disorder associated with high mortality and morbidity. Most deaths in patients with shock occur within the first few hours after presentation, and rapid diagnosis and treatment is therefore essential to save patients' lives. High-risk PE is an indication for thrombolytic therapy but has the potential for circulatory collapse and is therefore often a contraindication to thrombolysis. Large hospitals having an intensive care unit should preemptively establish diagnostic and therapeutic protocols and rehearse multidisciplinary management for patients with high-risk PE.

Abbreviations
aPTT: Activated partial thromboplastin time; CDT: Catheter-directed treatment; CT: Computed tomography; DVT: Deep vein thrombosis; ECMO: Extracorporeal membrane oxygenation; ICU: Intensive care unit; IVC: Inferior vena cava; LMWH: Low-molecular-weight heparin; LV: Left ventricular; PE: Pulmonary embolism; RV: Right ventricular; t-PA: Tissue plasminogen activator; UFH: Unfractionated heparin; VTE: Venous thromboembolism

Acknowledgements
The author thanks Angela Morben, DVM, ELS, from Edanz Group (http://www.edanzediting.co.jp) for editing a draft of this manuscript.

Funding
None.

Authors' contributions
TY searched literatures, drafted the manuscript, and approved the final manuscript.

Competing interests
The author declares that he has no competing interests.

References

1. Goldhaber SZ. Pulmonary embolism. In: Mann D, Zipes D, Libby P, Bonow R, editors. Braunwald's heart disease: a textbook of cardiovascular medicine. tenth ed. Philadelphia: Saunders; 2015. p. 1664–81.
2. Wood KE. Major pulmonary embolism: review of a pathophysiologic approach to the golden hour of hemodynamically significant pulmonary embolism. Chest. 2002;121:877–905.
3. Kucher N, Rossi E, De Rosa M, Goldhaber SZ. Massive pulmonary embolism. Circulation. 2006;113:577–82.
4. Sakuma M, Nakamura M, Nakanishi N, Miyahara Y, Tanabe N, Yamada N, Kuriyama T, Kunieda T, Sugimoto T, Nakano T, Shirato K. Inferior vena cava filter is a new additional therapeutic option to reduce mortality from acute pulmonary embolism. Circ J. 2004;68:816–21.
5. Kasper W, Konstantinides S, Geibel A, Olschewski M, Heinrich F, Grosser KD, Rauber K, Iversen S, Redecker M, Kienast J. Management strategies and determinants of outcome in acute major pulmonary embolism: results of a multicenter registry. J Am Coll Cardiol. 1997;30:1165–71.
6. Stein PD, Henry JW. Prevalence of acute pulmonary embolism among patients in a general hospital and at autopsy. Chest. 1995;108:978–81.
7. Yamamoto T, Sato N, Tajima H, Takagi H, Morita N, Akutsu K, Fujita N, Yasutake M, Tanaka K, Takano T. Differences in the clinical course of acute massive and submassive pulmonary embolism. Circ J. 2004;68:988–92.
8. Nakamura M, Miyata T, Ozeki Y, Takayama M, Komori K, Yamada N, Origasa H, Satokawa H, Maeda H, Tanabe N, Unno N, Shibuya T, Tanemoto K, Kondo K, Kojima T. Current venous thromboembolism management and outcomes in Japan. Circ J. 2014;78:708–17.
9. Geerts WH, Bergqvist D, Pineo GF, Heit JA, Samama CM, Lassen MR, Colwell CW. Prevention of venous thromboembolism: American College of Chest Physicians Evidence-Based Clinical Practice Guidelines (8th edition). Chest. 2008;133(Suppl):381–453.
10. Cook D, Crowther M, Meade M, Rabbat C, Griffith L, Schiff D, Geerts W, Guyatt G. Deep venous thrombosis in medical-surgical critically ill patients: prevalence, incidence, and risk factors. Crit Care Med. 2005;33:1565–71.
11. Pastores SM. Management of venous thromboembolism in the intensive care unit. J Crit Care. 2009;24:185–91.
12. Meyer G. Massive acute pulmonary embolism. In: Jeremias A, Brown D, editors. Cardiac intensive care. Philadelphia: Saunders; 2010. p. 398–404.
13. Torbicki A, Kurzyna M, Konstantinides S. Pulmonary embolism. In: Tubaro M, Vranckx P, Price S, Vrints C, editors. The ESC textbook of acute and intensive cardiac care, 2nd edition. Oxford: Oxford University Press; 2015. p. 634–44.
14. Stratmann G, Gregory GA. Neurogenic and humoral vasoconstriction in acute pulmonary thromboembolism. Anesth Analg. 2003;97:341–54.
15. Jardin F, Dubourg O, Gueret P, Delorme G, Bourdarias JP. Quantitative two-dimensional echocardiography in massive pulmonary embolism: emphasis on ventricular interdependence and leftward septal displacement. J Am Coll Cardiol. 1987;10:1201–6.
16. Belenkie I, Dani R, Smith ER, Tyberg JV. Ventricular interaction during experimental acute pulmonary embolism. Circulation. 1988;78:761–8.
17. Vlahakes GJ, Turley K, Hoffman JI. The pathophysiology of failure in acute right ventricular hypertension: hemodynamic and biochemical correlations. Circulation. 1981;63:87–95.
18. Sharma GV, McIntyre KM, Sharma S, Sasahara AA. Clinical and hemodynamic correlates in pulmonary embolism. Clin Chest Med. 1984;5:421–37.
19. Konstantinides SV, Torbicki A, Agnelli G, Danchin N, Fitzmaurice D, Galiè N, Gibbs JS, Huisman MV, Humbert M, Kucher N, Lang I, Lankeit M, Lekakis J, Maack C, Mayer E, Meneveau N, Perrier A, Pruszczyk P, Rasmussen LH, Schindler TH, Svitil P, Vonk Noordegraaf A, Zamorano JL, Zompatori M, Task Force for the Diagnosis and Management of Acute Pulmonary Embolism of the European Society of Cardiology (ESC). 2014 ESC guidelines on the diagnosis and management of acute pulmonary embolism. Eur Heart J. 2014;35:3033–69.
20. Burrowes KS, Clark AR, Tawhai MH. Blood flow redistribution and ventilation-perfusion mismatch during embolic pulmonary arterial occlusion. Pulm Circ. 2011;1:365–76.
21. Guidelines for the Diagnosis. Treatment and prevention of pulmonary thromboembolism and deep vein thrombosis (JCS 2009). Circ J. 2011;75: 1258–81.
22. Jaff MR, McMurtry MS, Archer SL, Cushman M, Goldenberg N, Goldhaber SZ, Jenkins JS, Kline JA, Michaels AD, Thistlethwaite P, Vedantham S, White RJ, Zierler BK. Management of massive and submassive pulmonary embolism, iliofemoral deep vein thrombosis, and chronic thromboembolic pulmonary hypertension: a scientific statement from the American Heart Association. Circulation. 2011;123:1788–830.
23. Taffoni MJ, Ravenel JG, Ackerman SJ. Prospective comparison of indirect CT venography versus venous sonography in ICU patients. AJR Am J Roentgenol. 2005;185:457–62.
24. Mercat A, Diehl JL, Meyer G, Teboul JL, Sors H. Hemodynamic effects of fluid loading in acute massive pulmonary embolism. Crit Care Med. 1999; 27:540–4.
25. Jardin F, Genevray B, Brun-Ney D, Margairaz A. Dobutamine: a hemodynamic evaluation in pulmonary embolism shock. Crit Care Med. 1985;13:1009–12.
26. Szold O, Khoury W, Biderman P, Klausner JM, Halpern P, Weinbroum AA. Inhaled nitric oxide improves pulmonary functions following massive pulmonary embolism: a report of four patients and review of the literature. Lung. 2006;184:1–5.
27. Munakata R, Yamamoto T, Hosokawa Y, Tokita Y, Akutsu K, Sato N, Murata S, Tajima H, Mizuno K, Tanaka K. Massive pulmonary embolism requiring extracorporeal life support treated with catheter-based interventions. Int Heart J. 2012;53:370–4.
28. Barritt DW, Jordan SC. Anticoagulant drugs in the treatment of pulmonary embolism. A controlled trial. Lancet. 1960;1:1309–12.
29. Hull RD, Raskob GE, Brant RF, Pineo GF, Valentine KA. Relation between the time to achieve the lower limit of the APTT therapeutic range and recurrent venous thromboembolism during heparin treatment for deep vein thrombosis. Arch Intern Med. 1997;157:2562–8.
30. Meyer G, Vieillard-Baron A, Planquette B. Recent advances in the management of pulmonary embolism: focus on the critically ill patients. Ann Intensive Care. 2016;6:19.
31. Dalla-Volta S, Palla A, Santolicandro A, Giuntini C, Pengo V, Visioli O, Zonzin P, Zanuttini D, Barbaresi F, Agnelli G, et al. PAIMS 2: alteplase combined with heparin versus heparin in the treatment of acute pulmonary embolism. Plasminogen activator Italian multicenter study 2. J Am Coll Cardiol. 1992; 20:520–6.
32. Goldhaber SZ, Haire WD, Feldstein ML, Miller M, Toltzis R, Smith JL, Taveira da Silva AM, Come PC, Lee RT, Parker JA, et al. Alteplase versus heparin in acute pulmonary embolism: randomised trial assessing right-ventricular function and pulmonary perfusion. Lancet. 1993;341:507–11.
33. Sharma GV, Burleson VA, Sasahara AA. Effect of thrombolytic therapy on pulmonary-capillary blood volume in patients with pulmonary embolism. N Engl J Med. 1980;303:842–5.
34. Meneveau N, Schiele F, Vuillemenot A, Valette B, Grollier G, Bernard Y, Bassand JP. Streptokinase vs alteplase in massive pulmonary embolism. A randomized trial assessing right heart haemodynamics and pulmonary vascular obstruction. Eur Heart J. 1997;18:1141–8.
35. Niwa A, Nakamura M, Harada N, Musha T. Observational investigation of thrombolysis with the tissue-type plasminogen activator monteplase for acute pulmonary embolism in Japan. Circ J. 2012;76:2471–80.
36. Yamamoto T, Murai K, Tokita Y, Kato K, Iwasaki YK, Sato N, Tajima H, Mizuno K, Tanaka K. Thrombolysis with a novel modified tissue-type plasminogen activator, monteplase, combined with catheter-based treatment for major pulmonary embolism. Circ J. 2009;73:106–10.

37. Meneveau N, Séronde MF, Blonde MC, Legalery P, Didier-Petit K, Briand F, Caulfield F, Schiele F, Bernard Y, Bassand JP. Management of unsuccessful thrombolysis in acute massive pulmonary embolism. Chest. 2006;129:1043–50.

38. Daniels LB, Parker JA, Patel SR, Grodstein F, Goldhaber SZ. Relation of duration of symptoms with response to thrombolytic therapy in pulmonary embolism. Am J Cardiol. 1997;80:184–8.

39. Jerjes-Sanchez C, Ramirez-Rivera A, de Lourdes GM, Arriaga-Nava R, Valencia S, Rosado-Buzzo A, Pierzo JA, Rosas E. Streptokinase and heparin versus heparin alone in massive pulmonary embolism: a randomized controlled trial. J Thromb Thrombolysis. 1995;2:227–9.

40. Wan S, Quinlan DJ, Agnelli G, Eikelboom JW. Thrombolysis compared with heparin for the initial treatment of pulmonary embolism: a meta-analysis of the randomized controlled trials. Circulation. 2004;110:744–9.

41. Chatterjee S, Chakraborty A, Weinberg I, Kadakia M, Wilensky RL, Sardar P, Kumbhani DJ, Mukherjee D, Jaff MR, Giri J. Thrombolysis for pulmonary embolism and risk of all-cause mortality, major bleeding, and intracranial hemorrhage: a meta-analysis. JAMA. 2014;311:2414–21.

42. Thabut G, Thabut D, Myers RP, Bernard-Chabert B, Marrash-Chahla R, Mal H, Fournier M. Thrombolytic therapy of pulmonary embolism: a meta-analysis. J Am Coll Cardiol. 2002;40:1660–7.

43. Fiumara K, Kucher N, Fanikos J, et al. Predictors of major hemorrhage following fibrinolysis for acute pulmonary embolism. Am J Cardiol. 2006;97:127–9.

44. Wang C, Zhai Z, Yang Y, Wu Q, Cheng Z, Liang L, Dai H, Huang K, Lu W, Zhang Z, Cheng X, Shen YH, China Venous Thromboembolism (VTE) Study Group. Efficacy and safety of low dose recombinant tissue-type plasminogen activator for the treatment of acute pulmonary thromboembolism: a randomized, multicenter, controlled trial. Chest. 2010;137:254–62.

45. Torbicki A, Galié N, Covezzoli A, Rossi E, De Rosa M, Goldhaber SZ, ICOPER Study Group. Right heart thrombi in pulmonary embolism: results from the International Cooperative Pulmonary Embolism Registry. J Am Coll Cardiol. 2003;41:2245–51.

46. Ferrari E, Benhamou M, Berthier F, Baudouy M. Mobile thrombi of the right heart in pulmonary embolism: delayed disappearance after thrombolytic treatment. Chest. 2005;127:1051–3.

47. Pierre-Justin G, Pierard LA. Management of mobile right heart thrombi: a prospective series. Int J Cardiol. 2005;99:381–8.

48. Agnelli G, Parise P. Bolus thrombolysis in venous thromboembolism. Chest. 1992;101(Suppl):172–82.

49. Lavonas EJ, Drennan IR, Gabrielli A, Heffner AC, Hoyte CO, Orkin AM, Sawyer KN, Donnino MW. Part 10: special circumstances of resuscitation: 2015 American Heart Association guidelines update for cardiopulmonary resuscitation and emergency cardiovascular care. Circulation. 2015; 132(Suppl2):501–18.

50. Engelberger RP, Kucher N. Catheter-based reperfusion treatment of pulmonary embolism. Circulation. 2011;124:2139–44.

51. Tajima H, Murata S, Kumazaki T, Nakazawa K, Abe Y, Komada Y, Niggemann P, Takayama M, Tanaka K, Takano T. Hybrid treatment of acute massive pulmonary thromboembolism: mechanical fragmentation with a modified rotating pigtail catheter, local fibrinolytic therapy, and clot aspiration followed by systemic fibrinolytic therapy. AJR Am J Roentgenol. 2004;183:589–95.

52. Kuo WT, Gould MK, Louie JD, Rosenberg JK, Sze DY, Hofmann LV. Catheter-directed therapy for the treatment of massive pulmonary embolism: systematic review and meta-analysis of modern techniques. J Vasc Interv Radiol. 2009;20:1431–40.

53. Kucher N, Boekstegers P, Müller OJ, Kupatt C, Beyer-Westendorf J, Heitzer T, Tebbe U, Horstkotte J, Müller R, Blessing E, Greif M, Lange P, Hoffmann RT, Werth S, Barmeyer A, Härtel D, Grünwald H, Empen K, Baumgartner I. Randomized, controlled trial of ultrasound-assisted catheter-directed thrombolysis for acute intermediate-risk pulmonary embolism. Circulation. 2014;129:479–86.

54. Takahashi H, Okada K, Matsumori M, Kano H, Kitagawa A, Okita Y. Aggressive surgical treatment of acute pulmonary embolism with circulatory collapse. Ann Thorac Surg. 2012;94:785–91.

55. Leacche M, Unic D, Goldhaber SZ, Rawn JD, Aranki SF, Couper GS, Mihaljevic T, Rizzo RJ, Cohn LH, Aklog L, Byrne JG. Modern surgical treatment of massive pulmonary embolism: results in 47 consecutive patients after rapid diagnosis and aggressive surgical approach. J Thorac Cardiovasc Surg. 2005;129:1018–23.

56. Fukuda I, Taniguchi S, Fukui K, Minakawa M, Daitoku K, Suzuki Y. Improved outcome of surgical pulmonary embolectomy by aggressive intervention for critically ill patients. Ann Thorac Surg. 2011;91:728–32.

57. Aklog L, Williams CS, Byrne JG, Goldhaber SZ. Acute pulmonary embolectomy: a contemporary approach. Circulation. 2002;105:1416–9.

58. Vohra HA, Whistance RN, Mattam K, Kaarne M, Haw MP, Barlow CW, Tsang GM, Livesey SA, Ohri SK. Early and late clinical outcomes of pulmonary embolectomy for acute massive pulmonary embolism. Ann Thorac Surg. 2010;90:1747–52.

59. Stein PD, Matta F, Keyes DC, Willyerd GL. Impact of vena cava filters on in-hospital case fatality rate from pulmonary embolism. Am J Med. 2012;125: 478–84.

60. Muriel A, Jime'nez D, Aujesky D, Bertoletti L, Decousus H, Laporte S, Mismetti P, Munoz FJ, Yusen R, Monreal M; RIETE investigators. Survival effects of inferior vena cava filter in patients with acute symptomatic venous thromboembolism and a significant bleeding risk. J Am Coll Cardiol 2014;63:1675–1683.

61. Hann CL, Streiff MB. The role of vena caval filters in the management of venous thromboembolism. Blood Rev. 2005;19:179–202.

62. StudyGroup PREPIC. Eight-year follow-up of patients with permanent vena cava filters in the prevention of pulmonary embolism: the PREPIC (Prevention du Risque d'Embolie Pulmonaire par Interruption Cave) randomized study. Circulation. 2005;112:416–22.

63. Mismetti P, Laporte S, Pellerin O, Couturaud F, Elias A, Falvo N, Meneveau N, Quere I, Roy PM, Sanchez O, Schmidt J, Seinturier C, Sevestre MA, Beregi JP, Tardy B, Lacroix P, Presles E, Leizorovicz A, Decousus H, Barral FG, Meyer G; PREPIC2 Study Group. Effect of a retrievable inferior vena cava filter plus anticoagulation vs anticoagulation alone on risk of recurrent pulmonary embolism: a randomized clinical trial. JAMA. 2015;313:1627–1635.

64. Duranteau J, Taccone FS, Verhamme P, Ageno W, ESA VTE. Guidelines Task Force. European guidelines on perioperative venous thromboembolism prophylaxis: intensive care. Eur J Anaesthesiol. 2017 Nov;6 [Epub ahead of print]

65. Yamamoto T, Nakamura M, Kuroiwa M, Tanaka K. Current prevention practice for venous thromboembolism in Japanese intensive care units. J Anesth. 2013;27:931–4.

66. Kabrhel C, Jaff MR, Channick RN, Baker JN, Rosenfield K. A multidisciplinary pulmonary embolism response team. Chest. 2013;144:1738–9.

23

Hepcidin predicts response to IV iron therapy in patients admitted to the intensive care unit

Edward Litton[1,2,14*] (ID), Stuart Baker[3], Wendy Erber[4], Shannon Farmer[5], Janet Ferrier[1], Craig French[6,7], Joel Gummer[8], David Hawkins[9], Alisa Higgins[10], Axel Hofmann[5], Bart De Keulenaer[1], Julie McMorrow[11], John K. Olynyk[12], Toby Richards[13], Simon Towler[1], Robert Trengove[8], Steve Webb[2,11], on behalf of the IRONMAN Study investigators and the Australian and New Zealand Intensive Care Society Clinical Trials Group

Abstract

Background: Both anaemia and red blood cell (RBC) transfusion are common and associated with adverse outcomes in patients admitted to the intensive care unit (ICU). The aim of this study was to determine whether serum hepcidin concentration, measured early after ICU admission in patients with anaemia, could identify a group in whom intravenous (IV) iron therapy decreased the subsequent RBC transfusion requirement.

Methods: We conducted a prospective observational study nested within a multicenter randomized controlled trial (RCT) of IV iron versus placebo. The study was conducted in the ICUs of four tertiary hospitals in Perth, Western Australia. Critically ill patients with haemoglobin (Hb) of < 100 g/L and within 48 h of admission to the ICU were eligible for participation after enrolment in the IRONMAN RCT. The response to IV iron therapy compared with placebo was assessed according to tertile of hepcidin concentration.

Results: Hepcidin concentration was measured within 48 h of ICU admission in 133 patients. For patients in the lower two tertiles of hepcidin concentration (< 53.0 μg), IV iron therapy compared with placebo was associated with a significant decrease in RBC transfusion requirement [risk ratio 0.48 (95% CI 0.26–0.85), $p = 0.013$].

Conclusions: In critically ill patients with anaemia admitted to an ICU, baseline hepcidin concentration predicts RBC transfusion requirement and is able to identify a group of patients in whom IV iron compared with placebo is associated with a significant decrease in RBC transfusion requirement.

Keywords: Anaemia, Critical care, Hepcidin, Intravenous iron, Red blood cell transfusion

Background

Anaemia is common in patients admitted to the intensive care unit (ICU) and is associated with adverse outcomes [1, 2]. Despite evidence to support a restrictive red blood cell (RBC) transfusion threshold, anaemia is also the most common indication for RBC transfusion in the ICU, itself associated with increased morbidity and mortality [3].

* Correspondence: ed.litton@health.wa.gov.au; ed_litton@hotmail.com
[1]Intensive Care Unit, Fiona Stanley Hospital, Perth, Western Australia 6065, Australia
[2]School of Medicine, University of Western Australia, Perth, Western Australia 6009, Australia
Full list of author information is available at the end of the article

In non-critically ill patients, intravenous (IV) iron therapy is effective in promoting erythropoiesis and decreasing RBC transfusion requirement [4]. However, recent randomized controlled trials (RCTs) of IV iron therapy in critically ill patients have not demonstrated benefit [5, 6]. This may be because critical illness results in an acute inflammatory response that confounds the interpretation of standard, clinically available measures of iron deficiency used in these studies. By contrast, the serum concentration of hepcidin, a key regulator of iron metabolism, decreases in response to iron-restricted erythropoiesis, even in the presence of inflammation [7]. Hepcidin is a small peptide secreted predominantly by the liver and acts by blocking duodenal iron absorption and decreasing availability of iron stored in hepatocytes and macrophages to red cell precursors. Although hepcidin may be more accurate in predicting an increase in red blood cell production in response to IV iron, prospective clinical data is lacking.

The primary aim of this study was to determine whether low serum hepcidin concentration could identify a subset of critically ill patients with anaemia in whom IV iron therapy was effective in reducing RBC transfusion requirement.

Methods

The study was a prospective cohort study, nested within the IRONMAN RCT, the protocol and primary results of which have previously been published [5, 8]. Briefly, the IRONMAN RCT enrolled adult patients who were within 48 h of admission to ICU, had a hemoglobin (Hb) of less than 100 g/L, and were anticipated to require ICU care beyond the next calendar day. Exclusion criteria included suspected or confirmed severe sepsis, a ferritin greater than 1200 ng/mL or transferrin saturation greater than 50%. Participants were randomised in a 1:1 ratio to receive either 500 mg IV ferric carboxymaltose or placebo and were followed up to hospital discharge. Human Research Ethics Committee approval was obtained at all sites prior to commencement, and prospective consent was obtained from all participants or their legal surrogates.

For this nested cohort study, blood was collected for serum hepcidin measurement immediately following enrolment and prior to study drug administration. Hepcidin-25 was isolated from blood for quantitation by liquid chromatography-quadrupole time-of-flight mass spectrometry (LC-qTOF-MS), using a Waters Synapt G2S (Waters, Manchester, UK) as previously described [9, 10]. Hepcidin was isolated by solid phase extraction following the initial addition of a synthetic human hepcidin ($^{13}C_{18}, ^{15}N_3$) peptide internal standard (Peptides International, Kentucky, USA) and removal of the more abundant polypeptides by organic solvent precipitation and centrifugation. The accurate mass measurement of the precursor hepcidin-25 $[M+5H]^{5+}$ ion was confirmed against a hepcidin-25 standard (Peptides International, Kentucky, USA) and further by MS/MS. Quantitation was by reference to a human hepcidin-25 ($^{13}C_{18}, ^{15}N_3$) calibration, prepared in human serum.

The primary objective was to determine whether hepcidin concentration could identify a group of critically ill patients for whom IV iron therapy was effective in decreasing the risk of RBC transfusion. The secondary objective was to develop a prognostic model for RBC transfusion quantity in patients admitted to the ICU.

Statistical analysis

Continuous variables were reported as mean (± SD) or median and interquartile range (IQR), with between-group differences analyzed using Student's t test or the Wilcoxon rank-sum test for apparently normal and

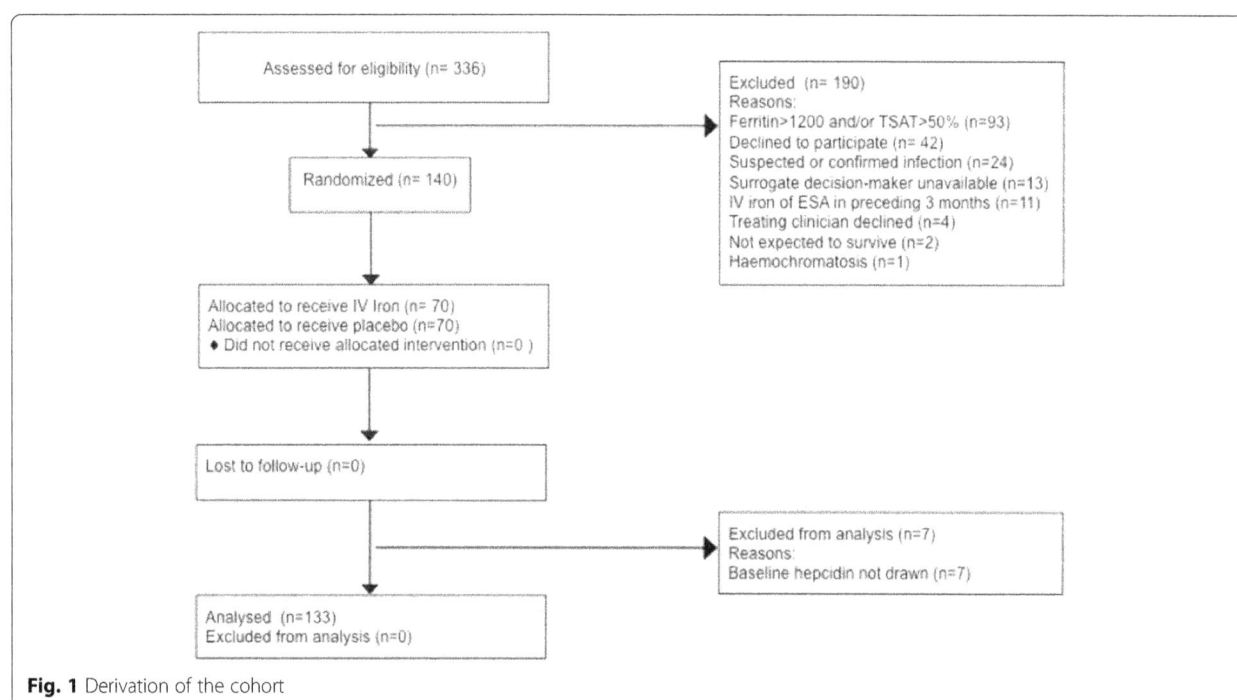

Fig. 1 Derivation of the cohort

non-normally distributed data respectively. Categorical variables were reported as proportion and analyzed using the χ^2 test or Fischer exact test as appropriate. Data was censored at 60 days after enrolment for RBC transfusion Hb concentration and vital status.

The relationship between hepcidin concentration and response to IV iron therapy was examined using similar methodology to a previously published RCT of IV iron in patients with chemotherapy-induced anaemia conducted by Steensma et al. [11]. Similar to this methodology, patients were first stratified by tertile of baseline hepcidin concentration then combined. The incident risk ratio for RBC transfusion was then compared between those who were randomized to receive IV iron and those who received placebo. The relationship between IV iron therapy and RBC transfusion quantity across the range of hepcidin values was further explored by locally weighted scatterplot smoothing (LOWESS) [12]. Receiver-operator characteristic curve analysis was not undertaken because the IRONMAN RCT demonstrated nearly identical overall proportions of patients transfused in the two groups.

The model to predict subsequent RBC transfusion quantity in patients admitted to the ICU was developed using negative binomial univariate and multivariate analyses. Variables with a p value of < 0.3 on univariate analysis were included in a multivariable analysis with backwards selection with an alpha of 0.05. Interaction was assessed using multivariable fractional polynomials to account for potential non-linear relationships. Significant interactions (p value of < 0.05) were examined graphically, and a final model was then produced. The relative prognostic value with and without baseline hepcidin concentration included was assessed using Akaike information criterion (AIC).

Outcome data was censored at 60 days after enrolment. A two-sided p value of 0.05 or less was considered to be statistically significant. All analyses were conducted with Stata Version 14 StataCorp College Station, TX77845, USA.

Results

Baseline hepcidin levels were available for 133 (95%) out of the 140 participants enrolled in the IRONMAN RCT. The flow of participants is presented in Fig. 1. The mean time from ICU admission to collection was 29 h [standard deviation (SD) 13], and median hepcidin concentration was 34.9 µg/L [interquartile range (IQR) 17.3–69.2, range 0–163.5]. The baseline characteristics of the population are provided in Table 1. There was no significant correlation between hepcidin concentration and baseline C reactive protein or iron indices (see Additional file 1).

Table 1 Baseline characteristics

Characteristic*	Outcome ($n = 133$)
Age—years	62 (41–73)
Male gender—no. (%)	91 (68)
ICU admission source—no (%)	
Emergency department	24 (18)
Hospital ward	8 (6)
Operating theater	97 (73)
Other hospital	4 (3)
ICU admission type—no (%)	
Medical	17 (13)
General surgical	20 (15)
Cardiothoracic	49 (37)
Trauma	42 (32)
Neurosurgical	5 (4)
APACHE II score	12 (9–17)
SOFA score	6 (4–9)
Prior RBC transfusion—no (%)	30 (23)
Haemoglobin—g/L	88 (81–94)
Mean corpuscular volume—fL	91 (88–94)
C reactive protein—mg/L	110 (48–170)
Iron—mcg/dL	3 (2–6)
Ferritin—ng/ml+	260 (161–437)
Transferrin—mg/dL	17 (15–20)
Transferrin saturation—%	9 (6–16)
Soluble transferrin receptor—mg/L	1.81 (1.28–2.44)
Hepcidin—µg/mL	34.9 (17.3–69.2)
Tertile 1—(0–20.08)	10.6 (4.2–15.6)
Tertile 2—(20.09–53.00)	34.9 (27.1–48.5)
Tertile 3—(53.01–163.46)	81.2 (69.2–97.9)

ICU intensive care unit, *APACHE* acute physiology and chronic health evaluation, *SOFA* sequential organ failure assessment, *RBC* red blood cell
*Median and interquartile range (IQR) unless otherwise reported
+ng/ml has a conversion factor of 1 to the standard international units mcg/ml

Hepcidin and prediction of response to IV iron

Of the 88 patients in the lower two tertiles of hepcidin concentration (0 to 53.0 µg/L), 44 received IV iron therapy and 44 received placebo. In patients with a low hepcidin concentration (≤ 53.0 µg/L), the relative risk (RR) of RBC transfusion associated with IV iron was 0.48 (95% CI 0.26–0.85), $p = 0.013$. In patients with a high hepcidin level (> 53.0 µg/L), there was no significant association between IV iron therapy and risk of RBC transfusion, RR 1.33 (95% CI 0.57–3.08), $p = 0.518$. The association between IV iron therapy and RBC transfusion by tertile of hepcidin concentration is provided in Table 2. The association between hepcidin concentration and RBC transfusion quantity in patients who received IV iron compared with placebo is represented by the LOWESS plot in Fig. 2.

Table 2 Hepcidin and risk of RBC transfusion with IV iron therapy

Variable	IV iron	Placebo	Risk ratio (95% CI)	p value
Hepcidin ≤ 53.0 µg/L				
Number RBC units/patients	38/44	80/44		
Median RBC units (IQR)	1 (0–2)	1 (0–3)	0.48 (0.26–0.85)	0.013
Hepcidin 1st tertile (0–20.1 µg/L)				
Number RBC units/number patients	23/22	35/21		
Median RBC units (IQR)	1 (0–2)	0 (0–2)	0.63 (0.26–1.50)	0.293
Hepcidin 2nd tertile (20.1–53.0 µg/L)				
Number RBC units/number patients	15/22	45/23		
Median RBC units (IQR)	0 (0–1)	1 (0–3)	0.35 (0.16–0.77)	0.009
Hepcidin 3rd tertile (> 53.0 µg/L)				
Number RBC units/number patients	43/22	34/23		
Median RBC units (IQR)	1 (0–3)	1 (0–3)	1.33 (0.57–3.08)	0.518

RBC red blood cell, *IQR* interquartile range

IV iron therapy compared with placebo was not associated with a significant increase in Hb for those in the lower two tertiles of hepcidin values [mean increase Hb 3 g/L (95% CI − 3–10), $p = 0.361$]. There was no significant correlation between hepcidin and concurrent Hb, ferritin, transferrin saturation, soluble transferrin receptor or C reactive protein. There was also no significant difference in iron, transferrin saturation, ferritin or transferrin receptor levels associated with lower versus higher hepcidin tertile (see Additional file 1).

Predicting RBC transfusion quantity

The complete list of variables assessed on univariate analysis and those added to the initial multivariable model is provided in Additional file 1. ICU admission related to trauma, baseline Hb < 80 g/L, lower transferrin saturation and lower hepcidin concentration were found to predict increased risk of RBC transfusion and were retained in the final multivariable model. There was a significant interaction between Hb and hepcidin concentrations in predicting the risk of RBC transfusion (likelihood ratio test for significance of interaction $p = 0.0462$), see Additional file 1: Figure S1. For patients with a Hb ≥ 80 g/L, each 10 µg/mL increase in hepcidin concentration was associated with a risk ratio of RBC transfusion of 1.09 (95% CI 1.01–1.18, $p = 0.034$). However, for patients with a Hb < 80 g/L, there was no significant association between hepcidin concentration and risk of RBC transfusion [RR 0.95 (95% CI 0.84–1.07), $p = 0.387$]. The variables included in the final model are

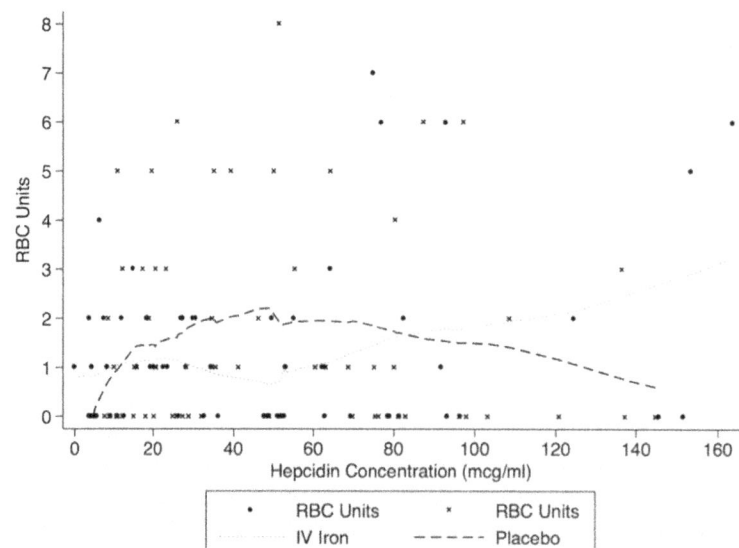

Fig. 2 Association between hepcidin concentration and Red Blood Cell units transfused for patients receiving IV iron and placebo

provided in Table 3. AIC with hepcidin in the model was 415.14 versus 468.16 with hepcidin removed.

Discussion

We found that serum hepcidin concentration identified a subset of anaemic, critically ill patients in whom IV iron therapy was effective in reducing RBC transfusion requirement. These findings are important when considering the dose-response relationship between increasing RBC transfusion quantity and worse clinical outcomes and also due to the scarcity and cost of RBC transfusion. In addition to predicting the effectiveness of IV iron in critically ill patients, we also found that hepcidin concentration was an independent predictor of RBC transfusion requirement but that the association was modified by Hb levels.

Although Lasocki et al. have described low hepcidin concentrations in some critically ill patients with anaemia, there is limited data exploring whether hepcidin can be used to guide treatment decisions [7]. Steensma et al. found that hepcidin concentration could predict response to IV iron therapy in patients with chemotherapy-induced anaemia [11]. In our study, the median C reactive protein was 110 mg/L but did not correlate with hepcidin concentration, suggesting that even in the presence of inflammation, measurement of hepcidin is useful in identifying critically ill patients in whom IV iron therapy is likely to reduce RBC transfusion requirement [13]. Our findings also support further investigation into the role of hepcidin antagonists in patients with elevated hepcidin [14].

Hepcidin synthesis is finely regulated and induced by both inflammation and iron overload [15]. Hepcidin levels have been shown to be the predominant predictor of erythrocyte iron incorporation in African children with anaemia [16]. Amongst adult patients admitted to the ICU, Tacke et al. have demonstrated an association between markers of increased iron availability and mortality [17]. It is plausible that using hepcidin concentration to target IV iron therapy in critically ill patients can also reduce the potential risk of initiating or exacerbating infection associated with both excessively high free iron levels and iron deficiency.

Accurate prediction of RBC transfusion quantity could provide an additional method to target IV iron therapy in critically ill patients. In the IRONMAN RCT, subgroup analysis did not suggest a differential effect of IV iron related to transferrin saturation or ferritin concentration [5]. Building on these findings, the current study found no significant difference in iron indices based on hepcidin tertile or correlation between iron indices and hepcidin. Although iron-restricted erythropoiesis is not present in all critical patients who require RBC transfusion, our study found that hepcidin was an independent predictor of subsequent transfusion. Although our model requires validation, a metric of observed versus predicted RBC transfusion may also be useful as a quality metric.

Future studies must also address the substantial variation that currently exists in hepcidin assays and reference ranges that makes comparison between studies difficult [14]. A reliable point of care hepcidin test is necessary to provide results in a clinically useful timeframe. The ongoing HEPCIDANE RCT (NCT02276690) of hepcidin-guided management of anaemia in critically ill patients will address some of these issues.

Limitations

Our study was limited to patients with an Hb < 100 g/L and did not enroll patients with sepsis. Whether hepcidin measurement is useful in these patients remains uncertain. Although soluble transferrin receptor levels were not found not to be predictive of RBC transfusion requirement in our study, other assays with potential diagnostic benefit including zinc protophoryn were not assessed. However, given the central role of hepcidin in iron metabolism, it is unlikely that other assays provide superior diagnostic utility. The relatively small number of participants precluded the use of methods to reduce the risk of over-fitting of the statistical models, and larger studies are required to validate the findings. Finally, the current study only assessed the use of hepcidin at a single point in time. Greater understanding is required of how hepcidin levels change over time including the effect interventions such as RBC transfusion and IV iron therapy.

Conclusion

In patients with anaemia admitted to the ICU, hepcidin measurement can identify a group of patients in whom IV iron therapy decreases RBC transfusion requirement.

Table 3 Final multivariate model—independent predictors of RBC transfusion

Characteristic (n = 133)	Coefficient (95% CI)	Risk ratio (95% CI)	p value
ICU admission type—trauma vs non trauma	0.833 (0.382–1.285)	2.30 (1.46–3.61)	< 0.001
Haemoglobin > 80 g/L*—yes vs no	− 0.99 (− 1.493 to − 0.493)	0.37 (0.22–0.61)	< 0.001
Transferrin saturation—per 10% increase	0.237 (0.082–0.391)	1.27 (1.09–1.48)	0.003
Hepcidin—per 10 µg/ml increase	0.086 (0.030–0.142)	1.09 (1.03–1.15)	0.002

CI confidence interval, ICU intensive care unit. Constant for model 0.088 (95% CI − 0.398–0.575)

*Likelihood ratio test for significance of interaction between haemoglobin as a continuous variable and hepcidin concentration in predicting the risk of RBC transfusion p = 0.0462. For patients with a haemoglobin < 80 g/L, there was no significant association between hepcidin concentration and risk of RBC transfusion [RR 0.95 (95% CI 0.84–1.07), p = 0.387]

Additional file

Additional file 1: Figure S1. Relationship between hepcidin concentration and RBC transfusion, moderated by haemoglobin concentration. Hb Haemoglobin, RBC red blood cell. **Table S1.** Iron indices according to hepcidin levels. **Table S2.** Univariate analysis of variables associated with risk of RBC transfusion. CI confidence interval, ICU intensive care unit, APACHE acute physiology and chronic health evaluation, SOFA sequential organ failure assessment. Variables in bold added to the initial multivariable model. (DOCX 108 kb)

Abbreviations
CI: Confidence interval; Hb: Haemoglobin; ICU: Intensive care unit; IQR: Interquartile range; IV: Intravenous; RBC: Red blood cell; RCT: Randomized controlled trial; RR: Risk ratio; SD: Standard deviation

Acknowledgements
The authors would like to thank Associate Professor KM Ho and the Centre for Applied Statistics, University of Western Australia for their review of the statistical aspects of the manuscript.
The IRONMAN RCT is part of the Blood – CRE, Centre of Research Excellence for Patient Blood Management in Critical Illness and Trauma.
The authors would also like to thank our collaborators Dr. Andy Chapman, Royal Perth Hospital, Perth, Western Australia, Ms. Elizabeth Jenkinson, Royal Perth Hospital, Perth, Western Australia, Ms. Anne Marie Palermo, Fremantle Hospital, Fremantle, WA, Ms. Brigit Roberts, and Sir Charles Gardner Hospital, Perth, Western Australia.
A list of additional IRONMAN study collaborators is provided as Additional file 1.

Funding
The IRONMAN RCT was funded by a SHRAC Research Translation Project Grant 2012 (Round 6) ref: F-AA-12440, Department of Health, Government of Western Australia. Study drug was provided by Vifor Pharma as in-kind support without any involvement in the design of the study, analysis of results or preparation of manuscripts.

Authors' contributions
EL designed the research study, performed the research, analyzed the data and wrote the paper. SB designed the research study, performed the research and assisted in re-drafting the paper. WE, SF, CF, AHi, AHo, JKO and TR designed the research study and assisted in re-drafting the paper. JF performed the research and assisted in re-drafting the paper. JG and RT contributed essential reagents and tools and assisted in writing the paper. DH, BDK, JM, ST and SW designed the research study, performed the research and assisted in re-drafting the paper. The ANZICS CTG provided critical appraisal, review and feedback of the IRONMAN programme of research and critical appraisal, feedback and editorial suggestions on the current manuscript. All authors read and approved the final manuscript.

Competing interests
AH has received industry-supplied funding for overseas lectures and travel from Vifor International AG and its subsidiaries of a total of approximately £60,000, from TEM International of a total of approximately £5000 and from UCB International of a total of approximately £9000 (all of it are not related to the subject matter). The other authors declare that they have no competing interests.

Author details
[1]Intensive Care Unit, Fiona Stanley Hospital, Perth, Western Australia 6065, Australia. [2]School of Medicine, University of Western Australia, Perth, Western Australia 6009, Australia. [3]Intensive Care Unit, Sir Charles Gardner Hospital, Perth, Western Australia 6009, Australia. [4]School of Patholody, University of Australia, Perth, Western Australia 6009, Australia. [5]Medical School, Faculty of Health and Medical Sciences, University of Western Australia, Perth, Western Australia 6009, Australia. [6]Western Health, Melbourne, Victoria, Australia. [7]University of Melbourne, Melbourne, Victoria, Australia. [8]Separation Science and Metabolomics Laboratory Metabolomics Australia (Western Australia node), Murdoch University, Perth, Western Australia, Australia. [9]Intensive Care Unit, Joondalup Health Campus, Joondalup, Western Australia, Australia. [10]Centre of Research Excellence for Patient Blood Management in Critical Illness and Trauma, Monash University, Melbourne, Victoria, Australia. [11]Intensive Care Unit, Royal Perth Hospital, Perth, Western Australia 6000, Australia. [12]School of Medicine, University of Western Australia, Perth, Western Australia 6009, Australia. [13]University College London, London, UK. [14]Intensive Care Unit, Fiona Stanley Hospital, Perth, Western Australia 6150, Australia.

References
1. Vincent JL, Baron JF, Reinhart K, Gattinoni L, Thijs L, Webb A, Meier-Hellmann A, Nollet G, Peres-Bota D, Investigators ABC. Anemia and blood transfusion in critically ill patients. JAMA. 2002;288(12):1499–507.
2. Hayden SJ, Albert TJ, Watkins TR, Swenson ER. Anemia in critical illness: insights into etiology, consequences, and management. Am J Respir Crit Care Med. 2012;185(10):1049–57.
3. Lelubre C, Vincent JL. Red blood cell transfusion in the critically ill patient. Ann Intensive Care. 2011;1:43.
4. Litton E, Xiao J, Ho KM. Safety and efficacy of intravenous iron therapy in reducing requirement for allogeneic blood transfusion: systematic review and meta-analysis of randomised clinical trials. Bmj. 2013;347:f4822.
5. Investigators I, Litton E, Baker S, Erber WN, Farmer S, Ferrier J, French C, Gummer J, Hawkins D, Higgins A, et al. Intravenous iron or placebo for anaemia in intensive care: the IRONMAN multicentre randomized blinded trial : a randomized trial of IV iron in critical illness. Intensive Care Med. 2016;42(11):1715–22.
6. Pieracci FM, Stovall RT, Jaouen B, Rodil M, Cappa A, Burlew CC, Holena DN, Maier R, Berry S, Jurkovich J, et al. A multicenter, randomized clinical trial of IV iron supplementation for anemia of traumatic critical illness. Crit Care Med. 2014;42(9):2048–57.
7. Lasocki S, Baron G, Driss F, Westerman M, Puy H, Boutron I, Beaumont C, Montravers P. Diagnostic accuracy of serum hepcidin for iron deficiency in critically ill patients with anemia. Intensive Care Med. 2010;36(6):1044–8.
8. Litton E, Baker S, Erber W, French C, Ferrier J, Hawkins D, Higgins AM, Hofmann A, Keulenaer BL, Farmer S, et al. The IRONMAN trial: a protocol for a multicentre randomised placebo-controlled trial of intravenous iron in intensive care unit patients with anaemia. Crit Care Resusc. 2014;16(4): 285–90.
9. Gummer J, Trengove R, Pascoe EM, Badve SV, Cass A, Clarke P, McDonald SP, Morrish AT, Pedagogos E, Perkovic V, et al. Association between serum hepcidin-25 and primary resistance to erythropoiesis stimulating agents in chronic kidney disease: a secondary analysis of the HERO trial. Nephrology (Carlton). 2017;7(22):548–54.
10. van Rijnsoever M, Galhenage S, Mollison L, Gummer J, Trengove R, Olynyk JK. Dysregulated erythropoietin, hepcidin, and bone marrow iron metabolism contribute to interferon-induced anemia in hepatitis C. J Interf Cytokine Res. 2016;36(11):630–4.
11. Steensma DP, Sasu BJ, Sloan JA, Tomita DK, Loprinzi CL. Serum hepcidin levels predict response to intravenous iron and darbepoetin in chemotherapy-associated anemia. Blood. 2015;125(23):3669–71.
12. May S, Bigelow C. Modeling nonlinear dose-response relationships in epidemiologic studies: statistical approaches and practical challenges. Dose-Response. 2006;3(4):474–90.
13. Lim J, Miles L, Litton E. Intravenous iron therapy in patients undergoing cardiovascular surgery: a narrative review. J Cardiothorac Vasc Anesth. 2018; 3(32):1439–51.
14. Girelli D, Nemeth E, Swinkels DW. Hepcidin in the diagnosis of iron disorders. Blood. 2016;127(23):2809–13.

The prognostic performance of qSOFA for community-acquired pneumonia

Fumiaki Tokioka[1]*[iD], Hiroshi Okamoto[2], Akio Yamazaki[1], Akihiro Itou[1] and Tadashi Ishida[1]

Abstract

Background: Quick Sepsis-related Organ Failure Assessment (qSOFA) is a new screening system for sepsis. The prognostic performance of qSOFA for patients with suspected infections outside the intensive care unit (ICU) is similar to that of full SOFA; however, its performance for community-acquired pneumonia (CAP) has not yet been evaluated in detail.

The objectives of the present study were to compare the prognostic performance of qSOFA with existing pneumonia severity scores, such as CURB-65 (confusion, blood urea nitrogen > 19 mg/dL, respiratory rate ≥ 30/min, systolic blood pressure < 90 mmHg, or diastolic blood pressure ≤ 60 mmHg, age ≥ 65 years) and the pneumonia severity index (PSI), and examine its usefulness for predicting mortality and ICU admission in patients with CAP of high severity and mortality that requires hospitalization.

Methods: We performed a secondary analysis of data from a prospective observational study of adult patients who were admitted to our hospital between October 2010 and June 2016. We compared the prognostic performance of qSOFA, CURB-65, and PSI for predicting in-hospital mortality and ICU admission using the C statistics.

Results: The median age of the 1045 enrolled patients was 77 (68–83) years, and 71.4% were males. The in-hospital mortality and ICU admission rates of the entire cohort were 6.1 and 7.9%, respectively. All scores were significantly higher in non-survivors and ICU admission patients than in survivors and non-ICU admission patients ($p < 0.001$). The C statistics of qSOFA for predicting in-hospital mortality was 0.69 (95% CI 0.63–0.75), and no significant differences were observed between CURB-65 (C statistics, 0.75; 95% CI 0.69–0.81) and PSI (C statistics, 0.74; 95% CI 0.69–0.80). The C statistics of qSOFA for predicting ICU admission was 0.76 (95% CI 0.71–0.80), and no significant differences were noted between CURB-65 (C statistics, 0.73; 95% CI 0.67–0.79) and PSI (C statistics, 0.72; 95% CI 0.66–0.78).

Conclusions: Regarding hospitalized CAP, the prognostic performance of qSOFA for in-hospital mortality and ICU admission was not significantly different from those of CURB-65 and PSI. qSOFA only requires a few items and vital signs, and, thus, may be particularly useful for emergency department or non-respiratory specialists.

Keywords: qSOFA, CURB-65, PSI, Pneumonia, Sepsis

Background

Sepsis-3, a new definition for sepsis, and its diagnostic criteria were published in 2016 [1]. Quick Sepsis-related Organ Failure Assessment (qSOFA) has been used to screen sepsis outside of the intensive care unit (ICU) [2]. Sepsis is diagnosed if at least two out of the three criteria are positive in patients with suspected infections. qSOFA is a very simple screening tool because it only has three evaluation items, does not require laboratory

examinations, and may be conducted at the bedside. Moreover, in the original study, the C statistics for the in-hospital mortality of qSOFA was 0.81 as a good indicator of prognosis, and its usefulness as a prognostic tool has been evaluated [3–5]; however, some studies have questioned its usefulness [6–8].

Community-acquired pneumonia (CAP) is a common infection, is frequently a causative disease for sepsis, and its mortality rate is between approximately 3 and 9% [1, 2, 9–13]. Therefore, the prognosis of CAP needs to be accurately assessed in order to select an appropriate treatment strategy.

* Correspondence: ft13419@kchnet.or.jp
[1]Department of Respiratory Medicine, Kurashiki Central Hospital, 1-1-1 Miwa, Kurashiki, Okayama 710-8602, Japan
Full list of author information is available at the end of the article

Few studies have examined the use of qSOFA for CAP [3, 10, 12]; however, one of these studies reported a high mortality rate [3], while another was a short report in a letter format [10]. Thus, there is currently no consensus as to whether qSOFA is an effective strategy.

A previous study comprehensively examined existing pneumonia severity scores for CAP and qSOFA [12]; however, relatively mild pneumonia that may be treated internally was incorporated and the patient background used was relatively young. The original clinical significance of severity scores was for pneumonia of high severity and mortality that requires hospitalization; however, it currently remains unclear whether qSOFA is useful as a prognostic tool for CAP that requires hospitalization.

The aims of the present study were to compare the prognostic accuracy of qSOFA with existing pneumonia severity scores (CURB-65 [Confusion, Urea, Respiratory Rate, Blood Pressure, and Age] [11] and the pneumonia severity index [PSI] [14]) and to examine the usefulness of qSOFA for CAP of high severity and mortality that requires hospitalization.

Methods
Study design and settings
We performed a secondary analysis of data from a prospective observational study of patients admitted to Kurashiki Central Hospital (1166-bed community hospital, Okayama, Japan) between October 2010 and June 2016.

Adult patients (age, ≥ 18 years) with pneumonia diagnosed by new infiltrates on chest imaging studies (radiography or computed tomography) and two or more symptoms consistent with pneumonia (including cough, dyspnea, fever, sputum production, breathlessness, and/or pleuritic chest pain) were enrolled at an emergency department or outpatient visit.

Exclusion criteria were as follows: age younger than 18 years, a resident of an extended care facility or nursing home, recently discharged from hospital within 90 days, an elderly or disabled individual receiving nursing care, and those receiving regular endovascular treatments as an outpatient (dialysis, antibiotic therapy, chemotherapy, and immunosuppressant therapy).

The present study was approved by the Kurashiki Central Hospital Ethics Committee. Informed consent was obtained from all patients at the time of admission.

Data collection
Data on demographic characteristics, vital signs, imaging, and laboratory test results of the enrolled patients were recorded upon hospital arrival at an emergency department or outpatient visit. All patients who were intubated immediately after hospital arrival also recorded vital signs before intubation. qSOFA, CURB-65, and PSI were calculated using data obtained at enrollment. All data were collected by a study team consisting of a four board-certificated pulmonologist.

Outcome variables
The primary outcome was in-hospital mortality and the secondary outcome was ICU admission.

Statistical analysis
We assessed the predictive performance of qSOFA, CURB-65, and PSI for the primary and secondary outcomes.

Data were presented as medians with interquartile ranges for continuous variables and as numbers and percentages for categorical variables. Variables with significant differences were tested by a binary logistic analysis together with the qSOFA score and presented with an odds ratio (OR) with a 95% confidence interval (CI). Categorical variables were compared using $\chi 2$ statistics. In order to assess the discriminatory power of the qSOFA score for predicting outcomes, we compared the C statistics of the qSOFA score with those of the CURB-65 and PSI scores. The C statistic is a summary measure of discrimination which quantifies the ability of the model to assign a high probability. C statistics are equivalent to the area under the receiver operating characteristic curve. C statistics range from 0.5 to 1.0; a measure of 0.5 indicates that the discrimination is caused by chance alone, and 1.0 indicates perfect discrimination. All p value analyses were two-sided and a p value of less than 0.05 was considered to be significant. All statistical analyses were performed with EZR (Saitama Medical Center, Jichii Medical University, Saitama, Japan), which is a graphical user interface for R (The R Foundation for Statistical Computing, Vienna, Austria). More precisely, it is a modified version of R commander designed to add statistical functions frequently used in biostatistics [15].

Results
Characteristics of the study cohort
A total of 1954 patients were evaluated in the enrollment period, and 909 were excluded, among which three were < 18 years, 133 were residents of an extended care facility or nursing home, 361 were recently discharged from hospital within 90 days, 301 were elderly or disabled and receiving nursing care, and 111 were receiving regular endovascular treatment as outpatients. Some patients fulfilled multiple items.

We ultimately enrolled 1045 patients with pneumonia, and their baseline characteristics are listed in Table 1. The median age of these patients was 77 (68–83) years, and 71.4% were males. The main comorbidities were respiratory diseases, such as chronic obstructive pulmonary disease (COPD) (25.5%) and bronchial asthma (13.8%), diabetes (19.5%), chronic heart failure (30.9%),

Table 1 Baseline characteristics of the study cohort

Variables	All encounters	In-hospital mortality			ICU admission		
		Non-survivors	Survivors	P value	ICU admission	Non-ICU	P value
Number of patients	1045	64 (6.1)	981 (93.9)		83 (7.9)	962 (92.1)	
Age, years	77 (68–83)	80 (74–85)	76 (68–83)	0.004	74 (66–82)	77 (68–84)	0.046
Male sex, %	746 (71.4)	51 (79.7)	697 (70.8)	0.15	64 (77.1)	682 (70.9)	0.26
Comorbidities, %							
COPD	266 (25.5)	26 (40.6)	240 (24.5)	0.007	24 (28.9)	242 (25.2)	0.51
Interstitial pneumonia	73 (7.0)	6 (9.4)	67 (6.8)	0.44	3 (3.6)	70 (7.3)	0.27
Old pulmonary tuberculosis	37 (3.5)	6 (9.4)	31 (3.2)	0.022	4 (4.8)	33 (3.4)	0.53
Asthma	144 (13.8)	5 (7.8)	139 (14.2)	0.19	10 (12.0)	134 (14.0)	0.74
Diabetes mellitus	203 (19.5)	14 (21.9)	189 (19.3)	0.63	22 (26.5)	181 (18.9)	0.11
Chronic liver disease	54 (5.2)	3 (4.7)	51 (5.2)	1.00	6 (7.2)	48 (5.0)	0.43
Congestive heart failure	323 (30.9)	22 (34.4)	301 (30.7)	0.58	29 (34.9)	294 (30.6)	0.46
Chronic kidney disease	94 (9.0)	5 (7.8)	89 (9.1)	1.00	5 (6.0)	89 (9.3)	0.43
Cerebrovascular disease	150 (14.3)	8 (12.5)	142 (14.5)	0.85	7 (8.4)	143 (14.9)	0.14
Malignancy	91 (8.7)	8 (12.5)	83 (8.5)	0.25	10 (12.0)	81 (8.4)	0.31
Vital signs							
Temperature, °C	37.8 (37.0–38.6)	37.1 (36.8–38.0)	38 (37.0–38.6)	0.001	38 (36.8–38.4)	38 (37.0–38.6)	0.07
Systolic blood pressure, mmHg	128 (111–148)	123 (105–143)	128(112–148)	0.21	120 (95–150)	128 (113–148)	0.032
Mean arterial pressure, mmHg	90 (78–103)	84 (76–100)	90 (78–103)	0.15	84 (69–103)	90 (78–103)	0.06
Respiratory rate, / min.	22 (20–26)	25 (20–30)	22 (19–26)	< 0.001	26 (23–30)	22 (19–25)	< 0.001
Heart rate, / min.	98 (84–111)	100 (84–115)	98 (84–111)	0.46	103 (89–124)	98 (84–110)	0.002
Mental confusion, %	134 (12.8)	24 (37.5)	110 (11.2)	< 0.001	32 (38.6)	102 (10.6)	< 0.001
Laboratory results							
Total protein, g/dl	6.6 (6.1–7.0)	6.1 (5.8–6.6)	6.6 (6.2–7.0)	< 0.001	6.1 (5.8–6.6)	6.6 (6.2–7.0)	< 0.001
Albumin, g/dl	3.2 (2.8–3.6)	2.8 (2.4–3.0)	3.3 (2.8–3.6)	< 0.001	2.9 (2.4–3.3)	3.2 (2.8–3.6)	< 0.001
AST, U/L	26 (20–39)	30 (22–44)	26 (19–39)	0.017	35 (22–58)	25 (19–37)	< 0.001
ALT, U/L	17 (12–28)	19 (11–33)	17 (12–27)	0.58	21 (14–36)	17 (12–27)	0.003
LDH, U/L	239 (195–293)	260 (211–342)	237 (195–290)	0.06	298 (240–383)	234 (193–284)	< 0.001
BUN, mg/dl	19 (14–27)	28 (20–38)	19 (14–26)	< 0.001	26 (18–41)	19 (14–25)	< 0.001
Na, mmol/L	137 (135–139)	137 (134–140)	137 (135–139)	0.90	137 (134–139)	137 (135–139)	0.35
Hgb, g/dl	12.4 (11.0–13.6)	12.2 (10.2–13.5)	12 (11.0–13.6)	0.33	13 (11.2–14.3)	12 (11.0–13.6)	0.049
WBC, $\times 10^9$/L	11.2 (8.1–15.2)	12.1 (8.2–15.9)	11 (8.1–15.2)	0.38	11 (7.3–15.9)	11 (8.1–15.1)	0.53
Platelets, $\times 10^9$/L	20.2 (15.0–26.6)	21.4 (16.4–27.6)	20 (14.9–26.5)	0.33	18 (13.3–23.7)	20 (15.3–26.9)	0.005
C-reactive protein, mg/dl	11.7 (5.5–18.8)	15.6 (11.4–24.0)	11.3 (5.2–18.3)	< 0.001	16.9 (9.3–27.9)	11.3 (5.2–17.8)	< 0.001
PCT, ng/mL	0.47 (0.14–2.22)	1.24 (0.31–6.79)	0.5 (0.13–2.11)	0.003	4.5 (0.80–17.56)	0.4 (0.13–1.84)	< 0.001
PaO_2/FIO_2 ratio, mmHg	265 (202–307)	178 (86–244)	267 (210–310)	< 0.001	116 (65–216)	271 (217–310)	< 0.001
$PaCO_2$, Torr	35.7 (32.0–40.2)	38.9 (31.9–52.3)	36 (32.0–40.0)	0.021	35 (30.7–47.4)	36 (32.0–40.0)	0.48
pH	7.45 (7.41–7.48)	7.4 (7.31–7.46)	7.5 (7.41–7.48)	< 0.001	7.4 (7.30–7.45)	7.5 (7.42–7.48)	< 0.001
Illness severity							
qSOFA	1 (0–1)	1 (1–2)	1 (0–1)	< 0.001	1 (1–2)	1 (0–1)	< 0.001
CURB-65	2 (1–2)	3 (2–3)	2 (1–2)	< 0.001	3 (2–4)	2 (1–2)	< 0.001
PSI points	97 (81–120)	130 (107–156)	96 (80–118)	< 0.001	128 (105–159)	96 (80–117)	< 0.001
PSI class	IV (III–IV)	IV (IV–V)	IV (III–IV)	< 0.001	IV (IV–V)	IV (III–IV)	< 0.001
SIRS	2 (1–3)	2 (1–3)	2 (1–3)	0.53	3 (2–3)	2 (1–3)	0.002

Table 1 Baseline characteristics of the study cohort *(Continued)*

Variables	All encounters	In-hospital mortality			ICU admission		
		Non-survivors	Survivors	*P* value	ICU admission	Non-ICU	*P* value
Outcomes							
Vasopressors, %	52 (5.0)	13 (20.3)	39 (4.0)	< 0.001	51 (61.4)	1 (0.1)	< 0.001
Respirator (including NPPV), %	89 (8.5)	26 (40.6)	63 (6.4)	< 0.001	69 (83.1)	20 (2.1)	< 0.001
ICU admission, %	83 (7.9)	22 (34.4)	61 (6.2)	< 0.001	–	–	
Hospital length of stay, days	11 (8–18)	11 (5–25)	11 (8–18)	0.21	21 (12–33)	11 (7–17)	< 0.001
28-day mortality, %	51 (4.9)	51 (79.7)	0 (0.0)	< 0.001	17 (20.5)	34 (3.5)	< 0.001
Hospital mortality, %	64 (6.1)	–	–		22 (26.5)	42 (4.4)	< 0.001

Data were expressed as a median (IQR) or number (%)
Abbreviations: *ALT* alanine aminotransferase, *AST* aspartate transaminase, *BUN* blood urea nitrogen, *COPD* chronic obstructive pulmonary disease, *CURB-65* confusion, urea, respiratory rate, blood pressure and age, *Hgb* hemoglobin, *ICU* intensive care unit, *IQR* interquartile range, *LDH* lactate dehydrogenase, *Na* sodium, *PSI* pneumonia severity index, *qSOFA* quick sequential (Sepsis-related) organ failure assessment, *SIRS* systemic inflammatory response syndrome, *WBC* white blood cell

and cerebrovascular diseases (14.3%). The median of qSOFA was 1 point (0–1), the median of CURB-65 was 2 points (1–2), and the median score of PSI was 97 (81–120) and its median class was class IV (III-IV).

The median duration of the hospital stay was 11 (8–18) days, the overall in-hospital mortality rate was 6.1%, the 28-day mortality rate was 4.9%, and the ICU admission rate was 7.9%.

Comparison between non-survivors and survivors

The median age (80 (74–85) vs 76 (68–83) years: $p = 0.004$) was significantly higher among non-survivors than survivors. Respiratory rates (25 (20–30) / min. vs 22 (19–26) / min.: $p < 0.001$) and mental confusion (37.5 vs 11.2%: $p < 0.001$) were significantly higher among non-survivors than survivors; however, no significant differences were noted in systolic blood pressure between the two groups ($p = 0.21$).

qSOFA, CURB-65, and PSI scores were significantly higher among non-survivors than survivors ($p < 0.001$) (Additional file 1: Figure S1-a).

Comparison between ICU and non-ICU admissions

Respiratory rates (26 (23–30) / min. vs 22 (19–25) / min.: $p < 0.001$) and mental confusion (38.6 vs 10.6%: $p < 0.001$) were significantly higher among ICU than non-ICU admissions. Systolic blood pressure was significantly lower among ICU than non-ICU admissions (120 vs 128 mmHg: $p = 0.032$).

qSOFA, CURB-65, and PSI scores were significantly higher among ICU than non-ICU admissions ($p < 0.001$) (Additional file 1: Figure S1-b).

In-hospital mortality and ICU admission rates according to each score

Among patients with pneumonia, 13.9% ($n = 145$) were screened with sepsis based on a qSOFA score ≥ 2 points.

In-hospital mortality rates were 2.1, 5.9, 17.3, and 16.7% for each of the qSOFA points. The mortality rate of a qSOFA score ≥ 2 points was significantly higher than that of a qSOFA score < 2 points (17.2 vs 4.3%, $p < 0.001$) (Fig. 1a).

ICU admission rates became higher as qSOFA scores increased. The ICU admission rate of a qSOFA score ≥ 2 points was significantly higher than that of a qSOFA score < 2 points (23.4 vs 5.4%: $p < 0.001$) (Fig. 1a).

Hospitalization was recommended for 60.8% ($n = 635$) and 59.9% ($n = 626$) of patients based on the CURB-65 score (≥ 2) and PSI class (≥ IV), respectively.

The hospital mortality and ICU admission rates of CURB-65 and PSI also became higher as qSOFA scores increased. The hospital mortality and ICU admission rates for patients with a CURB-65 score ≥ 2 points and PSI class ≥ IV were significantly higher than those with the lower cut-off values ($p < 0.001$) (Fig. 1b, c).

Score performance

The *C* statistics of qSOFA for predicting hospital mortality was 0.69 (95% CI, 0.63–0.75), and no significant differences were observed between CURB-65 (*C* statistics, 0.75; 95% CI 0.69–0.81; $p = 0.11$) and PSI (*C* statistics, 0.74; 95% CI, 0.69–0.80; $p = 0.18$) (Fig. 2a).

The *C* statistics of qSOFA for predicting ICU admission was 0.76 (95% CI 0.71–0.80), and no significant differences were noted between CURB-65 (*C* statistics, 0.73; 95% CI 0.67–0.79; $p = 0.41$) and PSI (*C* statistics, 0.72; 95% CI 0.66–0.78; $p = 0.21$) (Fig. 2b).

Sensitivity, specificity, and the likelihood ratio

A qSOFA score ≥ 2 points presented moderate sensitivity at 39% and high specificity at 88% for predicting hospital mortality. A CURB-65 score ≥ 2 points and PSI class ≥ IV presented high sensitivity, moderate specificity, and a high negative likelihood (Table 2).

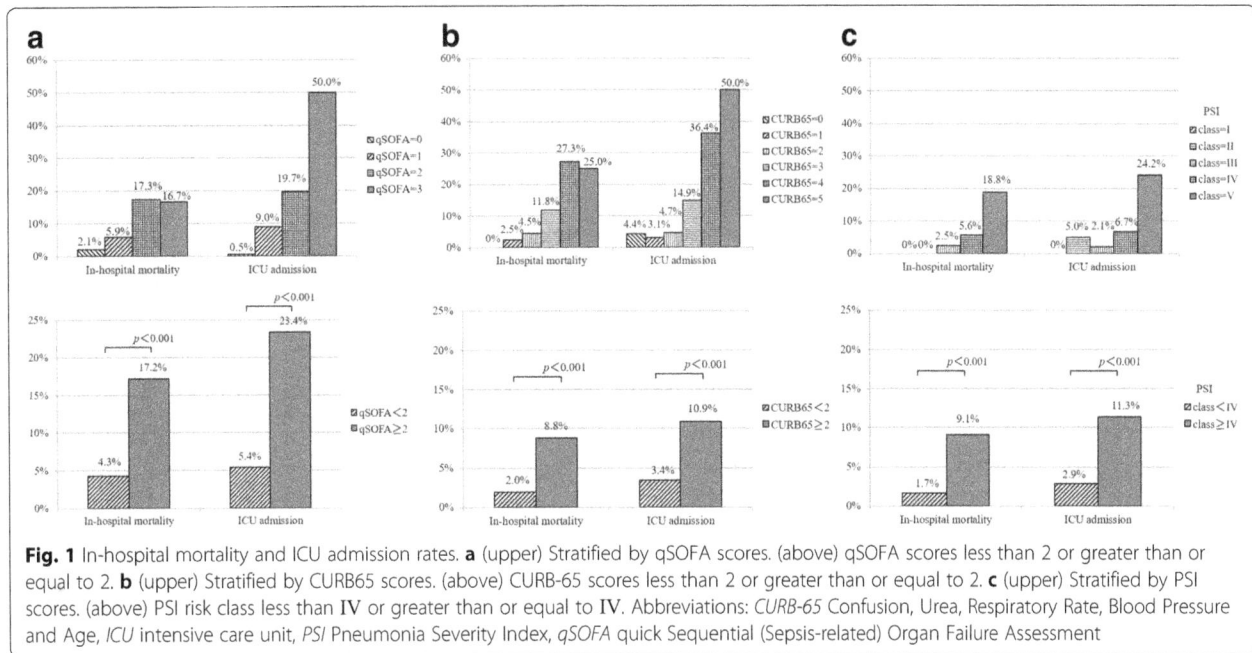

Fig. 1 In-hospital mortality and ICU admission rates. **a** (upper) Stratified by qSOFA scores. (above) qSOFA scores less than 2 or greater than or equal to 2. **b** (upper) Stratified by CURB65 scores. (above) CURB-65 scores less than 2 or greater than or equal to 2. **c** (upper) Stratified by PSI scores. (above) PSI risk class less than IV or greater than or equal to IV. Abbreviations: *CURB-65* Confusion, Urea, Respiratory Rate, Blood Pressure and Age, *ICU* intensive care unit, *PSI* Pneumonia Severity Index, *qSOFA* quick Sequential (Sepsis-related) Organ Failure Assessment

The prediction of ICU admission was similar, with a qSOFA score ≥ 2 points presenting moderate sensitivity and high specificity, and a CURB-65 score ≥ 2 points and PSI class ≥ IV presenting high sensitivity and moderate specificity (Table 3).

Discussion

The present study is the first to compare the prognostic performance of qSOFA with existing pneumonia severity scores (CURB-65 and PSI) for CAP of high severity and mortality that requires hospitalization. Regarding hospitalized CAP, the prognostic performance of qSOFA for in-hospital mortality did not significantly differ from the existing pneumonia severity scores (CURB-65 and PSI). Furthermore, no significant difference was observed in the prediction performance for ICU admission. PSI is the most famous severity classification of CAP [14], and it has been clearly shown to correlate with mortality. However, this index involves 20 evaluation items and its calculation is complex; therefore, its practical use in a busy clinical setting is limited. On the other hand, CURB-65 has been described as a convenient classification with only five items (confusion, urea, respiratory rate, blood pressure, and age) with high practicality and excellent prognostic accuracy [11]. However, "Urea > 7 mmol/L" requires a blood test. qSOFA has fewer evaluation items than CURB-65 and PSI, and because it involves tests that may be conducted at the bedside, it is regarded as a simpler prognostic tool than CURB-65 and PSI.

The prognostic performance of disease-specific severity scores is excellent because the severity classification was created using a database for each disease. CURB-65

and PSI were also created from a pneumonia database [11, 14]. Therefore, it was of interest that qSOFA, which was created for general infectious diseases, did not significantly differ from pneumonia-specific severity classifications, such as CURB-65 and PSI. The use of separate severity scores for each disease is considered to be burdensome. The present results demonstrated that qSOFA, which may be used for other diseases, may be substituted for existing severity scores for CAP and may be particularly useful for non-respiratory specialists.

Three previous studies were conducted on qSOFA for CAP: 1641 patients in China (28-day mortality rate: 33%, C statistics for predicting 28-day mortality: 0.655), 9327 patients in Germany (30-day mortality rate: 3.0%, C statistics for predicting 30-day mortality: 0.70), and 6874 patients in Spain (in-hospital mortality: 6.4%, C statistics for predicting in-hospital mortality: 0.649) [3, 10, 12]. Although mortality rates markedly varied among these studies, the C statistics of qSOFA for predicting mortality ranged between 0.655 and 0.70, with no significant differences being observed between studies. While our results revealed a 28-day mortality rate of 4.9% and in-hospital mortality rate of 6.1%, the C statistics of 0.69 for in-hospital mortality was in accordance with previous studies [3, 10, 12]. Therefore, qSOFA may be used for CAP irrespective of mortality, regional differences, and patient background differences.

The present study on patients with CAP showed that the C statistics of qSOFA for predicting in-hospital mortality was 0.69, which was lower than that of 0.81 in the original study [2]. Three previous studies on patients with CAP also showed C statistics for predicting

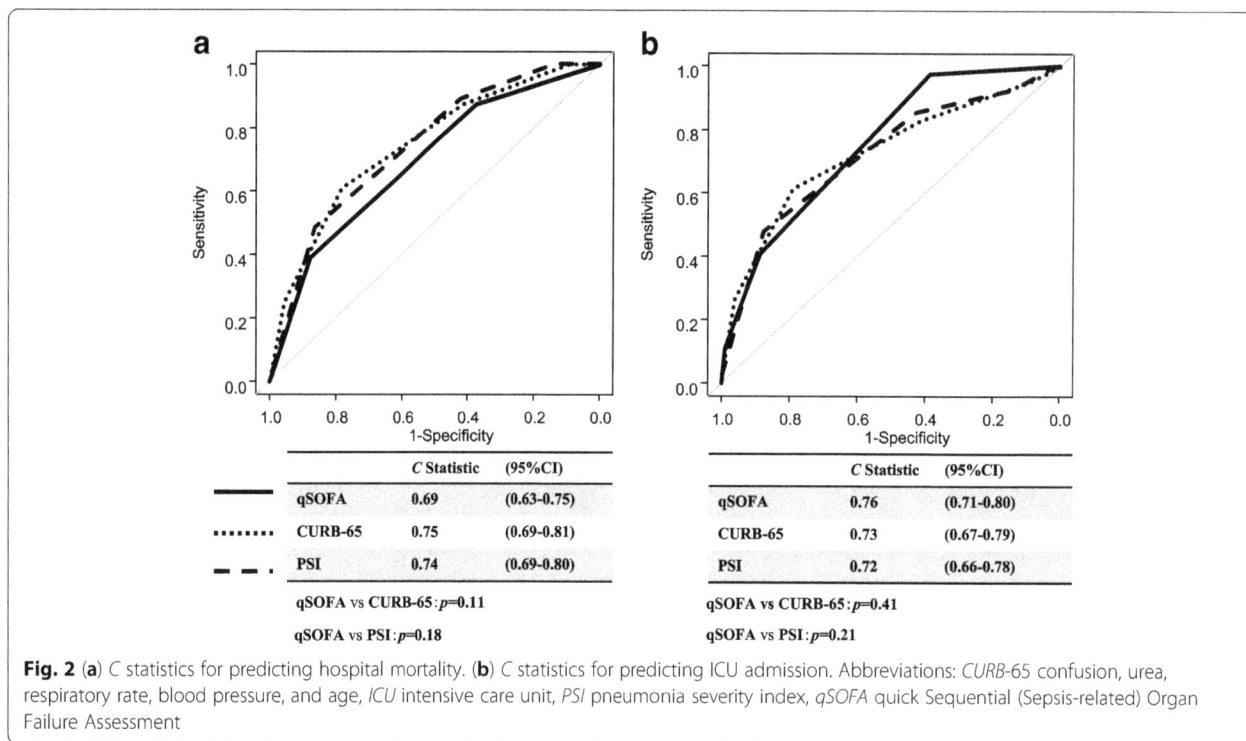

Fig. 2 (**a**) *C* statistics for predicting hospital mortality. (**b**) *C* statistics for predicting ICU admission. Abbreviations: *CURB*-65 confusion, urea, respiratory rate, blood pressure, and age, *ICU* intensive care unit, *PSI* pneumonia severity index, *qSOFA* quick Sequential (Sepsis-related) Organ Failure Assessment

mortality of between 0.655 and 0.70 [3, 10, 12]. The respiratory rate, which was one of the three qSOFA criteria evaluated in the present study, scored positive in at least 50% of the 1045 patients analyzed (Fig. 3). Since qSOFA only has three criteria, having a positive score for one of the criteria in more than 50% of patients may have decreased its reliability, thereby reducing the *C* statistics. The reason for the reduced *C* statistics may be the low cut-off value for the respiratory rate. Therefore, we changed the cut-off value for the respiratory rate in qSOFA to ≥ 30/min, which was the same as that in CURB-65 or PSI. However, no significant difference was observed, even though it changed from ≥ 22/min to ≥ 30/min (*C* statistics: qSOFA 0.69, qSOFA (RR ≥ 30/min) 0.71; $p = 0.28$) (Additional file 2: Figure S2).

Previous studies comparing qSOFA with CURB-65 and PSI were reviewed by the Spanish study [12] described above, in which qSOFA had a lower prognostic performance than CURB-65 and PSI. CURB-65 and PSI included age as an item of severity. The severity score in elderly patients was slightly high when measured by PSI

because a patient's age largely contributes to its scoring system. Since the median age of our study population was more than 10 years older than that of the Spanish study, patients in our study may have scored higher in PSI, thereby reducing the *C* statistics. Besides CURB-65 and PSI, many severity classifications include age as an evaluation item. Previous studies reported that it was not necessary to include age (older than 65 years) as one of the three items in qSOFA [3, 5]. In the present study, the addition of age to qSOFA did not affect the results obtained (qSOFA vs qSOFA + age ≥ 65: $p = 0.10$), although *C* statistics slightly increased to 0.71 (Additional file 3: Figure S3); therefore, the addition of age was unnecessary based on convenience.

In the present study, 13.9% of pneumonia cases were diagnosed with sepsis with a qSOFA score ≥ 2 points, and the mortality rate of a qSOFA score ≥ 2 points was 17.2%. This severity was close to "life-threatening organ dysfunction caused by a dysregulated host response to infection, in-hospital mortality rate 10%" defined as sepsis-3. As the score of qSOFA became higher,

Table 2 Performance of qSOFA for predicting hospital mortality

	Cut-off	Sensitivity	Specificity	PPV	NPV	OR	95%CI	
							5%	95%
qSOFA	≥ 2	39.1%	87.8%	17.2%	95.7%	4.61	2.57	8.12
CURB-65	≥ 2	87.5%	41.0%	8.8%	98.0%	4.89	2.29	12.01
PSI	$\geq IV$	89.1%	42.0%	9.1%	98.3%	5.88	2.64	15.46

Abbreviations: *CURB-65* Confusion, Urea, Respiratory Rate, Blood Pressure and Age; *ICU* intensive care unit; *PSI* Pneumonia Severity Index; *qSOFA* quick Sequential (Sepsis-related) Organ Failure Assessment; *PPV* positive predictive value; *NPV* negative predictive value; *OR* odds ratio

Table 3 Performance of qSOFA for predicting ICU admission

	Cut-off	Sensitivity	Specificity	PPV	NPV	OR	95%CI	
							5%	95%
qSOFA	≥ 2	41.0%	88.5%	23.4%	94.6%	5.30	3.18	8.80
CURB-65	≥ 2	83.1%	41.2%	10.9%	96.6%	3.44	1.89	6.72
PSI	≥ IV	85.5%	42.3%	11.3%	97.1%	4.33	2.29	8.90

Abbreviations: *CURB-65* Confusion, Urea, Respiratory Rate, Blood Pressure and Age; *ICU* intensive care unit; *PSI* Pneumonia Severity Index; *qSOFA* quick Sequential (Sepsis-related) Organ Failure Assessment; *PPV* positive predictive value; *NPV* negative predictive value; *OR* odds ratio

in-hospital mortality and ICU admission rates gradually increased, the in-hospital mortality rate for patients with a qSOFA score ≥ 2 points was fourfold higher than those with lower cut-off values, and the ICU admission rate was fivefold higher. Previous studies that investigated qSOFA in CAP showed high specificity, but moderate sensitivity, similar to the present study. On the other hand, CURB-65 and PSI showed high sensitivity and moderate specificity. *C* statistics were no significantly different between these predictive models; qSOFA might be used to screen severe pneumonia, because of its high specificity.

Limitations

The limitations of the present study were as follows. First, it was a single-center secondary analysis of data from a prospective observational study. The prospective observational study of qSOFA was only one study targeting all infectious diseases in the emergency department [4], and there has not yet been a prospective observational study on qSOFA for pneumonia. Therefore, multicenter prospective studies are needed in order to validate our results. Furthermore, although the *C* statistics of qSOFA for predicting mortality was similar to the three previous studies [3, 10, 12], there are still only four studies on pneumonia, including the present study; therefore, the evaluation of qSOFA for pneumonia is currently insufficient. In addition, it is unclear whether

qSOFA may be used reliably for patients in different regions or with varying backgrounds. Second, it was that the present study only considered hospitalized CAP. Pneumonia in patients with a poor performance status and hospital-acquired pneumonia also need to be considered. Third, the present study have the potential for the information bias given our retrospective study design. We attempted to reduce the information bias by using a prospectively collected data. Forth, the decision to enter the ICU is decided based on preset ICU admission criteria (such as, respiratory failure requiring mechanical ventilation, circulatory failure requiring vasopressor, confusion, etc.). However, potential selection bias existed, e.g., the decision of the physician might be biased by the score. Finally, if the period from emergency department visit to ICU admission was long, the meaning of the score at entry could be diminished. But in our study, the length from emergency department visit to ICU admission was all within 7 days except for two cases.

Conclusion

Regarding hospitalized CAP, the prognostic performance of qSOFA for in-hospital mortality and ICU admission was not significantly different to those of CURB-65 and PSI. Since qSOFA only requires a few items and vital signs, it may be particularly useful for emergency department or non-respiratory specialists.

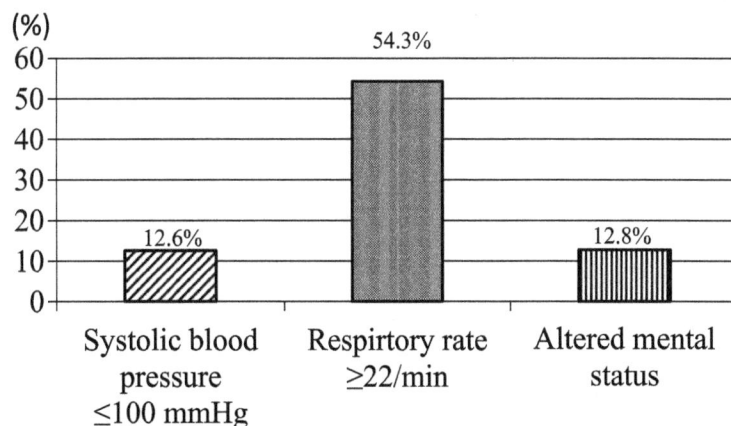

Fig. 3 Distribution of each criterion of qSOFA. Abbreviations: *qSOFA* quick Sequential (sepsis-related) Organ Failure Assessment

Additional files

Additional file 1: Figure S1. Distribution of illness severity. **a** Survivors and non-survivors. **b** Non-ICU admission and ICU admission. (PPTX 111 kb)

Additional file 2: Figure S2. C statistics for predicting hospital mortality (qSOFA [RR ≥ 30]). (PPTX 77 kb)

Additional file 3: Figure S3. C statistics for predicting hospital mortality (qSOFA + age ≥ 65). (PPTX 76 kb)

Abbreviations

CURB-65: Confusion, urea, respiratory rate, blood pressure, and age; ICU: Intensive care unit; PSI: Pneumonia Severity Index; qSOFA: Quick Sequential (sepsis-related) Organ Failure Assessment

Authors' contributions

HO analyzed and interpreted patient data. YW and AI managed data, including quality control. TI supervised the conduct of the trial and data collection. FT was a major contributor in writing the manuscript. All authors read and approved the final manuscript.

Competing interests

The authors declare that they have no competing interests.

Author details

[1]Department of Respiratory Medicine, Kurashiki Central Hospital, 1-1-1 Miwa, Kurashiki, Okayama 710-8602, Japan. [2]Center for Clinical Epidemiology, St. Luke's International University, Tokyo, Japan.

References

1. Singer M, Deutschman CS, Seymour CW, Shankar-Hari M, Annane D, Bauer M, et al. The third international consensus definitions for sepsis and septic shock (Sepsis-3). JAMA. 2016;315:801–10.
2. Seymour CW, Liu VX, Iwashyna TJ, Brunkhorst FM, Rea TD, Scherag A, et al. Assessment of clinical criteria for sepsis: for the third international consensus definitions for sepsis and septic shock (Sepsis-3). JAMA. 2016;315:762–74.
3. Chen YX, Wang JY, Guo SB. Use of CRB-65 and quick sepsis-related organ failure assessment to predict site of care and mortality in pneumonia patients in the emergency department: a retrospective study. Crit Care. 2016;20:167.
4. Freund Y, Lemachatti N, Krastinova E, Van Laer M, Claessens YE, Avondo A, Occelli C, et al. Prognostic accuracy of sepsis-3 criteria for in-hospital mortality among patients with suspected infection presenting to the emergency department. JAMA. 2017;317:301–8.
5. Wang JY, Chen YX, Guo SB, Mei X, Yang P. Predictive performance of quick sepsis-related organ failure assessment for mortality and ICU admission in patients with infection at the ED. Am J Emerg Med. 2016;34:1788–93.
6. Churpek MM, Snyder A, Han X, Sokol S, Pettit N, Howell MD, Edelson DP. Quick sepsis-related organ failure assessment, systemic inflammatory response syndrome, and early warning scores for detecting clinical deterioration in infected patients outside the intensive care unit. Am J Respir Crit Care Med. 2017;195:906–11.
7. Hwang SY, Jo IJ, Lee SU, Lee TR, Yoon H, Cha WC, et al. Low accuracy of positive qSOFA criteria for predicting 28-day mortality in critically ill septic patients during the early period after emergency department presentation. Ann Emerg Med. 2018;71:1–9.
8. Kim M, Ahn S, Kim WY, Sohn CH, Seo DW, Lee YS, Lim KS. Predictive performance of the quick sequential organ failure assessment score as a screening tool for sepsis, mortality, and intensive care unit admission in patients with febrile neutropenia. Support Care Cancer. 2017;25:1557–62.
9. Bone RC, Balk RA, Cerra FB, Dellinger RP, Fein AM, Knaus WA, et al. Definitions for sepsis and organ failure and guidelines for the use of innovative therapies in sepsis. The ACCP/SCCM consensus conference committee. American College of Chest Physicians/Society of Critical Care Medicine. Chest. 1992;101:1644–55.
10. Kolditz M, Scherag A, Rohde G, Ewig S, Welte T, Pletz M, Capnetz study group. Comparison of the qSOFA and CRB-65 for risk prediction in patients with community-acquired pneumonia. Intensive Care Med. 2016;42:2108–10.
11. Lim WS, van der Eerden MM, Laing R, Boersma WG, Karalus N, Town GI, Lewis SA, Macfarlane JT. Defining community acquired pneumonia severity on presentation to hospital: an international derivation and validation study. Thorax. 2003;58:377–82.
12. Ranzani OT, Prina E, Menendez R, Ceccato A, Cilloniz C, Mendez R, et al. New sepsis definition (Sepsis-3) and community-acquired pneumonia mortality. A validation and clinical decision-making study. Am J Respir Crit Care Med. 2017;196:1287–97.
13. Strehlow MC, Emond SD, Shapiro NI, Pelletier AJ, Camargo CA Jr, et al. National study of emergency department visits for sepsis, 1992 to 2001. Ann Emerg Med. 2006;48:326–31.
14. Fine MJ, Auble TE, Yealy DM, Hanusa BH, Weissfeld LA, Singer DE, et al. A prediction rule to identify low-risk patients with community-acquired pneumonia. N Engl J Med. 1997;336:243–50.
15. Kanda Y. Investigation of the freely-available easy-to-use software "EZR" (easy R) for medical statistics. Bone Marrow Transplant. 2013;48:452–8.

25

Immunosenescence in neurocritical care

Shigeaki Inoue*, Masafumi Saito and Joji Kotani

Abstract

Background: Several advanced and developing countries are now entering a superaged society, in which the percentage of elderly people exceeds 20% of the total population. In such an aging society, the number of age-related diseases such as malignant tumors, diabetes, and severe infections including sepsis is increasing, and patients with such disorders often find themselves in the ICU.

Main body: Age-related diseases are closely related to age-induced immune dysfunction, by which reductions in the efficiency and specificity of the immune system are collectively termed "immunosenescence." The most noticeable is a decline in the antigen-specific acquired immune response. The exhaustion of T cells in elderly sepsis is related to an increase in nosocomial infections after septicemia, and even death over subacute periods. Another characteristic is that senescent cells that accumulate in body tissues over time cause chronic inflammation through the secretion of proinflammatory cytokines, termed senescence-associated secretory phenotype. Chronic inflammation associated with aging has been called "inflammaging," and similar age-related diseases are becoming an urgent social problem.

Conclusion: In neuro ICUs, several neuro-related diseases including stroke and sepsis-associated encephalopathy are related to immunosenescence and neuroinflammation in the elderly. Several advanced countries with superaged societies face the new challenge of improving the long-term prognosis of neurocritical patients.

Keywords: Sepsis, Elderly, Immunosenescence, Immune paralysis

Background

Japan is facing the social problem of a declining birth rate and an aging population, in which it is estimated that people aged at least 65 will constitute 30% of the total population by 2030. The average age of citizens is rising not only in Japan but also in advanced regions such as Europe and the USA, as well as in many Asian countries such as China and South Korea. It is predicted that by 2050, most of the world's population except for Africa and the Middle East will be at least 65 years old. With the percentage of elderly people exceeding 20%, we are entering a superaged society [1]. In such an aging society, various diseases such as malignant tumors, diabetes, and severe infections are increasing, and patients with such disorders often find themselves in an intensive care unit (ICU). These diseases are closely associated with age-related immune dysfunction so-called immunosenescence.

What Is the immune system?

Immunity is the means by which multicellular organisms resist the attacks of harmful invading microorganisms. Such immunity is achieved by two systems: innate immunity and adaptive immunity.

The innate immune system mainly comprises innate immune cells (macrophages: neutrophils, dendritic cells) and complement factors. Innate immune cells are also called phagocytes because they phagocytose when they recognize foreign substances such as lipopolysaccharides (LPSs). Complement factors circulate in the blood and are activated by the membrane of the microorganism to directly destroy the pathogen or activate phagocytic cells indirectly to eliminate the pathogen. The innate immune system is activated within several hours of encountering pathogens, etc. However, the efficiency of this activation is not affected by previous infections.

In contrast, the adaptive immune system consists primarily of T and B cells and in theory can eliminate an infinite variety of targets. Although the acquired immune system functions as early as 2–4 days after encountering the pathogen, some T and B cells respond specifically to the invading microorganisms, even after the immune response has ended.

* Correspondence: inoues@med.kobe-u.ac.jp
Department of Disaster and Emergency Medicine, Kobe University Graduate
School of Medicine, Kusunoki-cho 7-5-2, Chuo-ward, Kobe 650-0017, Japan

The response is maintained as an immune memory and can be activated quickly when subsequent encounters with the same pathogen occur.

Because CD4 + T cells, which constitute the "control tower" of acquired immunity, cannot recognize microbial components such as LPSs, the acquired immunity response to microorganisms depends on the phagocytic cells of the innate immunity. This role is fulfilled by specialized cells called dendritic cells. When dendritic cells are activated by inflammatory cytokines such as LPSs and inflammatory cytokines produced by macrophages, they present fragments of pathogens digested intracellularly to T cells and induce the activation of antigen-specific T cells. During that process, naive T cells are stimulated and differentiated into effector T cells that can kill cells or activate other cells. Effector T cells activate B cells, so that B cells produce antibodies that recognize microorganisms.

Immunosenescence

Aging is a biological change that occurs in individuals over time and involves a decline in function and processes that is particularly apparent as the organism dies. This is a biological process that is common to all living things. Our bodies undergo functional deterioration with organic changes at various sites depending on aging. There are various theories about the aging mechanism, but telomere shortening always accompanies aging. Oxidative stress induced by molecular species such as active oxygen damages the genome, and somatic cells are thought to cause senescence-related protein accumulation and senescence. The immune system is similarly affected, and the immune response in normal individuals is dependent on aging. Because the prevalence of malignant tumors and infectious diseases increases with an age-related decline in immune function, it is presumed that there is some relationship between this reduction in immune function and the onset of these diseases.

The efficiency and specificity of the immune system decline with age. The most noticeable change in immune function associated with aging is a decrease in antigen-specific acquired immunity. Although elderly people generally retain pathogen-specific immune memory obtained when young, the efficiency of their response to new infections and vaccines is often low. Another characteristic is that senescent cells accumulate in body tissues over time and cause chronic inflammation. This is known as the senescence-associated secretory phenotype (SASP) and is described later [2]. The chronic inflammation accompanying such aging is called "inflammaging" (inflammation + aging), and its relationship with age-related disease is attracting increasing attention [3, 4]. The functional changes to the immune system that accompany aging are generally called immunosenescence. Hematopoietic stem cells are the source of all immune response cells, but their numbers in the bone marrow are not affected by aging. However,

the differentiation of hematopoietic stem cells into lymphoid common precursor cells decreases and shifts toward differentiation into myeloid-type common progenitor cells over time [5, 6]. Therefore, differentiation into lymphoid cells (T cells, B cells) decreases and differentiation into myeloid cells (granulocytes/monocytes) increases (Fig. 1). The roles of each immunocompetent cell and the changes associated with aging are described below.

Innate immunity (Fig. 2)
Neutrophils

Neutrophil is an essential part of the innate immune, which is chemotactic with regard to cytokines and pathogens such as bacteria and fungi. They infiltrate the inflamed region to engulf, disinfect, and decompose foreign substances including bacteria and fungi and are the main protagonist of inflammation and immunity in the early stages of infection. Neutrophils experience less pronounced changes than T cells with age, and there is no change in the expression level of receptors that are important for intracellular signal transduction factors such as neutrophil count, phagocytosis capability, and toll-like receptors 2 and 4. However, aging is accompanied by reduced superoxide and chemotaxin production and by a decline in bactericidal activity [7] (Fig. 2).

Macrophages

Macrophages are chemotactic phagocytes that move around the body like amoeba. They decompose and digest foreign bodies such as dead cells and their fragments, and invading bacteria. Macrophages have antigen-presenting capability and activate CD4 + T cells by fragmenting degraded foreign matter and presenting it to them. As with neutrophils, the number of macrophages is not affected by aging, but phagocytic activity, and the production of superoxide and nitric oxide (NO) do decline with age [8, 9]. Moreover, activation is impaired in the macrophages of elderly mice, i.e., the ability to present antigens to T cells is reduced [9, 10] and reactivity with interferon-γ (IFN-γ) declines [10].

Dendritic cells

Dendritic cells, which is a generic term for unspecified cells that exhibit dendritic morphology, have become widely known as antigen-presenting cells in recent years. They are present in tissues that come into contact with the exterior environment, including the skin, the nasal cavity, the lungs, the stomach, and the intestinal tract. They process antigens from microorganisms and promptly present them to CD4 + T cells, thereby acting as a link to acquired immunity. Recently, the observation that dendritic cells change with age has led to the suggestion that the number of Langerhans cells decreases in the elderly. The migration of dendritic cells to lymph nodes is impaired in elderly mice [11], and it has been reported that

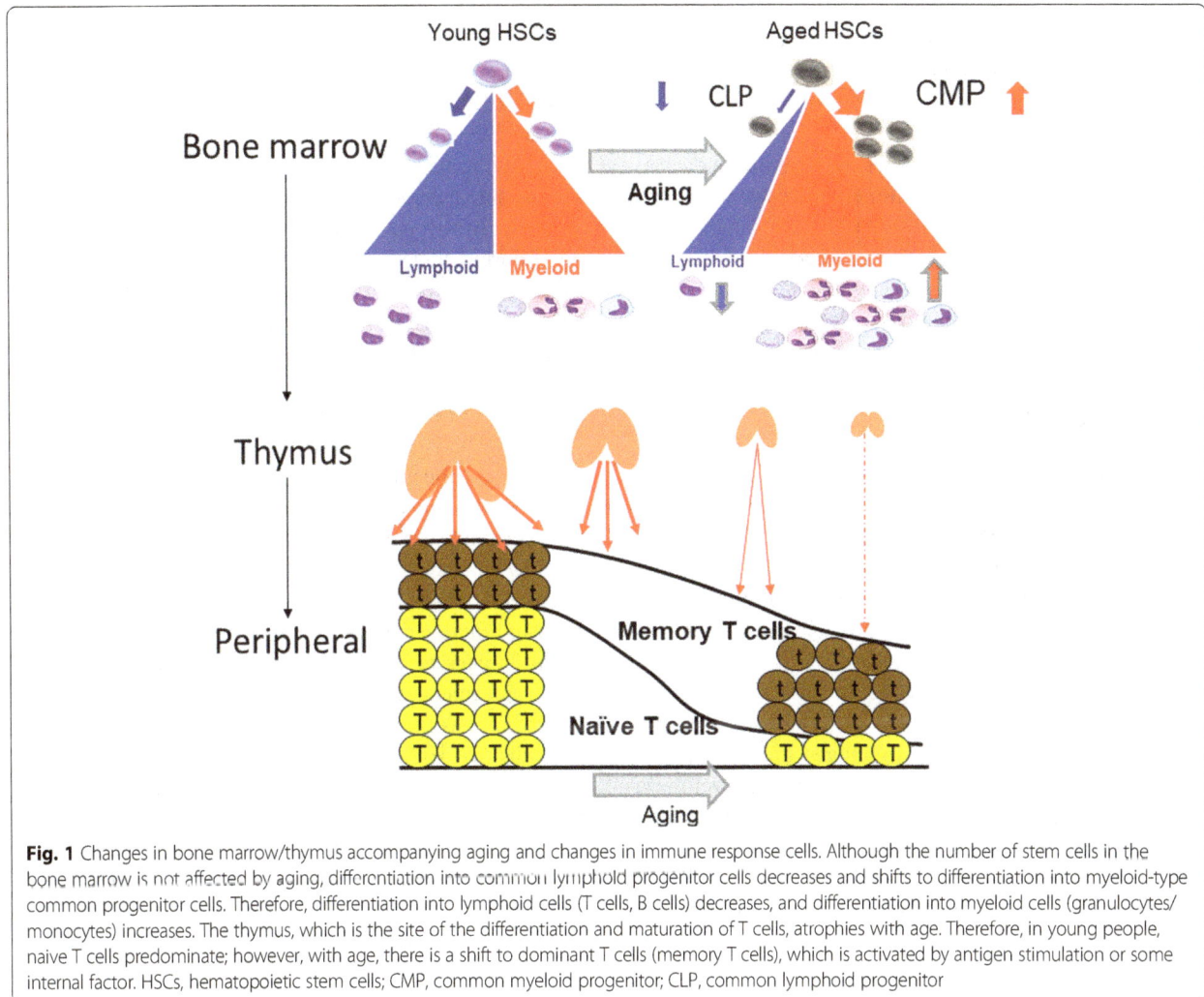

Fig. 1 Changes in bone marrow/thymus accompanying aging and changes in immune response cells. Although the number of stem cells in the bone marrow is not affected by aging, differentiation into common lymphoid progenitor cells decreases and shifts to differentiation into myeloid-type common progenitor cells. Therefore, differentiation into lymphoid cells (T cells, B cells) decreases, and differentiation into myeloid cells (granulocytes/monocytes) increases. The thymus, which is the site of the differentiation and maturation of T cells, atrophies with age. Therefore, in young people, naive T cells predominate; however, with age, there is a shift to dominant T cells (memory T cells), which is activated by antigen stimulation or some internal factor. HSCs, hematopoietic stem cells; CMP, common myeloid progenitor; CLP, common lymphoid progenitor

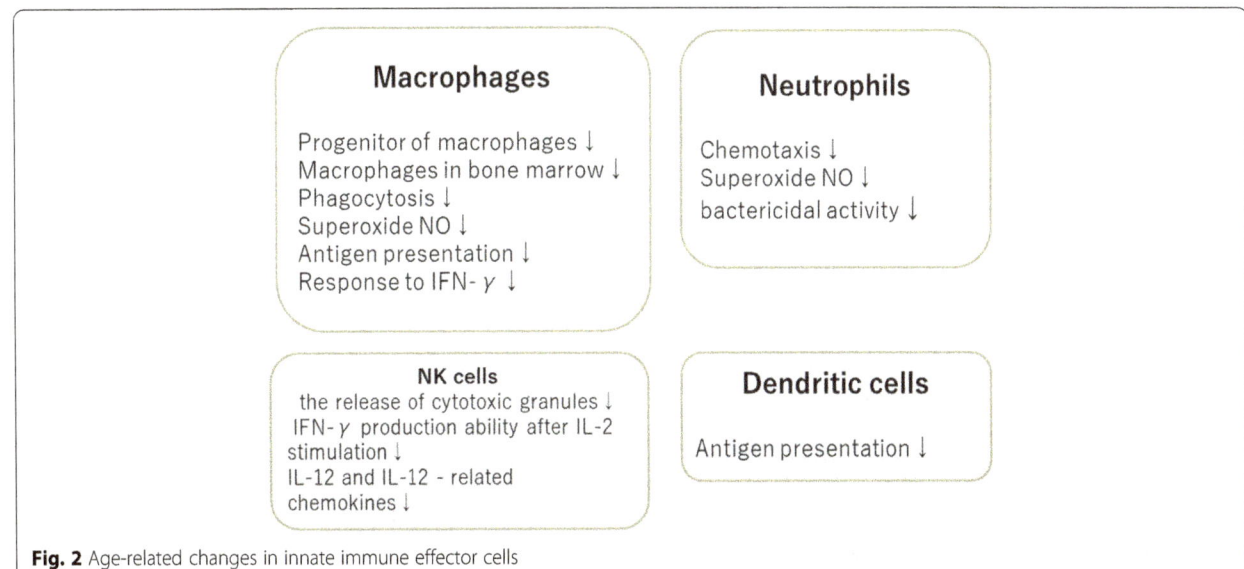

Fig. 2 Age-related changes in innate immune effector cells

major histocompatibility complex 2(MHC2), CD80/86, and other molecules are expressed less and have impaired antigen-presenting capability [12].

Natural killer (NK) cells

NK cells are cytotoxic lymphocytes that make an indispensable contribution to innate immunity. They are particularly important for eliminating tumors and virus-infected cells. Although it is not clear how the reduction in the number of NK cells is linked to aging, the release of cytotoxic granules and the decrease in IFN-γ production capability after stimulation with interleukin-2 (IL-2), IL-12, and IL-12-related chemokines [macrophage inflammatory proteins-1a (MIP-1a), regulated on activation, normal T cell expressed and secreted (RANTES), IL-8] reduce the production of NK cells [13]. Therefore, it is possible that virus removal in the early stages of infection may be impaired by aging [14]. A reduction in NK activity associated with aging has been reported in patients with oral candidiasis, and it has been suggested that aging is involved in the onset and progress of the disorder [15].

Adaptive immunity (Fig. 3)

B cells

B cells proliferate in response to antigen invasion and differentiate into plasma cells that produce antibodies (immunoglobulins). They are also affected by aging. For example, in the elderly, the ability to produce immunoglobulin M (IgM) antibodies decreases, and IgM antibody titers are also lower than that in healthy adults after ingesting pneumococcal vaccine [16, 17]. Antibody production capacity for influenza vaccines is also approximately 50% of that in healthy adults [18, 19]. The reason for this is that differentiation, proliferation, activation, and maintenance of memory B cells are impaired in the elderly [20] and, as described

above, functional disorders of CD4 + T cells associated with aging affect B cell activation [21] (Fig. 3).

T cells

The most dynamically age-dependent change with regard to immunity occurs in the thymus, which plays an important role in the differentiation and maturation of T cells. In humans, thymic epithelial tissues gradually become atrophied during adolescence, are replaced with adipose tissue, and become almost fatty remnants from maturity to old age. The thymus is a primary lymphoid organ that serves as a site of differentiation, maturation, and the selection of T cells from inflowing hematopoietic stem cells, suggesting that the generation of new functional mature T cells and their supply to the periphery is affected by age. This means that the activity of the thymus rapidly declines (Fig. 3). There is a greater proportion of naive T cells that have not yet received antigen stimulation in the young compared with T cells activated by antigen stimulation or some internal factor (memory T cells), which are predominant in the old. Furthermore, the length and activity of the telomeres within T cells, the responsiveness to cytokines that activate T cells such as IFN-γ and interleukin-2 (IL-2), and decreased proliferation of T cells are associated with aging [22, 23].

T cells are roughly divided into CD4 + T cells and CD8 + T cells. CD4 + T cells are activated by antigen presentation from macrophages, dendritic cells, etc., and act as controllers of the acquired immune system. During its activation, CD28—a surface antigen of T cells—plays an important role as a costimulatory molecule. CD4 + T cells are activated via CD28 to become effector T cells, but the prevalence of CD28 on T cells decreases with age [24], T cell activation disorder, viruses, etc. [25]. In contrast to the effects of CD28, T cell activity is suppressed via surface receptors such as

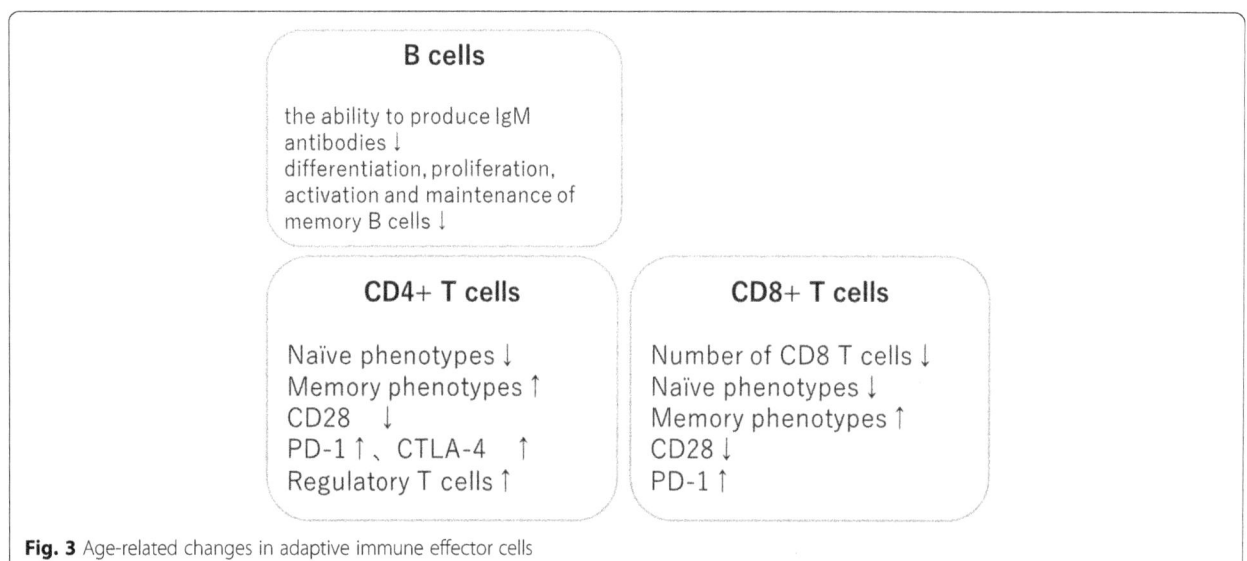

B cells

the ability to produce IgM antibodies ↓
differentiation, proliferation, activation and maintenance of memory B cells ↓

CD4+ T cells

Naïve phenotypes ↓
Memory phenotypes ↑
CD28   ↓
PD-1 ↑、CTLA-4   ↑
Regulatory T cells ↑

CD8+ T cells

Number of CD8 T cells ↓
Naïve phenotypes ↓
Memory phenotypes ↑
CD28 ↓
PD-1 ↑

Fig. 3 Age-related changes in adaptive immune effector cells

programmed cell death protein 1 (PD-1) and cytotoxic T-lymphocyte-associated protein 4 (CTLA-4).

T cell exhaustion in elderly patients with sepsis

Although the mechanism by which immunosuppression takes place after septicemia remains unclear, Hotchkiss et al. confirmed that the number of lymphocytes decreases owing to apoptosis in sepsis patients [26]. In addition to the lymphocyte count, attention has recently been focused on T cell dysfunction after sepsis, i.e., T cell exhaustion. T cell exhaustion means narrowing of the T cell antigen receptor (TCR) repertoire due to long-term exposure to antigens, decreased TCR signaling, and reduced levels of PD-1 and CTLA-4. The T cells are in a dysfunctional state as a result of the induction of various co-suppressive molecules, such as CTLA-4 and T cell immunoglobulin and mucin-domain containing-3 (TIM-3), and disorders in IL-2 production, activation, and proliferation [27–29].

In a previous study conducted by this research team, we found an increase in the level of PD-1-positive T cells and reduced IL-2 production, activation, and proliferation in elderly sepsis patients and older mouse sepsis models [30]. In the acute phase within 0–2 days after septicemia diagnosis, the rate of bacterial infection of the blood was similar in elderly and young patients, but 2 and 4 weeks after septicemia the rate of bacterial infection was higher in the elderly than in the young. In comparison, the opportunistic infection by attenuated pathogens such as *Acinetobacter* species, *Stenotrophomonas maltophilia*, and *Candida albicans* increased. Based on the above, we think that T cell exhaustion and death during subacute periods in elderly patients with sepsis are related to an increase in nosocomial infections after septicemia.

Aging and chronic inflammation

The SASP hypothesis, in which the senescent cells that accumulate in body tissues over time contribute to inflammation progression in the elderly, has recently been proposed [2]. First, during aging, the p53/RAS/pl6 signaling pathway is activated by DNA damage, reactive oxygen species (ROS) accumulation, telomere shortening, and cellular senescence. This produces the SASP phenotype, which secretes inflammatory cytokines such as IL-1β, IL-6, and IL-8, and vascular growth factors such as vascular endothelial growth factor. Further cell senescence and chronic inflammation of the surrounding cells are thought to be prolonged by this phenotype [2]. Persistent chronic inflammation that is not related to such infection is a fundamental pathology of various diseases such as obesity, diabetes, cancer, neurodegenerative diseases, and autoimmune disorders. The incidence of diseases associated with various chronic inflammatory pathologies increases with age (Fig. 4).

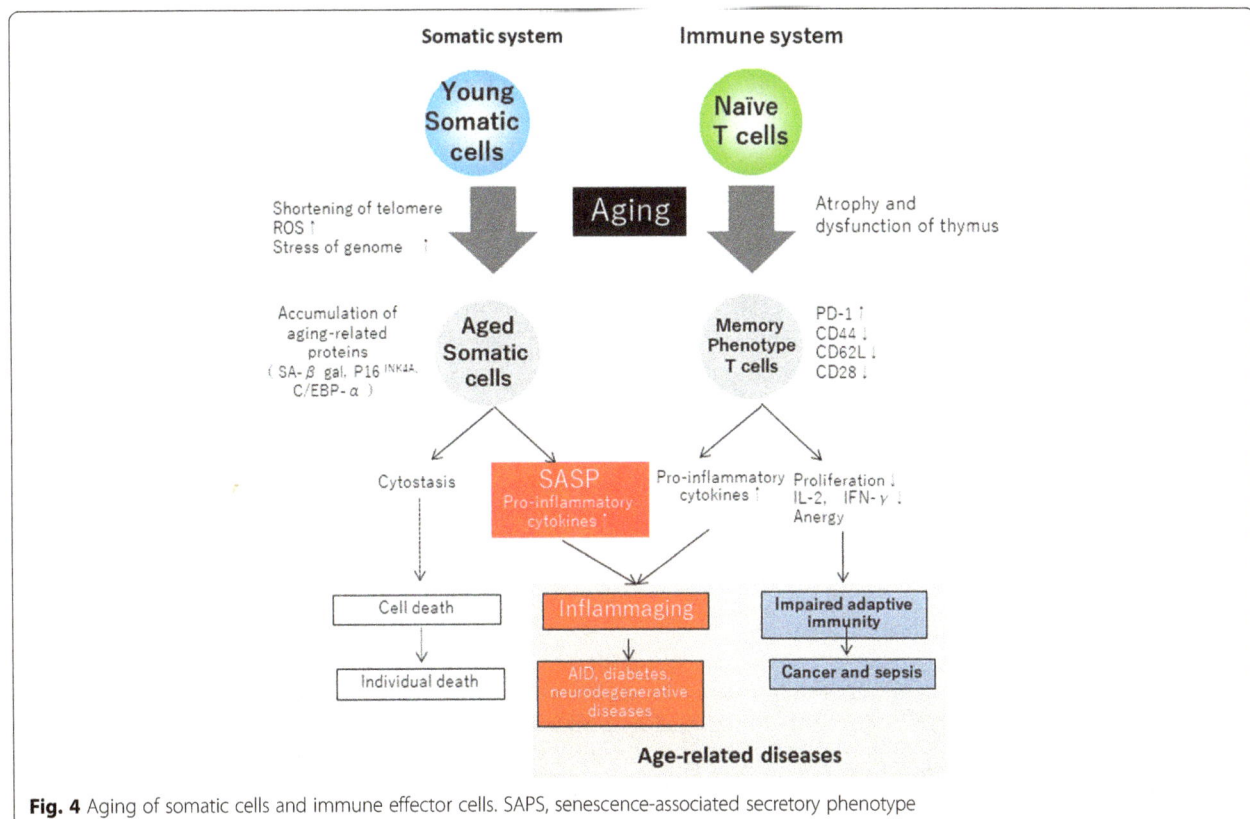

Fig. 4 Aging of somatic cells and immune effector cells. SAPS, senescence-associated secretory phenotype

Epidemiological studies of the elderly beginning in the 1990s have revealed that the prevalence of inflammatory markers such as C-reactive protein (CRP) increases with age and correlates with mortality and inflammaging. The relationship between age and disease has been noted. By specifically eliminating cells with p16^{INK4A}, which is a biomarker of aging, the development of age-related diseases can be delayed in the tissue (e.g., adipose and muscle tissue) of a senescence-promoting mouse model. Moreover, it is possible to directly cause aging of tissues and individuals [31, 32]. A long-term therapeutic strategy aimed at improving the quality of life of very old patients, which may involve molecular biology, will become increasingly important.

Aging in neurocritical care

Neurointensive care is an area of medicine that spans multiple fields and provides specialized care for critically ill patients with neurological illnesses [33, 34]. Neurointensivists are clinical professionals who orchestrate personnel including neurologists, neurosurgeons, consultants, therapists, pharmacists, nurses, and administrators in neurosciences intensive care units (NSICUs). Their role is important for the patient's health and clinical outcomes [35, 36]. Studies have shown that neurointensivists who manage NSICUs improve outcomes and documentation and shorten the length of stay of all neurocritically ill patients [37–41], including those suffering from ischemic stroke [41–46], subarachnoid hemorrhage [47, 48], traumatic brain injury [49, 50], intracerebral hemorrhage [51], and neuromuscular respiratory failure [52].

Stroke and T cell dysfunction

Stroke remains a leading cause of death and disability worldwide and is a major problem in neurocritical care. Ischemic stroke is characterized by the disruption of cerebral blood flow, which produces a central core of dead neurons surrounded by a penumbra of damaged but partially functional neurons [53].

T lymphocytes are central to the development of a sustained inflammatory response, and there is evidence that they accumulate in the post-ischemic brain within a few hours of reperfusion [54, 55]. Profound systemic immunodepression—or "stroke-induced immunodeficiency syndrome"—occurs as early as 12 h after ischemic stroke and may persist for several weeks [56–60]. This phenomenon is characterized by reduced numbers of T cells and other immune cells of the spleen, thymus, and lymph nodes and is mediated by hyperactivity of the sympathetic nervous system (SNS) and the hypothalamic–pituitary–adrenal axis (HPA) [60]. This leads to increased apoptosis of

immune cells in the spleen, thymus, and lymph nodes, and as a result, these secondary lymphatic organs undergo atrophy [59, 60]. Furthermore, there is a shift from the production of cytokine Th1 to that of Th2 [60, 61]. Infectious complications, predominantly chest and urinary tract infections, occur in many stroke patients within the first few days of the stroke, and the development of an infection soon after the stroke is associated with worse outcomes [62–64]. Several recent clinical studies have found evidence that SNS-mediated stroke-induced immunodepression and subsequent susceptibility to post-stroke infections also occur. In the PANTHERIS (Preventive Antibacterial Treatment in Acute Stroke) trial on the efficacy of short-term antibacterial therapy to prevent the development of post-stroke infections, Klehmet et al. confirmed that rapid loss and functional deactivation of T cells are common in stroke patients and are consistent with immunodepression following brain ischemia. Furthermore, a more pronounced decline in cellular immune responses and increased sympathetic activity following stroke are associated with a higher risk of infection [65]. Harms et al. conducted a post hoc analysis of the PANTHERIS trial by investigating the impact of distinct lesion patterns on SNS activation, immunodepression, and frequency of post-stroke infections [66]. Large stroke volume, lesions affecting distinct regions of the middle cerebral artery (MCA) cortex, and SNS activation (assessed by elevated norepinephrine levels) were all associated with impaired immune function and higher susceptibility to post-stroke infections. Whereas neither stroke severity nor stroke volume was independently associated with post-stroke infections, increased levels of norepinephrine and infarction of the anterior MCA cortex were both identified as independent risk factors for post-stroke infections [66]. A recent study by Hug et al. [67] found that reduced costimulatory efficacy of circulating costimulatory cells (i.e., splenic non-T cells) in mice is an important feature of stroke-induced immunodepression and, if confirmed in humans, points to such cells as potential targets for therapies to prevent secondary inflammatory damage to the brain after stroke. In addition to the well-established proinflammatory cytokine-mediated activation of the SNS and HPA, another pathway of communication between the nervous and immune systems, known as the vagal cholinergic anti-inflammatory pathway, has been identified. When the vagus nerve is activated by proinflammatory cytokines, it releases acetylcholine, which inhibits the release of more proinflammatory mediators by macrophages [68–70]. Experimental studies have shown that, according to various models of ischemia-reperfusion, vagal nerve signaling inhibits the release of proinflammatory cytokines and improves outcomes [70]. Taken together, the vagal cholinergic anti-inflammatory pathway is another potential mediator and therapeutic target of stroke-induced immunodepression.

Sepsis-associated encephalopathy (SAE)

Sepsis is one of the most common reasons for presentation to emergency departments and accounts for 6.4% of admissions [71, 72]. Sepsis and its attendant complications cause more deaths than prostate cancer, breast cancer, and HIV/AIDS combined and impose a major financial burden on healthcare systems.

Age increases the risk of mortality in sepsis patients [73]. Elderly people aged at least 65 account for approximately 60% of sepsis patients and approximately 80% of deaths due to sepsis [74]. The average age of sepsis patients in many developed countries is rising each year. In recent years, diseases closely related to physical dysfunction of the elderly, such as ICU-acquired weakness and post-intensive care syndrome, have also been proposed, and the subjects of intensive care in the twenty-first century are aging.

SAE is a multifactorial syndrome that is characterized by diffuse cerebral dysfunction induced by the systemic response to infection without clinical or laboratory evidence of direct brain infection or other types of encephalopathy (e.g., hepatic or renal encephalopathy). Brain dysfunction due to sepsis has been overlooked as a cause of delirium or altered mental status in critically ill patients. This is primarily because there are no precise, well-established clinical or biological markers of damage to assess brain dysfunction occurring because of sepsis [75]. However, the authors of recent studies have reported that SAE is a relatively common cause of altered mental status in critically ill patients admitted to ICUs, and its prevalence varies from 8 to 70% [76–78]. The clinical spectrum of SAE may range from mild inattentiveness or disorientation, agitation, and hypersomnolence to more severe disruption of consciousness, as seen in coma. Although there is no direct infection or invasion of the central nervous system (CNS), laboratory evidence of CNS dysfunction is common in SAE. The pathophysiology of SAE has not been established, but several likely mechanisms have been proposed [79]. SAE appears to involve direct cellular damage to the brain, mitochondrial and endothelial dysfunction, neurotransmission disturbances, and derangements of calcium homeostasis in brain tissue [80]. The direct local cerebral colonization of microorganisms and the formation of micro abscesses have been described in human SAE [78]. However, many cases of SAE without brain micro abscesses have been observed; there is no correlation between SAE and any microorganism, making it unlikely that microorganisms play a causative role in SAE.

Breakdown of blood–brain barrier (BBB) in SAE

Adequate function of the cerebral microcirculation and BBB is important for the maintenance of normal cerebral function. The BBB, which comprises endothelial cells, astrocytes, and pericytes, plays a central role in maintaining the vascular homeostasis of the CNS [81]. Experimental data indicate that, in the early phase of sepsis, endothelial nitric oxide synthase-derived NO exerts proinflammatory effects and contributes to the activation and dysfunction of cerebrovascular endothelial cells [82]. Secondly, LPSs and cytokines induce the expression of adhesion molecules on brain microvessel endothelial cells, which also contributes to BBB dysfunction. This breakdown of the BBB facilitates the passage of neurotoxic factors such as cytokines and accounts for the brain edema revealed by magnetic resonance imaging (MRI) in patients with SAE [83]. Inflammatory cytokines and the complement system constitute the final common pathway in the pathophysiology of brain dysfunction in SAE (Fig. 5). TNF-α appears to be one of the most significant inflammatory mediators in SAE. It induces neutrophil infiltration of the brain tissue, neuronal cell apoptosis, and brain edema (probably by inducing the expression of aquaporin-4) [84]. IL-6 also plays a crucial role in the pathogenesis of SAE. Excessive complement activation can cause altered expression of TLR4 and subsequent alterations in TNF-α, inducible nitric oxide synthetase (iNOS), and aquaporin-4, thereby causing edema, cell necrosis, or neuronal apoptosis [80, 85].

Aging induces breakdown of the BBB

In the aging population, common cardiovascular disorders such as hypertension [86], seizure [87], and stroke [88] contribute to BBB dysfunction. BBB permeability is altered by several factors including increased levels of inflammatory cytokines [89] and free radicals [90], which cause the increased influx of cytokines and immune cells into the brain. Moreover, dysfunction of the endothelial barrier facilitates extravasation of plasma proteins into the brain and subsequently triggers a variety of neuroinflammatory responses within the brain. Aging is associated with degeneration of the BBB/blood cerebrospinal fluid barrier, and the abnormal accumulation of albumin [91], fibrinogen, and IgG has been reported in the brains of patients with Alzheimer's disease [92]. Taken together, these observations suggest that aging induces the progression of SAE via BBB dysfunction in elderly patients with sepsis.

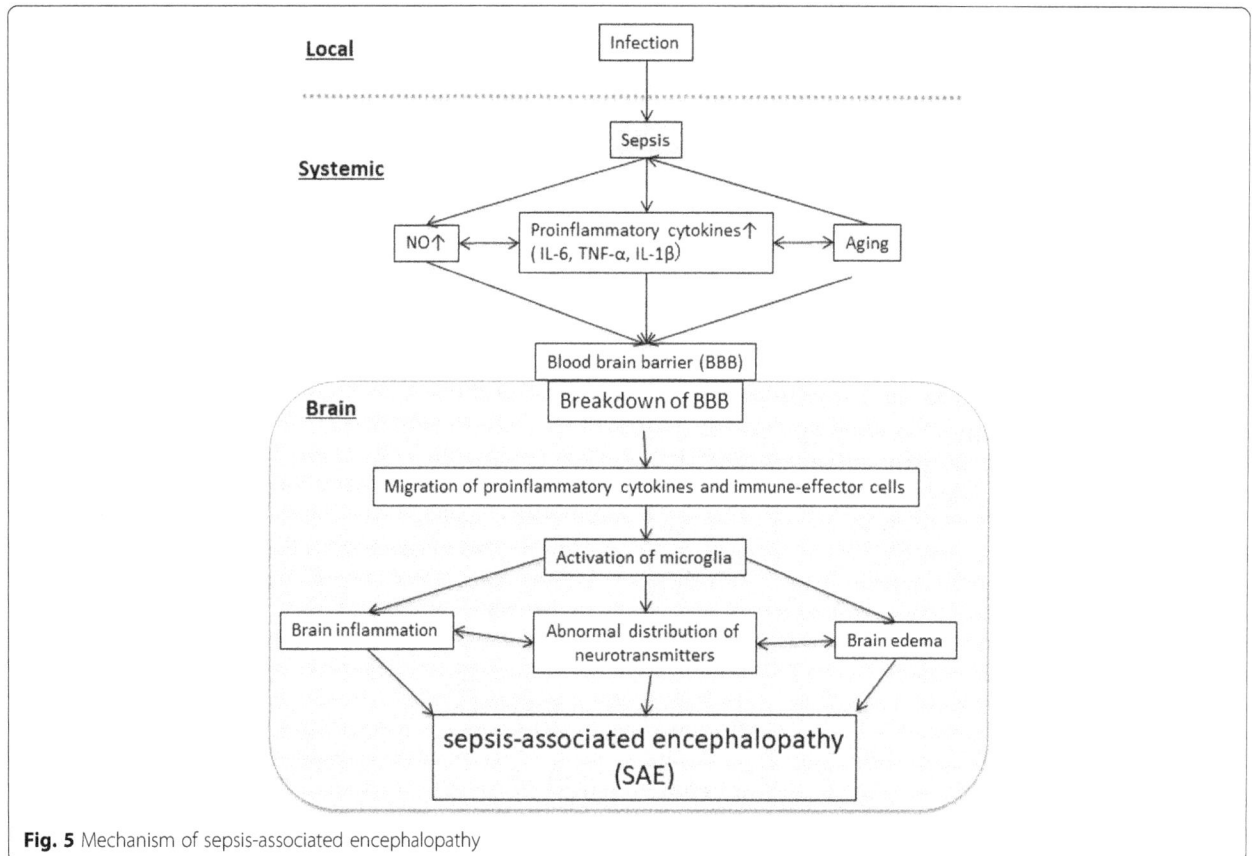

Fig. 5 Mechanism of sepsis-associated encephalopathy

Conclusions

Advances in medical science, especially developments in intensive care medicine, have increased the lifespan of human beings, and aging has become a global issue. Several diseases, including stroke and sepsis-induced encephalopathy, are closely related to aging-induced immune dysfunction, and the terms "immunosenescence" and "inflammaging" are sometimes used in neurocritical care units. Several advanced countries, which now have superaged societies, face the new problem of improving the long-term prognosis of neurocritical patients.

Abbreviations

BBB: Blood–brain barrier; CNS: Central nervous system; CRP: C-reactive protein; CTLA-4: Cytotoxic T-lymphocyte-associated protein 4; HPA: Hypothalamic–pituitary–adrenal axis; ICU: Intensive care unit; IFN-γ: Interferon-γ; IgM: Immunoglobulin M; IL-2: Interleukin-2; iNOS: Inducible nitric oxide synthetase; LPSs: Lipopolysaccharides; MCA: Middle cerebral artery; MHC2: Major histocompatibility complex 2; MIP-1a: Macrophage inflammatory proteins-1a; MRI: Magnetic resonance imaging; NSICUs: Neurosciences intensive care units; PD-1: Programmed cell death protein 1; RANTES: Regulated on activation, normal T cell expressed and secreted; ROS: Reactive oxygen species; SAE: Stroke and sepsis-associated encephalopathy; SASP: Senescence-associated secretory phenotype; SNS: Sympathetic nervous system; TCR: T cell antigen receptor; TIM-3: T cell immunoglobulin and mucin-domain containing-3

Authors' contributions

SI drafted and revised the manuscript. MS and JK contributed to arrange figures. All authors read and approved the final manuscript.

Competing interests

The authors declare that they have no competing interests.

References

1. Petsko GA. A seat at the table. Genome Biol. 2008;9:113.
2. Tchkonia T, Zhu Y, van Deursen J, Campisi J, Kirkland JL. Cellular senescence and the senescent secretory phenotype: therapeutic opportunities. J Clin Invest. 2013;123:966–72.
3. Prattichizzo F, De Nigris V, La Sala L, Procopio AD, Olivieri F, Ceriello A. "Inflammaging" as a druggable target: a senescence-associated secretory phenotype-centered view of type 2 diabetes. Oxidative Med Cell Longev. 2016;2016:1810327.
4. Baylis D, Bartlett DB, Patel HP, Roberts HC. Understanding how we age: insights into inflammaging. Longev Healthspan. 2013;2:8.
5. Rossi DJ, Bryder D, Weissman IL. Hematopoietic stem cell aging: mechanism and consequence. Exp Gerontol. 2007;42:385–90.
6. Rossi DJ, Bryder D, Zahn JM, Ahlenius H, Sonu R, Wagers AJ, Weissman IL. Cell intrinsic alterations underlie hematopoietic stem cell aging. Proc Natl Acad Sci U S A. 2005;102:9194–9.

7. Fulop T, Larbi A, Douziech N, Fortin C, Guerard KP, Lesur O, Khalil A, Dupuis G. Signal transduction and functional changes in neutrophils with aging. Aging Cell. 2004;3:217–26.

8. Gomez CR, Boehmer ED, Kovacs EJ. The aging innate immune system. Curr Opin Immunol. 2005;17:457–62.

9. Plowden J, Renshaw-Hoelscher M, Engleman C, Katz J, Sambhara S. Innate immunity in aging: impact on macrophage function. Aging Cell. 2004;3: 161–7.

10. Herrero C, Marques L, Lloberas J, Celada A. IFN-gamma-dependent transcription of MHC class II IA is impaired in macrophages from aged mice. J Clin Invest. 2001;107:485–93.

11. Cumberbatch M, Dearman RJ, Kimber I. Influence of ageing on Langerhans cell migration in mice: identification of a putative deficiency of epidermal interleukin-1beta. Immunology. 2002;105:466–77.

12. Shurin MR, Shurin GV, Chatta GS. Aging and the dendritic cell system: implications for cancer. Crit Rev Oncol Hematol. 2007;64:90–105.

13. Panda A, Arjona A, Sapey E, Bai F, Fikrig E, Montgomery RR, Lord JM, Shaw AC. Human innate immunosenescence: causes and consequences for immunity in old age. Trends Immunol. 2009;30:325–33.

14. Murasko DM, Jiang J. Response of aged mice to primary virus infections. Immunol Rev. 2005;205:285–96.

15. Oouchi M, Hasebe A, Hata H, Segawa T, Yamazaki Y, Yoshida Y, Kitagawa Y, Shibata KI. Age-related alteration of expression and function of TLRs and NK activity in oral candidiasis. Oral Dis. 2015;21:645–51.

16. Park S, Nahm MH. Older adults have a low capacity to opsonize pneumococci due to low IgM antibody response to pneumococcal vaccinations. Infect Immun. 2011;79:314–20.

17. Ademokun A, Wu YC, Martin V, Mitra R, Sack U, Baxendale H, Kipling D, Dunn-Walters DK. Vaccination-induced changes in human B-cell repertoire and pneumococcal IgM and IgA antibody at different ages. Aging Cell. 2011;10:922–30.

18. Sasaki S, Sullivan M, Narvaez CF, Holmes TH, Furman D, Zheng NY, Nishtala M, Wrammert J, Smith K, James JA, et al. Limited efficacy of inactivated influenza vaccine in elderly individuals is associated with decreased production of vaccine-specific antibodies. J Clin Invest. 2011;121:3109–19.

19. Remarque EJ, de Bruijn IA, Boersma WJ, Masurel N, Ligthart GJ. Altered antibody response to influenza H1N1 vaccine in healthy elderly people as determined by HI, ELISA, and neutralization assay. J Med Virol. 1998;55:82–7.

20. Kogut I, Scholz JL, Cancro MP, Cambier JC. B cell maintenance and function in aging. Semin Immunol. 2012;24:342–9.

21. Silva ML, Martins MA, Espirito-Santo LR, Campi-Azevedo AC, Silveira-Lemos D, Ribeiro JG, Homma A, Kroon EG, Teixeira-Carvalho A, Eloi-Santos SM, et al. Characterization of main cytokine sources from the innate and adaptive immune responses following primary 17DD yellow fever vaccination in adults. Vaccine. 2011;29:583–92.

22. Pawelec G, Akbar A, Caruso C, Solana R, Grubeck-Loebenstein B, Wikby A. Human immunosenescence: is it infectious? Immunol Rev. 2005;205:257–68.

23. Wang L, Xie Y, Zhu LJ, Chang TT, Mao YQ, Li J. An association between immunosenescence and CD4(+)CD25(+) regulatory T cells: a systematic review. Biomed Environ Sci. 2010;23:327–32.

24. Czesnikiewicz-Guzik M, Lee WW, Cui D, Hiruma Y, Lamar DL, Yang ZZ, Ouslander JG, Weyand CM, Goronzy JJ. T cell subset-specific susceptibility to aging. Clin Immunol. 2008;127:107–18.

25. Godlove J, Chiu WK, Weng NP. Gene expression and generation of CD28-CD8 T cells mediated by interleukin 15. Exp Gerontol. 2007;42: 412–5.

26. Hotchkiss RS, Karl IE. The pathophysiology and treatment of sepsis. N Engl J Med. 2003;348:138–50.

27. Linton PJ, Dorshkind K. Age-related changes in lymphocyte development and function. Nat Immunol. 2004;5:133–9.

28. Yi JS, Cox MA, Zajac AJ. T-cell exhaustion: characteristics, causes and conversion. Immunology. 2010;129:474–81.

29. Wherry EJ, Teichgraber V, Becker TC, Masopust D, Kaech SM, Antia R, von Andrian UH, Ahmed R. Lineage relationship and protective immunity of memory CD8 T cell subsets. Nat Immunol. 2003;4:225–34.

30. Inoue S, Suzuki K, Komori Y, Morishita Y, Suzuki-Utsunomiya K, Hozumi K, Inokuchi S, Sato T. Persistent inflammation and T cell exhaustion in severe sepsis in the elderly. Crit Care. 2014;18:R130.

31. Baker DJ, Childs BG, Durik M, Wijers ME, Sieben CJ, Zhong J, Saltness RA, Jeganathan KB, Verzosa GC, Pezeshki A, et al. Naturally occurring p16(Ink4a)-positive cells shorten healthy lifespan. Nature. 2016;530:184–9.

32. Baker DJ, Wijshake T, Tchkonia T, LeBrasseur NK, Childs BG, van de Sluis B, Kirkland JL, van Deursen JM. Clearance of p16Ink4a-positive senescent cells delays ageing-associated disorders. Nature. 2011;479:232–6.

33. Ward MJ, Shutter LA, Branas CC, Adeoye O, Albright KC, Carr BG. Geographic access to US neurocritical care units registered with the neurocritical care society. Neurocrit Care. 2012;16:232–40.

34. Wijdicks EFM, Worden WR, Miers AG, Piepgras DG. The early days of the neurosciences intensive care unit. Mayo Clin Proc. 2011;86:903–6.

35. Durbin CG Jr. Team model: advocating for the optimal method of care delivery in the intensive care unit. Crit Care Med. 2006;34:S12–S7.

36. Mirski MA, Chang CWJ, Cowan R. Impact of a neuroscience intensive care unit on neurosurgical patient outcomes and cost of care: evidence-based support for an intensivist-directed specialty ICU model of care. J Neurosurg Anesthesiol. 2001;13:83–92.

37. Sarpong Y, Nattanmai P, Schelp G. Importance of neurocritical care team in patient and family satisfaction in a neuroICU. Mayo Clinic First Annual Neuro and Intensive Care: Review and Hands-On Workshop 2016.

38. Sarpong Y, Nattanmai P, Schelp G. Importance of neurocritical care team in patient and family satisfaction in a neuroICU. Proceedings of the 14th Annual Neurocritical Care Society Meeting 2016.

39. Suarez JI, Zaidat OO, Suri MF, Feen ES, Lynch G, Hickman J, Georgiadis A, Selman WR. Length of stay and mortality in neurocritically ill patients: impact of a specialized neurocritical care team. Crit Care Med. 2004;32: 2311–7.

40. Varelas PN, Conti MM, Spanaki MV, Potts E, Bradford D, Sunstrom C, Fedder W, Bey LH, Jaradeh S, Gennarelli TA. The impact of a neurointensivist-led team on a semiclosed neurosciences intensive care unit. Crit Care Med. 2004;32:2191–8.

41. Varelas PN, Spanaki MV, Hacein-Bey L. Documentation in medical records improves after a neurointensivist's appointment. Neurocrit Care. 2005;3:234–6.

42. Dayno JM, Mansbach HH. Acute stroke units. J Stroke Cerebrovasc Dis. 1999; 8:160–70.

43. Gujjar AR, Deibert E, Manno EM, Duff S, Diringer MN. Mechanical ventilation for ischemic stroke and intracerebral hemorrhage: indications, timing, and outcome. Neurology. 1998;51:447–51.

44. Langhorne P. Collaborative systematic review of the randomised trials of organised inpatient (stroke unit) care after stroke. Br Med J. 1997;314:1151–9.

45. The European Ad Hoc Consensus G. Optimizing intensive care in stroke: a European perspective. Cerebrovasc Dis. 1997;7:113–28.

46. Varelas PN, Schultz L, Conti M, Spanaki M, Genarrelli T, Hacein-Bey L. The impact of a neuro-intensivist on patients with stroke admitted to a neurosciences intensive care unit. Neurocrit Care. 2008;9:293–9.

47. Enblad P, Persson L. Impact on clinical outcome of secondary brain insults during the neurointensive care of patient with subarachnoid haemorrhage: a pilot study. J Neurol Neurosurg Psychiatry. 1997;62:512–6.

48. Samuels O, Webb A, Culler S, Martin K, Barrow D. Impact of a dedicated neurocritical care team in treating patients with aneurysmal subarachnoid hemorrhage. Neurocrit Care. 2011;14:334–40.

49. Elf K, Nilsson P, Enblad P. Outcome after traumatic brain injury improved by an organized secondary insult program and standardized neurointensive care. Crit Care Med. 2002;30:2129–34.

50. Varelas PN, Eastwood D, Yun HJ, Spanaki MV, Bey LH, Kessaris C, Gennarelli TA. Impact of a neurointensivist on outcomes in patients with head trauma treated in a neurosciences intensive care unit. J Neurosurg. 2006;104:713–9.

51. Burns JD, Green DM, Lau H, Winter M, Koyfman F, Defusco CM, Holsapple JW, Kase CS. The effect of a neurocritical care service without a dedicated neuro-ICU on quality of care in intracerebral hemorrhage. Neurocrit Care. 2013;18:305–12.

52. Varelas PN, Chua HC, Natterman J, Barmadia L, Zimmerman P, Yahia A, Ulatowski J, Bhardwaj A, Williams MA, Hanley DF. Ventilatory care in myasthenia gravis crisis: assessing the baseline adverse event rate. Crit Care Med. 2002;30:2663–8.

53. Dirnagl U, Iadecola C, Moskowitz MA. Pathobiology of ischaemic stroke: an integrated view. Trends Neurosci. 1999;22:391–7.

54. Brait VH, Jackman KA, Walduck AK, Selemidis S, Diep H, Mast AE, Guida E, Broughton BRS, Drummond GR, Sobey CG. Mechanisms contributing to cerebral infarct size after stroke: gender, reperfusion, T lymphocytes, and Nox2-derived superoxide. J Cereb Blood Flow Metab. 2010;30:1306–17.

55. Jander S, Kraemer M, Schroeter M, Witte OW, Stoll G. Lymphocytic infiltration and expression of intercellular adhesion molecule-1 in

photochemically induced ischemia of the rat cortex. J Cereb Blood Flow Metab. 1995;15:42–51.

56. Gendron A, Teitelbaum J, Cossette C, Nuara S, Dumont M, Geadah D, Du Souich P, Kouassi E. Temporal effects of left versus right middle cerebral artery occlusion on spleen lymphocyte subsets and mitogenic response in Wistar rats. Brain Res. 2002;955:85–97.

57. Liesz A, Hagmann S, Zschoche C, Adamek J, Zhou W, Sun L, Hug A, Zorn M, Dalpke A, Nawroth P, et al. The spectrum of systemic immune alterations after murine focal ischemia: immunodepression versus immunomodulation. Stroke. 2009;40:2849–58.

58. Liesz A, Suri-Payer E, Veltkamp C, Doerr H, Sommer C, Rivest S, Giese T, Veltkamp R. Regulatory T cells are key cerebroprotective immunomodulators in acute experimental stroke. Nat Med. 2009;15:192–9.

59. Offner H, Subramanian S, Parker SM, Wang C, Afentoulis ME, Lewis A, Vandenbark AA, Hurn PD. Splenic atrophy in experimental stroke is accompanied by increased regulatory T cells and circulating macrophages. J Immunol. 2006;176:6523–31.

60. Prass K, Meisel C, Höflich C, Braun J, Halle E, Wolf T, Ruscher K, Victorov IV, Priller J, Dirnagl U, et al. Stroke-induced immunodeficiency promotes spontaneous bacterial infections and is mediated by sympathetic activation reversal by poststroke T helper cell type 1-like immunostimulation. J Exp Med. 2003;198:725–36.

61. Theodorou GL, Marousi S, Ellul J, Mougiou A, Theodori E, Mouzaki A, Karakantza M. T helper 1 (Th1)/Th2 cytokine expression shift of peripheral blood CD4 + and CD8+ T cells in patients at the post-acute phase of stroke. Clin Exp Immunol. 2008;152:456–63.

62. Aslanyan S, Weir CJ, Diener HC, Kaste M, Lees KR. Pneumonia and urinary tract infection after acute ischaemic stroke: a tertiary analysis of the GAIN International trial. Eur J Neurol. 2004;11:49–53.

63. Hilker R, Poetter C, Findeisen N, Sobesky J, Jacobs A, Neveling M, Heiss WD. Nosocomial pneumonia after acute stroke: implications for neurological intensive care medicine. Stroke. 2003;34:975–81.

64. Langhorne P, Stott DJ, Robertson L, MacDonald J, Jones L, McAlpine C, Dick F, Taylor GS, Murray G. Medical complications after stroke: a multicenter study. Stroke. 2000;31:1223–9.

65. Klehmet J, Harms H, Richter M, Prass K, Volk HD, Dirnagl U, Meisel A, Meisel C. Stroke-induced immunodepression and post-stroke infections: lessons from the preventive antibacterial therapy in stroke trial. Neuroscience. 2009;158:1184–93.

66. Harms H, Reimnitz P, Bohner G, Werich T, Klingebiel R, Meisel C, Meisel A. Influence of stroke localization on autonomic activation, immunodepression, and post-stroke infection. Cerebrovasc Dis. 2011;32:552–60.

67. Hug A, Liesz A, Muerle B, Zhou W, Ehrenheim J, Lorenz A, Dalpke A, Veltkamp R. Reduced efficacy of circulating costimulatory cells after focal cerebral ischemia. Stroke. 2011;42:3580–6.

68. Pavlov VA, Wang H, Czura CJ, Friedman SG, Tracey KJ. The cholinergic anti-inflammatory pathway: a missing link in neuroimmunomodulation. Mol Med. 2003;9:125–34.

69. Tracey KJ. The inflammatory reflex. Nature. 2002;420:853–9.

70. Tracey KJ. Physiology and immunology of the cholinergic antiinflammatory pathway. J Clin Investig. 2007;117:289–96.

71. Rezende E, Silva JM Jr, Isola AM, Campos EV, Amendola CP, Almeida SL. Epidemiology of severe sepsis in the emergency department and difficulties in the initial assistance. Clinics (Sao Paulo). 2008;63:457–64.

72. Vincent JL, Sakr Y, Sprung CL, Ranieri VM, Reinhart K, Gerlach H, Moreno R, Carlet J, Le Gall JR, Payen D, et al. Sepsis in European intensive care units: results of the SOAP study. Crit Care Med. 2006;34:344–53.

73. Martin GS, Mannino DM, Moss M. The effect of age on the development and outcome of adult sepsis. Crit Care Med. 2006;34:15–21.

74. Javadi P, Buchman TG, Stromberg PE, Turnbull IR, Vyas D, Hotchkiss RS, Karl IE, Coopersmith CM. Iron dysregulation combined with aging prevents sepsis-induced apoptosis. J Surg Res. 2005;128:37–44.

75. Iacobone E, Bailly-Salin J, Polito A, Friedman D, Stevens RD, Sharshar T. Sepsis-associated encephalopathy and its differential diagnosis. Crit Care Med. 2009;37:S331–6.

76. Kreger BE, Craven DE, McCabe WR. Gram-negative bacteremia. IV. Re-evaluation of clinical features and treatment in 612 patients. Am J Med. 1980;68:344–55.

77. Sprung CL, Peduzzi PN, Shatney CH, Schein RM, Wilson MF, Sheagren JN, Hinshaw LB. Impact of encephalopathy on mortality in the sepsis syndrome. The Veterans Administration Systemic Sepsis Cooperative Study Group. Crit Care Med. 1990;18:801–6.

78. Young GB, Bolton CF, Austin TW, Archibald YM, Gonder J, Wells GA. The encephalopathy associated with septic illness. Clin Invest Med. 1990;13:297–304.

79. Flierl MA, Rittirsch D, Huber-Lang MS, Stahel PF. Pathophysiology of septic encephalopathy--an unsolved puzzle. Crit Care. 2010;14:165.

80. Zhan RZ, Fujiwara N, Shimoji K. Regionally different elevation of intracellular free calcium in hippocampus of septic rat brain. Shock. 1996;6:293–7.

81. Ballabh P, Braun A, Nedergaard M. The blood-brain barrier: an overview: structure, regulation, and clinical implications. Neurobiol Dis. 2004;16:1–13.

82. Handa O, Stephen J, Cepinskas G. Role of endothelial nitric oxide synthase-derived nitric oxide in activation and dysfunction of cerebrovascular endothelial cells during early onsets of sepsis. Am J Physiol Heart Circ Physiol. 2008;295:H1712–9.

83. Sharshar T, Carlier R, Bernard F, Guidoux C, Brouland JP, Nardi O, de la Grandmaison GL, Aboab J, Gray F, Menon D, et al. Brain lesions in septic shock: a magnetic resonance imaging study. Intensive Care Med. 2007;33:798–806.

84. Alexander JJ, Jacob A, Cunningham P, Hensley L, Quigg RJ. TNF is a key mediator of septic encephalopathy acting through its receptor, TNF receptor-1. Neurochem Int. 2008;52:447–56.

85. Jacob A, Hensley LK, Safratowich BD, Quigg RJ, Alexander JJ. The role of the complement cascade in endotoxin-induced septic encephalopathy. Lab Investig. 2007;87:1186–94.

86. Hajjar I, Keown M, Frost B. Antihypertensive agents for aging patients who are at risk for cognitive dysfunction. Curr Hypertens Rep. 2005;7:466–73.

87. Janigro D. Blood-brain barrier, ion homeostasis and epilepsy: possible implications towards the understanding of ketogenic diet mechanisms. Epilepsy Res. 1999;37:223–32.

88. Mikulis DJ. Functional cerebrovascular imaging in brain ischemia: permeability, reactivity, and functional MR imaging. Neuroimaging Clin N Am. 2005;15:667–80.

89. Banks WA, Kastin AJ, Broadwell RD. Passage of cytokines across the blood-brain barrier. Neuroimmunomodulation. 1995;2:241–8.

90. Chan PH, Yang GY, Chen SF, Carlson E, Epstein CJ. Cold-induced brain edema and infarction are reduced in transgenic mice overexpressing CuZn-superoxide dismutase. Ann Neurol. 1991;29:482–6.

91. Pakulski C, Swiniarski A, Jaszczyk G. High subarachnoid block for severe bronchospasm. Eur J Anaesthesiol. 2000;17:594–5.

92. Ryu JK, McLarnon JG. A leaky blood-brain barrier, fibrinogen infiltration and microglial reactivity in inflamedAlzheimer's disease brain. J Cell Mol Med. 2009; 13(9A):2911–25.

26

How to manage various arrhythmias and sudden cardiac death in the cardiovascular intensive care

Yoshinori Kobayashi ⓘ

Abstract

In the clinical practice of cardiovascular critical care, we often observe a variety of arrhythmias in the patients either with (secondary) or without (idiopathic) underlying heart diseases. In this manuscript, the clinical background and management of various arrhythmias treated in the CCU/ICU will be reviewed.

The mechanism and background of lethal ventricular tachyarrhythmias vary as time elapses after the onset of MI that should be carefully considered to select a most suitable therapy. In the category of non-ischemic cardiomyopathy, several diseases are known to be complicated by the various ventricular tachyarrhythmias with some specific mechanisms. According to the large-scale registry data, the most common arrhythmia is atrioventricular block. It is essential for the decision of permanent pacemaker indication to rule out the presence of transient causes such as ischemia and electrolyte abnormalities.

The prevalence of atrial fibrillation (AF) is very high in the patients with heart failure (HF) and myocardial infarction (MI). AF and HF have a reciprocal causal relationship; thus, both are associated with the poor prognosis. Paroxysmal AF occurs in 5 to 20% during the acute phase of MI and triggered by several specific factors including pump failure, atrial ischemia, and autonomic instability.

After the total management of patients with various arrhythmias and basic heart diseases, the risk of sudden cardiac death should be stratified for each patient to assess the individual need for preventive therapies.

Finally, it is recommended that the modalities of the treatment and prophylaxis should be selected on a case-by-case basis in the scene of critical care.

Keywords: Cardiovascular intensive care, Arrhythmias, Electrical storm, Acute myocardial infarction, Congestive heart failure

Background

According to the registry of the Tokyo CCU Network of the patients hospitalized in the cardiovascular intensive care units (CCU/ICU) of 72 leading hospitals capable of advanced cardiovascular care in the Tokyo metropolitan area, approximately 10% received intensive care due to a variety of arrhythmias as a main cause of their admission. The arrhythmias were mainly comprised of idiopathic bradyarrhythmias, including atrioventricular conduction disturbances and sinus node dysfunction (Fig. 1 and Table 1), followed by ventricular tachycardia (VT) and atrial fibrillation (AF).

Further, we have a lot of patients transferred to the critical care for severely ill conditions such as cardiogenic shock or severe heart failure (HF) due to an acute myocardial infarction (MI) and/or an advanced stage of various cardiomyopathies. Such patients frequently have various arrhythmias that should be controlled to improve their cardiac performance and to decrease the prevalence of sudden cardiac death (SCD).

In this chapter, the clinical background and management of various arrhythmias treated in the cardiovascular critical care unit will be reviewed. The risk stratification and therapeutic strategies for the prevention of SCD will also be described.

Correspondence: yoshikoba@tokai-u.jp
Division of Cardiology, Tokai University Hachioji Hospital, 1838 Ishikawa-machi Hachioji-shi, Tokyo 192-0032, Japan

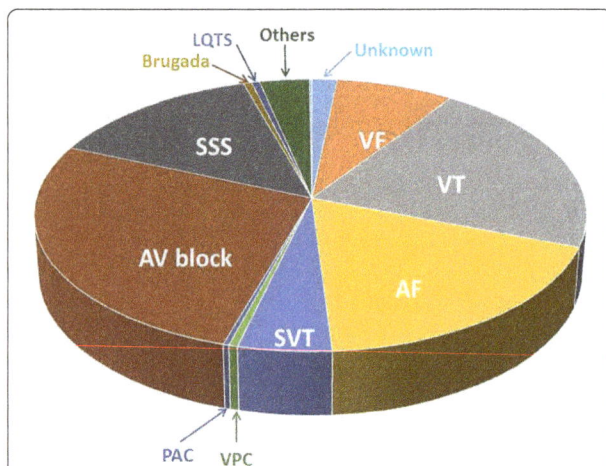

Fig. 1 The contents of the arrhythmias in the patients who were admitted to the CCU/ICU in the Tokyo CCU Network for the treatment of arrhythmias in 2014. Those correspond to approximately 10% of the total patients. The most common arrhythmia was AV block, which was followed by ventricular tachycardia and atrial fibrillation

Clinical features and management of VT/VF and electrical storms (ESs) in the CCU/ICU

About one fourth of the patients who are admitted to the CCU/ICU for the management of arrhythmias receive a diagnosis of VT or ventricular fibrillation (VF). They have a variety of underlying heart diseases, including ischemic

Table 1 Contents of arrhythmias as causes of admission

Cardiac arrest	22	
Ventricular fibrillation (VF)	103	
Ventricular tachycardia (VT)	277	
Sustained VT		198
Non-sustained VT		68
Torsade de points (TdP)		11
Atrial fibrillation (AF)	238	
Supraventricular tachycardia (SVT)	64	
Ventricular premature contraction(VPC)	8	
Atrial premature contraction (APC)	4	
AV block	351	
1st degree		1
2nd degree		65
Wenckebach		17
Morbitz II		48
3rd degree		285
Sick sinus syndrome (SSS)	184	
Brugada syndrome	7	
Long QT syndrome	7	
Others	43	
Unknown	2	

heart disease (IHD) and various cardiomyopathies. Using the database of the Tokyo CCU Network between 2012 and 2014, there were 1067 patients who were admitted to the CCU for the management of VT/VF as a main clinical manifestation [1]. Among them, 312 patients (29.2%) had IHD, 88 (8.2%) dilated cardiomyopathy (DCM), 78 (7.3%) hypertrophiccardiomyopathy (HCM), 25 (2.3%) cardiac sarcoidosis, and 18 (1.7%) arrhythmogenic right ventricular cardiomyopathy. However, approximately 40% of the patients diagnosed with idiopathic VT and idiopathic VF had no structural abnormalities found during the clinical check-ups. In this chapter, VT/VF and electrical storms (ESs) associated with and without structural heart disease, particularly during the acute phase of an MI, will be focused on.

VT/VF and ESs associated with acute MIs

Life-threatening ventricular tachyarrhythmias (VTAs), including VT and VF, can occur anytime from during the super-acute phase to during the remote phase of an MI. From the old days, the animal experimental studies such as the canine MI model (Harris Model) have shown that the characteristics and mechanisms of the VTAs dramatically vary as time elapses after the onset of an MI [2, 3]. Such a temporal variation in the mechanism of the VTAs obtained by experimental studies cannot totally be extrapolated to VTAs during an acute or subacute MI in humans, because there is a greater number of factors affecting the occurrence of VTAs in clinical practice as compared to the coronary ligation model. Those are spontaneous and intentional reperfusion and iatrogenic factors. Using the large data from the Tokyo CCU Network, we have elucidated the incidence, clinical features, background, and prognosis of patients with life-threatening VTAs during the acute or subacute phase of an MI and the time interval-dependent difference from the onset of the MI [4]. We analyzed the registry data from years 2011 and 2012 undertaken specifically in MI patients. The detailed individual data were provided from the allied hospitals for 2811 patients for 2011 and 3192 patients for 2012. After the perusal of the individual data, we judged that a total of 160 patients (141 males and 19 females, average age 66 ± 12 years) experienced ESs, either before or after the hospitalization, during the acute or subacute phase of an MI, if an ES was defined as two or more recurrent sustained VTAs during a 24-h period. The incidence of an ES was 160/6003 patients (2.67%). Among those, in 133 patients, the precise time of the onset of the MI could be obtained. Those 133 patients were then divided into three groups according to the time interval from the onset of the MI to the first episode of the VTA, that is, (1) the super-acute phase of the MI (MI-VTA interval ≤ 1 h: group A 63 patients), (2) acute phase of the MI (1 h < MI-VTA interval ≤ 24 h: group -B 51 patients), and (3) subacute phase of the MI (MI-VTA interval > 24 h: group C 19 patients). We also compared the demographic data and clinical parameters among those three groups (Table 2). In group A, the majority of the patients had ESs outside of the hospital before admission, whereas the ESs occurred in the catheter laboratory in the majority of patients in group B. On the other hand, the ESs emerged either in the CCU or general ward in group C. In the group A and group B patients, the main arrhythmia observed was VF, while it was VT in group C. In group A, the ESs were obviously associated with a large infarction size and severe hemodynamic deterioration, leading to a poor in-hospital mortality. In group B, the background of the ES patients varied rather widely, with a similar number of patients with a Killip-I and Killip-IV class and also anterior and inferior infarctions. The in-hospital mortality was relatively low as compared to that of group-A and group-C, however, it was still worse than that in the patients without ESs (6%). Finally, in group C, the status of the patients was not so severe on admission, in that there was a greater percentage of Killip-I patients and a relatively low peak-CK. Most of the ESs occurred during the subacute phase of the MI. The ESs themselves were more severe as the number of DC shocks applied were significantly greater than that in group A and group B. The short-term prognosis was worst in group C. As such, the background of the ESs was multi-factorial, but there were some periodic differences in the patient characteristics and contents of the arrhythmias.

Beta blockers [5], amiodarone [6], and nifekalant (a pure Ikr blocker) [7] have been shown to be effective in suppressing ESs during an acute MI. We often experience drug-refractory recurrent VTAs in patients with hemodynamic deterioration. For such patients, intra-aortic balloon pumping is a potent non-pharmacological therapy applied as the first choice and has been shown to be effective in suppressing ESs, probably by virtue of the improvement in both the hemodynamics and coronary perfusion [8]. For the patients complicated with cardiogenic shock, hypoxia due to severe pulmonary edema, and cardiac arrest, percutaneous cardiopulmonary support (PCPS) is also introduced [9]. There have been several reports in which a satellite ganglion block and renal sympathetic nerve ablation may have been

Table 2 Comparison of clinical background among 3 groups

	Group A MI-ES interval 0–1 h	Group B Interval 1–24 h	Group C Interval > 24 h	Statistics
Patient no.	63	51	19	
Average age (years)	65 ± 11	65 ± 13	71 ± 12	P < 0.1
Average MI-ES interval (hours)	0.3 ± 0.4	4.8 ± 5.1	204 ± 160	P < 0.001
Place of ES				
Out of hospital	54	10	0	P < 0.001
Emergency room	4	8	0	
Catheter laboratory	3	27	0	
CCU	2	6	16	
General ward	0	0	3	
MI site(9^6)	Anterior 75%	Anterior 52%	Anterior 74%	P < 0.01
	Inferopost 25%	Inferopost 48%	Inferopost 26%	
Killip class (pts no.)	I, 12; II, 6	I, 15; II, 6	I, 9; II, 4	P < 0.01
	III, 4; IV, 32	III, 7; IV, 17	III, 3; IV, 3	
Peak CK	6810 ± 6110	5780 ± 3700	3170 ± 3180	
Arrhythmia contents ES				
Cardiac arrest	3	1	0	
PEA	9	0	0	
VF only	13	22	3	
VF and VT	32	21	7	
VT only	4	7	9	
Number of DC	4.2 ± 2.5	4.3 ± 3.2	9.5 ± 14.0	P < 0.01
In-hospital mortality	49.2%	33.3%	57.9%	P < 0.01

MI myocardial infarction, *ES* electrical storm, *Pts* patients, *PEA* pulseless electrical activity, *DC* direct current shocks, *inferopost* inferoposterior

effective in suppressing the ES [6, 10]. When an ES could not be suppressed by drug therapy and cardiac support devices, catheter ablation procedures have occasionally been applied to rescue patients [11, 12]. In that case, a ventricular premature complex (VPC) triggering polymorphic VT or VF is one of the targets of the ablation. The triggering VPCs commonly originate from the surviving Purkinje network exhibiting a relatively narrow QRS configuration (Fig. 2). Radiofrequency deliveries at the earliest activation site where the local Purkinje potential precedes the QRS complex during the VPC usually result in the successful elimination of the incessant VTA.

VT/VF and ESs associated with non-ischemic heart disease
There are a variety of heart diseases in this category of patients, which is known to be complicated by VT and VF (Table 3). Accordingly, there are multiple electrophysiologic mechanisms of VT, including scar-related reentry (channel-dependent and isthmus-dependent), His bundle-Purkinje-related reentry (bundle-branch reentry, inter-fascicular reentry, and intra-fascicular reentry), and focal tachycardia (enhanced automaticity and triggered activity). It has been considered that bundle-branch

Table 3 Basic heart disease categorized in the non-ischemic heart disease and known to be complicated by VTAs

1) Degenerative disease
  a) Dilated cardiomyopathy (DCM)
  b) Arrhythmogenic right ventricularcardiomyopathy (ARVC)
2) Inflammatory disease
a) Acute myocarditis
b) Chronic myocarditis
c) Cardiac sarcoidosis
3) Hypertrophic disease
a) Hypertrophiccardiomyopathy (HCM)
b) Cardiac amyloidosis
4) Congestive heart disease and post-surgery (Tetralogy of Fallot)
5) Mitral valve prolapse
6) Pseudo ventricular aneurism
7) Neuro-muscular disease (myotonic dystrophy)

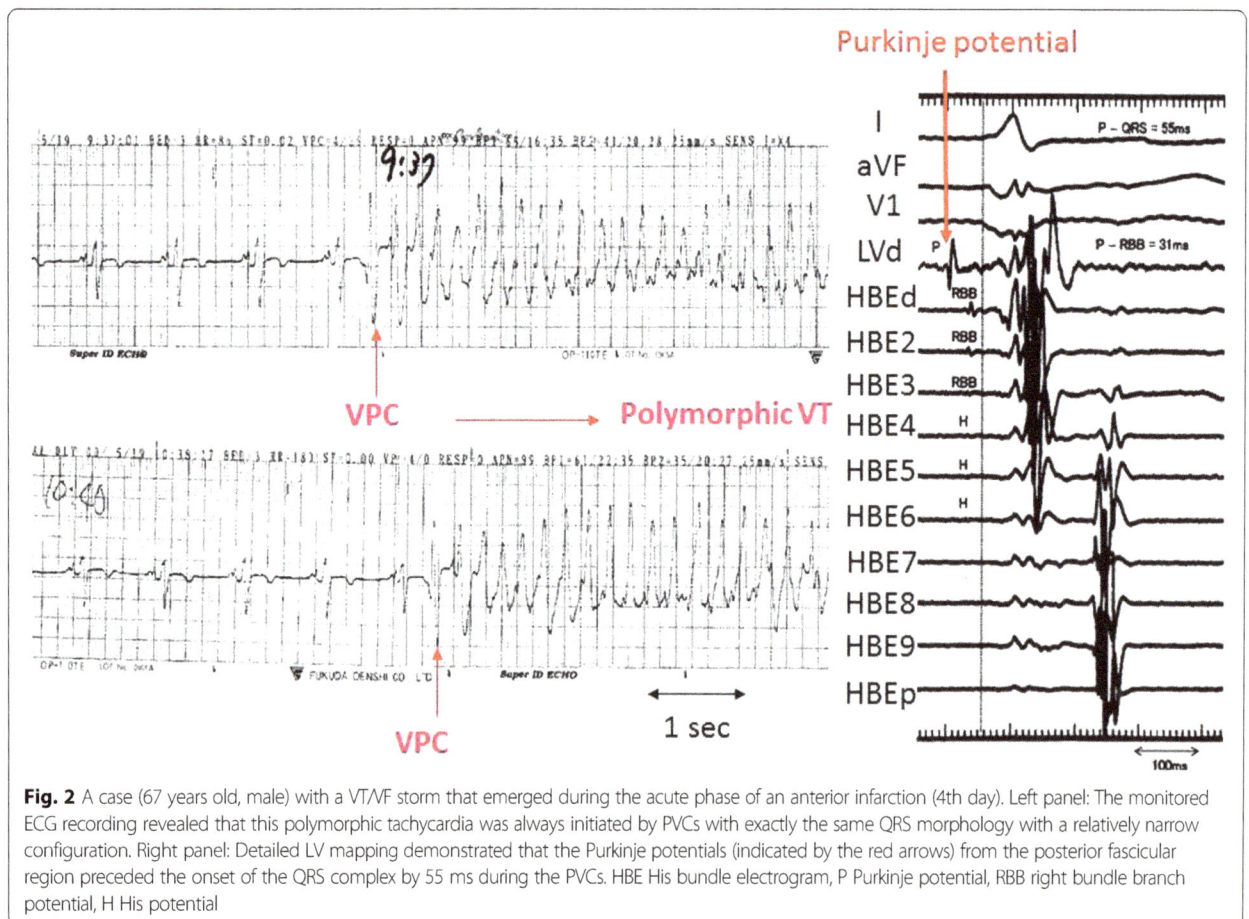

Fig. 2 A case (67 years old, male) with a VT/VF storm that emerged during the acute phase of an anterior infarction (4th day). Left panel: The monitored ECG recording revealed that this polymorphic tachycardia was always initiated by PVCs with exactly the same QRS morphology with a relatively narrow configuration. Right panel: Detailed LV mapping demonstrated that the Purkinje potentials (indicated by the red arrows) from the posterior fascicular region preceded the onset of the QRS complex by 55 ms during the PVCs. HBE His bundle electrogram, P Purkinje potential, RBB right bundle branch potential, H His potential

reentrant tachycardia (BBRT) is a specific arrhythmia observed in patients with DCM, whereas it is rarely observed in those with IHD. However, recent reports have clearly showed that this mechanism similarly causes the VTs in both categories of basic heart disease [13, 14]. During the advanced stage of non-ischemic CM, we sometimes experience multiple morphologies of the QRS complex that transform spontaneously or during pacing maneuvers. Such VTs, so-called "pleomorphic VTs," are attributable to complex degenerative ventricular lesions leading to the formation of multiple channels of slow conduction [15, 16]. The culprit lesions for sustained VTs have also been shown to more likely be located at epicardial sites in DCM as compared to IHD [16]. In patients with HCM, polymorphic VT or VF is a more common arrhythmia than monomorphic VT. Monomorphic VT is commonly observed in patients with an apical ventricular aneurysm formation resulting from a long-term mid-ventricular obstruction [17].

Cardiac sarcoidosis (CS) is observed with a greater prevalence in Japanese people (20%) than Caucasians and black Americans (2%) [18]. The prevalence of subclinical CS diagnosed by an autopsy study was also 70–80% in Japanese and 20% in Caucasians and black Americans, respectively. CS is complicated by various arrhythmias. The most common arrhythmia is AV block, followed by VT. A recent report showed that VT storms sometimes emerge in CS, particularly after the introduction of steroid therapy [19]. Most of the VTs associated with CS are due to scar-related reentry, which is located in the interventricular septum, right ventricular, or entire LV with patchy scarring. Storms are shown to be successfully suppressed by catheter ablation; however, the recurrence rate is relatively high (30–40% per year) [20].

In VTAs associated with non-ischemic CM, the first-line pharmacological therapy is amiodarone; however, the largest trial to date, that is, the Sudden Cardiac Death in Heart Failure Trial (SCD-HeFT), showed no significant difference in the mortality between the amiodarone treatment group and placebo group [21]. On the basis of that trial, it has been recommended that amiodarone not be used routinely in patients with DCM unless a specific arrhythmia indication exists [22]. Amiodarone is known to lengthen the tachycardia cycle length and reduce the frequency of implantable cardioverter defibrillator (ICD) shocks without worsening HF. Beta blockers are also shown to improve the prognosis of patients with DCM reducing both heart-failure-related death and sudden cardiac death [23, 24], and therefore, beta blockers are considered one of the standard medications for DCM. However, the introduction of those drugs should be done carefully in patients with severe HF because of their negative inotropic effects.

In patients with non-ischemic CM, aggravation of HF is usually the predisposing factor of the occurrence of arrhythmias and VT/VF storms. Therefore, the therapeutic target should simultaneously be addressed to improve the HF. That includes pharmacological therapies (diuretics, vasodilators, inhibitors of the renin-angiotensin system, positive inotropic agents, etc.) and non-pharmacological modalities (left ventricular assist devices, biventricular pacing, etc.) [25].

Idiopathic VT

As mentioned before, approximately 40% of patients who are admitted to the CCU/ICU for the management of VT are found not to have structural heart disease by screening check-ups [1]. Except for verapamil sensitive left VT (so-called fascicular VT), which has been shown to be caused by a reentrant mechanism probably involving the Purkinje network, idiopathic VT (IVT) commonly occurs due to a focal mechanism. The origins of focal IVTs are distributed in a variety of areas of the right (RV) and left (LV) ventricles. The most common site of origin is the outflow tract region of both the RV and LV. The mitral and tricuspid annular regions and papillary muscles are also the next most common sites of IVT origins [26].

Most IVTs usually present with a hemodynamically stable condition upon admission; however, IVT can occasionally appear as an unstable rapid VT in which prompt DC cardioversion is needed. Otherwise, drug therapy is the first choice to bail out any incessant form of VTs and for prophylactic purposes.

Verapamil is the most effective drug for the fascicular VT, which has a relatively narrow QRS configuration with CRBBB and both a superior axis (originating from the posterior fascicle) and inferior axis (originating from the anterior fascicle). There is another type of fascicular VT, that is, the upper septal type, which is reported to have a very narrow QRS complex with a QRS width of less than 120 ms. Catheter ablation can cure these tachycardias with a high success rate (> 90%) [27].

Furthermore, beta blockers are the first choice of drugs for focal IVTs following the administration of non-dihydropyridine calcium channel blockers such as verapamil. Class I and III drugs are also shown to be effective for focal IVTs [28]. Even though catheter ablation is also a very effective tool to eliminate these tachycardias, the consequence of the procedure deeply depends on the site of origin. The success rate for RV outflow origins is relatively high, while that for LV summit, papillary muscle, and so-called LV Crux VTs has not reached a satisfactory level [26, 28]. Therefore, the precise identification of the origin during the pre-ablation stage, while carefully examining the QRS morphology, is essential for a successful ablation. There are several diagnostic algorithms to determine the site of origin using the 12 lead ECG [29, 30].

QT prolongation and torsades de pointes (Tdp) polymorphic VT

The patients who are admitted to the ICU/CCU usually have several risk factors that can predispose them to QT prolongation and Tdp tachycardias [31]. Those include an elderly age, underlying heart disease (particularly MIs), the presence of HF, renal and hepatic dysfunction, electrolyte abnormalities, bradycardias, and various drugs such as diuretics, antiarrhythmic agents, and sedative agents that facilitate QT prolongation and hypokalemia (Table 4). It has been shown that a greater risk for the development of Tdp in the hospital setting occurs with the clustering of multiple recognizable risk factors in a single patient [31, 32].

The ECG signs as predictors of Tdp are (1) a QTc interval > 500 ms, (2) macroscopic T wave alternans, and (3) a prolonged QT interval with an increase in the terminal portion of the T wave ($T^{peak} - T^{end}$ interval) [31, 33]. Prior to the development of Tdp, a typical short-long-short sequence of the R-R interval is often

Table 4 Risk factors and drugs causing torsade de pointes in hospitalized patients

Clinically recognizable risk factors	List of drugs causing torsade de points
1) QTc > 500 ms	1) Antiarrhythmicdrugs
2) Use of QT-prolonging drug	i) Class la agents (disopyramide, cibenzoline)
3) Structural heart disease AMI and CHF	ii) Class III agents (amiodarone, bepridil, nifekalant)
4) Advanced age	2) Antidepressant (amitiptyline, desipramine)
5) Female sex	3) Antipsychotic agents (chlorpromazine, haloperidol)
6) Hypokalemia	4) Anticonvulsant (felbamate, fosphenytoin)
7) Hypomagnesemia	5) Sedative agents (droperidol)
8) Hypocalcemia	6) Antihistamine agent (astemizole, terfenadine)
9) Treatment with diuretics	7) Antibiotics (clarithromycin, erythromycin)
10) Impaired hepatic drug metabolism	8) Antiviral agents (foscarnet)
11) Bradycardia	9) Antimalarial agents (halofantrine, pentamidine)
Clinically silent risk factors	10) Antihypertensive agents (isradipine, nicardipine)
1) Latent congenital LQTS	11) Anticancer agent (tamoxifen, arsenic trioxide)
2) Genetic polymorphism	12) Anti-migraine agents (naratriptan, zolmitriptan)
	13) Lipid-lowering agent (probucol)

observed with a marked QT prolongation and T-U wave distortion with the last sinus beat (after the long pause) (Fig. 3).

Clinical features and management of bradyarrhythmias in the CCU/ICU
Atrioventricular (AV) block

AV block is the most common arrhythmia in critical care medicine. As shown in Fig. 1, approximately 27% of patients with various arrhythmias as the main cause of their admission to Tokyo CCU Network hospitals were due to AV block. Among them, most of the patients (81%) were diagnosed with complete AV block. The majority of the remaining patients had Mobitz type II second-degree AV block, while Wenckebach type second-degree AV block was relatively rare. The background of the appearance of AV block should be evaluated individually, because multiple factors may be associated with the AV conduction disturbance, including acute ischemia, chronic ischemic heart disease (IHD), degenerative disease, acute inflammatory disease (particularly fulminant myocarditis), chronic inflammatory disease (such as cardiac sarcoidosis), electrolyte disturbance (such as hyperkalemia), and the use of drugs suppressing the AV conduction, including Ca channel blockers, beta blockers, digitalis, and class I and III antiarrhythmic agents. In some patients, AV block seems to occur due to multiple factors. On the other hand, there are more patients in whom no cause of the AV block could be found, which is so-called idiopathic AV block (progressive cardiac conduction disease), which has been linked to a strong genetic background, i.e., gene mutations involving SCN5A and SCN1B [34]. It is essential in these patients, with obvious transient and reversible causes behind the AV block, to identify and improve, or eliminate, those causes by correcting any electrolyte abnormalities, cessation of the offending drugs, treatment of myocardial ischemia, and so on.

In the CCU/ICU, we occasionally experience paroxysmal AV block that is characterized by an abrupt and sustained AV block, usually in the absence of structural heart disease [35]. It is also commonly associated with long episodes of ventricular asystole resulting in syncope and even SCD. As an example, in the representative male case, shown in Fig. 2, he previously experienced several episodes of syncope, and the most recent episode caused a traumatic subarachnoid hemorrhage rendering the patient being admitted into the ICU. Before that episode, the ECG exhibited complete right bundle branch block; however, the PR interval was normal and a slight right anterior deviation was observed (Fig. 4a). The monitored ECG during the syncopal episode revealed the sudden onset of complete AV block without any escape rhythm (a long pause) (Fig. 4b). Paroxysmal AV block has been shown to be a unique phenotype of an

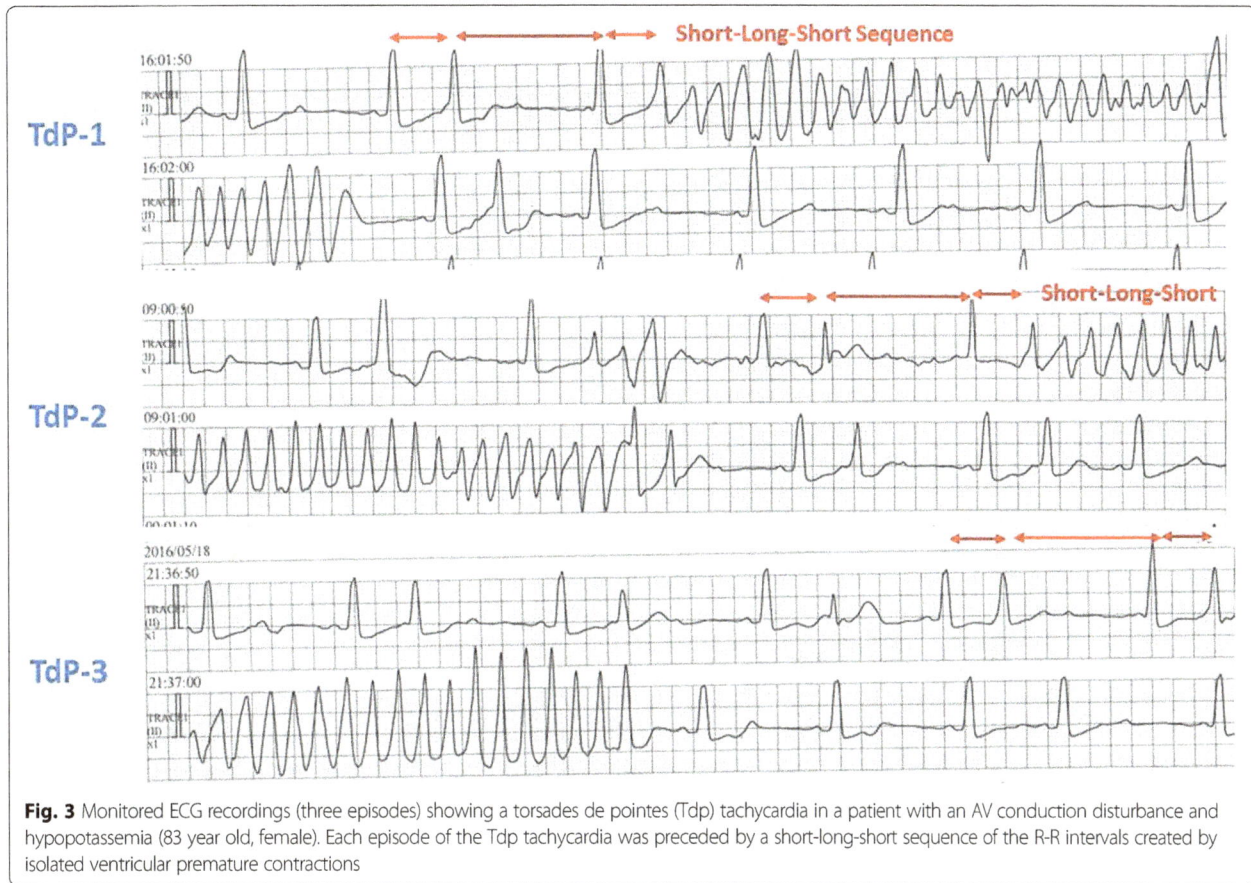

Fig. 3 Monitored ECG recordings (three episodes) showing a torsades de pointes (Tdp) tachycardia in a patient with an AV conduction disturbance and hypopotassemia (83 year old, female). Each episode of the Tdp tachycardia was preceded by a short-long-short sequence of the R-R intervals created by isolated ventricular premature contractions

infra-Hisian conduction disturbance. Because this is a rare and abrupt phenomenon, the diagnosis is sometimes difficult even when utilizing long-term Holter recordings and loop recorders. An electrophysiologic (EP) study with a provocation attempt using class I antiarrhythmic agents may play some role in the diagnosis of this entity [35].

Sinus node dysfunction (SND)
Out of the patients who are admitted for treating arrhythmias, approximately 14% are due to sick sinus syndrome (Fig. 1). As compared with AV block, SND is more of an intrinsic disorder localized to the sinus node and surrounding atrial tissue resulting in a variety of bradyarrhythmias (sinus bradycardia, sinus pauses, sinoatrial block, and tachycardia-bradycardia syndrome). The extrinsic factors facilitating SND include drug effects, an excessive vagal tone, electrical abnormalities, sleep apnea, and hypothyroidism [36]. Because most occurrences of SND become gradually more aggravated with the progression of idiopathic degenerative disorders, the patients are often asymptomatic or have only mild symptoms. The SND patients who are admitted into the CCU/ICU commonly have severe symptoms such as syncopal attacks and collapsing. Syncope is most likely to occur in patients with tachycardia bradycardia syndrome with prolonged sinus pauses.

Temporary pacing and permanent pacemaker implantations
Temporary pacing is sometimes required in patients with an acute MI. According to the guidelines for the management of an ST-Elevation Myocardial Infarction (STEMI), pacing is indicated (class I) for complete AV block, symptomatic bradyarrhythmias refractory to drug therapy, and tri-fascicular block, including alternating bundle branch block and bifascicular block with Mobitz type II second-degree AV block [37].

For patients with symptomatic AV block in the absence of a transient cause of the AV conduction disturbance, a permanent pacemaker (PM) is usually implanted. In patients with an acute MI, the necessity of a permanent PM is not that high, as the incidence of a PM implantation is shown to be needed in less than 1% of the total acute MI patients. Most AV block (even a high-degree block) has a transient nature, appearing only for a short term during the acute phase of an MI and is associated with an inferior MI and vagotony. Candidates for a PM implantation usually have an infra-Hisian block associated with an anterior MI rather than an inferior MI [38].

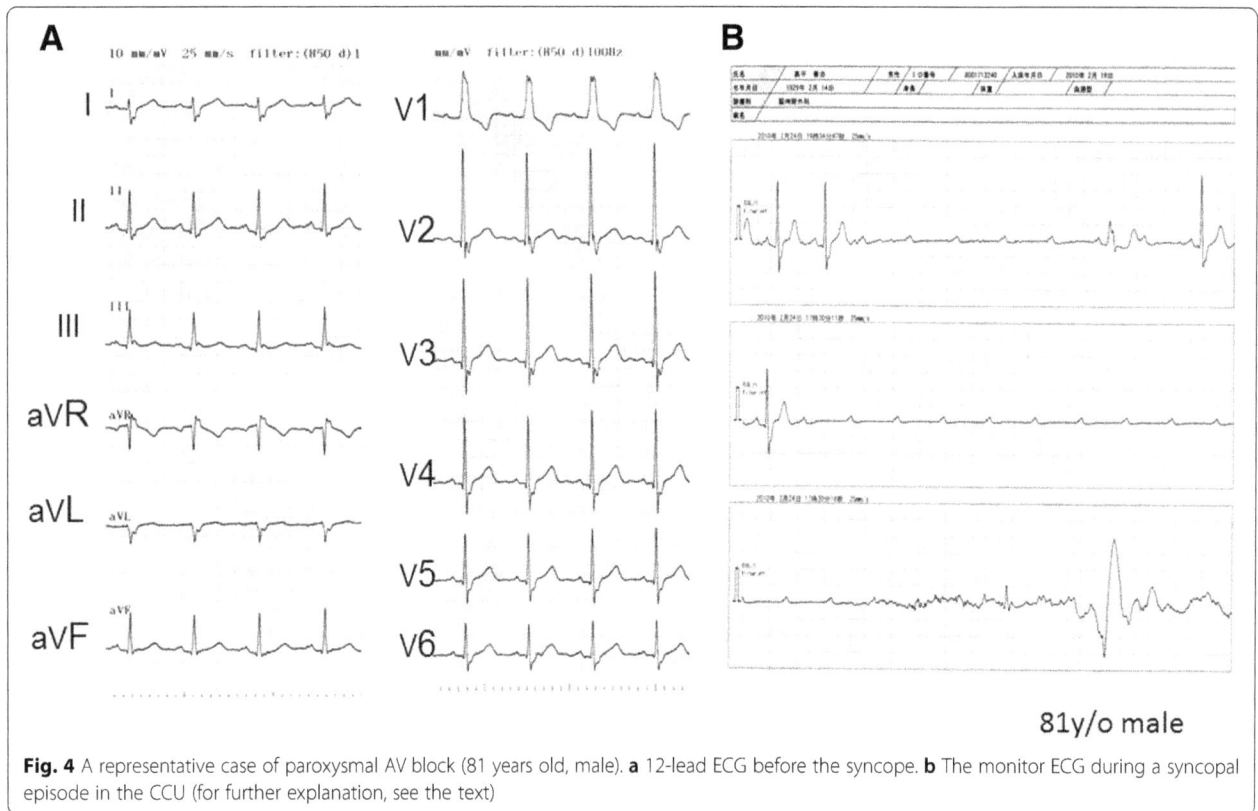

Fig. 4 A representative case of paroxysmal AV block (81 years old, male). **a** 12-lead ECG before the syncope. **b** The monitor ECG during a syncopal episode in the CCU (for further explanation, see the text)

Clinical features and management of AF in the CCU/ICU

AF is also one of the common arrhythmias observed in cardiovascular critical care. Approximately 18% of patients with various arrhythmias who are admitted to the CCU/ICU have AF (Fig. 1). AF is also frequently seen in the setting of HF and an MI (10–49%). In addition, a variety of pathogenic factors are associated with AF in clinical practice as shown in Table 5.

AF associated with HF

In patients with HF, various factors, including a volume overload in the atrium, increased intra-atrial pressure, hypoxia, and a neuro-humoral imbalance, contribute to the occurrence of arrhythmias. The severity of the HF has been shown to be well correlated with the prevalence of AF [39], and that prevalence in New York Heart Association (NYHA) class IV patients is more than 50% (Fig. 5), while that in class II patients is only 10–15%. Recently, the physicians' attention has been directed to HF associated with a preserved ejection fraction (HFpEF), particularly its pathophysiology, background, and prognosis. Campbell et al. [40] demonstrated in their review article on the previous clinical trials, evaluating the effects of various drug interventions on the outcome of HF patients, that the prevalence of AF is similar between the HFpEF patients and patients with HF with a reduced ejection fraction

(HFrEF). Thus, similar to systolic dysfunction, diastolic dysfunction is also shown to be an important factor underlying the occurrence of AF.

Both AF and HF are well known to have a reciprocal causal relationship, promoting the activities of each other, and together are associated with a significant increase in mortality and morbidity. A recent meta-analysis using 104 eligible cohort studies involving approximately one million participants [41] demonstrated that AF is associated with an increased risk of mortality (both all-cause mortality and cardiovascular mortality, including SCD), major cardiovascular events, ischemic strokes, IHD, HF, chronic

Table 5 Pathogenic factors associated with AF occurrence in critical care medicine

1) Heart failure: HFrEF, HEpEF
2) Cardiac ischemia: myocardial infarction
3) Inflammation: pericarditis myocarditis sepsis
4) Cardiac intervention: after cardiac surgery
5) Respiratory disorder: COPD
6) Bradyarrhythmias: sinus node dysfunction, post-PM implantation
7) Neuro-humoral imbalance: hyperthyroidism, heart failure, dehydration
8) Drug-induced: cathecolamine, teophylline, cilostazol, etc.
9) Intoxication: alcohol, CO
10) Chronic kidney disease (CKD)

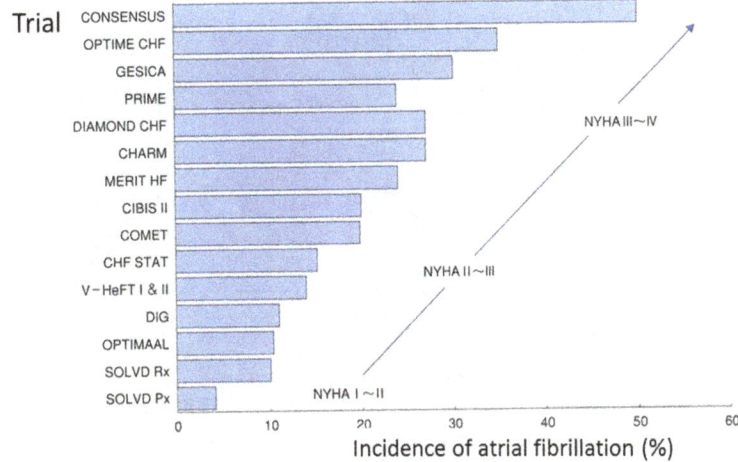

Fig. 5 The relationship between the severity of the CHF and the prevalence of AF. The data were collected from randomized trials of patients with CHF with various severities of heart failure (NYHA classification). The prevalence of AF is well correlated with the severity of CHF (cited from reference [39])

kidney disease, and peripheral arterial disease (Fig. 6). Among those endpoints, the highest absolute risk increase was observed for HF with a relative risk of up to 4.99 (CI 3.04–8.22). In terms of the stage of AF, new-onset AF is associated with HF progression with a greater degree than chronic AF [42].

AF associated with an acute MI
Paroxysmal AF (PAF) occurs in 5 to 20% during the acute phase of an MI [43–46]. The development of PAF is facilitated by a variety of factors including (1) anatomic factors: ischemia of atrial structures (sinus node, AV node, and the atrial musculature) and pericardial effusions (pericarditis), (2) autonomic factors: an enhanced vagal tone accompanying an infero-posterior infarction and a sympathomimetic reaction in patients

with a severe infarction, (3) hemodynamic factors: "pump failure" with left atrial hypertension, and (4) iatrogenic factors: digitalis, antiarrhythmic drugs, and sympathomimetic agents [47]. Among those factors, the most important factor underlying PAF is pump failure associated with a broad and severe MI [43–46]. Figure 7 shows comparative presentations of the hemodynamic variables between the patients with PAF (group 1) and those without PAF (group 2). Those variables were measured during sinus rhythm in both groups, within 24 h before the onset of PAF in group 1 and upon admission prior to various therapeutic interventions in group 2. Group 1 had a significantly higher pulmonary capillary wedge pressure (PCWP), higher central venous pressure (CVP), and lower blood pressure than group 2 [46]. It has been also shown that post-MI patients with a new

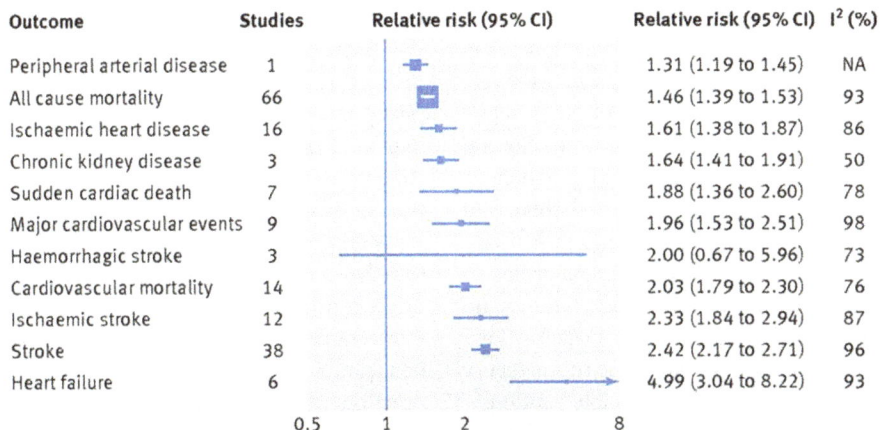

Fig. 6 Association between atrial fibrillation and the all-cause mortality and cardiovascular and renal disease, with a summary of the relative risks of each outcome examined (cited from reference [41])

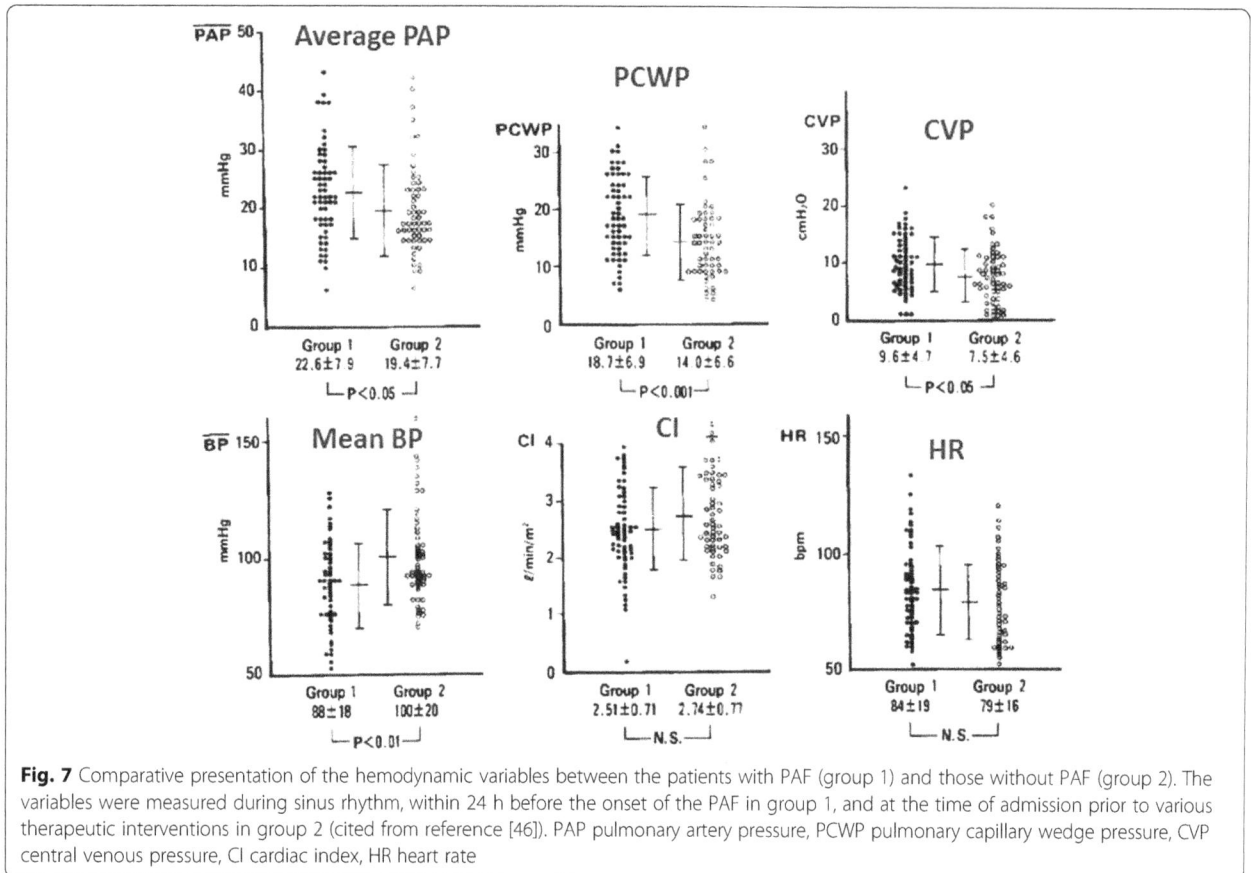

Fig. 7 Comparative presentation of the hemodynamic variables between the patients with PAF (group 1) and those without PAF (group 2). The variables were measured during sinus rhythm, within 24 h before the onset of the PAF in group 1, and at the time of admission prior to various therapeutic interventions in group 2 (cited from reference [46]). PAP pulmonary artery pressure, PCWP pulmonary capillary wedge pressure, CVP central venous pressure, CI cardiac index, HR heart rate

onset of AF have a higher in-hospital mortality than those without AF. Moreover, AF itself is one of the independent predictors of a poor prognosis [43–45]. Therefore, it is recommended that treatment should be directed toward the mechanism producing the arrhythmia (mostly pump failure) in patients with PAF, and the treatment should be simultaneously directed at terminating or controlling the arrhythmia.

Inflammation: sepsis
Recently it has been shown that AF commonly appears in critically ill patients with certain conditions, such as severe sepsis [47]. About 33% of critically ill patients with sepsis have AF, and 10% have new onset of AF [48]. Several pathogenic factors triggered by inflammation, such as hemodynamic compromise, cardiac injury, ischemia, and catecholamine surges, may promote the arrhythmia substrate. New onset of AF during a critical illness seems to be a marker of a poor prognosis, although there is no high-level evidence of this hypothesis [48]. Because there is little data in terms of how to manage AF in this category of patients, the management of AF in severely septic patients should be determined by a case-by-case fashion [49]. It is recommended that potentially reversible AF drivers, such as an electrolyte disturbance, acidemia, beta-

agonist medications, and hypoxia, be promptly found, and those predisposing factors should be resolved.

Management of AF in the critical care patients
Table 6 shows Japan's guideline for the treatment of AF [37] associated with an acute MI, which is quoted from the ACC/AHA/ESC practical guidelines [50].

When patients have a severe hemodynamic compromise or intractable ischemia, or when adequate rate control cannot be achieved with drug therapy, a direct-current (DC) cardioversion is recommended. Initially, a 200-J monophasic current or 120–200-J biphasic current is applied. If that is not successful, then energy current is increased by 50–100 J in a stepwise fashion. However, we sometimes experience new-onset AF with a very rapid ventricular response and hemodynamic deterioration that is refractory to DC cardioversion with the highest energy due to either failure of cardioversion to convert to sinus rhythm or an immediate re-initiation of AF. In this situation, the intravenous administration of class III drugs such as nifekalant can improve the patient outcome by decreasing the heart rate without decreasing the blood pressure during AF [51]. Moreover, nifekalant is shown to terminate AF and raise the success rate of DC cardioversion in some patients probably by reducing the defibrillation threshold.

Table 6 Recommendations in the management of atrial fibrillation in acute myocardial infarction

CLASS I

1. Direct-current cardioversion is recommended for patients with severe hemodynamic compromise or intractable ischemia, or when adequate rate control cannot be achieved with pharmacological agents in patients with acute MI and AF or AFL. *(Level of Evidence: C)*

2. Intravenous administration of amiodarone is recommended to slow a rapid ventricular response to AF and improve LV function in patients with acute MI. *(Level of Evidence: C) (Out of insurance coverage)*

3. Intravenous beta blockers and nondihydropyridine calcium antagonists are recommended to slow a rapid ventricular response to AF in patients with acute MI who do not display clinical LV dysfunction, bronchospasm, or AV block. *(Level of Evidence: C)*

4. For patients with AF and acute MI, administration of unfractionated heparin by either continuous intravenous infusion or intermittent subcutaneous injection is recommended in a dose sufficient to prolong the activated partial thromboplastin time to 1.5 to 2.0 times the control value, unless contraindications to anticoagulation exist. *(Level of Evidence: C)*

CLASS IIa

Intravenous administration of digitalis is reasonable to slow a rapid ventricular response and improve LV function in patients with acute MI and AF associated with severe LV dysfunction and HF. *(Level of Evidence: C)*

CLASS III

The administration of class IC antiarrhythmic drugs is not recommended in patients with AF in the setting of acute MI. *(Level of Evidence: C)*

For the rate control of AF to stabilize the hemodynamics, beta blockers and non-dihydropyridine calcium channel antagonists are used in patients who did not have either LV dysfunction or AV block. Due to the negative inotropic effects, these drugs are often intolerable in patients with HF. Intravenous amiodarone is a reasonable drug to improve this condition in that amiodarone may be expected to provide adequate rate control effects without any hemodynamic disturbance; however, the use of this drug for this aim is currently not under insurance coverage.

After the patient's condition stabilizes, we should carefully consider the need for rhythm control therapy and anticoagulation therapy. In a clinical randomized trial in patients with AF and congestive HF (AF-CHF), the rhythm control strategy using antiarrhythmic agents and electrical cardioversion did not improve the all-cause mortality or prevent worsening HF as compared to a rate control strategy [52]. The reason was considered to be that the side effects and proarrhythmic risk from antiarrhythmic drugs may offset any salutary effects from restoring and maintaining sinus rhythm [53]. Catheter ablation of AF has been demonstrated to decrease the mortality and hospitalization and to improve the quality of life as compared to pharmacological therapy mainly with amiodarone in patients with a severely reduced LV function [54].

Different diagnoses of tachycardia-induced cardiomyopathy (TICM) and tachycardia-mediated cardiomyopathy (TMCM) in AF patients

In clinical practice, we often see the patients with both persistent AF and significantly reduced LV function that might be associated with a rapid ventricular response, the so-called tachycardia-induced cardiomyopathy (TICM). In this condition, a disturbance in the LV contraction is commonly normalized by an adequate rate control therapy [55, 56]. In TICM patients, early recognition of the relationship of the culprit arrhythmia to a reduced LV function is paramount in selecting a suitable treatment, which is likely to improve the patient's condition. Figure 8 shows a diagnostic and therapeutic flowchart with the follow-up in the patients with TICM [57]. TICM can be classified into two categories, one in which the arrhythmia is the sole reason for the ventricular dysfunction (TICM) and another one in which the arrhythmia exacerbates the ventricular dysfunction and/or worsens the HF in patients with concomitant structural heart disease (TMCM). In either situation, the treatment modalities should be selected on a case-by-case basis targeting both the HF and AF itself. Then, if the HF resolves and LV function totally recovers, the patient can be diagnosed with TICM. When the HF resolves and the LV function somehow improves, it is confirmed to be TMCM. Finally, if there is no significant improvement in the LV function, it is neither TICM nor TMCM (see Fig. 8) [57]. Close surveillance is recommended in these patients, because the recurrence of AF can result in a rapid decline in the cardiac performance, even after normalization of the LV function by the initial treatment, and because there are several patient reports of SCD even in HF patients related to AF [55]. Since it has been shown that it takes 1–6 months for a complete recovery of the cardiac function [55, 56], the cardiac function should be re-evaluated using transthoracic echocardiography after a corresponding interval.

Risk stratification of sudden cardiac death and prevention therapy

After the critical management of patients with various cardiac diseases, the risk of sudden cardiac death (SCD) should be stratified for each patient to assess the individual need for preventive therapies. These are cardiac implantable electrical devices (CIEDs) incorporated with the function of an ICD, including cardiac resynchronization therapy defibrillators (CRT-Ds) and wearable ICDs.

Risk stratification of SCD in coronary artery disease

During the acute phase of an MI, the clinical significance of documented VTAs in terms of the predictive value of a future appearance of lethal VTAs varies as the time lapses [58, 59]. Non-sustained VT (NSVT) or VF, which

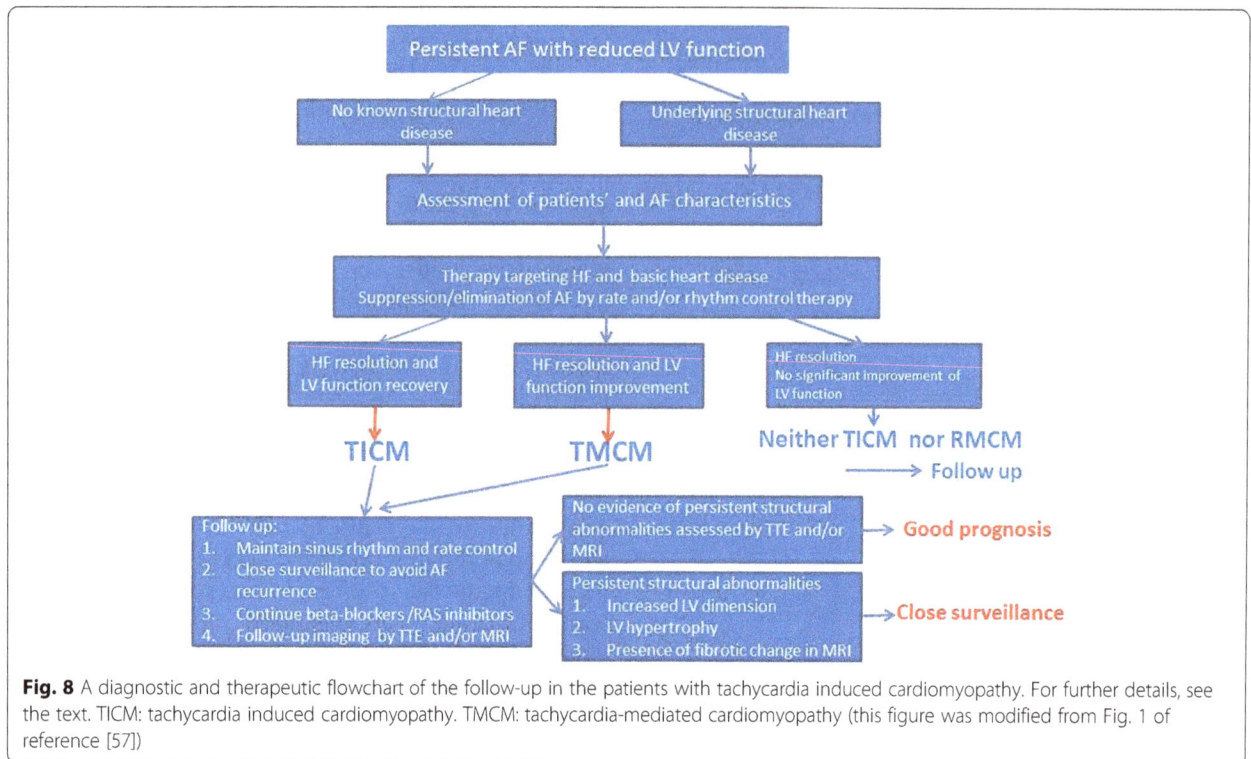

Fig. 8 A diagnostic and therapeutic flowchart of the follow-up in the patients with tachycardia induced cardiomyopathy. For further details, see the text. TICM: tachycardia induced cardiomyopathy. TMCM: tachycardia-mediated cardiomyopathy (this figure was modified from Fig. 1 of reference [57])

emerge within 48 h from the onset of the MI, do not necessarily predict the future occurrence of lethal arrhythmias. Although NSVT, which occurs after 24 h from the onset of an MI [60], has been shown to be a significant predictor of severe VTAs, the early application of an ICD after an MI does not improve the patient's prognosis [61, 62]. The benefit of an ICD (decrease in arrhythmic death) is offset by the increase in HF death, which is presumably caused by either appropriate or inappropriate shock deliveries [61]. Therefore, high-risk MI patients with SCD, such as those with a low left ventricular ejection fraction (LVEF) of ≤ 35%, should be monitored for at least 1 month after the onset of the MI according to the guidelines of the Japan Circulation Society [63]. If the patients have a transient high risk of lethal arrhythmias, a wearable ICD is recently indicated [64]. It can be expected to play a role as a bridge therapy to an ICD implantation and help the LV function recovery in patients at high risk for lethal VTAs, particularly during the acute phase of an MI and after a percutaneous coronary intervention (PCI). In patients with a remote MI, an ICD should be introduced if VF is clinically documented. Polymorphic VT, monomorphic (mono-) VT with hemodynamic compromise, drug refractory mono-VT, and mono-VT, which cannot be cured by catheter ablation, are also class I as indications for an ICD [63]. With regard to primary prevention, the criteria for a class I indication of an ICD includes an NYHA class II or III with an LVEF ≤ 35% and

NSVT under optimal medical therapies. In addition, an NYHA class I with an LVEF ≤ 35%, NSVT, and inducible sustained VTAs during the electrophysiological studies is another class I indication. On the other hand, the SCD-HeFT criteria in which only an NYHA class (II or III) and LVEF ≤ 35% are essential conditions are a class IIa indication. This is an important difference from the AHA/ACC/ESC guidelines [65] in which the SCD-HeFT criteria are ranked as a class I indication [45]. Recently, a report from the CHART-2 study [66] demonstrated that the prevalence of fatal arrhythmic events was 16.1% in patients categorized into a class I indication with the Japanese Circulation Society (JCS) guidelines, 8.9% in those with a class IIa indication, and 1.9% for those with no indication. Thus, the current JCS guidelines for prophylactic ICD usage have been validated at least for Japanese patients with CHF. Antiarrhythmic medical therapy (amiodarone, sotalol, and beta blockers) and catheter ablation are currently considered to be supplemental therapies for the reduction of appropriate and inappropriate shock deliveries by the ICD [67, 68]. Both shock therapies have been shown to aggravate the patient's prognosis [69, 70].

Risk stratification of SCD in non-ischemic cardiomyopathy

For patients with DCM, the risk stratification and indication of an ICD are analogous to that for a remote MI; however, the clinical significance of an inducible VTA in the risk stratification and the effect of the ICD in terms of mortality reduction are less in DCM as compared to IHD [63]. In the risk assessment for primary prevention in HCM, the thickness of the interventricular septum (≥ 30 mm), family history of SCD, an abnormality in the blood pressure response during exercise, and the presence of NSVT are important markers of a poor prognosis [71]. These are the essential conditions for a class IIa indication for an ICD in the JCS guidelines [63].

Risk stratification of SCD in the inherited channelopathies
This category includes long QT syndrome, idiopathic VF (Brugada syndrome, early repolarization syndrome, and short-coupled variant of torsade de points), catecholaminergic polymorphic ventricular tachycardia (CPVT), and short QT syndrome. Japan's guideline for ICD indication is currently available for long QT syndrome and Brugada syndrome. In brief, for the long QT syndrome, a history of either VF or cardiac arrest is class I indication of ICD, while a history of syncope and/or torsade de points which is refractory to beta blockers is class IIa indication. For Brugada syndrome, a history of aborted cardiac arrest and a documentation of VF or polymorphic VT are class I indications for ICD, while the patients with spontaneous coved type ST elevation in precordial leads who meet at least two criteria out of the following three criteria (history of syncope, family history of sudden cardiac death, and inducibility of VF by EP testing) (for details, please see the JCS guideline) [63, 72]. At the present time, the diagnostic role of the localization of responsible gene mutation is important; however, its role for the risk stratification remains unclarified.

Conclusion
In the practice of cardiovascular critical care, we often meet a variety of arrhythmias with a variety of clinical backgrounds. We should pay attention not only to the characteristics and mechanisms of the existing arrhythmias, but also to the upstream pathophysiology underlying the occurrence of those arrhythmias. We also have a lot of therapeutic options for the treatment of arrhythmias that often suppress them and improve the patient status. However, conversely, those therapies sometimes bring harmful results. Therefore, we should judge the necessity of the suppressive treatment of arrhythmias and select the most appropriate modality of treatment on a case-by-case basis.

Abbreviations
AF: Atrial fibrillation; APC: Atrial premature contraction; CCU: Coronary care unit; CIEDs: Cardiac implantable electrical devices; CS: Cardiac sarcoidosis; ES: Electrical storm; HF: Heart failure; HFpEF: Heart failure with preserved ejection fraction; HFrEF: Heart failure with reduced ejection fraction; ICD: Implantable cardioverter defibrillator; ICU: Intensive care unit; IHD: Ischemic heart disease; IVT: Idiopathic ventricular tachycardia; LQTS: Long QT syndrome; MI: Myocardial infarction; NSVT: Non-sustained ventricular tachycardia; PM: Pacemaker; SCD: Sudden cardiac death; SND: Sinus node dysfunction; SVT: Supraventricular tachycardia;

Tdp: Torsade de pointes; TICM: Tachycardia-induced cardiomyopathy; TMCM: Tachycardia-mediated cardiomyopathy; VF: Ventricular fibrillation; VPC: Ventricular premature contraction; VT: Ventricular tachycardia; VTA: Ventricular tachyarrhythmia

Acknowledgements
The author expresses his special gratitude to Mr. John Martin for his helpful linguistic assistance.

Funding
Not applicable.

Author's contribution
The author read and approved the final manuscript.

Competing interests
The author declares that he has no competing interests.

References
1. Ueno A, Kobayashi Y, Murata H et al The short-term prognosis of the patients with ventricular tachycardia and fibrillation: from the registry data of Tokyo CCU Network for 3 years. The proceedings of the 37th scientific meeting of Tokyo CCU Network. ICU and CCU 2018 (In press).
2. Harris AS. Delayed development of ventricular ectopic rhythms following experimental coronary occlusion. Circulation 1950;1:1318–1328.
3. Scherlag BJ, Lazzara R. In: Mandel WJ, editor. Ischemic arrhythmias: basic mechanisms. In cardiac arrhythmias. Their mechanisms, diagnosis, and management. Philaderphia: Lippincott Co; 1980. p. PP366–95.
4. Kobayashi Y. VT/VF storm in acute myocardial infarction (In japanese). Medical Topic Sesies Huseimyaku 2017 (Edited by Sugimoto K and Inoue H). Medical Review Co. Osaka Japan, 2017. P166-175.
5. Nademanee K, Taylor R, Bailey WE, et al. Treating electrical storm: sympathetic blockade versus advanced cardiac life support-guided therapy. Circulation. 2000;102:742–7.
6. Dorian P, Cass D, Schwartz B, et al. Amiodarone as compared with lidocaine for shock-resistent ventricular fibrillation. N Engl J Med. 2002;346:884–90.
7. Amino M, Inokuchi S, Nagao K, SOS-KANTO 2012 Study Group, et al. Nifekalant hydrochloride and amiodarone hydrochloride result in similar improvements for 24-hour survival in cardiopulmonary arrest patients: the SOS-KANTO 2012 study. J Cardiovasc Pharmacol. 2015;66:600–9.
8. Hanson EC, Levine FH, Kay HR, et al. Control of postinfarction ventricular irritability with the intraaortic balloon pump. Circulation. 1980;62(suppl I):I130–7.
9. Stretch R, Sauer CM, Yuh DD, et al. National trends in the utilization of short-term mechanical circulatory support: incidence, outcomes, and cost analysis. J Am Coll Cardiol. 2014;64:1407–15.
10. Armaganijan LV, Staico R, Moreira DA, et al. 6-month outcomes in patients with implantable cardioverter-defibrillators undergoing renal sympathetic denervation for the treatment of refractory ventricular arrhythmias. JACC Cardiovasc Interv. 2015;8:984–90.
11. Bänsch D, Oyang F, Antz M, et al. Successful catheter ablation of electrical storm after myocardial infarction. Circulation. 2003;108:3011–6.
12. Kobayashi Y, Iwasaki Y, Miyauchi Y, et al. The role of Purkinje fibers in the emergence of an incessant form of polymorphic ventricular tachycardia or ventricular fibrillation associated with ischemic heart disease. J Arrhythmia. 2008;24:200–8.

13. Blanck Z, Dhala A, Deshpande S, et al. Bundle branch reentrant ventricular tachycardia: cumulative experience in 48 patients. J Cardiovasc Electrophysiol. 1993;4:253–62.

14. Lopera G, Stevenson WG, Soejima K, et al. Identification and ablation of three types of ventricular tachycardia involving the his-purkinje system in patients with heart disease. J Cardiovasc Electrophysiol. 2004;15:52–8.

15. Dalal D, Jain R, Tandri H, Dong J, Eid SM, Prakasa K, Tichnell C, James C, Abraham T, Russell SD, Sinha S, et al. Long-term efficacy of catheter ablation of ventricular tachycardia in patients with arrhythmogenic right ventricular dysplasia/cardiomyopathy. J Am Coll Cardiol. 2007;50:432–40.

16. Soejima K, Stevenson WG, Sapp JL, et al. Endocardial and epicardial radiofrequency ablation of ventricular tachycardia associated with dilated cardiomyopathy: the importance of low-voltage scars. J Am Coll Cardiol. 2004;43:1834–42.

17. McKenna WJ, Elliott PM. In: Zipes DP, Jalife J, editors. Arrhythmia, sudden death and clinical risk stratification in hypertrophic cardiomyopathy. Cardiac electrophysiology from cell to bedside. 3rd ed. Philadelphia: WB Saunders; 2000. p. P555.

18. Kusano KF, Satomi K. Diagnosis and treatment of cardiac sarcoidosis. Heart. 2016;102:184–90.

19. Segawa M, Fukuda K, Nakano M, et al. Time course and factors correlating with ventricular tachyarrhythmias after introduction of steroid therapy in cardiac sarcoidosis. Circ Arrhythm Electrophysiol. 2016;9(6) https://doi.org/10.1161/CIRCEP.115.003353.

20. Kumar S, Barbhaiya C, Nagashima K, et al. Ventricular tachycardia in cardiac sarcoidosis: characterization of ventricular substrate and outcomes of catheter ablation. Circ Arrhythm Electrophysiol. 2015;8:87–93.

21. Bardy GH, Lee KL, Mark DB, et al. Sudden Cardiac Death in Heart Failure Trial (SCD-HeFT) investigators. Amiodarone or an implantable cardioverter-defibrillator for congestive heart failure. N Engl J Med. 2005;352:225–37.

22. Packer DL, Prutkin JM, Hellkamp AS, et al. Impact of implantable cardioverter-defibrillator, amiodarone, and placebo on the mode of death in stable patients with heart failure: analysis from the sudden cardiac death in heart failure trial. Circulation. 2009;120:2170–6.

23. Packer M, Bristow MR, Cohn JN, et al. The effect of carvedilol on morbidity and mortality in patients with chronic heart failure. U.S. Carvedilol Heart Failure Study Group. N Engl J Med. 1996;334:1349–55.

24. CIBIS-II Investigators and Committees*. The Cardiac Insufficiency Bisoprolol Study II (CIBIS-II): a randomised trial. Lancet. 1999;353:9–13.

25. Galvin JM, Ruskin JN. In: Zipes DP, Jalife J, editors. Ventricular tachycardia in patients with dilated cardiomyopathy. Cardiac electrophysiology from cell to bedside. 5th ed. Philadelphia: WB Saunders; 2009. p. P675.

26. Heeger CH, Hayashi K, Kuck KH, et al. Catheter ablation of idiopathic ventricular arrhythmias arising from the cardiac outflow tracts—recent insights and techniques for the successful treatment of common and challenging cases. Circ J. 2016;80:1073–86.

27. Nogami A. Verapamil sensitive idiopathic ventricular tachycardia. Purkinje arrhythmia. 1st edition, Nogami A, Kobayashi Y (eds) P2-36. IgakushoinTokyo: 2009.

28. Lerman BB. In: Zipes DP, Jalife J, editors. Ventricular tachycardia in patients with structurally normal heart. Cardiac electrophysiology from cell to bedside. 5th ed. Philadelphia: WB Saunders; 2009. p. P657.

29. Ito S, Tada H, Naito S, et al. Development and validation of an ECG algorithm for identifying the optimal ablation site for idiopathic ventricular outflow tract tachycardia. J Cardiovasc Electrophysiol. 2003;14:1280–6.

30. Yoshida N, Yamada T, Mcelderry HT, et al. A novel electrocardiographic criterion for differentiating a left from right ventricular outflow tract tachycardia origin: the V2S/V3R index. J Cardiovasc Electrophysiol. 2014;25:747–53.

31. Drew BJ, Ackerman MJ, Funk M, American Heart Association Acute Cardiac Care Committee of the Council on Clinical Cardiology; Council on Cardiovascular Nursing; American College of Cardiology Foundation, et al. Prevention of torsade de pointes in hospital settings: a scientific statement from the American Heart Association and the American College of Cardiology Foundation. J Am Coll Cardiol. 2010;55:934–47.

32. Roden DM. Drug-induced prolongation of the QT interval. N Engl J Med. 2004;350:1013–22.

33. Topilski I, Rogowski O, Rosso R, et al. The morphology of the QT interval predicts torsade de pointes during acquired bradyarrhythmias. J Am Coll Cardiol. 2007;49:320–8.

34. Gourraud JB, Kyndt F, Fouchard S, et al. Identification of a strong genetic background for progressive cardiac conduction defect by epidemiological approach. Heart. 2012;98:1305–10.

35. Lee S, Wellens HJJ, Josephson ME. Paroxysmal atrioventricular block. Heart Rhythm. 2009;6:1229–34.

36. Sinus node dysfunction (Chapter 8). Clinical arrhythmology and electrophysiology. A companion to Braunwald's Heart Disease (Edited by Issa ZF, Miller JM and Zipes DP). Philadelphia: Elsevier Saunders; 2012. pp. 164–174.

37. Guidelines for the management of patients with ST-elevation acute myocardial infarction (JCS 2013). http://www.j-circ.or.jp/guideline/pdf/JCS2013_kimura_h.pdf.

38. Atrioventricular conduction abnormalities (Chapter 9). Clinical arrhythmology and electrophysiology. A companion to Braunwald's Heart Disease (Edited by Issa ZF, Miller JM and Zipes DP). Philadelphia: Elsevier Saunders; 2012. pp. 175–193.

39. Savelieva I, Camm AJ. Atrial fibrillation and heart failure: natural history and pharmacological treatment. Europace. 2004;5:S5–S19.

40. Campbell RT, Jhund PS, Castagno D, et al. What have we learned about patients with heart failure and preserved ejection fraction from DIG-PEF, CHARM-preserved, and I-PRESERVE? J Am Coll Cardiol. 2012;60:2349–56.

41. Odutayo A, Wong CX, Hsiao AJ, et al. Atrial fibrillation and risks of cardiovascular disease, renal disease, and death: systematic review and meta-analysis. BMJ. 2016;354:i4482. https://doi.org/10.1136/bmj.i4482.

42. Aleong RG, Sauer WH, Davis G, et al. New-onset atrial fibrillation predicts heart failure progression. Am J Med. 2014;127:963–71.

43. Pizzetti F, Turazza FM, Franzosi MG, GISSI-3 Investigators, et al. Incidence and prognostic significance of atrial fibrillation in acute myocardial infarction: the GISSI-3 data. Heart. 2001;86:527–32.

44. Rathore SS, Berger AK, Weinfurt KP, et al. Acute myocardial infarction complicated by atrial fibrillation in the elderly: prevalence and outcomes. Circulation. 2000;101:969–74.

45. Behar S, Zahavi Z, Goldbourt U, et al. Long-term prognosis of patients with paroxysmal atrial fibrillation complicating acute myocardial infarction. SPRINT study group. Eur Heart J. 1992;13:45–50.

46. Kobayashi Y, Katoh T, Takano T, et al. Paroxysmal atrial fibrillation and flutter associated with acute myocardial infarction: hemodynamic evaluation in relation to the development of arrhythmias and prognosis. Jpn Circ J. 1992;56:1–11.

47. Walkey AJ, Hogarth DK, Lip GYH. Optimizing atrial fibrillation management: from ICU and beyond. Chest. 2015;148:859–64.

48. Walkey AJ, Greiner MA, Heckbert SR, et al. Atrial fibrillation among Medicare beneficiaries hospitalized with sepsis: incidence and risk factors. Am Heart J. 2013;165:949–55.

49. Arrigo M, Bettex D, Rudiger A. Management of atrial fibrillation in critically ill patients. Crit Care Res Pract. 2014;2014:840615.

50. Fuster V, Rydén LE, Cannom DS, et al. 2011 ACCF/AHA/HRS Focused updates incorporated into the ACC/AHA/ESC 2006 Guidelines for the management of patients with atrial fibrillation. A report of the American College of Cardiology Foundation /American Heart Association task force on practice guidelines. Circulation. 2011;123:e269–367.

51. Hayashi M, Tanaka K, Kato T, et al. Enhancing electrical cardioversion and preventing immediate reinitiation of hemodynamically deleterious atrial fibrillation with class III drug pretreatment. J Cardiovasc Electrophysiol. 2005; 16:740–7.

52. Roy D, Talajic M, Nattel S, Atrial Fibrillation and Congestive Heart Failure Investigators, et al. Rhythm control versus rate control for atrial fibrillation and heart failure. N Engl J Med. 2008;358:2667–77.

53. Corley SD, Epstein AE, DiMarco JP, AFFIRM Investigators, et al. Relationships between sinus rhythm, treatment, and survival in the Atrial Fibrillation Follow-Up Investigation of Rhythm Management (AFFIRM) study. Circulation. 2004;109:1509–13.

54. Hsu LF, Jaïs P, Sanders P, et al. Catheter ablation for atrial fibrillation in congestive heart failure. N Engl J Med. 2004;351:2373–83.

55. Nerheim P, Birger-Botkin S, Piracha L, et al. Heart failure and sudden death in patients with tachycardia-induced cardiomyopathy and recurrent tachycardia. Circulation. 2004;110:247–52.

56. Van Gelder IC, Crijns HJ, Blanksma PK, et al. Time course of hemodynamic changes and improvement of exercise tolerance after cardioversion of chronic atrial fibrillation unassociated with cardiac valve disease. Am J Cardiol. 1993;72:560–6.

57. Gopnathannair R, Etheridge SP, Marchlinski FE, et al. Arrhythmia-induced cardiomyopathies: mechanisms, recognition, and management. J Am Coll Cardiol. 2015;66:1714–28.

58. Mont L, Cinca J, Blanch P, et al. Predisposing factors and prognostic value of sustained monomorphic ventricular tachycardia in the early phase of acute myocardial infarction. J Am Coll Cardiol. 1996;28:1670–6.

59. Volpi A, Cavalli A, Santoro L, et al. Incidence and prognosis of early primary ventricular fibrillation in acute myocardial infarction—results of the Gruppo Italiano per lo Studio della Sopravvivenza nell'Infarto Miocardico (GISSI-2) database. Am J Cardiol. 1998;82:265–71.

60. Cheema AN, Sheu K, Packer M, et al. Nonsustained ventricular tachycardia in the setting of acute myocardial infarction. Tachycardia characteristics and their prognostic implication. Circulation. 1998;98:2030–2036.

61. Dorian P, Hohnloser SH, Thorpe KE, et al. Mechanisms underlying the lack of effect of implantable cardioverter-defibrillator therapy on mortality in high-risk patients with recent myocardial infarction: insights from the Defibrillation in Acute Myocardial Infarction Trial (DINAMIT). Circulation. 2010;122:2645–52.

62. Steinbeck G, Andresen D, Seidl K, et al. Defibrillator implantation early after myocardial infarction. New Engl J Med. 2009;361:1427–36.

63. Guidelines for non-pharmacotherapy of cardiac arrhythmias(JCS 2011) http://www.j-circ.or.jp/guideline/pdf/JCS2011_okumura_h.pdf.

64. Sasaki S, Shoji Y, Ishida Y, et al. Potential roles of the wearable cardioverter-defibrillator in acute phase care of patients at high risk of sudden cardiac death: a single-center Japanese experience. J Cardiol. 2017;69:359–63.

65. Zipes DP, Camm AJ, Borggrefe M, et al. ACC/AHA/ESC 2006 guidelines for management of patients with ventricular arrhythmias and the prevention of sudden cardiac death executive summary: a report of the American College of Cardiology/American Heart Association Task Force and the European Society of Cardiology Committee for Practice Guidelines. Circulation. 2006; 114:1088–132.

66. Satake H, Fukuda K, Sakata Y, CHART-2 investigators, et al. Current status of primary prevention of sudden cardiac death with implantable cardioverter defibrillator in patients with chronic heart failure–a report from the CHART-2 study. Circ J. 2015;79:381–90.

67. Connolly SJ, Dorian P, Roberts RS, Optimal Pharmacological Therapy in Cardioverter Defibrillator Patients (OPTIC) Investigators, et al. Comparison of beta-blockers, amiodarone plus beta-blockers, or sotalol for prevention of shocks from implantable cardioverter defibrillators: the OPTIC study: a randomized trial. JAMA. 2006;295:165–71.

68. Kuck KH, Schaumann A, Eckardt L, VTACH study group, et al. Catheter ablation of stable ventricular tachycardia before defibrillator implantation in patients with coronary heart disease (VTACH): a multicentre randomised controlled trial. Lancet. 2010;375:31–40.

69. Poole JE, Johnson GW, Hellkamp AS, et al. Prognostic importance of defibrillator shocks in patients with heart failure. N Engl J Med. 2008; 359:1009–17.

70. Daubert JP, Zareba W, Cannom DS, et al. Inappropriate implantable cardioverter-defibrillator shocks in MADIT II. J Am Coll Cardiol. 2008; 51:1357–65.

71. Maron BJ, Spirito P, Shen WK, et al. Implantable cardioverter-defibrillators and prevention of sudden cardiac death in hypertrophic cardiomyopathy. JAMA. 2007;298:405–12.

72. Guidelines for diagnosis and management of patients with long QT syndrome and Brugada syndrome(JCS 2012). http://www.j-circ.or.jp/guideline/pdf/JCS2013_aonuma_h.pdf

Permissions

All chapters in this book were first published in JIC, by BioMed Central; hereby published with permission under the Creative Commons Attribution License or equivalent. Every chapter published in this book has been scrutinized by our experts. Their significance has been extensively debated. The topics covered herein carry significant findings which will fuel the growth of the discipline. They may even be implemented as practical applications or may be referred to as a beginning point for another development.

The contributors of this book come from diverse backgrounds, making this book a truly international effort. This book will bring forth new frontiers with its revolutionizing research information and detailed analysis of the nascent developments around the world.

We would like to thank all the contributing authors for lending their expertise to make the book truly unique. They have played a crucial role in the development of this book. Without their invaluable contributions this book wouldn't have been possible. They have made vital efforts to compile up to date information on the varied aspects of this subject to make this book a valuable addition to the collection of many professionals and students.

This book was conceptualized with the vision of imparting up-to-date information and advanced data in this field. To ensure the same, a matchless editorial board was set up. Every individual on the board went through rigorous rounds of assessment to prove their worth. After which they invested a large part of their time researching and compiling the most relevant data for our readers.

The editorial board has been involved in producing this book since its inception. They have spent rigorous hours researching and exploring the diverse topics which have resulted in the successful publishing of this book. They have passed on their knowledge of decades through this book. To expedite this challenging task, the publisher supported the team at every step. A small team of assistant editors was also appointed to further simplify the editing procedure and attain best results for the readers.

Apart from the editorial board, the designing team has also invested a significant amount of their time in understanding the subject and creating the most relevant covers. They scrutinized every image to scout for the most suitable representation of the subject and create an appropriate cover for the book.

The publishing team has been an ardent support to the editorial, designing and production team. Their endless efforts to recruit the best for this project, has resulted in the accomplishment of this book. They are a veteran in the field of academics and their pool of knowledge is as vast as their experience in printing. Their expertise and guidance has proved useful at every step. Their uncompromising quality standards have made this book an exceptional effort. Their encouragement from time to time has been an inspiration for everyone.

The publisher and the editorial board hope that this book will prove to be a valuable piece of knowledge for researchers, students, practitioners and scholars across the globe.

List of Contributors

Miyuki H. Komachi
Division of Health Sciences, Graduate School of Health and Welfare Sciences, International University of Health and Welfare, 1-3-3 Minamiaoyama Aoyama 1-Chome Tower 4th and 5th floor, Minato-ku, Tokyo 107-0062, Japan

Kiyoko Kamibeppu
Department of Family Nursing, Division of Health Sciences and Nursing, Graduate School of Medicine, The University of Tokyo, 7-3-1 Hongo, Bunkyo-ku, Tokyo 113-0033, Japan

Stephen M. Vindigni
Division of Gastroenterology, Department of Medicine, University of Washington, 1959 NE Pacific Street, Box 356424, Seattle, WA 98195-6424, USA

Juan N. Lessing
Division of General Internal Medicine, Department of Medicine, University of Colorado, 13001 E 17th Place, Aurora, CO 80045, USA

David J. Carlbom
Division of Pulmonary, Critical Care and Sleep Medicine, Department of Medicine, University of Washington, 1959 NE Pacific Street, Seattle, WA 98195-6424, USA

Paolo Severgnini, Elena Contino, Elisa Serafinelli, Raffaele Novario and Maurizio Chiaranda
Department of Biotechnologies and Sciences of Life, Intensive Care Unit–ASST Sette Laghi–Ospedale di Circolo Fondazione Macchi, University of Insubria, Viale Luigi Borri 57, 21100 Varese, Italy

Paolo Pelosi
Largo R. Benzi 10, 16132 Genova, Italy

Bernt C. Hellerud, Hilde L. Orrem, Søren E. Pischke and Tom E. Mollnes
Department of Immunology, Oslo University Hospital Rikshospitalet, and K.G. Jebsen IRC, University of Oslo, N-0027 Oslo, Norway

Bernt C. Hellerud and Petter Brandtzæg
Department of Pediatrics, Oslo University Hospital Ullevål and University of Oslo, Oslo, Norway

Knut Dybwik
Department of Anesthesiology, Nordland Hospital and Nord University, Bodø, Norway

Albert Castellheim
Department of Anesthesiology and Intensive Care Unit, Institution of Clinical Science, Sahlgrenska Academy, University of Gothenburg, Gothenburg, Sweden

Hilde Fure, Grethe Bergseth, Dorte Christiansen and Tom E. Mollnes
Research Laboratory, Nordland Hospital, Bodø, Norway

Miles A. Nunn
Akari Therapeutics Plc, London, UK

Terje Espevik and Tom E. Mollnes
Centre of Molecular Inflammation Research and Department of Cancer Research and MolecularMedicine, Norwegian University of Science and Technology, Trondheim, Norway

Petter Brandtzæg
Institute of Clinical Medicine, Faculty of Medicine, University of Oslo, Oslo, Norway

Erik W. Nielsen and Tom E. Mollnes
Faculty of Health Sciences, K.G. Jebsen TREC, University of Tromsø, Tromsø, Norway

Gabriel Wardi
Department of Emergency Medicine and Division of Pulmonary, Critical Care and Sleep Medicine, UC San Diego Health System, 200 West Arbor Drive, San Diego, CA 92103, USA

Arvin R. Wali
University of California San Diego School of Medicine, 9500 Gilman Drive, La Jolla, CA 92093-0602, USA

Julian Villar
Division of Pulmonary and Critical Care Medicine, Stanford University School of Medicine, M121-L, Stanford, CA 94305-5119, USA

Vaishal Tolia
Department of Internal Medicine, University of California, San Diego, 200 West Arbor Drive, San Diego, CA 92103, USA

Vaishal Tolia, Christian Tomaszewski, Christian Sloane, Matthew Nolan and Daniel Lasoff
Department of Emergency Medicine, University of California, San Diego, 200 West Arbor Drive, San Diego, CA 92103, USA

Peter Fedullo, Jeremy R. Beitler and Rebecca E. Sell
Division of Pulmonary, Critical Care, and Sleep Medicine, University of California, San Diego, 200 W Arbor Drive, San Diego, CA 92103, USA

Joachim Marti
Centre for Health Policy, Imperial College London, Praed Street, London W2 1NY, UK

Peter Hall
Edinburgh Cancer Research Centre, University of Edinburgh, Crewe Road South, Edinburgh EH4 2XR, UK

Patrick Hamilton
Central Manchester University Hospitals NHS Foundation Trust, Manchester, UK

Sarah Lamb
Oxford Clinical Trials Unit, University of Oxford, Oxford, UK

Chris McCabe
Department of Emergency Medicine, University of Alberta, Alberta, Canada

Ranjit Lall
Warwick Clinical Trials Unit, University of Warwick, Coventry, UK

Julie Darbyshire and Duncan Young
Nuffield Department of Clinical Neurosciences, University of Oxford, Oxford, UK

Claire Hulme
Academic Unit of Health Economics, University of Leeds, Leeds, UK

Ryan R. Kroll, J. Gordon Boyd, Daniel Howes and David M. Maslove
Department of Critical Care Medicine, Queen's University and Kingston Health Sciences Centre, Kingston, Ontario, Canada

Erica D. McKenzie
School of Medicine, Queen's University, Kingston, Ontario, Canada

J. Gordon Boyd and David M. Maslove
Department of Medicine, Queen's University and Kingston Health Sciences Centre, Kingston, Ontario, Canada

Prameet Sheth
Department of Pathology and Molecular Medicine, Queen's University and Health Sciences Centre, Kingston, Ontario, Canada

Daniel Howes
Department of Emergency Medicine, Queen's University and Kingston Health Sciences Centre, Kingston, Ontario, Canada

Michael Wood
Department of Neuroscience, Queen's University, Kingston, Ontario, Canada

David M. Maslove
Kingston Health Sciences Centre, Kingston General Hospital, Davies 2, 76 Stuart St., Kingston, Ontario K7L 2V7, Canada

Lori J. Delaney and Marian J. Currie
Faculty of Nursing, University of Canberra, Canberra, Australia

Lori J. Delaney, Marian J. Currie and Frank Van Haren
College of Medicine, Biology and Environment, Australian National University, Canberra, Australia

Hsin-Chia Carol Huang
Respiratory and Sleep Medicine, Canberra Hospital, Canberra, Australia

Violeta Lopez
Alice Lee Centre for Nursing Studies, Yong Loo Lin School of Medicine, Singapore, Singapore

Violeta Lopez and Edward Litton
St. John of God Hospital, Subiaco Perth Australia, Subiaco, Australia

Edward Litton
School of Medicine and Pharmacology, University of Western Australia, Perth 6009, Australia

Frank Van Haren
Intensive Care Unit, Canberra Hospital, Canberra, Australia

Lori J. Delaney
Faculty of Health: Discipline of Nursing, University of Canberra, Canberra Act 2601, Australia

Gu Hyun Kang
Department of Emergency Medicine, Hallym University College of Medicine, Seoul, Republic of Korea

Hyun Youk, Kyoung Chul Cha, Yoonsuk Lee, Hyung Il Kim, Yong Sung Cha, Oh Hyun Kim, Hyun Kim, Kang Hyun Lee and Sung Oh Hwang
Department of Emergency Medicine, Yonsei University Wonju College of Medicine, 20 Ilsanro, Wonju, Republic of Korea

Keita Shibahashi, Kazuhiro Sugiyama, Masahiro Kashiura and Yuichi Hamabe
Department of Emergency and Intensive Care Center, Tokyo Metropolitan Bokutoh Hospital, 4-23-15, Kotobashi, Sumida-ku, Tokyo 130-8575, Japan

Young-Rock Ha
Emergency Department, Bundang Jesaeng Hospital, 20 Seohyeon-ro 180beongil, Bundang-gu, Seongnam-si, Gyeonggi-do, South Korea

Hong-Chuen Toh
Acute and Emergency Care Centre, Khoo Teck Puat Hospital, 90 Yishun Central, S768828 Singapore, Singapore

Ken Parhar, Victoria Millar, Vasileios Zochios, Emilia Bruton, Alain Vuylsteke and Alain Vuylsteke
Department of Anesthesia and Intensive Care, Papworth Hospital, Cambridge, England

Catherine Jaworksi and Nick West
Department of Interventional Cardiology, Papworth Hospital, Cambridge, England

Ken Parhar
Department of Critical Care Medicine, University of Calgary, ICU Administration - Ground Floor - McCaig Tower, Foothills Medical Center, 3134 Hospital Drive NW, Calgary, AB T2N 5A1, Canada

Vasileios Zochios
Department of Critical Care Medicine, University Hospitals of Birmingham NHS Foundation Trust, Queen Elizabeth Hospital, Birmingham, England

Takeshi Suzuki, Yuta Suzuki, Jun Okuda, Takuya Kurazumi, Tomohiro Suhara, Tomomi Ueda, Hiromasa Nagata and Hiroshi Morisaki
Department of Anesthesiology and General Intensive Care Unit, Keio University School of Medicine, 35 Shinanomachi, Shinjuku-ku, Tokyo 160-8582, Japan

Taku Tanaka
Medical Emergency and Disaster Center, Kawasaki Municipal Tama Hospital, 1-30-37 Shukugawara, Tama-ku, Kawasaki, Kanagawa 214-8525, Japan

Takeshi Kashimura, Marii Ise, Brandon D. Lohman and Yasuhiko Taira
Emergency and Critical Care Medicine, St. Marianna University School of Medicine, 2-16-1 Sugao, Miyamae-ku, Kawasaki, Kanagawa 216-8511, Japan

Anis Chaari, Karim Abdel Hakim, Kamel Bousselmi, Vipin Kauts, Mahmoud Etman and William Francis Casey
Critical Care Department, King Hamad University Hospital, Al Muharaq, Bahrain

Nevine Rashed
Gastroenterology Department, King Hamad University Hospital, Al Muharaq, Bahrain

Bruno François, Marc Clavel and Philippe Vignon
Medical-surgical Intensive Care Unit, Dupuytren University Hospital, 2 avenue Martin Luther King, 87042 Limoges, France

Bruno François
Inserm CIC 1435, Limoges University Hospital, Limoges, France

Pierre-François Laterre
Medical-surgical Intensive Care Unit, Cliniques Saint-Luc, Brussels, Belgium

Kimberley J. Hainess
Physiotherapy Department, Western Health, Furlong Road, St. Albans, VIC 3021, Australia

Kimberley J. Haines and Linda Denehy
Department of Physiotherapy, Melbourne School of Health Sciences, The University of Melbourne, 200 Berkeley Street, Parkville, VIC 3010, Australia

Sue Berney
Department of Physiotherapy, Austin Hospital, 145 Studley Road, Heidelberg, VIC 3084, Australia

Stephen Warrillow
Department of Intensive Care, Austin Hospital, 145 Studley Road, Heidelberg, VIC 3084, Australia

Simon Tilma Vistisen and Mikael Fink Vallentin
Research Centre for Emergency Medicine, Institute of Clinical Medicine, Aarhus University, Palle Juul-Jensens Boulevard 99, 8200 Aarhus N, Denmark

Simon Tilma Vistisen, Martin Buhl Krog, Thomas Elkmann and Christoffer Sølling
Department of Anesthesiology and Intensive Care, Aarhus University Hospitals, Aarhus, Denmark

Simon Tilma Vistisen and Thomas W. L. Scheeren
University Medical Center Groningen, Department of Anesthesiology, University of Groningen, Groningen, the Netherlands

Christoffer Sølling
Department of Anesthesiology and Intensive Care, Viborg Regional Hospital, Viborg, Denmark

Sushma Yerram, Nakul Katyal, Premkumar Nattanmai and Christopher R. Newey
Department of Neurology, University of Missouri, 5 Hospital Drive, CE 540, Columbia, MO 65211, USA

Keerthivaas Premkumar
Department of Biological Sciences, University of Missouri, Columbia, MO 65211, USA

Christopher R. Newey
Cleveland Clinic, Cerebrovascular Center, 9500 Euclid Avenue, Cleveland, OH 44195, USA

De Wen Zhang and Jian He
Department of Emergency and Critical Care Medicine, Eastern Hepatobiliary Surgery Hospital, Second Military Medical University, No. 700 North Moyu Road, Shanghai 201805, China

Fahad Alroumi, Ahmed Abdul Azim, Rachel Kergo, Yuxiu Lei and James Dargin
Department of Pulmonary and Critical Care Medicine, Lahey Hospital and Medical Center, Burlington, MA, USA

Fahad Alroumi, Ahmed Abdul Azim, Yuxiu Lei and James Dargin
Tufts University School of Medicine, Boston, MA, USA

Takeshi Yamamoto
Division of Cardiovascular Intensive Care, Nippon Medical School Hospital, 1-1-5 Sendagi, Bunkyo-ku, Tokyo 113-8603, Japan

Edward Litton
Intensive Care Unit, Fiona Stanley Hospital, Perth, Western Australia 6065, Australia
School of Medicine, University of Western Australia, Perth, Western Australia 6009, Australia
Intensive Care Unit, Fiona Stanley Hospital, Perth, Western Australia 6150, Australia

Stuart Baker
Intensive Care Unit, Sir Charles Gardner Hospital, Perth, Western Australia 6009, Australia

Wendy Erber
School of Patholody, University of Australia, Perth, Western Australia 6009, Australia

Alisa Higgins
Centre of Research Excellence for Patient Blood Management in Critical Illness and Trauma, Monash University, Melbourne, Victoria, Australia

Axel Hofmann
Medical School, Faculty of Health and Medical Sciences, University of Western Australia, Perth, Western Australia 6009, Australia

Toby Richards
University College London, London, UK

Simon Towler
Intensive Care Unit, Fiona Stanley Hospital, Perth, Western Australia 6065, Australia

Robert Trengove
Separation Science and Metabolomics Laboratory Metabolomics Australia (Western Australia node), Murdoch University, Perth, Western Australia, Australia

Fumiaki Tokioka, Akio Yamazaki, Akihiro Itou and Tadashi Ishida
Department of Respiratory Medicine, Kurashiki Central Hospital, 1-1-1 Miwa, Kurashiki, Okayama 710-8602, Japan

Hiroshi Okamoto
Center for Clinical Epidemiology, St.Luke's International University, Tokyo, Japan

Shigeaki Inoue, Masafumi Saito and Joji Kotani
Department of Disaster and Emergency Medicine, Kobe University Graduate School of Medicine, Kusunoki-cho 7-5-2, Chuo-ward, Kobe 650-0017, Japan

Yoshinori Kobayashi
Division of Cardiology, Tokai University Hachioji Hospital, 1838 Ishikawa-machi Hachioji-shi, Tokyo 192-0032, Japan

Index

A

Acute Myocardial Infarction, 91, 93-95, 98-101, 108-110, 223, 233, 235-237

Advanced Cardiac Life Support, 8, 235

Amylase, 128-130, 132-133

Anaemia, 199-201, 203-204

Anti-epileptic Drugs, 163, 167-168, 170

Ards, 42-43, 45-47, 49-50, 52, 85, 87-92, 95, 98, 134, 136, 138, 142-143, 145, 152, 188, 238-242, 244

Arrhythmias, 59, 223-225, 227-228, 230, 234-237

B

Behavioral Pain Scale, 16-18, 20-23

C

Cancer, 1-7, 31, 51, 80-81, 89, 142-143, 146, 188-189, 194-195, 212, 217, 219, 221

Carboxyhemoglobin, 120-121, 127

Cardiac Arrest, 14, 51, 60, 69-74, 82-83, 99, 102-104, 106-109, 147, 190, 194-195, 224-225, 235

Cardiopulmonary Resuscitation, 8, 11, 13-14, 69-70, 72-74, 198

Cardiovascular Intensive Care, 190, 223

Catheter-directed Treatment, 190, 194

Chemokines, 24, 29, 216

Chest Pain, 82-83, 85-86, 89, 91-93, 98-99, 206

Chest Tube, 69-70, 72-73, 85-86, 99

Code Blue, 8-9, 13

Cohb, 120-126

Congestive Heart Failure, 183, 188, 207, 223, 236

Continuous Electroencephalography, 163, 171

Cpr, 8-15, 69-73, 108

Critical Care Pain Observation Tool, 16-18, 20-21

Critical Illness, 7, 39, 51, 53-54, 56-58, 60, 145-146, 151-154, 199, 204, 232

Critically Ill Patients, 16-17, 21, 23, 40, 42-43, 51, 59-60, 80, 85, 99-100, 112, 118-119, 130-131, 133, 143-144, 154-156, 162-163, 169-170, 172, 189, 197-200, 203-204, 219, 232

Curb-65, 205-212

Cytokines, 24, 26, 28-32, 111-112, 115, 119, 174, 177, 186, 213-214, 216-219, 222

E

Ecmo, 106, 108, 193, 195-196

Ectopic Beat, 155-161

Endotoxin, 24, 31, 112-113, 118-119, 174, 176, 222

External Chest Compression, 69, 74

Extrasystole, 155-158, 161

F

Fluid Responsiveness, 89, 99, 155-157, 159-162

H

Hbo, 120-121, 124-126

Heart Rate Monitoring, 53, 58-60

Hemodynamic Monitoring, 155, 162

Hepcidin, 199-204

Hospital Rapid Response Teams, 8

Hyperbaric Oxygen, 120-121, 127

I

Icu, 1-7, 16-17, 19-23, 33-40, 42-46, 48-51, 53-68, 76-81, 101-110, 116-117, 128-139, 141-142, 145-153, 155-158, 160, 168-171, 173, 179-181, 184-188, 195-197, 199-213, 223-224, 235-236

Immune Paralysis, 213

Immune Response, 24, 29, 173, 177, 213-215

Immunoglobulin-like Transcript-4, 173, 177

Immunosenescence, 213-214, 220-221

Inflammation, 24, 31, 42, 113, 119, 173, 177, 179, 189, 199, 203, 213-214, 217, 221, 230, 232

Intensive Care, 1, 7, 15-17, 20, 22-24, 31, 33, 40, 42, 50-54, 59-61, 63-68, 74-77, 80-81, 98-99, 101-102, 106, 108-110, 116-119, 127-129, 142-147, 161-163, 173, 177, 180, 184, 192, 201, 208-213, 235

Interleukin (IL)-6, 173, 186

Intravenous Iron, 199, 204

Investigation Center, 134

L

Lactate, 33-39, 76-78, 111, 114, 118, 129-131, 133, 158, 183, 208

Lipase, 128-130, 132-133

Long-term Outcomes, 51, 145, 153

M

Major Histocompatibility Complex Class Ii, 173

Mechanical Ventilation, 14, 17, 21, 23, 35, 42-43, 50-52, 60, 86, 89, 99, 101-102, 106-109, 129-132, 154, 161, 179, 184-188, 192, 211, 221

Medical Emergency Teams, 8-9, 12

Medical Informatics, 53

Mhc-ii, 173-177

Mobile Health Technologies, 53

Monocytes, 30, 32, 173-177, 214-215

Mortality, 24, 30-34, 36-43, 45-46, 49-51, 58, 60, 67, 72, 74-81, 101-104, 106-111, 113-120, 127-132, 134, 143, 145-148, 153, 164, 168, 173, 179-181, 193, 203, 218-219, 225, 227, 230-233

Multi-organ Point-of-care Ultrasound, 82, 98

N
Neisseria Meningitidis, 24, 31-32
Normobaric, 120-121, 127

O
Occupational Medicine, 8
Oxyhemoglobin, 120-121

P
Pain Management, 16, 23
Pneumonia, 19, 34-36, 45-46, 49, 86, 89, 91-93, 102, 129, 133-134, 136, 142-144, 147, 158, 180-182, 185, 187-189, 205-212, 222
Posttraumatic Stress Disorder, 1, 6-7, 51, 154
Primary Percutaneous Coronary Intervention, 101, 108-109
Pulmonary Embolism, 88, 91, 93-94, 96, 98-100, 190-192, 196-198

Q
Qsofa, 205-212

R
Red Blood Cell Transfusion, 199, 204
Respiratory Difficulty, 82, 91

S
Sarcopenia, 75, 78-81
Seizure Prophylaxis, 163-167, 170-171

Sepsis-induced Cardiac Dysfunction, 110-114, 116, 118
Septic Shock, 24-26, 31-35, 37-41, 80, 89-90, 99, 110-111, 113-115, 118-119, 128-133, 143-144, 158, 162, 177, 179-181, 183-189, 212
Severe Sepsis, 25, 31-35, 37-40, 80-81, 110-111, 118-119, 133, 144, 152, 158, 162, 173, 177, 179-181, 183-188, 200, 222
Sleep Disturbance, 61, 67
Sleep Quality, 53-60, 65
Stroke Volume, 114, 116-117, 155-156, 158-161, 218
Surgical Embolectomy, 190, 195

T
Thoracostomy, 69
Thrombolytic Therapy, 109, 190, 193-198
Toll-like Receptor, 24, 29, 31

U
Unexpected Icu Transfer, 33, 35-39

V
Validation Study, 53, 212
Ventilator-associated Pneumonia, 134, 142

W
Wearable Devices, 53-54, 57-60

www.ingramcontent.com/pod-product-compliance
Lightning Source LLC
Chambersburg PA
CBHW080507200326
41458CB00012B/4124